Psychiatric Disorders: Causes, Symptoms and Management

Psychiatric Disorders: Causes, Symptoms and Management

Edited by Nathaniel Turner

STATES
ACADEMIC PRESS
www.statesacademicpress.com

States Academic Press,
109 South 5th Street,
Brooklyn, NY 11249, USA

Visit us on the World Wide Web at:
www.statesacademicpress.com

ISBN: 978-1-63989-450-5

Cataloging-in-Publication Data

Psychiatric disorders : causes, symptoms and management / edited by Nathaniel Turner.
p. cm.
Includes bibliographical references and index.
ISBN 978-1-63989-450-5
1. Psychology, Pathological. 2. Mental illness. 3. Mental illness--Etiology.
4. Mental illness--Treatment. 5. Psychiatry. 6. Psychotherapy. I. Turner, Nathaniel.
RC435 .P79 2022
616.89--dc23

Table of Contents

Preface

The mental or behavioral pattern which can result in considerable distress or difficulty in personal functioning is termed as a psychiatric disorder or a mental disorder. A few types of mental disorders are anxiety disorder, mood disorder, psychotic disorder, personality disorder, eating disorder and sleep disorder. A wide variety of factors can influence the likelihood of a person suffering from psychiatric disorder such as genetics, drug use, environment and personality traits. A psychiatric disorder's symptoms vary on the basis of the disorder, the social environment and the individual. The management of psychiatric disorders involves various methods which can be categorized into therapy, medication and lifestyle changes. This book attempts to understand the multiple psychiatric disorders as well as their causes, symptoms and management. Such selected concepts that redefine research on these disorders have been presented in it. The book is appropriate for students seeking detailed information in this area as well as for experts.

The information contained in this book is the result of intensive hard work done by researchers in this field. All due efforts have been made to make this book serve as a complete guiding source for students and researchers. The topics in this book have been comprehensively explained to help readers understand the growing trends in the field.

I would like to thank the entire group of writers who made sincere efforts in this book and my family who supported me in my efforts of working on this book. I take this opportunity to thank all those who have been a guiding force throughout my life.

Editor

Preface

1

A clinical review of the treatment of catatonia

Pascal Sienaert[1,2]*, Dirk M. Dhossche[3], Davy Vancampfort[4], Marc De Hert[4] and Gábor Gazdag[5,6]

[1] Department of Mood Disorders and Electroconvulsive Therapy, University Psychiatric Center, KU Leuven, Leuven, Belgium
[2] Department of Neurosciences, KU Leuven, Leuven, Belgium
[3] Department of Psychiatry, University of Mississippi Medical Center, Jackson, MS, USA
[4] University Psychiatric Center, KU Leuven, Leuven, Belgium
[5] Center for Psychiatry and Addiction Medicine, Szent István and Szent László Hospitals, Budapest, Hungary
[6] Department of Psychiatry and Psychotherapy, Faculty of Medicine, Semmelweis University, Budapest, Hungary

Edited by:
Mihaly Hajos, Yale University School of Medicine, USA

Reviewed by:
Mihaly Hajos, Yale University School of Medicine, USA
Sebastian Walther, University Hospital of Psychiatry, Switzerland
Manuel Morrens, University Antwerp, Belgium

***Correspondence:**
Pascal Sienaert, Department of Mood Disorders and Electroconvulsive Therapy, University Psychiatric Center, KU Leuven (University of Leuven), Campus Kortenberg, Leuvensesteenweg 517, Kortenberg 3070, Belgium
e-mail: pascal.sienaert@uc-kortenberg.be

Catatonia is a severe motor syndrome with an estimated prevalence among psychiatric inpatients of about 10%. At times, it is life-threatening especially in its malignant form when complicated by fever and autonomic disturbances. Catatonia can accompany many different psychiatric illnesses and somatic diseases. In order to recognize the catatonic syndrome, apart from thorough and repeated observation, a clinical examination is needed. A screening instrument, such as the Bush-Francis Catatonia Rating Scale, can guide the clinician through the neuropsychiatric examination. Although severe and life-threatening, catatonia has a good prognosis. Research on the treatment of catatonia is scarce, but there is overwhelming clinical evidence of the efficacy of benzodiazepines, such as lorazepam, and electroconvulsive therapy.

Keywords: catatonia, benzodiazepines, electroconvulsive therapy, glutamate antagonists, zolpidem, transcranial magnetic stimulation

INTRODUCTION

Catatonia is a severe motor syndrome with an estimated prevalence among psychiatric inpatients of about 10% (1, 2). Catatonia can accompany many different psychiatric illnesses and somatic diseases. A minority of catatonic patients suffers from schizophrenia (30%), while a majority has a bipolar disorder (43%) (1, 3, 4). Catatonia has also been linked to other psychiatric disorders, such as obsessive-compulsive disorder (5), post-traumatic stress disorder (6, 7), or withdrawal from alcohol (8) or benzodiazepines (9, 10). In up to 25% of cases, catatonia is related with general medical or neurologic conditions (1, 11). Recently, it was shown repeatedly that catatonic symptoms are observable in most patients diagnosed with anti-*N*-methyl-D-aspartate receptor (anti-NMDAR) encephalitis (12, 13). In adolescents and young adults with autism, catatonia is found in 12–17% (14). Pediatric catatonia also emerges in patients with tic disorders, and a variety of other (developmental) disorders (15). The same principles of evaluation and treatment seem to apply to pediatric patients as in adult patients (15, 16).

A life-threatening situation occurs when catatonia is accompanied by fever and autonomic abnormalities. Malignant catatonia, coined as "lethal catatonia" by Stauder in 1934 (17), presents as a constellation of catatonia, stuporous exhaustion, autonomic instability, respiratory failure, collapse, coma, and often death if left untreated. This clinical picture is very close to what is observed in neuroleptic malignant syndrome (NMS), which is considered by several experts to be a drug-induced form of catatonia (18).

EVALUATION, DIFFERENTIAL DIAGNOSIS, AND TREATMENT

An effective treatment starts with a swift and correct diagnosis. In any patient exhibiting marked deterioration in psychomotor function and overall responsiveness, catatonia should be considered. Moreover, any patient that is admitted to a psychiatric ward with a severe psychiatric disorder, such as depression, bipolar disorder, a psychotic disorder, or autism spectrum disorder, should be examined routinely (19). Some signs and symptoms are evident upon observation of the patient during a psychiatric interview. Other specific symptoms, however, such as automatic obedience, ambitendency, negativism should be elicited during a neuropsychiatric examination (19, 20). A rating scale can be used as a screening instrument and aid in the detection and quantification of catatonia. A number of rating scales have been found reliable, sensitive and specific: the Rogers Catatonia Scale, the Bush-Francis Catatonia Rating Scale (BFCRS) (and its revised version), the Northoff Catatonia Rating Scale, and the Braunig Catatonia Rating Scale (19). Early detection of catatonia is of great importance, since the presence of catatonic signs possesses significant prognostic and therapeutic value (19).

Unfortunately, no laboratory test specifically defines catatonia. The "diagnostic weight" of several proposed laboratory and imaging tests is limited (21). Possible laboratory tests, primarily to assess various underlying conditions, include a complete blood count and metabolic panel, erythrocyte sedimentation rate, blood urea nitrogen, creatinine, serum iron, and creatinine-phosphokinase, antinuclear antibodies, and urinalysis, and magnetic resonance imaging, electroencephalogram, cerebrospinal fluid analysis (4, 11). Given the frequent association with anti-NMDAR-encephalitis, detection of IgG antibodies to NMDAR in cerebrospinal fluid or serum is advisable (22). Since serum iron was found to be reduced in NMS compared to catatonia (23), some authors see low serum iron as a risk factor for developing NMS after using antipsychotics in a catatonic patient (24). A drug screen to detect common illicit and prescribed substances is necessary.

PROGNOSIS

Prognosis of catatonia is good, especially with early and aggressive treatment. In mood disorders, prognosis is probably better than in psychotic disorders. Kraepelin, who classified catatonia as a type of dementia praecox, wrote, in the 9th edition of his textbook, that almost half of catatonic attacks begin with a depressive phase and that these patients had a better prognosis. Hoch, in a monograph on benign stupors, reports good outcomes (*'remission and return to the community'*) in 13 patients with manic-depressive illness, and a poor outcome in 12 schizophrenics (25). In more recent studies, results are conflicting. Most of the available data confirm a worse prognosis in the context of schizophrenia. In a randomized double-blind, placebo-controlled trial in 18 patients with chronic schizophrenia, who also displayed enduring catatonic features, 6 mg lorazepam per day for 12 weeks did not have any effect on catatonic symptoms (26). In another recent study, 73% of 24 patients with catatonia remitted within 6 days after starting benzodiazepines: partial responders (6/24) all had schizophrenia (27). In a retrospective study ECT was only partially efficacious in 2 of 4 patients with schizophrenic catatonia, whereas 5 out of 5 patients with mood disorder fully recovered (28). In a small open study, however, lorazepam (4–12.5 mg/day) was reported ineffective in 5 of 20 patients; all 5 with mood disorders (29). In a recent retrospective chart study on the effects of lorazepam in 107 inpatients with a primary diagnosis of catatonia, there was no significant difference between patients with mood disorder and those with a non-affective psychotic disorder (30, 31). Similarly, in an ECT-study in 22 patients, 13 (59%) of which had a mood disorder, no statistically significant difference was found in the effectiveness of the resolution of catatonic symptoms in persons with mood disorder versus schizophrenia (32), although the authors stress that in the patients with mood disorders more catatonic symptoms resolved with ECT than in the other group.

A factor that might complicate the difference in reported response rates of affective versus schizophrenic catatonia is chronicity. At least part of the studies showing a worse response in the context of schizophrenia have included patients with chronic catatonia (4, 26, 33). Some authors have suggested that "chronic catatonia" in the context of schizophrenia is phenomenologically different and less responsive to either benzodiazepines or ECT (34), and thus carries a less favorable prognosis then the acute forms of catatonia. The fact that a longer duration of the episode has been reported to predict a worse response should not be seen as a reason to withhold adequate treatment in patients presenting with longstanding or resistant catatonic symptoms. Catatonia that is not effectively treated may persist for years, but should nevertheless be promptly treated upon detection. A number of cases are illustrative of the *overall* good prognosis, even in chronic and longstanding catatonic symptoms. A man with a 17-year history of catatonia responded swiftly to the administration of lorazepam (35); a 15-year-old girl with catatonic lupus, resistant to several treatments was successfully treated with ECT after 3 months (36). A man developing catatonia after myocardial infarction remained catatonic for 1.5 years until he was treated with ECT (37). A mentally retarded boy with catatonia of 5 year's duration improved with lorazepam (38). Both Ripley and Millson (39) and Salam et al. (40) reported positive response to lorazepam in two patients with psychogenic catatonia that lasted 2 1/2 years and 3 months, respectively. A long treatment delay should, however, be avoided since it can lead to a variety of serious medical complications, some of which may be lethal (41).

In the above mentioned retrospective lorazepam-study in 107 inpatients (30), predictors of response to lorazepam were examined. A longer illness duration, the presence of mutism, third-person auditory hallucinations and 'made phenomena' (in which the individual feels he is being made to do something) predicted a poor response, whereas the presence of waxy flexibility predicted a good response (30). It should be noted that low lorazepam doses (3–6 mg/day) were used. A longer illness duration also seemed to predict a worse outcome in the first 11 patients treated by László Meduna, who invented convulsive therapy in 1934 (42, 43). In a 1912 monograph, Urstein reports on 30 patients with catatonia, with various underlying conditions and a variable prognosis, being worse in patients with a higher number of episodes (44). Fink states that prognosis is especially favorable when the syndrome is dominated by stupor, hyperactivity, rapid, and pressured speech, and lability of mood, or if there is a previous episode with recovery, a rapid onset of the episode, and good social functioning prior to the episode (45, 46). Van Waarde and co-workers have examined predictors of response to ECT in 27 catatonic patients and found improvement to be significantly associated with younger age, and the presence of autonomic dysregulation, especially higher body temperature (47). There is anecdotal evidence that organic catatonia is less responsive, or does not respond at all, to ECT. Swartz and colleagues described four patients with a variety of neurological impairment (Alzheimer's disease, post-encephalitic mental retardation, cerebellar atrophy, epilepsy, and spinal injury). Patients showed only transient and partial improvement to ECT. The authors suggest that advanced pathological changes of the CNS might explain a diminished response and that these states require a particularly intensive treatment (48).

Raffin and coworkers (16) recently reported treatments used in 66 consecutively hospitalized children and adolescents between the ages 9–19 with catatonia. The most frequent comorbid conditions were schizophrenia ($N = 38$, 58%), pervasive developmental disorder ($N = 17$, 26%), medical conditions ($N = 16$, 24%), bipolar disorder ($N = 11$, 17%), and intellectual disability ($N = 8$, 12%). The naturalistic design of the study lists a wide range of treatments in various combinations. Average catatonia scores decreased and level of function increased during the admission. Fifty-one (77%) patients received benzodiazepines, in doses up to 15 mg of lorazepam per day, which were effective in 65% of cases. Twelve (18%) received ECT, in three cases as first-line treatment (of which two cases had malignant catatonia). One patient with schizophrenia received maintenance ECT. There was no association between sociodemographic variables, except gender (males improved less than females) or co-morbid (medical or psychiatric) condition, and treatment response. Lower catatonia scores on admission and acute onset were associated with better clinical response. Cases with posturing and mannerisms were found to have less improvement than other cases.

TREATMENT OF CATATONIA

SUPPORTIVE MEASURES

A broad range of complications of catatonia can occur, such as aspiration pneumonia, dehydration, muscle contractures, pressure ulcers, nutritional deficiencies, severe weight loss, thiamine deficiency, electrolyte disturbances, urinary tract infections, and venous thromboembolism (11, 49, 50), some of which can lead to life-threatening situations. Some patients will require a high level of nursing care, and IV fluids and/or nasogastric tube feeds, in order to reduce the risk of morbidity and mortality caused by immobility, poor nutrition and dehydration (11). Anticoagulant therapies can be used to prevent deep vein thrombosis/pulmonary embolism in immobile patients (50). Medical complications should be treated lege artis. Given the often dramatic and prompt improvement of motor immobility after treatment, the major measure in preventing complications is a prompt diagnosis, and a rapid initiation of an adequate treatment of the catatonic state.

ANTIPSYCHOTICS

All prescribed medications should be evaluated for their potential to induce catatonic symptoms and discontinued if possible. There is some ambiguity about the role of antipsychotics but it is generally encouraged to discontinue antipsychotic treatment in patients presenting with catatonia (46). In the presence of a catatonic state, both first and second generation antipsychotics (SGA) may contribute to maintaining or worsening the catatonic state and increase the risk of developing NMS (51–54). During a prospective follow-up of 82 patients that had received antipsychotics at some point when catatonic, NMS developed in three cases (3.6%) (4), a substantially higher incidence than the estimated incidence of 0.07–1.8% in all antipsychotics-treated patients (55). The risk of worsening catatonia appears greater with neuroleptics and antipsychotics with higher D2-blockade and a higher potential of causing extrapyramidal side effects (56), but a worsening of catatonia and precipitation of NMS has also been reported in association with, e.g., olanzapine (57, 58).

Although it is generally accepted that neuroleptics are ineffective in catatonia (59), the role of the SGA in the treatment of catatonia is more ambiguous, and based on cases mostly with schizophrenia (21). SGA have weak GABA-agonist activity and 5HT2-antagonism that could stimulate dopamine release in the prefrontal cortex and thus alleviate catatonic symptoms (11). Several authors have reported a beneficial effect of SGA, such as clozapine (60–63), olanzapine (64–66), risperidone (67–70), and quetiapine (71). In one randomized controlled trial, in 14 stuporous psychotic patients, risperidone (4–6 mg/day) was compared to ECT. ECT-treated patients showed significantly greater improvement than those receiving risperidone (72).

The use of antipsychotics in the presence of catatonia should be evaluated in any individual case. We support, however, the general notion to discontinue neuroleptics because of their inefficacy and their potential of aggravating the catatonic symptoms. Once treatment with benzodiazepines or ECT is started and catatonia improves, there may be a role for SGA to target residual psychotic symptoms such as delusions or hallucinations, especially in patients with schizophrenia (69), or as a prophylactic treatment in psychotic disorders and mood disorders. SGA with low D2 blockade (quetiapine, olanzapine) or with D2 partial agonism (aripiprazole) should be favored in these situations (54).

Patients presenting with both delirium and catatonia warrant special consideration (73, 74). Catatonia is a frequent feature of delirious mania, a severe syndrome characterized by the rapid onset of delirium, mania, and psychosis. Symptoms of catatonia and delirium overlap, complicating diagnosis. Moreover, DSM states that catatonia should not be diagnosed if it occurs during the course of a delirium. The issue is important because treatments for catatonia and delirium are different, albeit with overlap. While delirium is typically treated with (typical or atypical) antipsychotics, the emergence of catatonia may caution against the use of antipsychotics (75, 76). Moreover, if catatonia is not recognized in a delirious patient, the withdrawal or withholding of benzodiazepines sometimes thought to worsen delirium may induce catatonia or leave catatonia untreated. Further studies in delirious patients are needed to aid these treatment dilemmas (77).

DIAGNOSTIC TEST

Benzodiazepines are the mainstay of the treatment of catatonia and are also helpful as a diagnostic probe. A positive *Lorazepam Challenge Test* validates the diagnosis of catatonia. After the patient is examined for signs of catatonia, 1 or 2 mg of lorazepam is administered intravenously. After 5 minutes, the patient is re-examined. If there has been no change, a second dose is given, and the patient is again reassessed (46, 78). A positive response is a marked reduction (e.g., at least 50%) of catatonic signs and symptoms, as measured with a standardized rating scale. Favorable responses usually occur within 10 min (46). If lorazepam is given intramuscularly or *per os*, the interval for the second dose should be longer: 15′ and 30′, respectively. Many clinicians will share the experience that a "lorazepam test" not only confirms the diagnosis of catatonia but that it also makes the underlying psychopathology apparent "*by permitting mute patients to speak*" (79). Analogous to the lorazepam test, a *Zolpidem Challenge Test* was proposed (80, 81). In this test 10 mg of zolpidem is administered *per os* and after 30 min the patient is examined. A positive response is a reduction of at least 50% of the BFCRS-score. After a positive response, treatment can be initiated.

BENZODIAZEPINES

Benzodiazepines are the first-choice treatment for catatonia, regardless of the underlying condition. Benzodiazepines are positive allosteric modulators of GABA-A receptors and will correct deficient GABA-ergic function in the orbitofrontal cortex (11). Following a positive *Lorazepam Challenge Test*, repeated doses of benzodiazepines can be used as a treatment. Their use is safe, easy and effective, with remission rates reported to be as high as 70–80% (4, 27, 82–87). In a naturalistic study of 66 children and adolescents with catatonia, it was found that benzodiazepines improved catatonia in 65% of cases, that there was no relation between dose and level of improvement, that the dose was higher in some cases (up to 15 mg of lorazepam) than the dose recommended in pediatric patients, and that side effects were few (16). In a recent trial in 107 adult inpatients (49% with a psychotic disorder; 44% with a mood disorder), lower success rates were reported: two thirds responded but only one third of patients remitted (30). The authors argue that the lower remission rate could be explained by a delay between illness onset and treatment (30) but the doses used in the trial (3–6 mg per day) were inadequately low. As described above, it was shown repeatedly that chronic catatonia associated with schizophrenia is less responsive to benzodiazepines. Beckmann and colleagues, in a 5-year follow-up study, found benzodiazepines ineffective in the treatment of chronic catatonic schizophrenia (33). A comparable poor response (to lorazepam 6 mg per day) was shown in a randomized double-blind, placebo-controlled trial in 18 patients with chronic catatonia in schizophrenia (26).

Efficacy of benzodiazepines in catatonia is determined by dosage (75), and doses from 8 to 24 mg lorazepam per day are common and are tolerated without ensuing sedation, especially when instituted using daily incremental dosages (77). Most authors suggest starting at 1–2 mg of lorazepam every 4–12 h, and adjusting the dose in order to relieve catatonia without sedating the patient (11). With an adequate dose, response is usually seen within 3–7 days (75), but is some cases, response can be gradual and slow (38). If high dosages of lorazepam are used, patients should be monitored carefully for excessive sedation and respiratory compromise (77). The issue of whether some benzodiazepines are more efficacious in catatonia has not been cleared. Lorazepam is generally accepted to be a first-choice drug, demonstrating a 79% remission rate and the highest frequency of use (84). Successful use of diazepam (86–90), oxazepam (91), or clonazepam (27, 92–95) has also been reported. There is no consensus on how long benzodiazepines are to be continued, and generally they are discontinued once the underlying illness has remitted. In a number of cases, however, catatonic symptoms will emerge each time lorazepam is tapered off, urging the clinician to continue benzodiazepines for an extended period of time (96, 97).

ZOLPIDEM

Zolpidem, a positive allosteric modulator of GABA-A receptors, seems to be a safe and effective treatment alternative. To our knowledge, Mastain and colleagues were the first to report a dramatic durable improvement of catatonia, resistant to ECT and benzodiazepines, with zolpidem in a 56-year-old woman that was in a catatonic state secondary to a subcortical stroke (98). Two years later, the same group presented an open study with zolpidem in seven catatonic patients, observing remission of catatonic symptoms in five of them within 15–30 min after ingestion, lasting 2–5 h (99). They observed these therapeutic effects at a plasma concentration between 80 and 130 ng/L. They also published a case report about catatonia in a 21-year-old woman, resolving 15 min after administration of zolpidem as the plasma concentration reached a peak level of 90 ng/mL. Relapse occurred after 4 h when plasma concentrations fell below 90 ng/mL (80). In a subsequent publication of the same French group, the authors confirm a prompt response (i.e., reduction of at least 50% of symptoms) in all patients 20 min after the administration of 10 mg zolpidem, at a plasma level of 80–150 ng/L (29). These favorable results are replicated in a few case reports (100–102). In some instances, the beneficial response to zolpidem occurred after treatment with benzodiazepines and/or ECT had failed (98, 101, 102). These data have led to the proposition of a *Zolpidem Challenge Test* (see higher), and have urged some clinicians to continue treatment with zolpidem instead of benzodiazepines, using doses from 7.5 to 40 mg per day, without noticeable adverse effects. Even though the short-half life results in a transient effect on symptoms, long-term treatment with zolpidem has also been described (101, 102).

GLUTAMATE ANTAGONISTS

Because of its *N*-methyl-D-aspartic acid (NMDA) antagonist properties, amantadine (100–500 mg three times a day), and its derivative memantine (5–20 mg/day), have been tried in catatonia. Carroll and coworkers identified 25 cases of amantadine and memantine use in the treatment of catatonia (103). All cases (16/25 were psychotic disorders) were substantially improved, mostly after 1–7 days. It should be noted, however, that six of these cases were unpublished, and that seven other were cases experiencing a "*catatonia-parkinsonian syndrome*" while under treatment with the high-potency neuroleptic drugs haloperidol or fluphenazine. The symptoms diminished when neuroleptics were tapered and amantadine was added (104, 105). Since then, eleven additional cases describing the successful use of amantadine or memantine in catatonia have been published (58, 105–110). In one case, in an adolescent girl, catatonia that was resistant to ECT improved after the addition of amantadine (58). Only in a review of Hawkins and coworkers, a case is reported in which the use of amantadine remained without effect (84). It should be acknowledged, however, that negative cases are less likely to be published. Nevertheless, given these positive signals in the published literature, and evidence of its efficacy in treating the negative and cognitive symptoms of schizophrenia, amantadine should be further studied as a possible treatment option for catatonia.

OTHER AGENTS

There is anecdotal evidence from case-reports on the use of various other pharmacological agents, such as bromocriptine (111) and biperiden (112). Based on the GABA-hypothesis of catatonia, and the GABA-related working mechanism of several anti-convulsive mood stabilizers, these drugs have been proposed as a possible treatment option for the treatment of catatonia in bipolar patients. Only a few case-reports have been published. Valproate was used in several case reports (113–115), and found not only to have prophylactic effects but also "an ameliorating effect on the catatonic symptoms" (116). In a single case report, levetiracetam was advocated as a treatment for catatonia in bipolar disorder (117), given its possible mood stabilizing efficacy. It is of note, however, that levetiracetam has also been described to provoke catatonia (118). The use of topiramate (119) and carbamazepine (120) has also been reported. Although lithium has been anecdotally reported to have a beneficial effect on acute catatonic symptoms (121, 122), it is mostly described to be of use in the prevention of recurrent catatonia (121, 123–127), albeit with sometimes limited results (123).

ELECTROCONVULSIVE THERAPY

Electroconvulsive therapy should be started in a patient with catatonia that is not responding to benzodiazepines or when a decisive and rapid response is required in severe cases with life-threatening conditions such as malignant catatonia featuring high idiopathic fevers, tachycardia, severe blood pressure changes. If the underlying condition, e.g., psychotic depression, warrants ECT, this treatment may as well become the treatment of first choice.

The excellent efficacy of ECT in catatonia is generally acknowledged, even in the absence of randomized controlled evidence. The guidelines for the use of neurostimulation therapies in major depressive disorder of the Canadian Network for Mood and Anxiety Treatments define catatonia as one of the indications in which ECT should be considered as a first-line treatment (128).

Response rates in ECT are not systematically studied, but it is efficacy is described in hundreds of case reports and some small studies. In a review paper, Hawkins et al. reported an 85% (47/55) complete response rate (84). To our knowledge, only one randomized controlled ECT trial has been published. In this trial, the efficacy of ECT (BT, 3/W, $N = 8$) plus oral placebo was compared with sham ECT plus risperidone in lorazepam non-responsive non-affective catatonia. BFCRS scores reduced markedly, but the reduction was significantly more profound in the ECT group (72). Suzuki and co-workers studied both short- and long-term efficacy of ECT in intractable catatonic schizophrenia. In the acute phase, 100% of 11 patients responded to ECT. Relapse occurred in seven cases, and all occurred within 6 months. The 1-year recurrence rate was 63.6%, despite continuation pharmacotherapy (129). Relapsers received a second course of ECT followed by maintenance ECT for 1 year and four remained in remission (130). Those who relapsed again could be treated successfully with adjusting the frequency of treatment sessions (131). In another Japanese study, the efficacy of ECT was shown very clearly (132). Fifty patients presenting with catatonic symptoms, 23 of whom were diagnosed with schizophrenia, received either ECT or a benzodiazepine as first-line treatment. If benzodiazepines were ineffective, the next step was either ECT or an antipsychotic drug; if the latter failed, ECT was the last resort. Only 1 of 41 patients responded fully to benzodiazepines, and 19 responded partially. In contrast, all 17 patients who received ECT achieved remission. Payee and coworkers confirmed these favorable results: 8 of 9 (89%) lorazepam-non-responders responded to ECT (85). In another small (N = 9) prospective comparative study Escobar and colleagues (133) noted that catatonic symptoms remitted faster and to a greater extent in the depressed patients (4/9) than in those with schizophrenia (5/9).

In seven retrospective chart reviews, with a total of 222 patients, mostly benzodiazepine-non-responders, high response rates are confirmed (**Table 1**). The largest and most informative study included a chart review of 250 patients with catatonic schizophrenia, and was part of the Iowa 500 project (134). Eighty-five (40%) patients remitted (regardless of treatment used), while 53% of the 75 patients who had received ECT remitted. Another retrospective chart review was conducted in a university-affiliated inpatient unit. Seven of 19 patients presenting with catatonia were diagnosed with schizophrenia and ECT was used in four of them, experiencing partial ($N = 3$) or considerable ($N = 1$) improvement. In contrast, five out of five patients with mood disorder fully recovered after receiving ECT (28).

Rohland et al. reported ECT to be effective in 93% (26/28) of patients with catatonia admitted to an inpatient psychiatric unit (32). England et al. reported dramatic improvement in 10 of 12 (83%) patients with catatonia after 1–5 ECT sessions (63). In the largest study to date, 63 patients with catatonia (30% schizophrenia; 41% mood disorders) received bilateral ECT, thrice weekly, either as a first choice ($n = 6$), or after lorazepam had failed ($n = 57$). Fifty-six patients (89%) responded to ECT. Patients who responded in 4 sessions (31/56; 55%) had a lower duration of catatonia, a higher BFCRS-score, more often waxy flexibility and Gegenhalten, the involuntary resistance to passive movement of the extremities. Echophenomena predicted a slower response (136). The lowest response rates were reported in a retrospective study of 27 patients, treated with bitemporal ECT, often daily during the first week (47). Response rates were 59%. Probably, the smaller proportion of patients with a primary mood disorder, a significant treatment delay (a mean time interval of 2 months) may have negatively influenced treatment response. Another possible explanation is the fact that one third of the patients had been exposed to antipsychotics before ECT, which was reported earlier to be related to a decreased effectiveness (84).

The successful use of ECT in chronic catatonia has been described in a few case reports (137–140). Duration of catatonia varied from 3 months to 12 years, and in some cases protracted courses of bitemporal ECT (e.g., 17–68 treatments (138, 140) were needed to achieve a response. In several of these chronic cases, the catatonic symptoms reappeared when ECT was stopped. Some patients with chronic catatonia in schizophrenia will respond to a

Table 1 | ECT in catatonia: retrospective chart reviews.

Author(s), year	ECT EP/Schedule	Mood (%)/psychotic disorder (%)	N responders/*N* total	Responders (%)
Morrison (134)	NA/NA	0/100	40/75	53
Pataki (28)	BT/NA	56/44	6/9	67
McCall (135)	BT/NA	75/12	7/8	88
Rohland (33)	BT/3*W	59/23	26/28	93
van Waarde (47)	BT (93%)/daily [first week (56%)]	48/44	16/27	59
England (63)	BT/NA	NA	10/12	83
Raveendranathan (136)	BT/3*W	41/30	56/63	89

EP, electrode position; BT, bitemporal; N, number; NA, not available.

combination of ECT and clozapine. In a retrospective study, this combination resulted in sound clinical improvement as measured with the clinical global impression (CGI) in 22 patients (141).

A recent systematic review of treatment of (severe) autistic catatonia identified 12 cases with autism and catatonic symptoms of a few months to around 6 years' duration, treated with ECT-courses that ranged from 7 to 29 sessions. Almost all cases reported a dramatic improvement with ECT, usually after relatively few sessions. A few papers report a more mixed response to ECT. Several cases reported rapid recurrence of symptoms when ECT was discontinued or suspended (142). Consoli et al collected 59 cases of children and adolescents with catatonia treated with ECT. Response to ECT was favorable for 45 patients (76%), with partial improvement noted in 3 (5%) and a lack of response in only one (143).

Recently, several authors report on the successful use of unilateral ECT in a total number of 21 cases (36, 144), 15 of which were treated with an ultra-brief pulse (UB) width (139, 145, 146). In a case-series of 5 patients with catatonia, resistant to benzodiazepines, 4 patients experienced a full response with unilateral ECT; one patient achieved only partial response, and was switched to bitemporal without experiencing any additional benefit (144). In the largest case-series to date, of 13 catatonic patients treated, 11 had rapid symptom resolution with UB right-unilateral (RUL) ECT with minimal adverse effects. Two patients who did not improve with RUL ECT were switched to bilateral ECT, which provided no additional symptom benefit (146). These favorable results probably reflect the high responsiveness of catatonia to ECT, whatever technique is used. Most authors, however, strongly recommend bilateral ECT at substantially suprathreshold stimulus dosing in severely ill patients, arguing that there is substantially more evidence, and that transient cognitive impairment is a secondary consideration in patients with severe catatonia (41, 147).

It is generally advised to stop psychopharmacological agents prior to initiation of ECT. When there was a partial response with benzodiazepine treatment, it might be unwise to abruptly discontinue this treatment, because of possible interference with seizure threshold and the risk of aggravating the catatonic state. Lorazepam and ECT can be given concurrently. If lorazepam interferes with eliciting seizures, flumazenil, a partial benzodiazepine antagonist, can be given just before the anesthetic (75).

The number of treatments, before substantial and sustained improvement becomes obvious, cannot be predicted. Often, a rapid response is seen, after one or a few treatment sessions (63, 136), but sometimes catatonia seems to require more treatments than is necessary for the relief of major depression (138, 140). Therefore, ECT treatment must be individually tailored. In severe or malignant catatonia, daily ("en bloc") treatments for three to 5 days may be necessary. Maintenance-ECT may be useful for sustained symptom-remission.

TRANSCRANIAL MAGNETIC STIMULATION

The successful use of rTMS was reported in four cases, after 7–10 high-frequency stimulation sessions of the dorso-lateral prefrontal cortex (148–151). In one case, a 45-year-old man with schizophrenia, previously recovering from catatonia with ECT failed to improve with rTMS (152).

CONCLUSION

Catatonia is a severe psychomotor syndrome with an excellent prognosis if recognized and treated appropriately. The treatment of catatonia in children and adolescents should follow the same principles as in adults. Great care should be taken to avoid (medical) complications. Although a number of pharmacological agents have been tried successfully in catatonia, rarely, if ever, the effect is as immediate and dramatic as seen with benzodiazepines. If lorazepam is not available, zolpidem can be used as a diagnostic probe, and probably as a treatment alternative. If benzodiazepines fail (inadequate or transient response, excessive sedation), ECT should be started without delay. If the underlying condition warrants ECT-treatment, or in life-threatening situations like malignant catatonia or NMS, ECT is the treatment of first choice. It is advised to choose the most efficacious technique, i.e., bilateral standard-pulse ECT with a stimulus dose that is substantially above the seizure threshold.

REFERENCES

1. Pommepuy N, Januel D. [Catatonia: resurgence of a concept. A review of the international literature]. *Encephale* (2002) **28**(6 Pt 1):481–92.
2. Francis A, Fink M, Appiani F, Bertelsen A, Bolwig TG, Braunig P, et al. Catatonia in diagnostic and statistical manual of mental disorders, fifth edition. *J ECT* (2010) **26**(4):246–7. doi:10.1097/YCT.0b013e3181fe28bd
3. Abrams R, Taylor MA. Catatonia: a prospective clinical study. *Arch Gen Psychiatry* (1976) **33**(5):579–81. doi:10.1001/archpsyc.1976.01770050043006
4. Rosebush PI, Mazurek MF. Catatonia and its treatment. *Schizophr Bull* (2010) **36**(2):239–42. doi:10.1093/schbul/sbp141
5. Fontenelle LF, Lauterbach EC, Telles LL, Versiani M, Porto FH, Mendlowicz MV. Catatonia in obsessive-compulsive disorder: etiopathogenesis, differential diagnosis, and clinical management. *Cogn Behav Neurol* (2007) **20**(1):21–4. doi:10.1097/WNN.0b013e31802e3bc6
6. Shiloh R, Schwartz B, Weizman A, Radwan M. Catatonia as an unusual presentation of posttraumatic stress disorder. *Psychopathology* (1995) **28**(6):285–90. doi:10.1159/000284940
7. Moskowitz AK. "Scared stiff": catatonia as an evolutionary-based fear response. *Psychol Rev* (2004) **111**(4):984–1002. doi:10.1037/0033-295X.111.3.808
8. Geoffroy PA, Rolland B, Cottencin O. Catatonia and alcohol withdrawal: a complex and underestimated syndrome. *Alcohol Alcohol* (2012) **47**(3):288–90. doi:10.1093/alcalc/agr170
9. Parameswaran R, Moore K, Hannan T, Austin M. Catatonia associated with temazepam withdrawal. *Aust N Z J Psychiatry* (2011) **45**(11):1006–7. doi:10.3109/00048674.2011.607131
10. Sivakumar T, Yadav A, Sood M, Khandelwal SK. Lorazepam withdrawal catatonia: a case report. *Asian J Psychiatr* (2013) **6**(6):620–1. doi:10.1016/j.ajp.2013.05.008
11. Daniels J. Catatonia: clinical aspects and neurobiological correlates. *J Neuropsychiatry Clin Neurosci* (2009) **21**(4):371–80. doi:10.1176/appi.neuropsych.21.4.371
12. Dalmau J, Gleichman AJ, Hughes EG, Rossi JE, Peng X, Lai M, et al. Anti-NMDA-receptor encephalitis: case series and analysis of the effects of antibodies. *Lancet Neurol* (2008) **7**(12):1091–8. doi:10.1016/S1474-4422(08)70224-2
13. Gulyayeva NA, Massie MJ, Duhamel KN. Anti-NMDA receptor encephalitis: psychiatric presentation and diagnostic challenges from psychosomatic medicine perspective. *Palliat Support Care* (2014) **12**(2):159–63. doi:10.1017/S1478951513000515
14. Wing L, Shah A. Catatonia in autistic spectrum disorders. *Br J Psychiatry* (2000) **176**:357–62. doi:10.1192/bjp.176.4.357
15. Dhossche D, Goetz M, Gazdag G, Sienaert P. New DSM-5 category 'unspecified catatonia' is a boost for pediatric catatonia: review and case reports. *Neuropsychiatry* (2013) **3**(4):401–10. doi:10.2217/npy.13.42
16. Raffin M, Zugaj-Bensaou L, Bodeau N, Milhiet V, Laurent C, Cohen D, et al. Treatment use in a prospective naturalistic cohort of children and adolescents with catatonia. *Eur Child Adolesc Psychiatry* (2014). doi:10.1007/s00787-014-0595-y

17. Stauder KH. Die todliche Katatonie. *Arch Psychiatr Nervenkr* (1934) **102**:614–34. doi:10.1007/BF01813829
18. Sienaert P, Dhossche DM, Gazdag G. Adult catatonia: etiopathogenesis, diagnosis and treatment. *Neuropsychiatry* (2013) **3**(4):391–9. doi:10.2217/npy.13.41
19. Sienaert P, Rooseleer J, De Fruyt J. Measuring catatonia: a systematic review of rating scales. *J Affect Disord* (2011) **135**(1–3):1–9. doi:10.1016/j.jad.2011.02.012
20. Rooseleer J, Willaert A, Sienaert P. [Rating scales for assessing catatonia; which ones are the best?]. *Tijdschr Psychiatr* (2011) **53**(5):287–98.
21. Gazdag G, Sienaert P. Diagnosing and treating catatonia: an update. *Curr Psychiatry Rev* (2013) **9**(2):130–5. doi:10.2174/1573400511309020007
22. Lazar-Molnar E, Tebo AE. Autoimmune NMDA receptor encephalitis. *Clin Chim Acta* (2014) **438C**:90–7. doi:10.1016/j.cca.2014.08.010
23. Rosebush PI, Mazurek MF. Serum iron and neuroleptic malignant syndrome. *Lancet* (1991) **338**(8760):149–51. doi:10.1016/0140-6736(91)90138-F
24. Lee JW. Serum iron in catatonia and neuroleptic malignant syndrome. *Biol Psychiatry* (1998) **44**(6):499–507. doi:10.1016/S0006-3223(98)00109-7 Epub 1998/10/20.,
25. Hoch A, MacCurdy JT. *Benign Stupors; A Study of a New Manic-Depressive Reaction Type.* New York, NY: The Macmillan Company (1921). 284 p.
26. Ungvari GS, Chiu HF, Chow LY, Lau BS, Tang WK. Lorazepam for chronic catatonia: a randomized, double-blind, placebo-controlled cross-over study. *Psychopharmacology (Berl)* (1999) **142**(4):393–8. doi:10.1007/s002130050904
27. Lee JW, Schwartz DL, Hallmayer J. Catatonia in a psychiatric intensive care facility: incidence and response to benzodiazepines. *Ann Clin Psychiatry* (2000) **12**(2):89–96. doi:10.3109/10401230009147094
28. Pataki J, Zervas IM, Jandorf L. Catatonia in a university inpatient service (1985-1990). *Convuls Ther* (1992) **8**(3):163–73.
29. Thomas P, Cottencin O, Rascle C, Vaiva G, Goudemand M, Bieder J. Catatonia in French psychiatry: implications for the Zolpidem challenge test. *Psychiatr Ann* (2007) **37**(1):45–54.
30. Tibrewal P, Narayanaswamy J, Zutshi A, Srinivasaraju R, Math SB. Response rate of lorazepam in catatonia: a developing country's perspective. *Prog Neuropsychopharmacol Biol Psychiatry* (2010) **34**(8):1520–2. doi:10.1016/j.pnpbp.2010.08.017
31. Narayanaswamy JC, Tibrewal P, Zutshi A, Srinivasaraju R, Math SB. Clinical predictors of response to treatment in catatonia. *Gen Hosp Psychiatry* (2012) **34**(3):312–6. doi:10.1016/j.genhosppsych.2012.01.011
32. Rohland BM, Carroll BT, Jacoby RG. ECT in the treatment of the catatonic syndrome. *J Affect Disord* (1993) **29**(4):255–61. doi:10.1016/0165-0327(93)90015-C
33. Beckmann H, Fritze J, Franzek E. The influence of neuroleptics on specific syndromes and symptoms in schizophrenics with unfavourable long-term course. A 5-year follow-up study of 50 chronic schizophrenics. *Neuropsychobiology* (1992) **26**(1–2):50–8. doi:10.1159/000118896
34. Ungvari GS, Caroff SN, Gerevich J. The catatonia conundrum: evidence of psychomotor phenomena as a symptom dimension in psychotic disorders. *Schizophr Bull* (2010) **36**(2):231–8. doi:10.1093/schbul/sbp105
35. Singh LK, Praharaj SK. Immediate response to lorazepam in a patient with 17 years of chronic catatonia. *J Neuropsychiatry Clin Neurosci* (2013) **25**(3):E47–8. doi:10.1176/appi.neuropsych.12070181
36. Mon T, L'Ecuyer S, Farber NB, White AJ, Baszis KW, Hearn JK, et al. The use of electroconvulsive therapy in a patient with juvenile systemic lupus erythematosus and catatonia. *Lupus* (2012) **21**(14):1575–81. doi:10.1177/0961203312464803
37. Bulbul F, Unal A, Copoglu US, Alpak G, Savas HA. Persistent catatonia for 1.5 years finally resolved with electroconvulsive therapy. *J ECT* (2013) **29**(1):e1. doi:10.1097/YCT.0b013e318257c8fe
38. Gaind GS, Rosebush PI, Mazurek MF. Lorazepam treatment of acute and chronic catatonia in two mentally retarded brothers. *J Clin Psychiatry* (1994) **55**(1):20–3.
39. Ripley TL, Millson RC. Psychogenic catatonia treated with lorazepam. *Am J Psychiatry* (1988) **145**(6):764–5.
40. Salam SA, Pillai AK, Beresford TP. Lorazepam for psychogenic catatonia. *Am J Psychiatry* (1987) **144**(8):1082–3.
41. Nazarian RS, Liebman LS, Kellner CH. Electroconvulsive therapy (ECT) for catatonia: delay may be risky. *Lupus* (2013) **22**(3):336. doi:10.1177/0961203313476362
42. Meduna L. *Die Konvulsionstherapie der Schizophrenie.* Halle: Carl Marhold Verlagsbuch-Handlung (1937).
43. Gazdag G, Bitter I, Ungvari GS, Baran B, Fink M. Laszlo Meduna's pilot studies with camphor inductions of seizures: the first 11 patients. *J ECT* (2009) **25**(1):3–11. doi:10.1097/YCT.0b013e31819359fc
44. Urstein M. *Manisch-depressives und periodisches Irresein als Erscheinungsform der Katatonie.* Berlin: Urban und Schwarzenberg (1912).
45. Fink M. Catatonia: syndrome or schizophrenia subtype? Recognition and treatment. *J Neural Transm* (2001) **108**(6):637–44. doi:10.1007/s007020170041
46. Fink M, Taylor MA. *Catatonia: A Clinician's Guide to Diagnosis and Treatment.* New York, NY: Cambridge University Press (2003). 256 p.
47. van Waarde JA, Tuerlings JH, Verwey B, van der Mast RC. Electroconvulsive therapy for catatonia: treatment characteristics and outcomes in 27 patients. *J ECT* (2010) **26**(4):248–52. doi:10.1097/YCT.0b013e3181c18a13
48. Swartz CM, Acosta D, Bashir A. Diminished ECT response in catatonia due to chronic neurologic condition. *J ECT* (2003) **19**(2):110–4. doi:10.1097/00124509-200306000-00010
49. Rosebush PI. Perspectives on catatonia: 2 decades of personal clinical experience. *10th World Congress of Biological Psychiatry.* Prague: (2011).
50. Clinebell K, Azzam PN, Gopalan P, Haskett R. Guidelines for preventing common medical complications of catatonia: case report and literature review. *J Clin Psychiatry* (2014) **75**(6):644–51. doi:10.4088/JCP.13r08870
51. White DA, Robins AH. Catatonia: harbinger of the neuroleptic malignant syndrome. *Br J Psychiatry* (1991) **158**:419–21. doi:10.1192/bjp.158.3.419
52. White DA. Catatonia and the neuroleptic malignant syndrome – a single entity? *Br J Psychiatry* (1992) **161**:558–60. doi:10.1192/bjp.161.4.558
53. Braunig P, Kruger S, Hoffler J. [Exacerbation of catatonic symptoms in neuroleptic therapy]. *Nervenarzt* (1995) **66**(5):379–82.
54. Carroll BT, Lee JWY, Appiani F, Thomas C. The pharmacotherapy of catatonia. *Prim psychiatry* (2010) **17**(4):41–7. doi:10.1097/YCT.0b013e3181fe28bd
55. Adityanjee, Aderibigbe YA, Mathews T. Epidemiology of neuroleptic malignant syndrome. *Clin Neuropharmacol* (1999) **22**(3):151–8.
56. Lee JW. Neuroleptic-induced catatonia: clinical presentation, response to benzodiazepines, and relationship to neuroleptic malignant syndrome. *J Clin Psychopharmacol* (2010) **30**(1):3–10. doi:10.1097/JCP.0b013e3181c9bfe6
57. Lewis AL, Pelic C, Kahn DA. Malignant catatonia in a patient with bipolar disorder, B12 deficiency, and neuroleptic malignant syndrome: one cause or three? *J Psychiatr Pract* (2009) **15**(5):415–22. doi:10.1097/01.pra.0000361282.95962.9f
58. Goetz M, Kitzlerova E, Hrdlicka M, Dhossche D. Combined use of electroconvulsive therapy and amantadine in adolescent catatonia precipitated by cyber-bullying. *J Child Adolesc Psychopharmacol* (2013) **23**(3):228–31. doi:10.1089/cap.2012.0045
59. Ungvari GS, Kau LS, Wai-Kwong T, Shing NF. The pharmacological treatment of catatonia: an overview. *Eur Arch Psychiatry Clin Neurosci* (2001) **251**(Suppl 1):I31–4. doi:10.1007/PL00014198
60. Naber D, Holzbach R, Perro C, Hippius H. Clinical management of clozapine patients in relation to efficacy and side-effects. *Br J Psychiatry Suppl* (1992) **161**(17):54–9.
61. Rommel O, Tegenthoff M, Widdig W, Braunig P, Malin JP. Organic catatonia following frontal lobe injury: response to clozapine. *J Neuropsychiatry Clin Neurosci* (1998) **10**(2):237–8.
62. Hung YY, Yang PS, Huang TL. Clozapine in schizophrenia patients with recurrent catatonia: report of two cases. *Psychiatry Clin Neurosci* (2006) **60**(2):256–8. doi:10.1111/j.1440-1819.2006.01495.x
63. England ML, Ongur D, Konopaske GT, Karmacharya R. Catatonia in psychotic patients: clinical features and treatment response. *J Neuropsychiatry Clin Neurosci* (2011) **23**(2):223–6. doi:10.1176/appi.neuropsych.23.2.223
64. Cassidy EM, O'Brien M, Osman MF, Finucane J, O'Keane V. Lethal catatonia responding to high-dose olanzapine therapy. *J Psychopharmacol* (2001) **15**(4):302–4. doi:10.1177/026988110101500412
65. Martenyi F, Metcalfe S, Schausberger B, Dossenbach MR. An efficacy analysis of olanzapine treatment data in schizophrenia patients with catatonic signs and symptoms. *J Clin Psychiatry* (2001) **62**(Suppl 2):25–7.
66. Numata S, Kato O, Misawa H. Treatment of catatonia with olanzapine. *German J Psychiatr* (2002) **5**:115–6.
67. Kopala LC, Caudle C. Acute and longer-term effects of risperidone in a case of first-episode catatonic schizophrenia. *J Psychopharmacol* (1998) **12**(3):314–7. doi:10.1177/026988119801200312

68. Valevski A, Loebl T, Keren T, Bodinger L, Weizman A. Response of catatonia to risperidone: two case reports. *Clin Neuropharmacol* (2001) **24**(4):228–31. doi:10.1097/00002826-200107000-00006
69. Van Den Eede F, Van Hecke J, Van Dalfsen A, Van den Bossche B, Cosyns P, Sabbe BG. The use of atypical antipsychotics in the treatment of catatonia. *Eur Psychiatry* (2005) **20**(5–6):422–9. doi:10.1016/j.eurpsy.2005.03.012
70. Grenier E, Ryan M, Ko E, Fajardo K, John V. Risperidone and lorazepam concomitant use in clonazepam refractory catatonia: a case report. *J Nerv Ment Dis* (2011) **199**(12):987–8. doi:10.1097/NMD.0b013e3182392d7e
71. Yoshimura B, Hirota T, Takaki M, Kishi Y. Is quetiapine suitable for treatment of acute schizophrenia with catatonic stupor? A case series of 39 patients. *Neuropsychiatr Dis Treat* (2013) **9**:1565–71. doi:10.2147/NDT.S52311
72. Girish K, Gill NS. Electroconvulsive therapy in lorazepam non-responsive catatonia. *Indian J Psychiatry* (2003) **45**(1):21–5.
73. Detweiler MB, Mehra A, Rowell T, Kim KY, Bader G. Delirious mania and malignant catatonia: a report of 3 cases and review. *Psychiatr Q* (2009) **80**(1):23–40. doi:10.1007/s11126-009-9091-9
74. Lee BS, Huang SS, Hsu WY, Chiu NY. Clinical features of delirious mania: a series of five cases and a brief literature review. *BMC Psychiatry* (2012) **12**:65. doi:10.1186/1471-244X-12-65
75. Fink M, Taylor MA. Neuroleptic malignant syndrome is malignant catatonia, warranting treatments efficacious for catatonia. *Prog Neuropsychopharmacol Biol Psychiatry* (2006) **30**(6):1182–3. doi:10.1016/j.pnpbp.2006.03.029
76. Seitz DP, Gill SS. Neuroleptic malignant syndrome complicating antipsychotic treatment of delirium or agitation in medical and surgical patients: case reports and a review of the literature. *Psychosomatics* (2009) **50**(1):8–15. doi:10.1176/appi.psy.50.1.8
77. Dhossche DM, Wachtel LE, Goetz M, Sienaert P. Catatonia in psychiatric illnessess. In: Fatemi H, Clayton P, editors. *The Medical Basis of Psychiatry*. New York: Springer (2014).
78. Bush G, Fink M, Petrides G, Dowling F, Francis A. Catatonia. II. Treatment with lorazepam and electroconvulsive therapy. *Acta Psychiatr Scand* (1996) **93**(2):137–43. doi:10.1111/j.1600-0447.1996.tb09815.x
79. McEvoy JP. Relief from catatonic immobility can be maintained. *J Clin Psychopharmacol* (1986) **6**(2):126–7. doi:10.1097/00004714-198604000-00025
80. Thomas P, Rascle C, Mastain B, Maron M, Vaiva G. Test for catatonia with zolpidem. *Lancet* (1997) **349**(9053):702. doi:10.1016/S0140-6736(05)60139-0
81. Cottencin O, Warembourg F, de Chouly de Lenclave MB, Lucas B, Vaiva G, Goudemand M, et al. Catatonia and consultation-liaison psychiatry study of 12 cases. *Prog Neuropsychopharmacol Biol Psychiatry* (2007) **31**(6):1170–6. doi:10.1016/j.pnpbp.2007.04.006
82. Rosebush PI, Hildebrand AM, Furlong BG, Mazurek MF. Catatonic syndrome in a general psychiatric inpatient population: frequency, clinical presentation, and response to lorazepam. *J Clin Psychiatry* (1990) **51**(9):357–62.
83. Rosebush PI, Hildebrand AM, Mazurek MF. The treatment of catatonia: benzodiazepines of ECT? *Am J Psychiatry* (1992) **149**(9):1279–80.
84. Hawkins JM, Archer KJ, Strakowski SM, Keck PE. Somatic treatment of catatonia. *Int J Psychiatry Med* (1995) **25**(4):345–69. doi:10.2190/X0FF-VU7G-QQP7-L5V7
85. Payee H, Chandrasekaran R, Raju GV. Catatonic syndrome: treatment response to Lorazepam. *Indian J Psychiatry* (1999) **41**(1):49–53.
86. Hung YY, Huang TL. Lorazepam and diazepam rapidly relieve catatonic features in major depression. *Clin Neuropharmacol* (2006) **29**(3):144–7. doi:10.1097/01.WNF.0000221908.56361.C7
87. Huang YC, Lin CC, Hung YY, Huang TL. Rapid relief of catatonia in mood disorder by lorazepam and diazepam. *Biomed J* (2013) **36**(1):35–9. doi:10.4103/2319-4170.107162
88. McEvoy JP, Lohr JB. Diazepam for catatonia. *Am J Psychiatry* (1984) **141**(2):284–5.
89. Huang TL. Lorazepam and diazepam rapidly relieve catatonic signs in patients with schizophrenia. *Psychiatry Clin Neurosci* (2005) **59**(1):52–5. doi:10.1111/j.1440-1819.2005.01331.x
90. Hung YY, Huang TL. Lorazepam and diazepam for relieving catatonic features in multiple sclerosis. *Prog Neuropsychopharmacol Biol Psychiatry* (2007) **31**(7):1537–8. doi:10.1016/j.pnpbp.2007.06.016
91. Schmider J, Standhart H, Deuschle M, Drancoli J, Heuser I. A double-blind comparison of lorazepam and oxazepam in psychomotor retardation and mutism. *Biol Psychiatry* (1999) **46**(3):437–41. doi:10.1016/S0006-3223(98)00312-6
92. Clothier JL, Pazzaglia P, Freeman TW. Evaluation and treatment of catatonia. *Am J Psychiatry* (1989) **146**(4):553–4.
93. Martenyi F, Harangozo J, Mod L. Clonazepam for the treatment of stupor in catatonic schizophrenia. *Am J Psychiatry* (1989) **146**(9):1230.
94. Benazzi F. Parenteral clonazepam for catatonia. *Can J Psychiatry* (1991) **36**(4):312.
95. Kumar R. Acute severe catatonia in a young woman with chronic schizophrenia responding to parenteral clonazepam. *Aust N Z J Psychiatry* (2001) **35**(3):391. doi:10.1046/j.1440-1614.2001.0905i.x
96. Manjunatha N, Saddichha S, Khess CR. Idiopathic recurrent catatonia needs maintenance lorazepam: case report and review. *Aust N Z J Psychiatry* (2007) **41**(7):625–7. doi:10.1080/00048670701400032
97. Grover S, Aggarwal M. Long-term maintenance lorazepam for catatonia: a case report. *Gen Hosp Psychiatry* (2011) **33**(1):e1–3. doi:10.1016/j.genhosppsych.2010.06.006
98. Mastain B, Vaiva G, Guerouaou D, Pommery J, Thomas P. [Favourable effect of zolpidem on catatonia]. *Rev Neurol (Paris)* (1995) **151**(1):52–6.
99. Rascle C, Thomas P, Maron M, Mastain B, Guesdon I, Cottencin O, et al. Catatonia relief with zolpidem: an open study. *Eur Neuropsychopharmacol* (1997) **7**(Suppl 2):S277. doi:10.1016/S0924-977X(97)88920-1
100. Zaw ZF, Bates GD. Replication of zolpidem test for catatonia in an adolescent. *Lancet* (1997) **349**(9069):1914. doi:10.1016/S0140-6736(05)63915-3
101. Peglow S, Prem V, McDaniel W. Treatment of catatonia with zolpidem. *J Neuropsychiatry Clin Neurosci* (2013) **25**(3):E13. doi:10.1176/appi.neuropsych.11120367
102. Hlal H, Kettani N, Berhili N, Rammouz I, Aalouane R. Place du zolpidem dans le traitement des catatonies résistantes aux benzodiazépines. À propos d'un cas. *Presse Med* (2014) **43**(9):1018–20. doi:10.1016/j.lpm.2013.11.023
103. Carroll BT, Goforth HW, Thomas C, Ahuja N, McDaniel WW, Kraus MF, et al. Review of adjunctive glutamate antagonist therapy in the treatment of catatonic syndromes. *J Neuropsychiatry Clin Neurosci* (2007) **19**(4):406–12. doi:10.1176/appi.neuropsych.19.4.406
104. Gelenberg AJ, Mandel MR. Catatonic reactions to high-potency neuroleptic drugs. *Arch Gen Psychiatry* (1977) **34**(8):947–50. doi:10.1001/archpsyc.1977.01770200085010
105. Obregon DF, Velasco RM, Wuerz TP, Catalano MC, Catalano G, Kahn D. Memantine and catatonia: a case report and literature review. *J Psychiatr Pract* (2011) **17**(4):292–9. doi:10.1097/01.pra.0000400268.60537.5e
106. Babington PW, Spiegel DR. Treatment of catatonia with olanzapine and amantadine. *Psychosomatics* (2007) **48**(6):534–6. doi:10.1176/appi.psy.48.6.534
107. Muneoka K, Shirayama Y, Kon K, Kawabe M, Goto M, Kimura S. Improvement of mutism in a catatonic schizophrenia case by add-on treatment with amantadine. *Pharmacopsychiatry* (2010) **43**(4):151–2. doi:10.1055/s-0029-1242821
108. Hervey WM, Stewart JT, Catalano G. Treatment of catatonia with amantadine. *Clin Neuropharmacol* (2012) **35**(2):86–7. doi:10.1097/WNF.0b013e318246ad34
109. de Lucena DF, Pinto JP, Hallak JE, Crippa JA, Gama CS. Short-term treatment of catatonia with amantadine in schizophrenia and schizoaffective disorder. *J Clin Psychopharmacol* (2012) **32**(4):569–72. doi:10.1097/JCP.0b013e31825ebf6e
110. Ene-Stroescu V, Nguyen T, Waiblinger BE. Excellent response to amantadine in a patient with bipolar disorder and catatonia. *J Neuropsychiatry Clin Neurosci* (2014) **26**(1):E43. doi:10.1176/appi.neuropsych.13020038
111. Mahmood T. Bromocriptine in catatonic stupor. *Br J Psychiatry* (1991) **158**:437–8. doi:10.1192/bjp.158.3.437
112. Franz M, Gallhofer B, Kanzow WT. Treatment of catatonia with intravenous biperidene. *Br J Psychiatry* (1994) **164**(6):847–8. doi:10.1192/bjp.164.6.847b
113. DelBello MP, Foster KD, Strakowski SM. Case report: treatment of catatonia in an adolescent male. *J Adolesc Health* (2000) **27**(1):69–71. doi:10.1016/S1054-139X(00)00109-9
114. Kruger S, Braunig P. Intravenous valproic acid in the treatment of severe catatonia. *J Neuropsychiatry Clin Neurosci* (2001) **13**(2):303–4. doi:10.1176/appi.neuropsych.13.2.303
115. Bowers R, Ajit SS. Is there a role for valproic acid in the treatment of catatonia? *J Neuropsychiatry Clin Neurosci* (2007) **19**(2):197–8. doi:10.1176/appi.neuropsych.19.2.197

116. Yoshida I, Monji A, Hashioka S, Ito M, Kanba S. Prophylactic effect of valproate in the treatment for siblings with catatonia: a case report. *J Clin Psychopharmacol* (2005) **25**(5):504–5. doi:10.1097/01.jcp.0000177850.23534.69
117. Muneer A. Catatonia in a patient with bipolar disorder type I. *J Neurosci Rural Pract* (2014) **5**(3):314–6. doi:10.4103/0976-3147.133652
118. Chouinard MJ, Nguyen DK, Clement JF, Bruneau MA. Catatonia induced by levetiracetam. *Epilepsy Behav* (2006) **8**(1):303–7. doi:10.1016/j.yebeh.2005.04.016
119. McDaniel WW, Spiegel DR, Sahota AK. Topiramate effect in catatonia: a case series. *J Neuropsychiatry Clin Neurosci* (2006) **18**(2):234–8. doi:10.1176/appi.neuropsych.18.2.234
120. Rankel HW, Rankel LE. Carbamazepine in the treatment of catatonia. *Am J Psychiatry* (1988) **145**(3):361–2.
121. Wald D, Lerner J. Lithium in the treatment of periodic catatonia: a case report. *Am J Psychiatry* (1978) **135**(6):751–2.
122. Pheterson AD, Estroff TW, Sweeney DR. Severe prolonged catatonia with associated flushing reaction responsive to lithium carbonate. *J Am Acad Child Psychiatry* (1985) **24**(2):235–7. doi:10.1016/S0002-7138(09)60454-4
123. Gjessing LR. Lithium citrate loading of a patient with periodic catatonia. *Acta Psychiatr Scand* (1967) **43**(4):372–5. doi:10.1111/j.1600-0447.1967.tb05774.x
124. Petursson H. Lithium treatment of a patient with periodic catatonia. *Acta Psychiatr Scand* (1976) **54**(4):248–53. doi:10.1111/j.1600-0447.1976.tb00118.x
125. Looper KJ, Milroy TM. Catatonia 20 years later. *Am J Psychiatry* (1997) **154**(6):883.
126. Sugahara Y, Tsukamoto H, Sasaki T. Lithium carbonate in prophylaxis of reappearing catatonic stupor: case report. *Psychiatry Clin Neurosci* (2000) **54**(5):607–9. doi:10.1046/j.1440-1819.2000.00762.x
127. Padhy SK, Subodh B, Bharadwaj R, Arun Kumar K, Kumar S, Srivastava M. Recurrent catatonia treated with lithium and carbamazepine: a series of 2 cases. *Prim Care Companion CNS Disord* (2011) **13**(1). doi:10.4088/PCC.10l00992
128. Kennedy SH, Milev R, Giacobbe P, Ramasubbu R, Lam RW, Parikh SV, et al. Canadian network for mood and anxiety treatments (CANMAT) clinical guidelines for the management of major depressive disorder in adults. iv. neurostimulation therapies. *J Affect Disord* (2009) **117**(Suppl 1):S44–53. doi:10.1016/j.jad.2009.06.039
129. Suzuki K, Awata S, Matsuoka H. One-year outcome after response to ECT in middle-aged and elderly patients with intractable catatonic schizophrenia. *J ECT* (2004) **20**(2):99–106. doi:10.1097/00124509-200406000-00005
130. Suzuki K, Awata S, Takano T, Ebina Y, Iwasaki H, Matsuoka H. Continuation electroconvulsive therapy for relapse prevention in middle-aged and elderly patients with intractable catatonic schizophrenia. *Psychiatry Clin Neurosci* (2005) **59**(4):481–9. doi:10.1111/j.1440-1819.2005.01402.x
131. Suzuki K, Awata S, Takano T, Ebina Y, Shindo T, Harada N, et al. Adjusting the frequency of continuation and maintenance electroconvulsive therapy to prevent relapse of catatonic schizophrenia in middle-aged and elderly patients who are relapse-prone. *Psychiatry Clin Neurosci* (2006) **60**(4):486–92. doi:10.1111/j.1440-1819.2006.01536.x
132. Hatta K, Miyakawa K, Ota T, Usui C, Nakamura H, Arai H. Maximal response to electroconvulsive therapy for the treatment of catatonic symptoms. *J ECT* (2007) **23**(4):233–5. doi:10.1097/yct.0b013e3181587949
133. Escobar R, Rios A, Montoya ID, Lopera F, Ramos D, Carvajal C, et al. Clinical and cerebral blood flow changes in catatonic patients treated with ECT. *J Psychosom Res* (2000) **49**(6):423–9. doi:10.1016/S0022-3999(00)00190-2
134. Morrison JR. Catatonia: prediction of outcome. *Compr Psychiatry* (1974) **15**(4):317–24. doi:10.1016/0010-440X(74)90053-4
135. McCall WV. The response to an amobarbital interview as a predictor of therapeutic outcome in patients with catatonic mutism. *Convuls Ther* (1992) **8**(3):174–8.
136. Raveendranathan D, Narayanaswamy JC, Reddi SV. Response rate of catatonia to electroconvulsive therapy and its clinical correlates. *Eur Arch Psychiatry Clin Neurosci* (2012) **262**(5):425–30. doi:10.1007/s00406-011-0285-4
137. Malur C, Pasol E, Francis A. ECT for prolonged catatonia. *J ECT* (2001) **17**(1):55–9. doi:10.1097/00124509-200103000-00012
138. Ozgen H, Wijkstra J, Vorstman J. Successful electroconvulsive therapy in a young woman with chronic catatonia. *Primary Care Companion CNS Disord* (2012) **14**(3). doi:10.4088/PCC.11l01328
139. Cupina D, Patil S, Loo C. Chronic catatonic schizophrenia treated successfully with right unilateral ultrabrief pulse electroconvulsive therapy: case report. *J ECT* (2013) **29**(2):134–6. doi:10.1097/YCT.0b013e31827659e4
140. de Silva VA, Lakmini WD, Gunawardena HN, Hanwella R. Chronic catatonia treated with electroconvulsive therapy: a case report. *J Med Case Reports* (2013) **7**:219. doi:10.1186/1752-1947-7-219
141. Gazdag G, Kocsis-Ficzere N, Tolna J. The augmentation of clozapine treatment with electroconvulsive therapy. *Ideggyogy Sz* (2006) **59**(7–8):261–7.
142. DeJong H, Bunton P, Hare DJ. A systematic review of interventions used to treat catatonic symptoms in people with autistic spectrum disorders. *J Autism Dev Disord* (2014) **44**(9):2127–36. doi:10.1007/s10803-014-2085-y
143. Consoli A, Benmiloud M, Wachtel L, Dhossche D, Cohen D, Bonnot O. Electroconvulsive therapy in adolescents with the catatonia syndrome: efficacy and ethics. *J ECT* (2010) **26**(4):259–65. doi:10.1097/YCT.0b013e3181fb3924
144. Cristancho P, Jewkes D, Mon T, Conway C. Successful use of right unilateral ECT for catatonia: a case series. *J ECT* (2014) **30**(1):69–72. doi:10.1097/YCT.0b013e31829a01d3
145. Rhoads JC, Votolato NA, Young JL, Gilchrist RH. The successful use of right unilateral ultra-brief pulse electroconvulsive therapy in an adolescent with catatonia. *Brain Stimul* (2010) **3**(1):51–3. doi:10.1016/j.brs.2009.07.003
146. Kugler JL, Hauptman AJ, Collier SJ, Walton AE, Murthy S, Funderburg LG, et al. Treatment of catatonia with ultrabrief right unilateral electroconvulsive therapy: a case series. *J ECT* (2014). doi:10.1097/YCT.0000000000000185
147. Kellner CH, Popeo DM, Aloysi AS. Electroconvulsive therapy for catatonia. *Am J Psychiatry* (2010) **167**(9):1127–8. doi:10.1176/appi.ajp.2010.10020261
148. Grisaru N, Chudakov B, Yaroslavsky Y, Belmaker RH. Catatonia treated with transcranial magnetic stimulation. *Am J Psychiatry* (1998) **155**(11):1630.
149. Saba G, Rocamora JF, Kalalou K, Benadhira R, Plaze M, Aubriot-Delmas B, et al. Catatonia and transcranial magnetic stimulation. *Am J Psychiatry* (2002) **159**(10):1794. doi:10.1176/appi.ajp.159.10.1794
150. Di Michele V, Bolino F. A novel treatment option of bipolar depression with psychotic and catatonic features. *Gen Hosp Psychiatry* (2006) **28**(4):364–5. doi:10.1016/j.genhosppsych.2006.05.003
151. Kate MP, Raju D, Vishwanathan V, Khan FR, Nair, Thomas SV. Successful treatment of refractory organic catatonic disorder with repetitive transcranial magnetic stimulation (rTMS) therapy. *J Neuropsychiatry Clin Neurosci* (2011) **23**(3):E2–3. doi:10.1176/appi.neuropsych.23.3.E2
152. Trojak B, Meille V, Bonin B, Chauvet-Geliner J-C. Repetitive transcranial magnetic stimulation for the treatment of catatonia: an alternative treatment to electroconvulsive therapy? *J Neuropsychiatry Clin Neurosci* (2014) **26**(2):E42–3. doi:10.1176/appi.neuropsych.13050102

2

Neurological abnormalities in recent-onset schizophrenia and Asperger-syndrome

Dusan Hirjak [1]*, Robert Christian Wolf [1,2], Sabine C. Koch[3], Laura Mehl [1], Janna K. Kelbel [1], Katharina Maria Kubera [1], Tanja Traeger [4], Thomas Fuchs [1] and Philipp Arthur Thomann [1]

[1] *Department of General Psychiatry, Center for Psychosocial Medicine, University of Heidelberg, Heidelberg, Germany*
[2] *Department of Psychiatry, Psychotherapy and Psychosomatics, Saarland University, Homburg, Germany*
[3] *Department of Dance Movement Therapy, Faculty of Therapeutic Sciences, SRH University Heidelberg, Heidelberg, Germany*
[4] *Personality, Psychological Assessment, and Psychological Methods, Department of Psychology, University of Koblenz Landau, Landau, Germany*

Edited by:
Sebastian Walther, University Hospital of Psychiatry of Bern, Switzerland

Reviewed by:
Einar Patrick Wilder-Smith, National University of Singapore, Singapore
Tobias Bracht, Cardiff University Brain Research Imaging Centre, UK
Lise Docx, University of Antwerp, Belgium

****Correspondence:***
Dusan Hirjak, Department of General Psychiatry, Center for Psychosocial Medicine, University of Heidelberg, Voßstraße 4, D-69115 Heidelberg, Germany
e-mail: dusan.hirjak@med.uni-heidelberg.de

Background: Neurological abnormalities including a variety of subtle deficits such as discrete impairments in sensory integration, motor coordination (MOCO), and sequencing of complex motor acts are frequently found in patients with schizophrenia (SZ) and commonly referred to as neurological soft signs (NSS). Asperger-syndrome (AS) is characterized by sensory-motor difficulties as well. However, the question whether the two disorders share a common or a disease-specific pattern of NSS remains unresolved.

Method: A total of 78 age- and education-matched participants [26 patients with recent-onset SZ, 26 individuals with AS, and 26 healthy controls (HC)] were recruited for the study. Analyses of covariance (ANCOVAs), with age, years of education, and medication included as covariates, were used to examine group differences on total NSS and the five subscale scores. Discriminant analyses were employed to identify the NSS subscales that maximally discriminate between the three groups.

Results: Significant differences among the three groups were found in NSS total score and on the five NSS subscales. The clinical groups differed significantly in the NSS subscale MOCO. The correct discriminant rate between patients with SZ and individuals with AS was 61.5%. The correct discriminant rate was 92.3% between individuals with AS and HC, and 80.8% between SZ patients and HC, respectively.

Conclusion: Our findings provide new evidence for the presence of NSS in AS and lend further support to previously reported difficulties in movement control in this disorder. According to the present results, SZ and AS seem to be characterized by both quantitative and qualitative NSS expression.

Keywords: NSS, motor abnormalities, recent-onset schizophrenia, Asperger-syndrome

INTRODUCTION

Neurological soft signs (NSS) are neurological abnormalities including a variety of subtle deficits such as discrete impairments in sensory integration, motor coordination, sequencing of complex motor acts, clumsiness, and occurrence of primitive reflexes (1–3). A higher prevalence of NSS has been consistently demonstrated not only in patients with clinically manifest schizophrenia (SZ) but also in their non-psychotic first-degree relatives (4). Recent studies indicated that NSS are not only restricted to SZ but are also present in bipolar disorders, depression, obsessive–compulsive disorders (OCD), and other forms of psychosis (5). Nevertheless, previous studies have assessed the power of NSS to discriminate between SZ and other neuropsychiatric disorders. In particular, SZ patients have significantly higher NSS levels than individuals with OCD (6, 7), alcohol dependence (8), bipolar disorders (9, 10), depression (11), and mixed psychiatric diagnoses (12). From a neurobiological point of view, the prefix "soft" indicates that NSS refer to a non-specific or global cerebral dysfunction rather than to impairments of specific or distinct brain regions. Recent magnetic resonance imaging (MRI) studies on SZ found that increased NSS levels are related to aberrant brain morphology within cortical (13–15) and subcortical regions (13, 16–20). Furthermore, the aforementioned studies converge on the conclusion that NSS should be discussed as potential endophenotypes for SZ (4).

In 1911, a renowned German psychiatrist named Eugen Bleuler introduced the concept of accessory and fundamental symptoms in SZ (21, 22). Accessory symptoms were non-specific state phenomena and comprised hallucinations, delusions, and catatonic signs (21). The fundamental symptoms were more specific to SZ and included autism, formal thought disorders, ambivalence, disorders of volition, affective-emotional, and affect-expressive changes (21, 22). Furthermore, when Bleuler (21) described the "autistic core" in SZ patients, he spoke about the withdrawal within the own inner world: "*The most severe schizophrenics, who have no more contact with the outside world live in a world of their own. They have encased themselves with their desires and wishes [...]; they have cut themselves off as much as possible from any contact with the external world. This detachment from reality with the relative and absolute predominance of the inner life, we term autism"* [(21, 23), p. 1122]. In general, the schizophrenic autism is characterized by a rich variety of clinical phenomena such as poor ability to interact with others, inaccessibility, negativistic tendencies, indifference, rigid attitudes, and behaviors, private hierarchy of values and goals, inappropriate expression and behavior, and idiosyncratic logic and thinking, respectively (22). Taken together, from the historical standpoint, SZ, and autism have been regarded as part of the same spectrum (24, 25).

In the early 40s, Kanner's (26) and Asperger's (27) use of the term autism changed it in the direction of its present meaning of disturbed social cognition. Subsequently, with the introduction of DSM-III in the late 1970s, autism became an independent diagnostic entity not being part of the diagnostic concept of SZ. However, problems with interpersonal contact, interaffective attunement, and perspective-taking, are core to both pathologies, though appearing in different forms, and hence, several studies provided empirical evidence for a diagnostic overlap in both disorders (28). Furthermore, clinical studies have shown that negative/deficit, disorganized, and motor symptoms are present in both individuals with autism and patients with SZ (29–31). More recently, before introduction of DSM-5, some authors even discussed an autism dimension for SZ (25). This suggests that distinguishing between both spectrum disorders remains a diagnostic challenge. Such diagnostic overlaps might confound the diagnosis and delay appropriate treatment of these patients. As a matter of fact, the symptoms overlap could at least partially account for the inconsistent findings in previous scientific studies.

Asperger-syndrome (AS) belongs to pervasive developmental disorders and is characterized by interaction and communication difficulties, and repetitive, stereotype, and restricted patterns of behavior. In fact, several clinical studies observed motor abnormalities in individuals with AS including involuntary dyskinesia, rigidity, hypotonia, abnormal posture and gait, clumsiness, reduced coordination of locomotor skills, and unstable balance, respectively (32–35). Some authors even consider motor abnormalities as a putative endophenotype for autism spectrum disorders (36). In the last decade, clinical research interest on motor abnormalities in autism has extended to the investigation of NSS in AS. However, there are only two studies which have investigated NSS prevalence in individuals diagnosed with AS (33, 34) and we are still lacking a profound understanding of NSS in AS.

Overall, the above mentioned clinical studies suggest that motor abnormalities are a typical characteristic of SZ and AS. Hence, there is a stimulating debate whether these disorders share similar sensory-motor features or not (37). Regarding subtle neurological deficits in autism, however, only Mayoral et al. (34) compared NSS in early-onset SZ and AS. Therefore, at present it is difficult to highlight a potential difference in subtle sensory-motor abnormalities in patients with SZ and individuals with AS. The precise evaluation of subtle sensory-motor neurological signs in SZ and AS is of potential clinical significance, since the assessment of NSS might allow for more accurate disease classification. Also, this approach might help to overcome the missing conceptual clarity and better delineate a precise phenotype in order to identify endophenotypes underpinning SZ and AS.

The purpose of this investigation was twofold. First, we were interested in whether there is a difference between NSS severity in patients with SZ and individuals with AS. Second, we sought to identify characteristic NSS, which are either unique or shared by both disorders. Based on the findings of a previous study in juveniles (34) and on our clinical observation, it was hypothesized that individuals with AS would show NSS scores at least as high as patients with SZ. Further, we expected AS individuals being predominantly susceptible to NSS that involve gross motor skills. Finally, we employed a descriptive and predictive linear discrimination analysis (LDA) in order to examine if both total NSS and subscale scores are able to discriminate between the three groups.

MATERIALS AND METHODS

SUBJECTS

The study sample consisted of 26 clinically stable patients with recent-onset SZ, 26 individuals with AS, and 26 healthy controls (HC) who participated in a larger study at the Department of General Psychiatry in Heidelberg, Germany as part of the Toward an Embodied Science of Intersubjectivity-Project (TESIS). The study sample was consecutively recruited between 2010 and 2013 from the Department of General Psychiatry in Heidelberg, Germany and from SALO GmbH in Ludwigshafen, Germany, a professional rehabilitation institution of education for autistic individuals. All participants were Caucasians. Study participants were excluded if: (1) they were aged <18 or >35 years, (2) they had a history of brain trauma or neurological disease, (3) they had a comorbid Axis-I- or -II-Disorder according to ICD-10 or DSM-IV, (4) they had shown alcohol/substance abuse or dependence within 24 months prior to participation, or (5) they had an IQ < 70. Diagnoses of SZ and AS were made by specialized clinicians (DH and PAT) corresponding to DSM-IV criteria and supplemented by an extensive neuropsychological assessment. Clinical symptom determinations and structured clinical diagnostic interviews were conducted by trained clinical raters (Dusan Hirjak, Laura Mehl, and Janna K. Kelbel) and senior diagnosticians (Sabine C. Koch, Philipp Arthur Thomann). In particular, all study individuals were assessed for lifetime psychiatric diagnoses by trained psychiatrists (Dusan Hirjak and Philipp Arthur Thomann) via the German version of the Structured Clinical Interview for DSM-IV (38) and reviews of hospital case notes. All participants in the AS group had previously received a clinical diagnosis of AS (F84.5) from an independent clinician according to standard criteria (a valid diagnosis of autism is an admission criterion for SALO GmbH). In addition, diagnoses of the participants with AS were confirmed with the Autism Diagnostic Observation Schedule [ADOS; (39)] administered by a trained and clinically experienced psychiatrist (Dusan Hirjak). In addition, IQ of individuals with AS (F84.5) has been systematically assessed with the German version of the *Culture Fair Intelligence Test* (CFT-20-R) (40). The intelligence in SZ patients and HC was not explicitly assessed, but clinically judged to be average or above average. Both patients with SZ and HC were required to have a leaving certificate from one of the secondary schools – Hauptschule (9 years), Realschule (10 years), or Gymnasium (13 years) – in order to participate in our study. The demographics and psychiatric history of the two clinical samples were retrieved from medical records. To examine the possible effect of medications on NSS, we standardized the dosage of antipsychotic medications chlorpromazine equivalents (CPZ). In healthy individuals, we used the PRIME early psychosis screening test [prevention through risk identification, management, and education (PRIME)] to screen for the presence of early psychotic symptoms, including information on any contact or treatment for any mental or psychological disorder (41). All study participants gave informed consent to participation, and the study has been approved by the local ethics committee of the Medical Faculty, University of Heidelberg, Germany.

CLINICAL ASSESSMENTS

Neurological soft signs were assessed using the Heidelberg Scale (2) that consists of five items assessing motor coordination (MOCO) (Ozeretski's test, diadochokinesia, pronation/supination, finger-to-thumb opposition, speech articulation), three items assessing integrative functions (IF) (station and gait, tandem walking, two-point discrimination), two items assessing complex motor tasks (COMT) (finger-to-nose test, fist-edge-palm test), four items assessing right/left and spatial orientation (RLSO) (right/left orientation, graphesthesia, face-hand test, stereognosis), and two items assessing hard signs (HS) (arm holding test, mirror movements). Items were rated on a 0 (no prevalence) to 3 (marked prevalence) point scale. All items, with the exception of station and gait, tandem walking, right/left orientation, speech articulation, primitive reflexes, and Ozeretzki's test were rated separately on the right and left side. A sufficient internal reliability (Cronbach's alpha 0.83) and high test-retest reliability (0.88) have been established previously (2, 42). In the study conducted by Schröder and colleagues (2), to test the interrater reliability of the NSS scale, 42 patients and HC were simultaneously evaluated by two raters. The internal reliability of the scale was assessed by calculating Cronbach's α. The testing procedure was generally standardized, but the explanations and the time required to complete the tasks were adjusted to the condition of the patients. In the present study, the NSS assessment has been conducted by two raters (Janna K. Kelbel and Laura Mehl) trained and supervised by the same psychiatrist (Dusan Hirjak). Both raters were blind to the main hypothesis of the study and investigated study participants independent of their diagnosis. Handedness was assessed on the Edinburgh Inventory (43). The severity of psychopathological symptoms was assessed with the Brief Psychiatric Rating Scale (BPRS) (44), the Scale for the Assessment of Positive Symptoms (SAPS) (45), and the Scale for the Assessment of Negative Symptoms (SANS) (46). Predictors of outcome were rated on the Strauss-Carpenter Scale (SCS) (47). The social, occupational, and psychological functioning in individuals with AS was assessed with the Global Assessment of Functioning (GAF) scale (48).

CHARACTERISTICS OF PARTICIPANTS

The three groups of participants were matched according to age and education. Level of IQ among individuals with AS ranged from 71 to 124 (mean IQ: 99.0 ± 18.5) according to CFT-20-R (40). Patients with SZ according to DSM-IV had an initial onset of psychosis within 2 years prior to study entry with a mean duration of illness of 7.15 months (range 2–15 months). SZ subtypes were distributed as follows: paranoid $n = 12$, disorganized $n = 4$, and undifferentiated $n = 10$. At the time of inclusion, all SZ patients were clinically stable with consistent medication doses for 4 weeks or longer. They were receiving treatment with a single second-generation antipsychotic agent according to their psychiatrists' choice. Patients were treated on average for 2.33 ± 1.44 months throughout the course of illness. Potential extrapyramidal side effects were excluded before study entry by an experienced psychiatrist who was not directly involved in the study. Individuals with AS and HC did not take any antipsychotic, mood stabilizing, anti-cholinergic, or antidepressive medications. SZ patients had low or no prevalence of positive and negative symptoms, as measured by SAPS (range: 0–74), SANS (range: 0–70), and BPRS. At the time of clinical and NSS assessment, no SZ patients manifested psychotic symptoms (two or more of the positive symptom items >3 or a total SAPS score >40).

DATA ANALYSIS

Data were analyzed using the Statistical Package of the Social Sciences (SPSS version 21.0, SPSS Inc., Chicago, IL, USA). Sociodemographic and clinical variables were described and compared between the three groups with unpaired *t-test* or chi-square test for categorical variables using conventional significance levels ($p < 0.05$). To test for differences in NSS performance between the three study subgroups, we conducted an analysis of covariance (ANCOVA) including the potentially distorting factors age, years of education, and CPZ. Gender comparisons on NSS performance within each study group and between the three groups used *t-tests* and analysis of covariance (ANCOVA). Further, p values of the identified NSS subscales were corrected for the number of tested NSS subscales in our main analysis using the Bonferroni method. To this end, α was set to $p = 0.05/N$, where n (=18) equaled the number of correlations (classical Bonferroni correction). For this reason, the corrected threshold was set to $p = 0.0027$ [$\alpha = 0.05/18$ tests (total NSS + five subscale scores × three groups)]. In a second step, a series of ANCOVAs considering age, years of education, and CPZ as covariates was conducted to further examine the differences between groups if a significant main effect was identified. Further, p values of the identified NSS subscales were corrected for the number of tested NSS subscales using the Bonferroni method. To this end, α was set to $p = 0.05/N$, where n (=12) equaled the number of correlations (classical Bonferroni correction). For this reason, the corrected threshold was set to $p = 0.0041$ [$\alpha = 0.05/12$ tests (total NSS + five subscale scores × two groups)]. Correlative analyses of SAPS, SANS, BPRS, and CPZ with total scores and subscores of NSS were conducted with the Pearson correlation coefficient.

To examine the ability of NSS to discriminate among the three groups, both descriptive and predictive LDAs were used (11, 49, 50). The aim of this analysis was to determine whether NSS subscales would discriminate between patients with SZ and those with AS. In this study, total NSS and the five subscale scores were treated as "within subject variable" (independent variables), whereas the diagnostic group was treated as the "between subject factor" (grouping variable). However, only those NSS scores that reached statistical significance in the ANCOVAs were used as predictive variables.

RESULTS

Demographic characteristics of the patient groups and the HC are summarized in **Table 1**. Comparison of the three groups revealed a significant difference in gender (chi-square test: $\chi^2 = 8.35$; df = 2; $p = 0.015$) and CPZ [$F(2, 75) = 85.16$; $p < 0.001$]. There were no significant differences in age [$F(2, 75) = 0.55$; $p = 0.577$] and years of education [$F(2, 75) = 2.63$; $p = 0.078$] among the three groups. There was also no significant difference for BPRS scores between SZ patients and individuals with AS [$F(1, 50) = 2.9$; $p = 0.094$]. There were no significant differences between male and female participants in NSS performance among the three groups. In addition, we found no significant differences between male and female individuals in the control group in any of NSS scores (**Table 3**). But, there was a significant gender difference in the performance on NSS subscale COMT in both individuals with AS and SZ patients (**Table 3**). However, this effect is most likely driven by the influence of confounders such as age, education, and medication, since a significant gender effect diminished after covarying for these factors.

GROUP DIFFERENCE IN NSS SCORES (ANCOVA: CONTROLLING FOR AGE, YEARS OF EDUCATION, AND MEDICATION)

Table 1 shows the prevalence of NSS across the three groups. Significant differences after controlling for age, years of education, and CPZ were found in NSS total score [$F(5, 72) = 14.7$; $p < 0.001$] and on the five NSS subscales MOCO [$F(5, 72) = 11.5$; $p < 0.001$], IF [$F(5, 72) = 3.41$; $p = 0.008$], COMT [$F(5, 72) = 8.9$; $p < 0.001$], RLSO [$F(5, 72) = 4.02$; $p = 0.003$] and HS [$F(5, 72) = 3.2$; $p = 0.012$] among the three groups (**Figure 1**; **Table 2**). Further, p values of the identified NSS subscales were corrected for the number of tested NSS subscales in our main analysis using the Bonferroni method ($p < 0.0027$). NSS total and two subscale scores (MOCO and COMT) hold Bonferroni correction for multiple testing.

AS VS. SZ

The ANCOVA showed that compared with SZ patients, the individuals with AS showed significantly higher NSS total scores [$F(4, 47) = 3.63$; $p = 0.012$] and higher scores on the subscale COMT [$F(4, 47) = 4.2$; $p = 0.005$]. However, individuals with AS showed lower scores on the NSS subscale MOCO [$F(4, 47) = 4.38$; $p = 0.004$] when compared to SZ patients. Further, p values of the two identified NSS subscales were corrected for the number of tested NSS subscales in our main analysis using the Bonferroni method ($p < 0.0041$). Only the NSS subscale, MOCO hold Bonferroni correction for multiple testing. No significant difference was found between individuals with AS and SZ patients on the

Table 1 | Descriptive summary of the sociodemographic and clinical variables of all participants.

Variable	Asperger-syndrome ($n = 26$)	Schizophrenia ($n = 26$)	Healthy controls ($n = 26$)
Mean age, years (SD)	22.76 ± 3.81	23.38 ± 3.87	23.58 ± 3.77
Gender, *n*			
Male	18 (69.2%)	9 (34.7%)	9 (34.7%)
Female	8 (30.8%)	17 (65.3%)	17 (65.3%)
Handedness, *n*			
Right	23 (88.4%)	26 (100%)	26 (100%)
Left	3 (11.6%)	0 (0%)	0 (0%)
Mean education, years (SD)	12.03 ± 1.84	12.07 ± 1.32	12.8 ± 0.63
Mean duration of illness, months (SD)	–	7.15 ± .31	–
Mean antipsychotic dose(CPZ) (SD)	0	435.11 ± 240.4	0
Mean NSS score (SD)	16.19 ± 6.71 (median = 14.5)	14.92 ± 7.54 (median = 16.0)	5.57 ± 3.08 (median = 5.5)
MOCO	6.23 ± 3.31	6.79 ± 3.91	2.11 ± 1.55
IF	2.61 ± 1.62	1.92 ± 1.38	1.42 ± 1.06
COMT	2.84 ± 1.68	1.61 ± 1.67	0.61 ± 0.89
RLSO	3.07 ± 2.41	1.65 ± 1.89	0.8 ± 1.05
HS	1.42 ± 1.65	1.73 ± 1.34	0.61 ± 0.89
Mean ADOS[a] (SD)	13.61 ± 3.27	–	–
Mean SAPS[b] (SD)	–	20.11 ± 13.98	–
Mean SANS[c] (SD)	41.07 ± 15.78	30.69 ± 18.81	–
Mean BPRS[d] (SD)	29.34 ± 15.49	23.0 ± 10.94	–
Mean SCS[e] (SD)	–	39.0 ± 15.72	–
Mean GAF[f] (SD)	63.96 ± 10.67	–	–

Mean ± standard deviation (SD).

[a]Autism Diagnostic Observation Schedule.

[b]Scale for the assessment of negative symptoms.

[c]Scale for the assessment of positive symptoms.

[d]Brief Psychiatric Rating Scale.

[e]Strauss-Carpenter Scale.

[f]Global Assessment of Functioning.

Table 2 | Group differences in NSS perfomance.

NSS measure	AS vs. SZ vs. HC		AS vs. SZ		AS vs. HC		SZ vs. HC	
	$F(5, 72)$	p	$F(4, 47)$	p	$F(3, 48)$	p	$F(4, 47)$	p
NSS total score	**14.7**	**<0.001**	3.63	0.012	**24.5**	**<0.001**	**12.9**	**<0.001**
MOCO	**11.5**	**<0.001**	**4.38**	**0.004**	**15.29**	**<0.001**	**11.33**	**<0.001**
COMT	**8.9**	**<0.001**	4.2	0.005	**17.81**	**<0.001**	2.45	0.059
IF	3.41	0.008	2.51	0.054	3.71	0.018	2.59	0.048
RLSO	4.02	0.003	1.5	0.217	**6.21**	**0.001**	1.56	0.2
HS	3.2	0.012	1.1	0.364	3.25	0.03	**4.48**	**0.004**

ANCOVA = controlling for age, years of education and medication (CPZ); MOCO, motor coordination; COMT, complex motor tasks; IF, integrative function; RLSO, right/left and spatial orientation; HS, hard signs; AS, Asperger-syndrome; SZ, schizophrenia patients; HC, healthy controls. Differences surviving Bonferroni correction in bold.

Table 3 | Gender differences in NSS performance (two-tailed t-tests).

NSS measures	Asperger-syndrome				Schizophrenia				Healthy controls			
	Male ($n = 18$)	Female ($n = 8$)	t (df = 24)	p	Male ($n = 9$)	Female ($n = 17$)	t (df = 24)	p	Male ($n = 9$)	Female ($n = 17$)	t (df = 24)	p
NSS total score	16.5 ± 6.86	15.5 ± 6.76	−0.34	0.73	11.66 ± 7.77	16.64 ± 7.04	1.65	0.11	5.88 ± 3.10	5.41 ± 3.16	−0.36	0.71
MOCO	6.55 ± 3.72	5.5 ± 2.13	−0.74	0.46	5.44 ± 4.15	7.47 ± 3.71	1.27	0.21	2.11 ± 1.69	2.11 ± 1.53	0.01	0.99
COMT	3.27 ± 1.70	1.87 ± 1.14	−2.08	**0.04**	0.66 ± 1.65	2.11 ± 1.49	2.26	**0.03**	0.66 ± 1.0	0.58 ± 087	−0.2	0.83
IF	2.50 ± 1.72	2.87 ± 1.45	0.53	0.59	1.55 ± 1.01	2.11 ± 1.53	0.98	0.33	1.66 ± 1.11	1.29 ± 1.04	−0.84	0.40
RLSO	2.77 ± 1.80	3.75 ± 3.49	0.94	0.35	1.44 ± 1.87	1.76 ± 1.95	0.4	0.69	0.55 ± 0.88	0.94 ± 1.14	0.87	0.38
HS	1.38 ± 1.81	1.50 ± 1.30	0.15	0.87	1.33 ± 1.0	1.94 ± 1.47	1.1	0.28	0.88 ± 1.16	0.47 ± 0.71	−1.13	0.26

Mean ± SD; MOCO, motor coordination; COMT, complex motor tasks; IF, integrative function; RLSO, right/left and spatial orientation; HS, hard. Bold font indicates significant differences ($p < 0.05$).

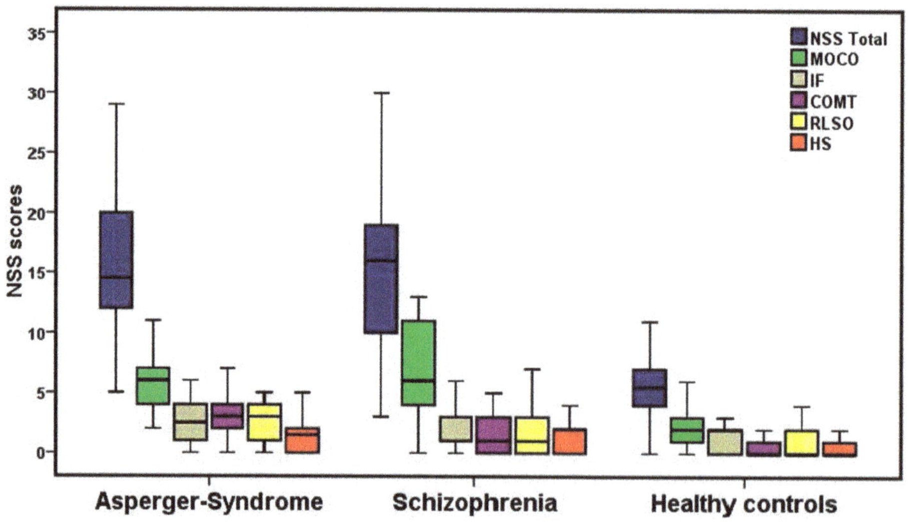

FIGURE 1 | Neurological soft signs total scores and NSS scores on the five subscales among the three groups. The bottom and top of the box represent the first and third quartile, and the band inside the box is the second quartile (the median). The ends of the whiskers indicate the minimum and maximum of the NSS performance. MOCO, motor coordination; COMT, complex motor tasks; IF, integrative functions; RLSO, right/left and spatial orientation; HS, hard signs.

subscales IF [$F(4, 47) = 2.51$; $p = 0.054$], RLSO [$F(4, 47) = 1.5$; $p = 0.217$], and HS [$F(4, 47) = 1.1$; $p = 0.364$].

AS VS. HC

Compared with HC, individuals with AS showed significantly higher NSS total scores [$F(3, 48) = 24.50$; $p < 0.001$] and elevated NSS on the subscales MOCO [$F(3, 48) = 15.29$; $p < 0.001$], IF [$F(3, 48) = 3.71$; $p = 0.018$], COMT [$F(3, 48) = 17.81$; $p < 0.001$], RLSO [$F(3, 48) = 6.21$; $p = 0.001$], and HS [$F(3, 48) = 3.25$; $p = 0.03$]. NSS total and three subscale scores (MOCO, COMT, and RLSO) hold Bonferroni correction for multiple testing ($p < 0.0041$).

SZ VS. HC

Compared with HC, SZ patients showed significantly more total NSS signs [$F(4, 47) = 12.90$; $p < 0.001$] and higher NSS scores on the subscale MOCO [$F(4, 47) = 11.33$; $p < 0.001$], IF [$F(4, 47) = 2.59$; $p = 0.048$], and HS [$F(4, 47) = 4.48$; $p = 0.004$]. NSS total and two subscale scores (MOCO and HS) hold Bonferroni correction for multiple testing ($p < 0.0041$). Additionally, no significant difference was found between SZ patients and HC on the subscale COMT [$F(4, 47) = 2.45$; $p = 0.059$] and RLSO [$F(4, 47) = 1.56$; $p = 0.2$].

CLINICAL COMPARISONS

In patients with SZ, SAPS, SANS, and BPRS scores were not significantly associated with total score and five subscores of NSS at the conventional significance level ($p < 0.05$). In individuals with AS, BPRS scores were not associated with total score and five subscores of NSS at the conventional significance level ($p < 0.05$).

DISCRIMINANT ANALYSES OF NSS PERFORMANCE

In this study, we conducted a LDA (11, 49, 50), to examine the ability of the total NSS and five subscale scores to discriminate between the three groups. With this method, we also tested for the possibility of predicting the correct diagnosis solely based on NSS performance. Only the NSS subscales that reached statistical significance in *post hoc* analysis and survived the Bonferroni correction were used as predictive variables.

Using predictive LDA, we found that 71.8% of the cases were correctly classified in terms of the group as a function of the total NSS and two subscale scores (MOCO and COMT). The individual discriminant rates for each diagnostic group were 92.3% for HC, 69.2% for individuals with AS, and 53.8% for SZ patients. The results of the descriptive LDA revealed the emergence of two significant linear discriminant functions: function 1 (Wilks' $\lambda = 0.495$; $\chi^2 = 52.106$; $p < 0.001$; eigenvalue: 0.627; canonical correlation = 0.621) could explain 72.1% of the variance, while function 2 (Wilks' $\lambda = 0.805$; $\chi^2 = 16.084$; $p < 0.001$; eigenvalue: 0.243; canonical correlation = 0.442) could only explain 27.9% of the variance. The distribution of the three groups is shown in **Figure 2** and function 1 and function 2 are illustrated.

In this study, predictive LDA was also conducted for group–group comparison. All three analyses showed significant results.

AS VS. SZ

One of them was between individuals with AS and SZ patients. In this analysis, only the NSS subscale MOCO that reached statistical significance in the *post hoc* analysis and survived the Bonferroni correction was used as predictor variable. The total correct discriminant rate was 61.5%. The results of the descriptive LDA revealed the emergence of non-significant linear discriminant function (Wilks' $\lambda = 0.994$; $\chi^2 = 0.283$; $p = 0.595$; eigenvalue: 0.006; canonical correlation = 0.076). Because of the non-significant discriminant function between individuals with AS and patients with SZ, we re-ran the LDA by adding two more NSS variables, which did not survive the Bonferroni correction (11). After including the NSS total score and the NSS subscale COMT in the LDA, the correct discriminant rate elevated from 61.5 to 71.2% (Wilks' $\lambda = 0.774$; $\chi^2 = 12.438$; $p = 0.006$; eigenvalue: 0.292; canonical correlation = 0.476). The correct rate of AS individuals was 65.4%, while the correct rate of SZ patients was 76.9%.

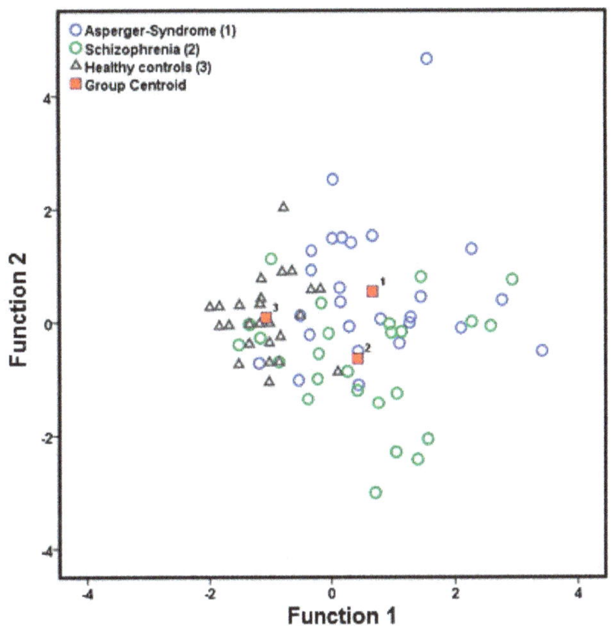

FIGURE 2 | Canonical discriminant functions of neurological soft signs (total score, MOCO, and COMT), which are prevalence for patients with AS, schizophrenia, and healthy controls. MOCO, motor coordination; COMT, complex motor tasks.

AS VS. HC

The other was between individuals with AS and HC. In this analysis, total NSS and three subscale scores (MOCO, COMT, and HS) that reached statistical significance in the *post hoc* analysis and survived the Bonferroni correction were used as predictor variables. The total correct discriminant rate was 92.3%. The descriptive LDA revealed the emergence of one significant linear discriminant function (Wilks' $\lambda = 0.445$; $\chi^2 = 37.746$; $p < 0.001$; eigenvalue: 1.195; canonical correlation = 0.738).

SZ VS. HC

The remaining predictive LDA was between SZ patients and HC. In this analysis, total NSS and three subscale scores (MOCO and HS) that reached statistical significance in the *post hoc* analysis and survived the Bonferroni correction were used as predictor variables.

The total correct discriminant rate was 80.8%. The results of the descriptive LDA revealed the emergence of one significant linear discriminant function (Wilks' $\lambda = 0.569$; $\chi^2 = 27.334$; $p < 0.001$; eigenvalue: 0.757; canonical correlation = 0.656).

POTENTIAL INFLUENCE OF MEDICATION

In patients with SZ, NSS total scores ($r = 0.335$; $p = 0.095$) and scores on the subscales MOCO ($r = 0.262$; $p = 0.228$), COMT ($r = 0.133$; $p = 0.547$), HS ($r = 0.255$; $p = 0.240$), IF ($r = 0.289$; $p = 0.182$), and RLSO ($r = 0.140$; $p = 0.523$) were not associated with CPZ equivalents at the conventional significance level ($p < 0.05$).

DISCUSSION

This study assessed and compared NSS levels in both patients with SZ and AS. Two main findings emerged: first, patients with SZ show significantly higher NSS score on the subscale MOCO when compared to individuals with AS. Second, SZ patients can be distinguished from those with AS by only one NSS subscale (MOCO). These findings were consistent across the analyses of prevalence and in the LDA.

Previous studies on motor abnormalities in AS clearly underestimated the prevalence of NSS in this syndrome and focused exclusively on rather complex movement disorders. In fact, only two previous studies investigated the severity of NSS in AS (33, 34). In the study conducted by Tani (33), individuals with AS had significantly higher NSS total and complex motor acts scores when compared to the control group. The authors concluded that NSS represent a non-specific vulnerability factor for AS (33). More recently, Mayoral (34) investigated 30 patients with early-onset SZ and 29 individuals with AS. In agreement with our results, they found that individuals with AS have higher NSS scores than HC. Second, however, the authors concluded that there are no significant differences between both patient groups in any of the NSS scores. However, it is possible that the discordant findings reported by Mayoral (34) were due to large differences in sociodemographic variables among the study participants. In fact, the IQ levels in the control group were significantly higher than in SZ patients and individuals with AS. Hence, some patients with AS were taking antipsychotic medication, a fact that may have biased particular NSS tasks in this group. Last but not least, recent research indicates that only 5% of SZ patients have a psychosis onset before age of 15 years (51). Therefore, investigating young patients with early-onset SZ does not allow making inferences for the whole SZ spectrum, because NSS might be instable in subgroups of young patients with incomplete brain maturation. Thus, the above mentioned findings cannot be generalized to the whole autism spectrum.

To some extent, our findings are consistent with the two above mentioned NSS studies. In line with results presented by Tani (33), we found that individuals with AS exhibit higher NSS levels on the subscale MOCO, COMT, and RLSO when compared to HC. However, we did not find any significant difference between NSS levels on the subscale HS. In contrast to Mayoral (34), who found no differences between SZ and patients with AS, we observed significantly higher NSS scores on the subscale MOCO in SZ when compared to individuals with AS. Compared with both previous studies, our findings are likely to be more robust because of three reasons: first, individuals with AS were free of psychotropic medication. Though all our SZ patients were medicated, the negative results in correlations between NSS and CPZ further reduces potential concerns that our findings might be confounded by antipsychotic drug treatment. Furthermore, the duration of exposure to second-generation antipsychotic medication in SZ patients was rather low. A second strength of our study is that individuals with SZ and AS had low prevalence of acute psychiatric symptoms and, in addition, did not differ in BPRS scores as measures of psychopathology. We believe this to be important, as SZ patients with more severe psychotic symptoms have been shown to score higher on the NSS scale in comparison with SZ patients without any negative or positive symptoms (3). In fact, recent studies showed that patients with negative symptoms are characterized by more severe neurological abnormalities including different sensory-motor functions (52). For instance, a number of reports have also noted that SZ patients with negative symptoms exhibit higher prevalence of spontaneous movements (53, 54) or NSS (55–59) . In conclusion, there is an association between NSS and negative symptoms in SZ. However, our SZ sample scored rather low on SANS and SAPS. Third, SZ patients and individuals with AS were of similar educational level. Given the large body of evidence in individuals with AS and SZ suggesting a significant relationship between intelligence and movement (60), we used years of education as a covariate when analyzing differences in NSS scores. In contrast to both aforementioned studies, our study sample comprised mainly young adults in a clinically stable disease state and rather advanced brain maturation. However, for the interpretation of the present results, it is important to bear in mind that the human brain undergoes a highly dynamic development, which continues into adulthood (61). While the majority of longitudinal studies on brain growth in autism focused on children, the trend of brain development in adolescence, and adulthood remains unidentified (62). Our data might support the hypothesis of developmental deficits in AS during adolescence and adulthood.

Several lines of scientific evidence suggest that AS and SZ have both unique and similar sensory-motor features. In particular, there is a stimulating debate whether these disorders are related conditions or not (37). The findings of our present study provide support for both positions. SZ patients exhibited significantly higher NSS levels on the subscale MOCO when compared to individuals with AS. The NSS subscale MOCO comprises both, tasks which involve small muscles of the hand, and tasks which necessitate a tight link between one's own bodily movement and the spatial–temporal constraints. This finding is of particular interest given recent evidence of individuals with SZ showing poor levels of motor dexterity (63). As such, this action is based on visual perception and fine motor precision. Therefore, our first finding supports the hypothesis that patients with SZ exhibit serious problems when using sensory information to guide and time fine finger and hand movements. Moreover, there is some evidence that abnormalities of fine MOCO have a developmental origin and manifest even in a group of clinical at-risk mental state individuals (64, 65). In fact, research on NSS in ultra-high risk (UHR) conditions for developing mental illness might also provide important clues for the understanding of motor abnormalities in psychotic disorders. Nevertheless, to date, only few studies investigated NSS in UHR individuals (66, 67). Leask and colleagues (67) concluded that NSS might precede SZ, but are not caused by infectious illness in early childhood. In the pioneer longitudinal neuroimaging study on UHR individuals, Mittal and colleagues (68) suggested a significant relationship between NSS and longitudinal cerebellar-thalamic tract integrity. As such, NSS might provide insight into the role of cognitive dysmetria in the high-risk period. These results are supported by previous research on infant motor development that considered childhood neuromotor dysfunction as a risk factor for SZ spectrum disorders (64, 69). In summary, NSS might be considered as an intrinsic part of vulnerability to psychosis and should be discussed as markers of disordered neurodevelopment in SZ (70).

After Bonferroni correction, no significant differences were found between SZ and AS in total NSS and four subscales comprising rather gross motor skills such as stait and gait, tandem walking, finger-to-nose test or right/left orientation. There are several explanations for the particular deficit in gross motor skills in both disorders. In order to properly perform gross bodily actions, the interaction of motor cortex, basal ganglia, and thalamus is critical. Recently, altered gray matter volumes within the limbic basal ganglia loop system (e.g., left thalamus, putamen) were found to be common in both SZ and autism (37, 71). We believe that these findings lend support to the theory of a disrupted basal ganglia loop system in both disorders and suggest that SZ and AS share a number of neurobiological similarities. Hence, our results provide arguments against the theory that SZ and AS are diametrically opposite ends of a continuum (72).

The present study employed LDA in order to test for unique disease related patterns of NSS and to explore the degree of accuracy to which these patterns could be used to statistically discriminate between SZ and AS. Although the NSS subscale MOCO was found to be the most important predictor involved in discriminating, among the two clinical groups, it only accounted for an overall 61.5% correct classification. These results implicate that the level of abnormalities in perception-action coupling as described by MOCO may serve as a valuable predictor when trying to differentiate between patients with SZ and AS. However, it is noteworthy that by combining the NSS subscale MOCO with the total NSS and COMT subscale score the correct discriminant rate elevated to 71.2% and revealed significant discriminant function. Because of our modest sample size, some findings diminished more than it would have probably been the case with a larger study group. Although the LDA consisting NSS total scores was significant, NSS subscales tended to fall below our cut-off of 0.05 as the determinant of significance. Still, our observation that the subscale MOCO has a significant discriminant power between SZ patients and individuals with AS supports earlier assumptions that abnormalities of motor dexterity *per se* might be a major characteristic of SZ (73). According to our results, especially motor tests evaluating fine motor skills and manual dexterity might be helpful when classifying and differentiating patients with SZ and individuals with AS.

LIMITATIONS

We acknowledge several potential limitations of this study such as the possible differences in IQ levels among the study participants. It is thus possible that we missed small between-group effects due to missing IQ scores in SZ patients and the control group. Apart from this, deficits in global measures of cognition such as intelligence are common in SZ patients (74, 75). On the other side, it is a well-established finding that IQ levels do not change over the course of illness and that lower IQ is a stable trait in patients suffering from SZ (76–78). Furthermore, variables such as education, occupation, and age can contribute significantly to IQ values (79). In other words, we believe the recent evidence to clearly suggest years of education as being an appropriate and stable indicator of global cognition in SZ. Second, the relatively small number of participants in each study group limits the power of the LDA. Third, statistical analysis of the three groups revealed a significant difference in gender. According to Cai (80) and colleagues, higher NSS levels were observed in 14- and 15-years-old boys when compared with girls of the same age. Since the differences in NSS performance declined with increasing age, the authors concluded that young boys might experience a delay of brain maturation when compared to girls of similar age, and hence, this might cause higher NSS scores in the male group (80). In our study, there were no differences for age distribution among the three groups and the majority of our study subjects were young adults with completed brain maturation. Further, there were no significant differences between male and female participants in NSS performance among the three groups. Therefore, uneven gender distribution across diagnostic groups might have not directly impact upon results of the statistical analysis in this study. Fourth, all SZ patients had been exposed to antipsychotic medication. In order to partial out a putative dose-dependent effect of second-generation antipsychotics on NSS performance, SZ patients' CPZ were considered as potential confounders in the present study. Although CPZ doses were included as covariates in the statistical analyses, we cannot completely rule out the possibility that antipsychotic medication might have influenced the NSS performance to some degree. Still, an influence of medication in our study is unlikely as every SZ patient was treated with atypical neuroleptics, the duration of treatment was relatively short, and none of the subjects showed serious medication side effects. Furthermore, none of the individuals with AS was treated with second- or first-generation antipsychotics. Correspondingly, second-generation antipsychotic treatment or medication side effects seem to have no effect on NSS performance in SZ (81). Fifth, healthy participants were not explicitly screened for AS by means of a standardized test. However, no signs of autistic traits were observed in healthy subjects during clinical and diagnostic (DSM-IV) interviewing. Last but not least, our study sample comprised patients suffering from different subtypes of SZ, a point that might complicate the interpretation of our results (82). However, subgroups were too small to test for this potential influence. Moreover, it is important to bear in mind that our findings are preliminary and that they need to be replicated in larger samples.

CONCLUSION

Sensory-motor abnormalities in SZ and AS might manifest as NSS. Since NSS are present in both, individuals with SZ and AS, they may represent a putative neuromotor marker across the traditional diagnostic categorization. Understanding the role of NSS could help to gain further insight into the neurobiological underpinnings of SZ and AS. To this end, future studies should ideally combine thorough clinical, neurological, and psychopathological assessments with multi-modal neuroimaging techniques in order to elucidate how the respective factors relate to each other.

AUTHOR CONTRIBUTIONS

Dusan Hirjak, Philipp Arthur Thomann, Sabine C. Koch, and Thomas Fuchs designed the study and were involved in the interpretation of the results. Dusan Hirjak, Robert Christian Wolf, Katharina Maria Kubera, and Tanja Traeger performed statistical analyses. Dusan Hirjak, Philipp Arthur Thomann, Laura Mehl, and Janna K. Kelbel undertook neurological, psychopathological and psychometric assessments. Dusan Hirjak, Philipp Arthur Thomann, Katharina Maria Kubera and Robert Christian Wolf wrote the manuscript. All authors contributed to and have approved the final manuscript.

ACKNOWLEDGMENTS

The authors cordially thank all patients and healthy controls for participating in this study. This work was supported by the Marie-Curie Initial Training Network TESIS: "Toward an Embodied Science of InterSubjectivity" (FP7-PEOPLE-2010-ITN, 264828). We also acknowledge financial support by Deutsche Forschungsgemeinschaft (DFG) and University of Heidelberg within the funding program "Open Access Publishing".

REFERENCES

1. Heinrichs DW, Buchanan RW. Significance and meaning of neurological signs in schizophrenia. *Am J Psychiatry* (1988) **145**:11–8.
2. Schroder J, Niethammer R, Geider FJ, Reitz C, Binkert M, Jauss M, et al. Neurological soft signs in schizophrenia. *Schizophr Res* (1991) **6**:25–30. doi:10.1016/0920-9964(91)90017-L
3. Jahn T, Hubmann W, Karr M, Mohr F, Schlenker R, Heidenreich T, et al. Motoric neurological soft signs and psychopathological symptoms in schizophrenic psychoses. *Psychiatry Res* (2006) **142**:191–9. doi:10.1016/j.psychres.2002.12.003
4. Chan RC, Xu T, Heinrichs RW, Yu Y, Wang Y. Neurological soft signs in schizophrenia: a meta-analysis. *Schizophr Bull* (2010) **36**:1089–104. doi:10.1093/schbul/sbp011
5. Bombin I, Arango C, Buchanan RW. Significance and meaning of neurological signs in schizophrenia: two decades later. *Schizophr Bull* (2005) **31**:962–77. doi:10.1093/schbul/sbi028
6. Bolton D, Gibb W, Lees A, Raven P, Gray JA, Chen E, et al. Neurological soft signs in obsessive compulsive disorder: standardised assessment and comparison with schizophrenia. *Behav Neurol* (1998) **11**:197–204. doi:10.1155/1999/639045
7. Jaafari N, Baup N, Bourdel MC, Olie JP, Rotge JY, Wassouf I, et al. Neurological soft signs in OCD patients with early age at onset, versus patients with schizophrenia and healthy subjects. *J Neuropsychiatry Clin Neurosci* (2011) **23**:409–16. doi:10.1176/appi.neuropsych.23.4.409
8. Mohr F, Hubmann W, Cohen R, Bender W, Haslacher C, Honicke S, et al. Neurological soft signs in schizophrenia: assessment and correlates. *Eur Arch Psychiatry Clin Neurosci* (1996) **246**:240–8. doi:10.1007/BF02190275
9. Kinney DK, Yurgelun-Todd DA, Woods BT. Neurologic signs of cerebellar and cortical sensory dysfunction in schizophrenics and their relatives. *Schizophr Res* (1999) **35**:99–104. doi:10.1016/S0920-9964(98)00121-2
10. Rigucci S, Dimitri-Valente G, Mandarelli G, Manfredi G, Comparelli A, Filippis SD, et al. Neurological soft signs discriminate schizophrenia from bipolar disorder. *J Psychiatr Pract* (2014) **20**:147–53. doi:10.1097/01.pra.0000445250.20875.0e
11. Zhao Q, Ma YT, Lui SS, Liu WH, Xu T, Yu X, et al. Neurological soft signs discriminate schizophrenia from major depression but not bipolar disorder. *Prog Neuropsychopharmacol Biol Psychiatry* (2013) **43**:72–8. doi:10.1016/j.pnpbp.2012.12.006
12. Krebs MO, Gut-Fayand A, Bourdel M, Dischamp J, Olie J. Validation and factorial structure of a standardized neurological examination assessing neurological soft signs in schizophrenia. *Schizophr Res* (2000) **45**:245–60. doi:10.1016/S0920-9964(99)00206-6
13. Thomann PA, Wustenberg T, Santos VD, Bachmann S, Essig M, Schroder J. Neurological soft signs and brain morphology in first-episode schizophrenia. *Psychol Med* (2009) **39**:371–9. doi:10.1017/S0033291708003656
14. Hirjak D, Wolf RC, Stieltjes B, Hauser T, Seidl U, Schroder J, et al. Cortical signature of neurological soft signs in recent onset schizophrenia. *Brain Topogr* (2014) **27**:296–306. doi:10.1007/s10548-013-0292-z
15. Zhao Q, Li Z, Huang J, Yan C, Dazzan P, Pantelis C, et al. Neurological soft signs are not "soft" in brain structure and functional networks: evidence from ALE meta-analysis. *Schizophr Bull* (2014) **40**:626–41. doi:10.1093/schbul/sbt063
16. Dazzan P, Morgan KD, Orr KG, Hutchinson G, Chitnis X, Suckling J, et al. The structural brain correlates of neurological soft signs in AESOP first-episode psychoses study. *Brain* (2004) **127**:143–53. doi:10.1093/brain/awh015
17. Janssen J, Diaz-Caneja A, Reig S, Bombin I, Mayoral M, Parellada M, et al. Brain morphology and neurological soft signs in adolescents with first-episode psychosis. *Br J Psychiatry* (2009) **195**:227–33. doi:10.1192/bjp.bp.108.052738
18. Thomann PA, Roebel M, Dos Santos V, Bachmann S, Essig M, Schroder J. Cerebellar substructures and neurological soft signs in first-episode schizophrenia. *Psychiatry Res* (2009) **173**:83–7. doi:10.1016/j.pscychresns.2008.07.006
19. Hirjak D, Wolf RC, Stieltjes B, Seidl U, Schroder J, Thomann PA. Neurological soft signs and subcortical brain morphology in recent onset schizophrenia. *J Psychiatr Res* (2012) **46**:533–9. doi:10.1016/j.jpsychires.2012.01.015
20. Hirjak D, Wolf RC, Stieltjes B, Hauser T, Seidl U, Thiemann U, et al. Neurological soft signs and brainstem morphology in first-episode schizophrenia. *Neuropsychobiology* (2013) **68**:91–9. doi:10.1159/000350999
21. Bleuler E. *Dementia Praecox or the Group of Schizophrenias. Zinkin J, Trans.* New York, NY: International Universities Press (1950).
22. Parnas J. The core Gestalt of schizophrenia. *World Psychiatry* (2012) **11**:67–9. doi:10.1016/j.wpsyc.2012.05.002
23. Parnas J. A disappearing heritage: the clinical core of schizophrenia. *Schizophr Bull* (2011) **37**:1121–30. doi:10.1093/schbul/sbr081
24. Cappon D. Clinical manifestations of autism and schizophrenia in childhood. *Can Med Assoc J* (1953) **69**:44–9.
25. Pelletier AL, Mittal VA. An autism dimension for schizophrenia in the next Diagnostic and Statistical Manual? *Schizophr Res* (2012) **137**:269–70. doi:10.1016/j.schres.2012.01.033
26. Kanner L. Early infantile autism. *J Pediatr* (1944) **25**:211–7. doi:10.1016/S0022-3476(44)80156-1
27. Asperger H. Die "Autistischen Psychopathen" im kindesalter. *Arch Psychiatr Nervenkr* (1944) **117**:76–136. doi:10.1007/BF01837709
28. Barneveld PS, Pieterse J, De Sonneville L, Van Rijn S, Lahuis B, Van Engeland H, et al. Overlap of autistic and schizotypal traits in adolescents with Autism Spectrum Disorders. *Schizophr Res* (2011) **126**:231–6. doi:10.1016/j.schres.2010.09.004
29. Konstantareas MM, Hewitt T. Autistic disorder and schizophrenia: diagnostic overlaps. *J Autism Dev Disord* (2001) **31**:19–28. doi:10.1023/A:1005605528309
30. Bevan Jones R, Thapar A, Lewis G, Zammit S. The association between early autistic traits and psychotic experiences in adolescence. *Schizophr Res* (2012) **135**:164–9. doi:10.1016/j.schres.2011.11.037
31. Waris P, Lindberg N, Kettunen K, Tani P. The relationship between Asperger's syndrome and schizophrenia in adolescence. *Eur Child Adolesc Psychiatry* (2013) **22**:217–23. doi:10.1007/s00787-012-0338-x
32. Rinehart NJ, Tonge BJ, Bradshaw JL, Iansek R, Enticott PG, Mcginley J. Gait function in high-functioning autism and Asperger's disorder: evidence for basal-ganglia and cerebellar involvement? *Eur Child Adolesc Psychiatry* (2006) **15**:256–64. doi:10.1007/s00787-006-0530-y
33. Tani P, Lindberg N, Appelberg B, Nieminen-Von Wendt T, Von Wendt L, Porkka-Heiskanen T. Clinical neurological abnormalities in young adults with Asperger syndrome. *Psychiatry Clin Neurosci* (2006) **60**:253–5. doi:10.1111/j.1440-1819.2006.01494.x
34. Mayoral M, Merchan-Naranjo J, Rapado M, Leiva M, Moreno C, Giraldez M, et al. Neurological soft signs in juvenile patients with Asperger syndrome, early-onset psychosis, and healthy controls. *Early Interv Psychiatry* (2010) **4**:283–90. doi:10.1111/j.1751-7893.2010.00197.x
35. Whyatt C, Craig C. Sensory-motor problems in Autism. *Front Integr Neurosci* (2013) **7**:51. doi:10.3389/fnint.2013.00051

36. Esposito G, Pasca SP. Motor abnormalities as a putative endophenotype for Autism Spectrum Disorders. *Front Integr Neurosci* (2013) **7**:43. doi:10.3389/fnint.2013.00043
37. Cheung C, Yu K, Fung G, Leung M, Wong C, Li Q, et al. Autistic disorders and schizophrenia: related or remote? An anatomical likelihood estimation. *PLoS One* (2010) **5**:e12233. doi:10.1371/journal.pone.0012233
38. Wittchen HU, Wunderlich U, Gruschwitz S, Zaudig M. *SKID-I: Strukturiertes Klinisches Interview für DSM-IV*. Göttingen: Hogrefe (1997).
39. Lord C, Rutter M, Goode S, Heemsbergen J, Jordan H, Mawhood L, et al. Autism diagnostic observation schedule: a standardized observation of communicative and social behavior. *J Autism Dev Disord* (1989) **19**:185–212. doi:10.1007/BF02211841
40. Weiß RH, editor. *CFT 20-R Grundintelligenztest Skala 2 – Revision*. Göttingen: Hogrefe (2006).
41. Miller TJ, Mcglashan TH, Rosen JL, Cadenhead K, Cannon T, Ventura J, et al. Prodromal assessment with the structured interview for prodromal syndromes and the scale of prodromal symptoms: predictive validity, interrater reliability, and training to reliability. *Schizophr Bull* (2003) **29**:703–15. doi:10.1093/oxfordjournals.schbul.a007040
42. Bachmann S, Bottmer C, Schroder J. Neurological soft signs in first-episode schizophrenia: a follow-up study. *Am J Psychiatry* (2005) **162**:2337–43. doi:10.1176/appi.ajp.162.12.2337
43. Oldfield RC. The assessment and analysis of handedness: the Edinburgh inventory. *Neuropsychologia* (1971) **9**:97–113. doi:10.1016/0028-3932(71)90067-4
44. Overall JE, Gorham DR. The brief psychiatric rating scale. *Psychol Rep* (1962) **10**:799–812. doi:10.2466/pr0.1962.10.3.799
45. Andreasen NC. *The Scale for the Assessment of Positive Symptoms (SAPS)*. Iowa City: University of Iowa (1984).
46. Andreasen NC. *The Scale for the Assessment of Negative Symptoms (SANS)*. Iowa City: University of Iowa (1983).
47. Strauss JS, Carpenter WT Jr. The prediction of outcome in schizophrenia. II. Relationships between predictor and outcome variables: a report from the WHO international pilot study of schizophrenia. *Arch Gen Psychiatry* (1974) **31**:37–42. doi:10.1001/archpsyc.1974.01760130021003
48. Hall RC. Global assessment of functioning. A modified scale. *Psychosomatics* (1995) **36**:267–75. doi:10.1016/S0033-3182(95)71656-5
49. Fisher RA. The use of multiple measurements in taxonomic problems. *Ann Hum Genet* (1936) **7**:179–88.
50. Arango C, Bartko JJ, Gold JM, Buchanan RW. Prediction of neuropsychological performance by neurological signs in schizophrenia. *Am J Psychiatry* (1999) **156**:1349–57.
51. Pakyurek M, Yarnal R, Carter C. Treatment of psychosis in children and adolescents: a review. *Adolesc Med State Art Rev* (2013) **24**:420–32, ix.
52. Galderisi S, Maj M. Deficit schizophrenia: an overview of clinical, biological and treatment aspects. *Eur Psychiatry* (2009) **24**:493–500. doi:10.1016/j.eurpsy.2009.03.001
53. Chen EY, Lam LC, Chen RY, Nguyen DG. Negative symptoms, neurological signs and neuropsychological impairments in 204 Hong Kong Chinese patients with schizophrenia. *Br J Psychiatry* (1996) **168**:227–33. doi:10.1192/bjp.168.2.227
54. Telfer S, Shivashankar S, Krishnadas R, Mccreadie RG, Kirkpatrick B. Tardive dyskinesia and deficit schizophrenia. *Acta Psychiatr Scand* (2011) **124**:357–62. doi:10.1111/j.1600-0447.2011.01751.x
55. Buchanan RW, Kirkpatrick B, Heinrichs DW, Carpenter WT Jr. Clinical correlates of the deficit syndrome of schizophrenia. *Am J Psychiatry* (1990) **147**:290–4.
56. Galderisi S, Maj M, Mucci A, Cassano GB, Invernizzi G, Rossi A, et al. Historical, psychopathological, neurological, and neuropsychological aspects of deficit schizophrenia: a multicenter study. *Am J Psychiatry* (2002) **159**:983–90. doi:10.1176/appi.ajp.159.6.983
57. Peralta V, Moreno-Izco L, Sanchez-Torres A, Garcia De Jalon E, Campos MS, Cuesta MJ. Characterization of the deficit syndrome in drug-naive schizophrenia patients: the role of spontaneous movement disorders and neurological soft signs. *Schizophr Bull* (2014) **40**:214–24. doi:10.1093/schbul/sbs152
58. Buchanan RW, Breier A, Kirkpatrick B, Elkashef A, Munson RC, Gellad F, et al. Structural abnormalities in deficit and nondeficit schizophrenia. *Am J Psychiatry* (1993) **150**:59–65.
59. Arango C, Kirkpatrick B, Buchanan RW. Neurological signs and the heterogeneity of schizophrenia. *Am J Psychiatry* (2000) **157**:560–5. doi:10.1176/appi.ajp.157.4.560
60. Dziuk MA, Gidley Larson JC, Apostu A, Mahone EM, Denckla MB, Mostofsky SH. Dyspraxia in autism: association with motor, social, and communicative deficits. *Dev Med Child Neurol* (2007) **49**:734–9. doi:10.1111/j.1469-8749.2007.00734.x
61. Giedd JN, Blumenthal J, Jeffries NO, Castellanos FX, Liu H, Zijdenbos A, et al. Brain development during childhood and adolescence: a longitudinal MRI study. *Nat Neurosci* (1999) **2**:861–3. doi:10.1038/13158
62. Hua X, Thompson PM, Leow AD, Madsen SK, Caplan R, Alger JR, et al. Brain growth rate abnormalities visualized in adolescents with autism. *Hum Brain Mapp* (2013) **34**:425–36. doi:10.1002/hbm.21441
63. Sasayama D, Hori H, Teraishi T, Hattori K, Ota M, Matsuo J, et al. Benzodiazepines, benzodiazepine-like drugs, and typical antipsychotics impair manual dexterity in patients with schizophrenia. *J Psychiatr Res* (2014) **49**:37–42. doi:10.1016/j.jpsychires.2013.10.019
64. Cannon M, Jones P, Huttunen MO, Tanskanen A, Huttunen T, Rabe-Hesketh S, et al. School performance in Finnish children and later development of schizophrenia: a population-based longitudinal study. *Arch Gen Psychiatry* (1999) **56**:457–63. doi:10.1001/archpsyc.56.5.457
65. Tamagni C, Studerus E, Gschwandtner U, Aston J, Borgwardt S, Riecher-Rossler A. Are neurological soft signs pre-existing markers in individuals with an at-risk mental state for psychosis? *Psychiatry Res* (2013) **210**:427–31. doi:10.1016/j.psychres.2013.06.016
66. McGorry PD, Mcfarlane C, Patton GC, Bell R, Hibbert ME, Jackson HJ, et al. The prevalence of prodromal features of schizophrenia in adolescence: a preliminary survey. *Acta Psychiatr Scand* (1995) **92**:241–9. doi:10.1111/j.1600-0447.1995.tb09577.x
67. Leask SJ, Done DJ, Crow TJ. Adult psychosis, common childhood infections and neurological soft signs in a national birth cohort. *Br J Psychiatry* (2002) **181**:387–92. doi:10.1192/bjp.181.5.387
68. Mittal VA, Dean DJ, Bernard JA, Orr JM, Pelletier-Baldelli A, Carol EE, et al. Neurological soft signs predict abnormal cerebellar-thalamic tract development and negative symptoms in adolescents at high risk for psychosis: a longitudinal perspective. *Schizophr Bull* (2014). doi:10.1093/schbul/sbt199
69. Murray GK, Jones PB, Moilanen K, Veijola J, Miettunen J, Cannon TD, et al. Infant motor development and adult cognitive functions in schizophrenia. *Schizophr Res* (2006) **81**:65–74. doi:10.1016/j.schres.2005.08.016
70. Dazzan P, Murray RM. Neurological soft signs in first-episode psychosis: a systematic review. *Br J Psychiatry Suppl* (2002) **43**:s50–7. doi:10.1192/bjp.181.43.s50
71. Hirjak D, Wolf RC, Wilder-Smith EP, Kubera KM, Thomann PA. Motor abnormalities and basal ganglia in schizophrenia: evidence from structural magnetic resonance imaging. *Brain Topogr* (2014). doi:10.1007/s10548-014-0377-3
72. Crespi B, Badcock C. Psychosis and autism as diametrical disorders of the social brain. *Behav Brain Sci* (2008) **31**:241–261;discussion261–320. doi:10.1017/S0140525X08004214
73. Midorikawa A, Hashimoto R, Noguchi H, Saitoh O, Kunugi H, Nakamura K. Impairment of motor dexterity in schizophrenia assessed by a novel finger movement test. *Psychiatry Res* (2008) **159**:281–9. doi:10.1016/j.psychres.2007.04.004
74. Keefe RS, Fenton WS. How should DSM-V criteria for schizophrenia include cognitive impairment? *Schizophr Bull* (2007) **33**:912–20. doi:10.1093/schbul/sbm046
75. Irani F, Kalkstein S, Moberg EA, Moberg PJ. Neuropsychological performance in older patients with schizophrenia: a meta-analysis of cross-sectional and longitudinal studies. *Schizophr Bull* (2011) **37**:1318–26. doi:10.1093/schbul/sbq057
76. Mockler D, Riordan J, Sharma T. Memory and intellectual deficits do not decline with age in schizophrenia. *Schizophr Res* (1997) **26**:1–7.
77. Hijman R, Hulshoff Pol HE, Sitskoorn MM, Kahn RS. Global intellectual impairment does not accelerate with age in patients with schizophrenia: a cross-sectional analysis. *Schizophr Bull* (2003) **29**:509–17. doi:10.1093/oxfordjournals.schbul.a007023
78. Hedman AM, Van Haren NE, Van Baal GC, Brans RG, Hijman R, Kahn RS, et al. Is there change in intelligence quotient in chronically ill schizophrenia patients? A longitudinal study in twins discordant for schizophrenia. *Psychol Med* (2012) **42**:2535–41. doi:10.1017/S0033291712000694
79. Dragovic M, Waters FA, Jablensky A. Estimating premorbid intelligence in schizophrenia patients: demographically based approach. *Aust N Z J Psychiatry* (2008) **42**:814–8. doi:10.1080/00048670802277214

80. Cai L, Zhu X, Yi J, Bai M, Wang M, Wang Y, et al. Neurological soft signs and their relationship with measures of executive function in Chinese adolescents. *J Dev Behav Pediatr* (2013) **34**:197–203. doi:10.1097/DBP.0b013e3182825c41
81. Gupta S, Andreasen NC, Arndt S, Flaum M, Schultz SK, Hubbard WC, et al. Neurological soft signs in neuroleptic-naive and neuroleptic-treated schizophrenic patients and in normal comparison subjects. *Am J Psychiatry* (1995) **152**: 191–6.
82. Walther S, Horn H, Razavi N, Koschorke P, Muller TJ, Strik W. Quantitative motor activity differentiates schizophrenia subtypes. *Neuropsychobiology* (2009) **60**:80–6. doi:10.1159/000236448

3

Psychological effects of implantable cardioverter defibrillator shocks

Gian Mauro Manzoni[1,2]*, Gianluca Castelnuovo[1,2], Angelo Compare[3], Francesco Pagnini[2], Vidal Essebag[4] and Riccardo Proietti[5]

[1] *Psychology Research Laboratory, Istituto Auxologico Italiano IRCCS, Verbania, Italy*
[2] *Department of Psychology, Catholic University of Milan, Milano, Italy*
[3] *Department of Psychology, University of Bergamo, Bergamo, Italy*
[4] *McGill University Health Center, Montreal, QC, Canada*
[5] *Cardiology Department, Luigi Sacco Hospital, Milano, Italy*

Edited by:
Sayyed Mohsen Fatemi, Harvard University, USA

Reviewed by:
Valentina Ieraci, University of Turin, Italy
Mingna Liu, Northwestern University, USA

****Correspondence:***
Gian Mauro Manzoni, Psychology Research Laboratory, Istituto Auxologico Italiano IRCCS, Via Cadorna 90, 28824 Piancavallo (Oggebbio), Verbania, Italy
e-mail: gm.manzoni@auxologico.it

Background: The implantable cardioverter defibrillator (ICD) saves lives but clinical experience suggests that it may have detrimental effects on mental health. The ICD shock has been largely blamed as the main offender but empirical evidence is not consistent, perhaps because of methodological differences across studies.

Objective: To appraise methodologies of studies that assessed the psychological effects of ICD shock and explore associations between methods and results.

Data Sources: A comprehensive search of English articles that were published between 1980 and 30 June 2013 was applied to the following electronic databases: PubMed, EMBASE, NHS HTA database, PsycINFO, Sciencedirect and CINAHL.

Review Methods: Only studies testing the effects of ICD shock on psychological and quality of life outcomes were included. Data were extracted according to a PICOS pre-defined sheet including methods and study quality indicators.

Results: Fifty-four observational studies and six randomized controlled trials met the inclusion criteria. Multiple differences in methods that were used to test the psychological effects of ICD shock were found across them. No significant association with results was observed.

Conclusions: Methodological heterogeneity of study methods is too wide and limits any quantitative attempt to account for the mixed findings. Well-built and standardized research is urgently needed.

Keywords: implantable cardioverter defibrillator, ICD shock, quality of life, anxiety, depression, review

INTRODUCTION

The implantable cardioverter defibrillator (ICD) has become the treatment of choice for both primary and secondary prevention of sudden cardiac death (SCD) due to ventricular arrhythmias (VA). Major clinical trials have consistently shown the ICD to be superior to antiarrhythmic drugs in patients at high risk (Buxton et al., 1999; Kuck et al., 2000; Connolly et al., 2000a,b; Moss et al., 2002; Bardy et al., 2005). As ICDs can avoid SCD but cannot affect the underlying cardiac substrate, the prolonged lifespan enjoyed by patients with significant heart disease is thus shifting the clinical burden to the resulting increase in heart failure events (Sears et al., 2006; Mishkin et al., 2009) and to the possibility of repeated shocks (Barnay et al., 2007). Reported rates of appropriate ICD shocks range from 60% in the 3-year secondary prevention AVID study (Anderson et al., 1999) to 20% in the 2-year primary prevention MADIT II trial (Moss et al., 2002).

As many patients who receive a shock develop some form of psychological distress in the aftermath (Sears and Kirian, 2010), the possible relation between ICD shocks and psychological distress/disorders or reduced QoL was assessed with particular attention. Investigations of such relationship were largely confined to descriptive or observational studies because of the clear impossibility to control the shock factor and thus to use randomized designs. Despite these limitations, an amount of studies attempted to test the hypothesis that ICD shocks are responsible for the occurrence of psychological distress/disorders and the reduction of QoL in ICD patients. However, findings were promptly discordant (Sears et al., 1999; Burke et al., 2003) and the supposed negative effect of ICD shock on patients' QoL and psychological health is still an object of debate (Pedersen and Van Den Broek, 2008; Pedersen et al., 2010b).

In order to examine whether such mixed findings might depend on design and methodological differences, we reviewed and critically appraised all quantitative studies that statistically assessed the effect of ICD shocks on psychological variables such as QoL, anxiety, depression, psychological stress or well-being and post-traumatic stress disorder (PTSD) in patients implanted with an ICD for primary and secondary prevention.

METHODS

STUDY ELIGIBILITY CRITERIA

Types of studies

Quantitative studies that statistically assessed the association between ICD shock and psychological outcomes were included. Qualitative and single-case or case-series reports were not considered. Studies were selected irrespective of designs, aims, hypotheses, time from ICD implantation and length of follow-up. Studies that explicitly assessed the causal effect of psychosocial factors on ICD shock occurrence were not considered.

Types of participants

Patients of age ≥18 implanted with an ICD for primary or secondary prevention of SCD were considered. No restriction was made on patients' clinical and demographic characteristics with the exception of age. Young patients of age <18 were not considered.

Types of intervention

Only automatic ICD shock therapy was considered. No restriction was made on appropriateness (both appropriate and misappropriate shocks were considered), duration, electric power and the absolute or relative number of delivered shocks (isolated shocks, electric storms and shock clusters were considered).

Types of outcome measures

Only valid and reliable standardized measures of psychological and quality of life outcomes were considered. Anxiety, depression, PTSD and health-related quality of life measures were specified in advance and documented in the review protocol. However, no restriction was made on any other psychological outcomes that were measured in a valid and reliable manner.

REPORT ELIGIBILITY CRITERIA

Only English articles that were published in indexed journals were considered. Abstracts, letters, unpublished data and gray literature in general were not searched nor considered.

DATA SOURCES

A comprehensive search of English articles that were published between 1980 and 30 June 2013 was applied to the following electronic databases: PubMed, EMBASE, NHS HTA database, PsycINFO, Sciencedirect and CINAHL. Since the first ICD implantation took place in 1980, it was unnecessary to search records predating that year. Bibliographies of included studies were screened for further references.

LITERATURE SEARCH

A two-step search strategy was used. We arbitrarily defined four time intervals (1980–1996, 1997–2003, 2004–2007, 2008–2011) and randomly assigned each of them to one of four independent reviewers who had been previously instructed about the search protocol. We first searched online databases for the following terms in article titles or abstracts: ICD, implant*, defib*, cardiover*, (internal near defib*), (internal near cardiover*), (implant* near cardiover*), (implant* or internal), (cardiac near defib*), (implant* and defib*), (internal and defib*), (cardiac and defib*). We recorded results in a reference database (EndNote X2, the Thomson Corporation). The second step refined the first search by filtering for the following terms: mood, quality of life, QOL, health, health-related quality of life, adjust*, psych*, anx*, depress*, stress, well-being.

STUDY SELECTION

Studies identified by the whole search strategy were assessed for inclusion through three stages. First, three independent reviewers (GMM, RP, and GC) screened titles and abstracts of papers to exclude irrelevant records. Full-texts of remaining papers were obtained and assessed against eligibility criteria by the same independent reviewers at the second stage. Any differences in opinion were resolved through discussion with a forth independent reviewer at the third stage.

DATA COLLECTION

All included studies were randomly and equally assigned to three review authors (GMM, RP, SC) who independently extracted and coded data in accordance to a refined sheet. Information was extracted on: (1) design and aim of study, (2) ICD indication (primary, secondary or both) and programming (only shock or shock and pacing); (3) demographic characteristics of participants implanted with an ICD (age and sex); (4) inclusion and exclusion criteria; (5) number of participants included in the analysis and lost to follow-up; (6) shock therapy; (7) timing of psychological assessments and length of follow-up; (8) outcome measures; (9) statistical analysis; (10) results.

RISK OF BIAS ASSESSMENT

The Cochrane data collection form for non-randomized studies and the Newcastle-Ottawa scale for assessing quality of cohort studies were used to assess risk of bias and to ascertain the validity of studies. Both templates were retrieved from the Cochrane Handbook for Systematic Reviews of Interventions, Chapter 13, Supplementary Material (retrieved at www.cochrane.org/training/cochrane-handbook). The same three review authors (GMM, RP, and GC) who extracted data determined also the adequacy of: (1) ascertainment of shock exposure; (2) demonstration that outcomes of interest was not present before ICD implantation; (3) control for confounding; (4) assessment of outcomes (self-report or interview); (5) validity and reliability of outcome measures; (6) completeness of data set. Furthermore, the review authors appraised the method used for identifying relevant confounders and the method used for controlling relevant confounders.

DATA ANALYSIS

Wide methodological differences were promptly observed across studies during the review process. The feasibility of standardizing individual study results and combining them in a meta-analysis was thus discussed several times during the first intermediate meetings and no consensus was established before the middle of the review process when we decided not to perform any meta-analysis. As reported extensively in the results section, included studies differ in many characteristics, in particular analytical and operationalizing methods, and statistical combination of data from two or more similar studies in a meta-analysis may be neither necessary nor desirable (Liberati et al., 2009). Hence, the extracted data were only qualitatively analyzed and tabulated. Despite the danger of poor validity associated to quasi-quantitative methods such as vote counting, we decided also to perform subgroup analyses in order to explore if significant results depend on the methodological factors we specified in advance. Publication bias or selective reporting bias were not systematically assessed because we did not specify this possibility before starting the review and, even if we observed some clues of selective reporting in a number of articles, we decided not to investigate further.

RESULTS

STUDY SELECTION

A total of 60 studies were identified for inclusion in the review (**Table 1**). The first-step search of electronic databases provided a huge amount of records that were then drastically reduced with the filtering for the second-step search terms. Of these records, a large part was discarded in accordance to the report eligibility criteria and because, after screening the abstracts, it appeared that these studies clearly did not assess a statistical association between ICD shock and the outcomes of interest. No further article was discarded after examining the full text of the remaining 60 records. No additional study was identified by checking the references of relevant papers, by searching for studies that have cited these papers or by contacting the principal authors of the field.

CHARACTERISTICS OF INCLUDED STUDIES

Designs

Study designs were coded considering only the part of study in which an association between ICD shock and outcomes of interest was assessed. According to criterion, 32 studies out of 60 were classified as cross-sectional, 27 as prospective and 1 as randomized controlled trial (RCT). Hence, prospective cohort studies that evaluated the effect of shock cross-sectionally (e.g., Mark et al., 2008) were coded as cross-sectional. Only cohort studies that assessed the effect of ICD shock on change in psychological variables and quality of life along time were considered prospective. Six of the included studies are randomized controlled trials (Namerow et al., 1999; Irvine et al., 2002; Schron et al., 2002; Strickberger et al., 2003; Wathen et al., 2004; Mark et al., 2008) but three out of them were classified as cross-sectional (Namerow et al., 1999; Strickberger et al., 2003; Mark et al., 2008) and two as prospective (Irvine et al., 2002; Schron et al., 2002) because assessment of the shock effect was a sub-analysis performed only on patients randomized to the ICD condition. Only the PainFREE Rx II trial (Wathen et al., 2004) was coded as RCT because the ICD shock was partially manipulated. In fact, patients with ICDs were randomized into two treatment conditions that differed only for the delivering of shock therapy or anti-tachycardia pacing.

Participants with ICDs

The included studies vary a lot with respect to sample sizes. The study with the smaller sample involved 15 ICD patients and has a prospective design (Dougherty, 1995), while the study with the larger sample included 816 ICD patients and was coded as cross-sectional although it is an RCT comparing amiodarone vs. ICD in heart failure patients (Mark et al., 2008). Considering only patients with an ICD whose data were included in statistical analyses and contributed to results, the whole number of participants considered in this review is 10558. The average of the mean ages of patients across the included studies is 61.2 with a standard deviation (SD) of 3.6 (range: 53–69.1), while the average of the relative SDs is 12.1 (range: 6.3–16). Patients included in the studies were mainly males. Percentages of females varied from 0% (Keren et al., 1991; Burgess et al., 1997; Goodman and Hess, 1999) to 81% (Pedersen et al., 2008b) with a mean of only 20% (SD 10.9%).

ICD indication

As expected, studies that involved only patients with a secondary ICD indication are more frequent than studies that recruited only patients with a primary ICD indication (22 vs. 10). Samples were heterogeneous (both patients with a primary indication and patients with a secondary prevention were recruited) in 22 studies, while in 6 papers no information about ICD indication was reported and relative studies were thus not classified (see **Table 1** for details).

ICD Shock therapy

Twenty-seven studies operationalized number of ICD shocks in a dichotomized variable with patients who received 1 or more shocks classified in one category and patients who did not receive any shock assigned to the other one. Across 22 out of 27 studies that operationalized ICD shocks in this manner (no shock vs. ≥1 shocks), 38.5% of patients received at least 1 shock on average. The smallest percentage of patients who received 1 or more shocks (4.2%) was found in the study of Van Den Broek et al. (2009), while the higher (64%) was found in the study of Crossmann et al. (2007), followed by Jacq et al. (2009) and Bilge et al. (2006) with 61.5% shocked patients. In five of the articles describing the studies that we classified in this category (no shock vs. ≥1 shocks), data about percentage of patients who received 1 or more shock from their ICD were lacking (Keren et al., 1991; Kamphuis et al., 2002; Wathen et al., 2004; Cuculi et al., 2006; Piotrowicz et al., 2007). Indeed, some articles reported only the number, the mean or the median of ICD shocks delivered during the study period. Furthermore, we found that two articles classified in this category (no shock vs. ≥1 shocks) described two studies whose aims and hypotheses were different but shared the same sample (Pedersen et al., 2004, 2005). Two studies operationalized number of ICD shocks in a dichotomized variable with patients who received 5 or more shocks classified in one category and patients who received between 0 and 4 shocks assigned to the other one. In Luderitz et al.'s study (1993), 57.9% of ICD patients received 5 or more shocks during a 12-month follow-up, while in the Von Känel et al.'s study (2011), 8.4% received 5 or more shocks before baseline assessment (24.4 ± 20.7 months post ICD-implantation) and 19.3 % received 5 or more shocks between the baseline and the end of follow-up (65.5 ± 27.4 months post ICD-implantation). Nine studies categorized ICD shocks in multiple groups and eight different categorizations were used. Three studies out of them created an extreme group of patients who had received ten or

Table 1 | Characteristics of studies.

Source	Indication	Sample[1]	Age (mean ± SD)	Age (range)	Gender (% females)	Inclusion criteria	Exclusion criteria
Keren et al., 1991	Secondary	18	62	Not reported	0%	Not reported	History of organic brain syndrome Psychiatric hospitalizations Anxiolytic, antidepressant or neuroleptic medications at the time of the initial clinical evaluation
Morris et al., 1991	Secondary	20	60.9	Not reported	35%	Not reported	Not reported
Luderitz et al., 1993	Unclear	57	59 ± 13	Not reported	12%	Third-generation ICD ATP device	Not reported
Dougherty, 1995	Secondary	15	57	Not reported	13.4%	Cardiac arrest from primary VF	Physiologically or neurologically compromised AMI in conjunction with SCA or a cardiac arrest for reasons not related to cardiovascular causes
Chevalier et al., 1996	Primary	32	54.5	22–73	12.5%	Not reported	Not reported
Burgess et al., 1997	Not declared	25	65	29–80	0%	Not reported	Not reported
Herrmann et al., 1997	Both	63	61 ± 13	Not reported	21%	Not reported	Not reported
Heller et al., 1998	Primary	58	64 ± 11	37–84	28%	Not reported	Not reported
Dunbar et al., 1999	Both	163	59.6 ± 13	24–85	17%	Intact cognitive status	History of psychiatric disorder
Dunbar et al., 1999	Both	176	59.8 ± 13	25–85	18%	Intact cognitive status	History of psychiatric illness requiring medication, psychotherapy or hospitalization
Goodman and Hess, 1999	Not declared	25	65	29–80	0%	Not reported	Not reported
Herbst et al., 1999	Not declared	49	65 ± 11.7	Not reported	12%	Not reported	Major cardiac surgery (i.e., heart transplantation or CABG) or pacemaker implantation LVEF < 35% NYHA Class < III
Namerow et al., 1999	Primary	262	63.6 ± 9.2	Not reported	15%	Scheduled CABG LVEF <0.36 Abnormal signal-averaged ECG	Participation in the enrolling center's ICD support group meetings
Pauli et al., 1999	Both	61	55.7 ± 9	25–65	20%	Not reported	Not reported
Duru et al., 2001	Not declared	76	57 ± 13	Not reported	15.8%	Not reported	Not reported
Godemann et al., 2001	Secondary	72	69.1 ± 10.4	Not reported	13.9%	Intellectual and physical fit for participation	Not reported

(Continued)

Table 1 | Continued

Source	Indication	Sample[1]	Age (mean ± SD)	Age (range)	Gender (% females)	Inclusion criteria	Exclusion criteria
Irvine et al., 2002	Secondary	86	64.4 ± 8.6	Not reported	12.1%	CISD	Not reported
Schron et al., 2002	Secondary	373	64.3 ± 10.5	Not reported	18.7%	AVID	Not reported
Wallace et al., 2002	Secondary	58	67	Not reported	24%	Not reported	Not reported
Kamphuis et al., 2002	Secondary	133	55.24 ± 13.7	Not reported	26.3%	Out-of-hospital cardiac arrest	Not reported
Kamphuis et al., 2003	Secondary	132	55.24 ± 13.7	Not reported	26.5%	Not reported	Not reported
Newman et al., 2003	Primary	150	62 ± 12	Not reported	27%	2 symptomatic AF or atrial flutter episodes in the 3 months before implantation and to have failed at least 1 antiarrhythmic drug because of inefficacy or toxicity	History of sustained ventricular tachyarrhythmias or class IV heart failure
Strickberger et al., 2003	Primary	51	58 ± 11	Not reported	33%	NIDCM LVEF = 0.35 asymptomatic NSVT NYHA functional class I to III	Syncope, pregnancy, a contraindication to Amiodarone or defibrillator therapy or concomitant therapy with a Class I antiarrhythmic drug
Godemann et al., 2004a	Secondary	90	59.5 ± 11.1	Not reported	13.3%	Intact cognitive status	ICD implantation <1 year previously
Godemann et al., 2004b	Secondary	93	59.7 ± 11.2	29–81	14%	Intact cognitive status	ICD implantation <1 year previously
Pedersen et al., 2004	Secondary	182	62 ± 13	Not reported	19%	Not reported	Terminally ill, brain damage, too many missing values on questionnaires
Wathen et al., 2004	Both	55	67 ± 11	Not reported	21%	Not reported	Hypertrophic cardiomyopathy, long-QT syndrome or Brugada syndrome
Carroll and Hamilton, 2005	Secondary	59	60	21–84	28.8%	Intact cognitive status	Not reported
Pedersen et al., 2005	Secondary	182	62 ± 13	Not reported	19%	Not reported	Terminally ill, brain damage, too many missing values on questionnaires
Sears et al., 2005	Secondary	60	65.3	22–89		Not reported	Cognitive impairment
Bilge et al., 2006	Both	91	53 ± 14	18–86	13.2%	Not reported	Significant psychiatric illness and recent ICD implantation (<3 months)
Cuculi et al., 2006	Both	55	61.6	30–81	23.3%	Recalled and potentially flawed ICD	Not reported
Leosdottir et al., 2006	Not reported	41	61.8 ± 14.2	25–85	31.7%	Not reported	Major mental or physical disabilities

(Continued)

Table 1 | Continued

Source	Indication	Sample[1]	Age (mean ± SD)	Age (range)	Gender (% females)	Inclusion criteria	Exclusion criteria
Luyster et al., 2006	Both	100	67.9 ± 11.7	35–85	19%	Not reported	Not reported
Crossmann et al., 2007	Both	35	57 ± 6.3	35–65	14%	LVEF <0.36 Abnormal signal-averaged electrocardiogram	Participation in the enrolling center's ICD support group meetings
Passman et al., 2007	Primary	227	59 ± 14	Not reported	27%	LVEF ≤ 35% not caused by CAD History of symptomatic heart failure Either non-sustained ventricular tachycardia or 10 or more premature ventricular depolarizations per hour	Not reported
Pedersen et al., 2007	Secondary	154	58.5 ± 12.5	Not reported	18.8%	Not reported	Life expectancy <1 year, history of psychiatric illness other than affective/anxiety disorders, on the waiting list for heart transplantation
Piotrowicz et al., 2007	Primary	390	Unclear	Not reported	Unclear	MADIT-II	Not reported
Sossong, 2007	Both	90	65.4 ± 10.6	36–88	22.2%	ICD for at least 2 months since implantation Intact cognitive status	Not reported
Johansen et al., 2008	Secondary	610	62.4	18–85	18%	Not reported	First ICD implant within the last 3 months, HTX, death or ICD removed, cognitive impairment, overall insufficient data quality, procedural error
Ladwig et al., 2008	Both	147	59.9 ± 13	Not reported	15%	Time since implantation longer than 3 months Rapid onset of the CHD condition	Not reported
Mark et al., 2008	Primary	816	59.9 ± 11.9	Not reported	22.9%	NYHA chronic and stable class II or III congestive heart failure LVEF ≤ 35%	Not reported
Pedersen et al., 2008a	Secondary	566	61.9 ± 14.3	18–85	18%	Not reported	First ICD implant within the last 3 months, HTX, death or ICD removed, cognitive impairment, overall insufficient data quality, procedural error
Pedersen et al., 2008b	Both	176	59	Not reported	80.7%	LVEF <0.36 Abnormal signal-averaged electrocardiogram	Life expectancy <1 year, history of psychiatric illness other than affective/anxiety disorders, on the waiting list for heart transplantation
Van Den Broek et al., 2008	Both	308	62.6 ± 10.1	Not reported	18%	Not reported	Not reported

(Continued)

Table 1 | Continued

Source	Indication	Sample[1]	Age (mean ± SD)	Age (range)	Gender (% females)	Inclusion criteria	Exclusion criteria
Jacq et al., 2009	Both	65	59.8 ± 14.8	Not reported	13.8%	Not reported	Previous medical or surgical problem at the time of interview
Noyes et al., 2009	Primary	601	64.6	Not reported	17%	Prior AMI and a LVEF ≤ 0.30	Experience of an ICD shock before baseline HRQOL data collection
Pedersen et al., 2009	Secondary	557	61.9 ± 14.3	Not reported	18.1%	Not reported	First ICD implant within the last 3 months, HTX, death or ICD removed, cognitive impairment, overall insufficient data quality, procedural error
Spindler et al., 2009	Secondary	535	61.5 ± 14.4	Not reported	18.1%	Not reported	First ICD implant within the last 3 months, HTX, death or ICD removed, cognitive impairment, overall insufficient data quality, procedural error
Thomas et al., 2009	Primary	57	59.8 ± 11.8	Not reported	18%	NYHA class II or III LVEF ≤ 35%	History of ventricular arrhythmias or cardiac arrest.
Van Den Broek et al., 2009	Both	165	62.1 ± 10.6	Not reported	12.7%	Not reported	Cognitive impairment (e.g., dementia), severe comorbidities (e.g., cancer)
Kapa et al., 2010	Both	223	66 ± 12	Not reported	17.9%	Not reported	Not reported
Pedersen et al., 2010a	Both	348	57.7 ± 12.1	Not reported	21%	Not reported	Life expectancy <1 year, history of psychiatric illness other than affective/anxiety disorders, on the waiting list for heart transplantation
Redhead et al., 2010	Secondary	100	69	41–88	17%	ICD already implanted over a 3-year period	Not reported
Suzuki et al., 2010	Both	90	57 ± 16	Not reported	28%	new implantation of ICD or CRT-D devices, an existing ICD/CRT-D, upgrade from ICD to CRT-D, generator replacement, electrical storm or acute decompensated heart failure	Not reported
Versteeg et al., 2010	Secondary	300	57.9 ± 12	Not reported	19.7%	MIDAS	Not reported
Dickerson et al., 2010	Both	76	62.4 ± 11.5	32–84	23.8%	Not reported	History of acute psychiatric disorders

(Continued)

Table 1 | Continued

Source	Indication	Sample[1]	Age (mean ± SD)	Age (range)	Gender (% females)	Inclusion criteria	Exclusion criteria
Habibovic et al., 2012	Both	395	62.8 ± 10.3	Not reported	19%	Not reported	Cognitive impairments (e.g., dementia), psychiatric history (other than affective disorders), life-threatening comorbidities (e.g., cancer), life expectancy <1 year
Pedersen et al., 2011	Both	284	61.2 ± 10.2	Not reported	21.1%	Not reported	Significant cognitive impairments (e.g., dementia), life-threatening comorbidities (e.g., cancer), history of psychiatric illness other than affective/anxiety disorders
Von Känel et al., 2011	Both	107	57.2 ± 14.2	Not reported	38.3%	Time since implantation longer than 3 months	Not reported

[1] Number of ICD patients whose data were analyzed.

more shocks (Herrmann et al., 1997; Ladwig et al., 2008; Suzuki et al., 2010), while three studies grouped also patients who had received electrical storms (Kapa et al., 2010; Redhead et al., 2010; Suzuki et al., 2010). Three studies operationalized ICD shocks in units of time. Morris et al. (1991) divided the number of delayed ICD shocks by length of follow-up (in months) to generate a frequency rate per unit of time; Jacq et al. (2009) divided the number of shocks received since implantation by the time elapsed since implantation (ratio shock) in order to take into account the significant difference in time elapsed since implantation between participants who did or did not experience ICD shock; Pauli et al. (1999) calculated the relative number of ICD shocks per year. Finally, six studies calculated the number of ICD shocks that were delivered within a fixed length of time or since last assessment (Kamphuis et al., 2003; Bilge et al., 2006; Mark et al., 2008; Noyes et al., 2009; Dickerson et al., 2010; Suzuki et al., 2010). In all the other studies, the absolute number of ICD shocks that each patient received was considered for the analysis.

Outcomes

The most prevalent outcomes are measures of anxiety, depression and health-related quality of life. In particular, anxiety was measured in 36 studies, depression in 30 studies and health-related quality of life (both mental and physical) in 29 studies. Anxiety and depression were mostly measured with self-report questionnaires. In only three studies (two of them used also a self-report questionnaire) anxiety was assessed with a clinical interview (Van Den Broek et al., 2008, 2009; Jacq et al., 2009), while depression was evaluated with a diagnostic interview in only one study (Jacq et al., 2009). With respect to the self-report measure of anxiety as an outcome of ICD shocks, the Hospital Anxiety and Depression Scale (HADS) was the most used psychometric questionnaire (13 studies out of 35, i.e., the total number of studies that used a self-report measure of anxiety, used the HADS). The second most used measure is the Spielberger State-Trait Anxiety Inventory (STAI), which was used in ten studies. The remaining self-report questionnaires that were used to measure anxiety are the Hamilton Anxiety Scale (1 study), the Beck Anxiety Inventory (1 study) and the anxiety index of the Symptom Checklist 90 (1 study). The Hamilton Rating Scale for Anxiety was used in two of the three studies that assessed anxiety with a clinical interview. Differently, Jacq et al. (2009) used the Mini International Neuropsychiatric Interview. With respect to the self-report measure of depression as an outcome of ICD shocks, the Hospital Anxiety and Depression Scale (HADS) was again the most used psychometric questionnaire (13 studies out of 30, i.e., the total number of studies that used a self-report measure of depression, used the HADS). The second most used measure is the Beck Depression Inventory (version 1 or 2) which was used in 6 studies. The remaining self-report questionnaires that were used to measure depression are the Zung Self-Rating Depression Scale (1 study), the Centre for Epidemiologic Studies Depression Scale (1 study) and the depression index of the Symptom Checklist 90 (1 study). The only study that assessed depression symptoms with a clinical interview used the Mini International Neuropsychiatric Interview (Jacq et al., 2009). General mental disorders were assessed in four studies (Morris et al., 1991; Chevalier et al., 1996; Godemann et al., 2001, 2004a). All of them used a semi-structured psychiatric interview according to the DSM-III-R criteria. Health-related quality of life was mostly measured with the SF-36 (15 studies) and the SF-12 (4 studies). Few other studies used the Health Utility Index 3 (Noyes et al., 2009), the Health Complaints Scale (Van Den Broek et al., 2009), the RAND-36 Health Survey (Kamphuis et al., 2002, 2003), the Ferrans and Powers Quality of Life Index (Carroll and Hamilton, 2005; Sossong, 2007; Dickerson et al., 2010), the General Health Questionnaire and the Icelandic Quality of Life Questionnaire (Leosdottir et al., 2006), the RAND-38 Mental Health Inventory and the Nottingham Health Profile (Irvine et al., 2002), and the Quality of Well Being Schedule (Strickberger et al., 2003). Further psychological outcomes are Post-Traumatic Stress Disorder (PTSD) or PTSD symptomatology, ICD acceptance and ICD concerns. PTSD was evaluated in five studies. The Impact of Event Scale-R was used in three studies (Ladwig et al., 2008; Kapa et al., 2010; Von Känel et al., 2011), while the Posttraumatic Stress Diagnostic Scale was administered in the other ones (Versteeg et al., 2010; Habibovic et al., 2012). ICD acceptance was analyzed as an outcome of ICD shocks in three studies (Pedersen et al., 2008a; Spindler et al., 2009; Keren et al., 2011). The Florida Patient Acceptance Survey was used in all of them. Finally, ICD concerns were assessed as an outcome of ICD shocks in two studies (Spindler et al., 2009; Van Den Broek et al., 2009). The ICD Concerns questionnaire was used in both ones.

Timing of outcome assessment and follow-up

Included studies vary a lot with respect to the timing of outcome assessment and follow-up. The first sharp distinction concerns study design. However, even considering cross-sectional and prospective studies separately, a large amount of variability remains in each category. In real cross-sectional studies, in which patients were assessed only once, a great heterogeneity in time from ICD implantation was observed both within and between studies. For example, the average of the mean times from ICD implantation across the 19 cross-sectional studies that reported time data on a continuous scale is 32 months with a SD of 18.2 (range: −60). The briefer mean time from ICD implantation was found in Namerow et al.' study (1999), while the longer one was found in Pedersen, Spindler, Johansen and Mortensen study (2009). In Jacq et al.'s study (2009), mean time from ICD implantation was divided between patients who received 1 or more shocks (37.4 months ±31.9) and patients who did not receive any shock (17.9 months ±16), while in 2 studies (Bilge et al., 2006; Redhead et al., 2010) patients were divided into multiple sub-groups according to fixed time intervals. In prospective studies, in which patients were assessed at least twice along the follow-up (repeated measures), differences and heterogeneities were observed in four factors: (1) baseline assessment (before ICD implantation or after ICD implantation); (2) time before ICD implantation; (3) timing of repeated measurements from ICD implantation; (4) length of follow-up. Baseline was clearly assessed before ICD implantation in 14 studies, but in only 3 out of them the baseline time-point was explicitly reported, i.e., 1 day before ICD implantation (Pedersen et al., 2007, 2008a, 2010a). However, these 3 studies are not independent because patients who comprised the three samples participated in the same study (MIDAS—Mood and personality as precipitants of arrhythmia in patients with an ICD: A prospective Study). Baseline was assessed before ICD implantation also in other 3 studies but not for all participants, some of whom were evaluated just after the implantation before hospital discharge (Dunbar et al., 1999; Irvine et al., 2002; Suzuki et al., 2010). Baseline was clearly assessed after ICD implantation in 8 studies but the timing of first assessment was highly heterogeneous both between and within them. For example, in some studies patients were evaluated few days after ICD implantation or at hospital discharge, while in other studies patients were firstly assessed after months from surgery. Finally, if baseline assessment was performed before or after the ICD implantation was impossible to establish in three studies because the respective articles do not report sufficient information. Prospective studies are quite heterogeneous also with respect to the number and timing of repeated measurements from ICD implantation and length of follow-up. For example, in only 19 out of 28 studies patients were followed for at least 12 months (see **Table 2** for details).

Statistical analysis

Last but not least, studies vary quite a lot with respect to the statistical analyses that were performed to test the effect of ICD shocks on patients' psychological health and quality of life. Clearly, much of this heterogeneity is explained by the ways outcomes and ICD shocks were operationalized and also by study designs. However, two main analytical solutions were identified: (1) classifying patients in two or more shock-groups in accordance with different numerical criteria and testing the simple or adjusted effect of such dichotomized or categorized shock variable by univariate or multivariate analyses and (2) regressing outcome on number of shocks by multivariate regression analyses. Furthermore, in few studies patients were classified in different outcome-groups according to criteria such as psychiatric diagnoses, outcome change patterns or outcome distribution cut-offs and then compared on number of shocks. Finally, in only two studies intra-individual changes from pre-shock to post-shock assessments were analyzed by hierarchical regression models.

The heterogeneity of analytical approaches can be further explained by three factors: (1) the outcome variable scale (dichotomous, dichotomized or continuous); (2) the operationalization of ICD shocks (see previous paragraph) and (3) the number and kind of covariates/predictors that were entered into the statistical models. A fourth factor that pertains only to multivariate regression models concerns the importance of the ICD shock variable within the analysis. In fact, some of the studies that were included in the review did not handle the ICD shock variable as the main explaining factor but treated it as a potential covariate or controlling predictor. In these studies, the leading role was given to other psychological or medical factors (for example, type-D personality, concerns about the ICD, device acceptance and disease severity) and the ICD shock variable was mainly used as a competing predictor in the statistical explanation of patients' psychological distress.

Table 2 | Study methods.

Source	Study name	Design	Timing of outcome assessment	Self-report measures	Outcomes	Shock operationalization	Shock analysis
Keren et al., 1991		Cross-sectional	18 months post-ICD implantation (range 4–34)	Self-report: - STAI-Y[10] - BDI[11] - *Ad-hoc* questionnaire	State-anxiety Trait-anxiety Depression ICD Experiences	Dicothomized (yes/no)	Shock as grouping variable
Morris et al., 1991		Cross-sectional	7.5 months post-ICD implantation (range 3–21)	Semi-structured psychiatric interview (DSM-III-TR)	Mental disorders	Shock ratio (Shock frequency devided by lenght of follow-up)	Shock ratio as test variable Mental disorder as grouping variable (3 groups)
Luderitz et al., 1993		Prospective	Before and 1, 3, 6, 12 months post-ICD implantation	Self-report: - STAI-Y[10] - *Ad-hoc* questionnaire	State-anxiety ICD appraisal	Dicothomized (0–4/≥5)	Shock as grouping variable
Dougherty, 1995		Prospective	At hospital discharge and 6, 12 months after	Self-report: - POMS[12] - STAI-Y[10] - the Distancing Subscale of the Ways of Coping Checklist-Revised - The Dyadic Adjustment Scale - The F-COPES	State-anxiety-tension Depression Anger Stress Denial	Dicothomized (yes/no)	Shock as grouping variable
Chevalier et al., 1996		Cross-sectional	25 ± 1.6 months post-ICD implantation (range 1–54)	Interviewer: - Diagnostic interview (DSM-III-TR) Self-report: - Hamilton Anxiety scale - BDI[11] - MMPI[13] - *Ad-hoc* ICD-QoL	Depression symptoms Anxiety symptoms ICD-related QoL Mental disorders	Dicothomized (yes/no)	Shock as grouping variable
Burgess et al., 1997		Cross-sectional	Unclear	Self-report: - SCL-90-R - demographics questionnaire (premorbid medical and psychiatric self-report health histories. Life-style changes)	Psychological distress	Shock frequency	Shock as predictor variable

(Continued)

Table 2 | Continued

Source	Study name	Design	Timing of outcome assessment	Self-report measures	Outcomes	Shock operationalization	Shock analysis
Herrmann et al., 1997		Cross-sectional	510 ± 408 days since implantation	Self-report: - HADS[14] - Quality-of-Life Profile for the Chronically ill (PLC) - Unstandardized items dealing with patients' attitudes toward the ICD	Anxiety symptoms Depression symptoms QoL	Categorized (0–4/5–9/≥10)	Shock as grouping variable
Heller et al., 1998		Cross-sectional	20 ± 14 months post-ICD implantation	Self-report: - BDI[11] - STAI-Y[10] - Cook-Medley subscale of the MMPI- questions examining attitudes toward the ICD experience and cardiac illness	Emotional states	Dichotomized (0–4/5–9)	Shock as predictor variable
Dunbar et al., 1999		Prospective	Before (for 7% soon after implantation) and 1, 3 months post-ICD implantation	Self-report: - Life Orientation Test (LOT) - Threat and Challenge subscales from the Meaning in Illness Questionnaire (MIQ) - The symptom and fear components from the ICD Concerns Questionnaire - The Jalowiec Coping Scale (JCS) - POMS[12] - Heart Failure Functional Status Inventory (HFFSI)	Total mood disturbance	Shock frequency	Shock as predictor variable
Dunbar et al., 1999		Prospective	Before and 1, 3, 6, 9 months post-ICD implantation	Self-report: - POMS[12] - STAI-Y[10] - the Distancing Subscale of the Ways of Coping Checklist-Revised - The Dyadic Adjustment Scale - The F-COPES	Emotional states	Shock occurrence	Shock as within-subject factor

(Continued)

Table 2 | Continued

Source	Study name	Design	Timing of outcome assessment	Self-report measures	Outcomes	Shock operationalization	Shock analysis
Goodman and Hess, 1999		Cross-sectional	Unclear	Self-report: - SCL-90-R - demographics questionnaire (premorbid medical and psychiatric self-report health histories)	Anxiety symptoms Depression symptoms	Shock frequency	Shock as predictor variable
Herbst et al., 1999		Cross-sectional	31.2 ± 16.8 months post-ICD implantation	Self-report: - SF-36 - Brief Symptom Inventory - demographics questionnaire (premorbid medical and psychiatric self-report health histories)	QoL Psychological distress	Dicothomized (yes/no)	Shock as grouping variable
Namerow et al., 1999	CABG Patch Trial	RCT Cross-sectional	6 months after CABG surgery	Self-report: - SF-36 - demographics questionnaire (premorbid medical and psychiatric self-report health)	QoL	Dicothomized (yes/no)	Shock as grouping variable
Pauli et al., 1999		Cross-sectional	22.8 ± 19.2 months post-ICD implantation (range 2–89)	Self-report: - AICD-questionnaire (anxiety related to future shocks) - The ACQ (catastrophizing cognitions) - The BSQ (anxiety of bodily symptoms) - STAI-Y[10] - BAI[15] - BDI[11]	Shock-related anxiety	Shocks frequency Shock ratio (Shock frequency devided by lenght of follow-up) Dichotomized (yes/no)	Shock as predictor variable Shock as fixed factor
Duru et al., 2001		Cross-sectional	≥6 months post-ICD implantation (2.3 years on average)	Self-report: - SF-36 - HADS[14] - *Ad-hoc* questionnaire (perceptions of ICD)	Anxiety symptoms Depression symptoms ICD appraisal	Dicothomized (yes/no)	Shock as grouping variable

(Continued)

Table 2 | Continued

Source	Study name	Design	Timing of outcome assessment	Self-report measures	Outcomes	Shock operationalization	Shock analysis
Godemann et al., 2001		Cross-sectional	3.4 ± 1.8 years post-ICD implantation	Interviewer: - Semi-structured interview (DIPS) Self-report: - SCL-90-R	Mental disorders	Shock frequency	Shock as predictor variable
Irvine et al., 2002	CISD[9]	RCT Prospective	Before or soon after randomization and 2, 6, 12 months post-ICD implantation	Self-report: - Rand Corporation's 38-item Mental Health Inventory - Nottingham Health Profile	QoL	Categorized (0/1–4/≥5)	Shock as fixed factor
Schron et al., 2002	AVID[8]	RCT Prospective	Before randomization and 3, 6, 12 months after randomization	Self-report: - SF-36 - Patient concerns checklist - The cardiac version of the QoL index	QoL	Dichotomized (yes/no and <3/≥3)	Shock as fixed factor
Wallace et al., 2002		Cross-sectional	12–24 (70.6%), 25–36 (27.4%) and 37–48 (2%) months post-ICD implantation	Self-report: -State Trait Personality Inventory - Interpersonal Support Evaluation List - Disease-specific QoL AVID checklist - SF-12	QoL	Shocks frequency	Shock as predictor variable
Kamphuis et al., 2002		Prospective	Few days before and 1, 6, 12 months post-discharge	Self-report: - Rand 36-item Health Survey - The Heart Patients Psychological Questionnaire (HPPQ) - CES-D[16] - STAI-Y[10]	QoL State-Anxiety Depression symptoms Psychological well-being	Dicothomized (yes/no)	Shock as fixed factor
Kamphuis et al., 2003		Prospective	after admission (before cardiac evaluation) and 1, 6, 12 months after discharge	Self-report: - RAND-36 - Heart Patient Psychological Questionnaire (HPPQ) - STAI-Y[10] - CES-D[16]	QoL State-Anxiety Depression symptoms Psychological well-being	Categorized (Shocks in both time intervals/Shocks exclusively during the first 6 months/Shocks exclusively during the last 6 months/No shocks during first year)	Shock as fixed factor

(Continued)

Table 2 | Continued

Source	Study name	Design	Timing of outcome assessment	Self-report measures	Outcomes	Shock operationalization	Shock analysis
Newman et al., 2003		Prospective	At baseline (?) and 3, 6 months post-baseline	Self-report: - SF-36 - The Symptom Checklist - AF symptoms.	QoL	Categorized (0/1–4/≥5 shocks)	Shock as fixed factor
Strickberger et al., 2003	AMIOVIRT[7]	Cross-sectional	Before and 2 ± 1.3 years post-ICD implantation (range 0.1–4.8 years)	Self-report: - Quality of Well Being Schedule - STAI-Y[10]	State-Anxiety	Dicothomized (yes/no)	Shock as grouping variable
Godemann et al., 2004a		Cross-sectional	3.5 ± 2.0 years post-ICD implantation	Interviewer: - Diagnostic Interview of Psychiatric Disorders -DSM-III-R Self-report: - Cognitive coping with shocks	Mental disorders	Shock frequency	Shock as predictor variable
Godemann et al., 2004b		Cross-sectional	3.4 ± 2.8 years post-ICD implantation (range 1–11)	Self-report: - SF-12 - The Freiburg Questionnaire on Disease Coping (short version) - SCL-90-R	QoL	Shock frequency	Shock as predictor variable
Pedersen et al., 2004	MIDAS[2]	Cross-sectional	55 ± 35 months post-ICD implantation (range 8–132)	Self-report: - HADS[14] - Type D Personality Scale (DS14) - The Perceived Social Support Scale (PSSS)	Anxiety symptoms Depression symptoms	Dichotomized (yes/no)	Shock as predictor variable (direct and interaction effects)
Wathen et al., 2004	PainFREE Rx II[6]	RCT Prospective	Before and 1 year post-ICD implantation	Self-report: - SF-36	QoL	Not applicable	ATP treatment vs. shock treatment
Carroll and Hamilton, 2005		Prospective	From time of ICD implantation to 1 year after implantation	Self-report: - Ferrans and Powers Quality of Life Index - SF-36 - POMS[12] - Brodsky ICD Questionnaire	QoLEmotional states ICD concerns	Dicothomized (yes/no)	Shock as grouping variable

(Continued)

Table 2 | Continued

Source	Study name	Design	Timing of outcome assessment	Self-report measures	Outcomes	Shock operationalization	Shock analysis
Pedersen et al., 2005	MIDAS[2]	Cross-sectional	55 ± 35 months post-ICD implantation (range 8–132)	Self-report: - The ICDC Questionnaire (concerns) - HADS[14]	Anxiety symptoms Depression symptoms	Dichotomized (yes/no)	Shock as predictor variable
Sears et al., 2005		Prospective	During hospitalization, 6–9 and 12–15 months after ICD implantation	Interviewer: - The Schedule for Affective Disorders and Schizophrenia (DSM-IV) Self-report: - Interpersonal Support Evaluation List - Short-Form - The Life Orientation Test - STAI-Y[10] - SF-36 - The Seattle Angina Questionnaire	QoL	Dichotomized (yes/no)	Shock as predictor variable
Bilge et al., 2006		Cross-sectional	3–6 months (15.4%), 6 months–1 year (2.2%), 1–5 years (68.1%), >5 years (14.3%) post-ICD implantation	Self-report: - HADS[14]	Anxiety symptoms Depression symptoms	Dichotomized (Yes/No) Shock frequency	Shock as predictor variable
Cuculi et al., 2006		Cross-sectional	Not reported	Self-report: - Brief Symptom Inventory	Psychological distress	Dicothomized (yes/no)	Shock as grouping variable
Leosdottir et al., 2006		Cross-sectional	37.8 ± 28.6 months post-ICD implantation (range 11.6–154.9)	Self-report: - BAI[15] - BDI[11] - The General Health Questionnaire - 30-item - The Icelandic Quality of Life Questionnaire (IQL) - ICD Psychosocial Index	Anxiety symptoms Depression symptoms QoL	Dicothomized (yes/no)	Shock as grouping variable
Luyster et al., 2006		Cross-sectional	1.9 ± 1.8 years post-ICD implantation (range 0.07–8.8)	Self-report: - The ENRICHD Social Support Inventory - The Duke Activity Status Index	Depression symptomsTrait-anxiety	Dichotomized (yes/no)	Shock as predictor variable

(Continued)

Table 2 | Continued

Source	Study name	Design	Timing of outcome assessment	Self-report measures	Outcomes	Shock operationalization	Shock analysis
				- The Conservation of Resources Evaluation (COR-E) - BDI[11] - Brief Patient Health Questionnaire - STAI-Y[10]			
Crossmann et al., 2007		Prospective	25.5 ± 19.2 months post-ICD implantation (range 1.5–88) and 30.3 months after first assessment (range 29.6–31.2)	Self-report: - The ACQ (catastrophizing cognitions) - The BSQ (anxiety of bodily symptoms) - STAI-Y[10] - BAI[15] - The Mobility Inventory (avoidance behavior)	Trait-anxiety Anxiety symptoms Anxiety related to bodily symptoms	Dicothomized (yes/no)	Shock as grouping variable
Passman et al., 2007		Prospective	Baseline (?), 1 and 3 months after randomization and every 3 months thereafter up to 63 months	Self-report: - SF-12 - the Minnesota Living with Heart Failure Questionnaire	QoL	Shock occurrence	Shock as within-subject factor
Pedersen et al., 2007	MIDAS[2]	Prospective	1 day prior to implantation and 3 months post-ICD implantation	Self-report: - Type D Personality Scale (DS14) - SF-36	QoL	Shock frequency	Shock as covariate
Piotrowicz et al., 2007	MADIT-II[3]	Prospective	At baseline (before randomization) and at 12-month follow-up	Self-report: - SF-12	QoL	Dicothomized (yes/no)	Shock as grouping variable
Sossong, 2007		Cross-sectional	15.9 ± 13 months post-ICD implantation (range 2.1–56.1)	Self-report: - The Sossong ICD Knowledge Questionnaire - Mishel Uncertainty in Illness Scale (MUIS-Adult) - Ferrans and Powers Quality of Life Index - Cardiac Version IV	QoL	Shock frequency	Shock as predictor variable

(Continued)

Table 2 | Continued

Source	Study name	Design	Timing of outcome assessment	Self-report measures	Outcomes	Shock operationalization	Shock analysis
Johansen et al., 2008		Cross-sectional	4.8 years post-ICD implantation (range 0.4–15.9)	Self-report: - HADS[14] - SF-36 - The Minnesota living with heart failure questionnaire	Anxiety symptoms Depression symptoms QoL	Shock frequency	Shock as predictor variable
Ladwig et al., 2008	LICAD[1]	Cross-sectional	27 ± 21 months post ICD implantation (range 3–142)	Self-report: - Impact of Event Scale-R	PTSD symptoms	Categorized (0/1–4/5–9/≥10)	Shock as crossing variable
Mark et al., 2008	SCD-HeFT[4]	RCT Cross-sectional	3, 12, and 30 months post-ICD implantation	Self-report: - SF-36 - Mental Health Inventory 5	QoL	Dicothomized (yes/no) within different time intervals (within 1 month and 2 months before a scheduled QoL assessment and at any time along follow-up)	Shock as grouping variable
Pedersen et al., 2008a		Cross-sectional	4.7 ± 3.3 years post-ICD implantation (range 0.4–15.9)	Self-report: - the Florida Patient Acceptance Survey	ICD Acceptance	Shock frequency	Shock as predictor variable
Pedersen et al., 2008b	MIDAS[2]	Prospective	1 day prior and 6 months post-ICD implantation	Self-report: - HADS[14]	Anxiety symptoms Depression symptoms	Shock frequency	Shock as covariate
Van Den Broek et al., 2008		Prospective	0 and 3 weeks after ICD implantation and 2 months after	Self-report: - STAI-Y[10] Interviewer: - Hamilton Rating Scale for Anxiety	Anxiety symptoms	Dicothomized (yes/no)	Shock as fixed factorShock as predictor variable
Jacq et al., 2009		Cross-sectional	Shock: 37.4 ± 31.9 months (range 6–44) No shock: 17.9 ± 16 months (range 6–66)	Self-report: - HADS[14] - SF-36 Interviewer:- Mini International Neuropsychiatric Interview	Anxiety symptoms Depression symptoms QoL	Dichotomized (Yes/No) Shock ratio (Shock frequency/time elapsed since implantation)	Shock as grouping variable Shock as crossing variable Shock ratio as correlational variable
Noyes et al., 2009	MADIT-II[3]	Prospective	0, 3, 12, 24, 36 months post-ICD implantation	Self-report: - Health Utility Index 3	QoL	Shock occurrence	Shock as within-subject factor

(Continued)

Table 2 | Continued

Source	Study name	Design	Timing of outcome assessment	Self-report measures	Outcomes	Shock operationalization	Shock analysis
Pedersen et al., 2009		Cross-sectional	4.9 ± 3.2 years post-ICD implantation	Self-report: - HADS[14] - The 18-item Florida Patient Acceptance Survey - Type D Personality Scale (DS14)	Anxiety symptoms Depression symptoms	Shock frequency	Shock as covariate
Spindler et al., 2009		Cross-sectional	4.6 ± 3.2 years post-ICD implantation	Self-report: - HADS[14] - The ICD Concerns questionnaire (8 item) - The 18-item Florida Patient Acceptance Survey - SF-36	Anxiety symptoms Depression symptoms ICD concerns Device acceptance QoL	Dicothomized (yes/no)	Shock as covariate
Thomas et al., 2009	SCD-HeFT/PFOS[5]	Prospective	At entry, 1, 6, 12, 18, and 2 years after ICD implantation	Self-report: - BDI-2 - STAI-Y[10] - The Social Support Questionnaire-6	State-anxiety Depression symptoms	Dicothomized (yes/no)	Shock as predictor variable
Van Den Broek et al., 2009		Prospective	7.7 ± 6.8 days and 2 months after ICD implantation	Self-report: - STAI-Y[10] - The 18-item Cardiac Anxiety Questionnaire - The Health Complaints Scale - the ICD-Concerns questionnaire (8 item) Interviewer: - The Hamilton Rating Scale for Anxiety	Anxiety symptoms ICD concerns Health complaints	Dicothomized (yes/no)	Shock as predictor variable
Kapa et al., 2010		Prospective	Within 2 months after ICD implantation, 6 and 12 months following baseline	Self-report: - HADS[14] - Impact of Events Scale-Revised - SF-36	PTSD symptoms Anxiety symptoms Depression symptoms QoL	Categorized (0/≥1/electrical storm)	Shock as fixed factor

(Continued)

Table 2 | Continued

Source	Study name	Design	Timing of outcome assessment	Self-report measures	Outcomes	Shock operationalization	Shock analysis
Pedersen et al., 2010a	MIDAS[2]	Prospective	1 day prior to ICD implantation (baseline) and 10 days, 3 months, 6 months and 1 year post-ICD implantation.	Self-report: - STAI-Y[10] - the ICD-Concerns questionnaire (8 item) - Type D Personality Scale (DS14) - Multidimensional Scale of Perceived Social Support	State-anxiety Trait-anxiety ICD concerns	Shock frequency	Shock as predictor variable
Redhead et al., 2010		Cross-sectional	6-month "time windows": 6–12, 12–18, 18–24, 24–30, and 30–36 months post-ICD implantation	Self-report: - HADS[14] - SF-36	Anxiety symptoms Depression symptoms QoL	Categorized (0/≥1/storm)	Shock as crossing variable
Suzuki et al., 2010		Prospective	Within 7 days before implantation or 8 ± 5 days after admission and 2 years later	Self-report: - Zung Self-Rating Depression Scale	Depression	Dichotomized (yes/no) Dichotomized (within 6 months /beyond 6 months) Categorized (0, 1–9, ≥10)	Shock as test variable Depressed patients vs. non-depressed patients
Versteeg et al., 2010	MIDAS[2]	Prospective	3 and 6 months post-ICD implantation	Self-report: - The Posttraumatic Stress Diagnostic Scale	PTSD symptoms	Shock frequency	Shock as predictor variable
Dickerson et al., 2010		Prospective	Before and 1 and 3 months after ICD implantation	Self-report: - STAI-Y[10] - the Ferrans and Powers Quality of Life Index, Cardiac Version	State-anxiety	Shock frequency	Shock as test variable Comparison of QoL-change patterns
Habibovic et al., 2012		Cross-sectional	0–3 weeks and 18 months post-ICD implantation	Self-report: - STAI-Y[10] - the Posttraumatic Stress Diagnostic Scale - Type D Personality Scale (DS14)	PTSD symptoms	Shock frequency	Shock as predictor variable
Pedersen et al., 2011	MIDAS[2]	Prospective	0–3 weeks and 12 months post-ICD implantation	Self-report: - STAI-Y[10] - Type D Personality Scale (DS14)	Chronic anxiety	Shock frequency	Shock as predictor variable

(Continued)

Table 2 | Continued

Von Känel et al., 2011	LICAD[1]	Prospective	24.4 ± 20.7 months post ICD-implantation (baseline) 65.5 ± 27.4 months post-implantation (follow-up) 41.1 ± 18.2 months from baseline to follow-up	Self-report: - Impact of Events Scale-Revised - Toronto Alexithymia Scale - HADS[14] Interviewer: - Peri-traumatic Dissociative Experiences Questionnaire	PTSD symptoms	Dichotomized (Yes/No and 0–4/≥5)	Shock as predictor variable

[1] *Living with an implanted cardioverter defibrillator study.*

[2] *Mood and personality as precipitants of arrhythmia in patients with an ICD, A prospective Study.*

[3] *Multicenter Automatic Defibrillator Trial-II.*

[4] *Sudden Cardiac Death in Heart Failure.*

[5] *Sudden Cardiac Death in Heart Failure/Psychosocial Factors Outcome Study in Sudden Cardiac Death.*

[6] *Pacing Fast Ventricular Tachycardia Reduces Shock Therapies Trial.*

[7] *Amiodarone vs. Implantable Cardioverter-Defibrillator: Randomized Trial in Patients With Non-ischemic Dilated Cardiomyopathy and Asymptomatic Non-sustained Ventricular Tachycardia.*

[8] *Antiarrhythmics vs. Implantable Defibrillators.*

[9] *Canadian Implantable Defibrillator Study.*

[10] *Spielberger State-Trait Anxiety Inventory – Y form.*

[11] *Beck Depression Inventory.*

[12] *Profile of Mood States Questionnaire.*

[13] *Minnesota Multiphasic Personality Inventory.*

[14] *Hospital Anxiety and Depression Scale.*

[15] *Beck Anxiety Inventory.*

[16] *The Center for Epidemiological Studies Depression Scale.*

RISK OF BIAS WITHIN STUDIES

All papers that were included in the review were screened in search of some potential biases that could affect the validity of results. In particular, we searched for the systematic biases that can affect the internal validity of cross-sectional and cohort studies. In this kind of non-randomized studies, the major threat to internal validity concerns all the systematic differences that may exist between groups over and beyond the difference determined by the factor of interest and that may confound its effect. One of the methods that can protect against this bias consists in statistically controlling for the effects of all confounding variables that are related to the outcome and/or to the factor. A further method consists in matching subjects between groups according to some variables (for example, age, sex, type of heart disease, LVEF, NYHA Functional Class, etc.) but this procedure was used in only one study (Keren et al., 1991). All the other studies that attempted to reduce the risk of such a bias used the multiple regression method (35 out of 60). However, the number and kind of confounding variables that were selected and controlled for vary significantly across studies. The effect of the ICD shock was indeed adjusted for heterogeneous confounders and this may partially explain why results are discordant. A further major threat to the internal validity of cross-sectional and cohort studies is the presence of the outcome of interest before the occurrence of the event that hypothetically causes it. This bias, when uncontrolled, may affect seriously the causal meaning of an association and, for example, may lead to the wrong conclusion that the ICD shock caused the development of psychological disorders when the reverse was true. The most robust method that may protect against this bias consists in starting the evaluation of patients quite before the ICD implantation and in collecting short-spaced repeated measures along the follow-up. This was fully accomplished in only 18 prospective studies, in which patients were evaluated for the first time few days before surgery. In all the other prospective studies, the baseline was assessed after the ICD implantation. Anyway, for the issue of the review, i.e., the critical appraisal of methods that were adopted in studies on the psychological effect of ICD shock, the most important part of the procedure is clearly the short-spaced timing of repeated measurements that, combined with the hierarchical analysis of intra-individual pre- to post-shock changes, represents for us the best methodology for enhancing the internal validity of cohort studies whose aim is to evaluate the negative effect of ICD shock on patient's health. Another method that was used in few studies consists in evaluating patients retrospectively. However, this approach is prone to biases (e.g., the recall bias and the response shift) that may affect seriously the validity and reliability of patients' responses and that should be avoided. According to the Newcastle-Ottawa checklist, further threats to the internal validity of cross-sectional and cohort studies are the self-reported exposure to the event, the self-reported assessment of outcome, the low validity and reliability of outcome measures and the incompleteness of data set. Except for this last bias, which may seriously affect the validity of results as much as the previous major ones, all the other items were considered minor threats because of their relative low and negligible impact on the validity of results.

RESULTS OF STUDIES AND SUBGROUP ANALYSIS

Because of the great heterogeneity that was observed in methods across the included studies, a statistical meta-analysis of effects and moderators was deemed unfeasible and was not performed. Further, no attempt was made to describe each study in a narrative manner because of two reasons: (1) the large number of studies that were included and (2) the review aim to focus mainly on methods and to explore cross-sectionally their effects on results. Hence, key methodological features and results of each study were only coded and tabulated (**Tables 2, 3**). For example, results were coded with 1 when a significant effect of ICD shock was found and with 0 otherwise. We established the statistical significance of effects only on the basis of final results (in studies where both bivariate and multivariate analyses were performed, we considered only the adjusted effects). A series of subgroup analyses according to study design, shock operationalization, shock analysis and multivariate controlling was then performed only on outcomes for which at least 20 studies were available (twenty units were deemed sufficient to test cross-sectional associations between methodological factors and results). Findings are described in the following paragraphs for each outcome of interest.

Anxiety

Patients' anxiety was assessed as an outcome in 35 studies and it was mainly measured by self-report questionnaires. In RCTs that were included in the review, anxiety was never measured. A statistically significant effect of ICD shocks on self-reported anxiety was found in 17 studies, while a significant effect of shocks on interviewer-rated anxiety was found in only 1 study out of 3. Subgroup analyses (Fisher's exact test) did not demonstrate any significant association between the methodological factors and the statistical significance of the shock effect on anxiety.

Depression

Patients' depression was assessed as an outcome in 29 studies and, as for anxiety, it was mainly measured by self-report questionnaires. Even depression was never measured in the RCTs included in the review. A statistically significant effect of ICD shocks on self-reported depression was detected in 10 studies, while a non-significant result was found in the only study in which depression was rated by a clinical interview. Subgroup analyses did not demonstrate any significant association between the methodological factors and the statistical significance of the shock effect on depression.

Health-related quality of life

Patients' health-related quality of life was assessed as an outcome in 30 studies and was always measured with self-report questionnaires. In most studies, both mental and physical components were evaluated, while in few studies only mental health (4 studies) or physical health (3 studies) were evaluated. With respect to mental health or psychological well-being, a statistically significant effect of ICD shock was found in 12 studies out of 27, while a statistically significant effect of ICD shock on physical health was detected in 11 studies out of 26. Subgroup analyses did not

Table 3 | Statistical analyses and results of studies.

Source	Statistical analysis	Anxiety	Anxiety interview	Depression	Depression interview	PTSD	QoL-mental	QoL-physical	Psychiatric disorders	ICD acceptance	ICD concerns
Keren et al., 1991	*T*-test	0		0							
Morris et al., 1991	ANOVA								1		
Luderitz et al., 1993	*T*-test	1									
Dougherty, 1995	Mann-Whitney U Test	1		0							
Chevalier et al., 1996	*T*-test	0		0					0		
Burgess et al., 1997	Stepwise Multiple Regression	1		1							
Herrmann et al., 1997	ANOVA	0		1			1				
Heller et al., 1998	Multiple logistic regression	1		1							
Dunbar et al., 1999	Hierarchical multiple regression	0		0				0			
Dunbar et al., 1999	Paired *t*-test	0		0							
Goodman and Hess, 1999	Regression	0		0							
Herbst et al., 1999	MANCOVA	1		1			0	0			
Namerow et al., 1999	ANOVA						0	0			
Pauli et al., 1999	Multiple regression MANOVA	0		0							
Duru et al., 2001	ANOVA	0		0			0	0			
Godemann et al., 2001	Logistic regression								1		
Irvine et al., 2002	ANCOVA						1				
Schron et al., 2002	Generalized estimating equations						1	1			
Wallace et al., 2002	Stepwise regression analysis						1				
Kamphuis et al., 2002	MANOVA						0	1			
Kamphuis et al., 2003	MANOVA for repeated measures	1		1			1	1			
Newman et al., 2003	MANOVA for repeated measures						0	0			
Strickberger et al., 2003	*T*-test	0					0				
Godemann et al., 2004a	Multiple regression								1		
Godemann et al., 2004b	Multiple regression						0	0			
Pedersen et al., 2004	Logistic univariate and multivariate regression	0		0							
Wathen et al., 2004	Wilconxon test						1	1			
Carroll and Hamilton, 2005	Mann-Whitney U test	1		0			0	0			
Pedersen et al., 2005	Logistic univariate and multivariate regression	0		0							1
Sears et al., 2005	Hierarchical multiple regression						1	1			
Bilge et al., 2006	Multiple regression	1		0							
Cuculi et al., 2006	Mann-Whitney U Test	0		0							
Leosdottir et al., 2006	*T*-test	0		0			0	0			
Luyster et al., 2006	Hierarchical multiple regression	0		1							

(Continued)

Table 3 | Continued

Source	Statistical analysis	Anxiety	Anxiety interview	Depression	Depression interview	PTSD	QoL-mental	QoL-physical	Psychiatric disorders	ICD acceptance	ICD concerns
Crossmann et al., 2007	Mann-Whitney U test	0									
Passman et al., 2007	Mixed-effects hierarchical linear regression						1	0			
Pedersen et al., 2007	ANCOVA						0	0			
Piotrowicz et al., 2007	*T*-test						0	1			
Sossong, 2007	Multiple regression						0	0			
Johansen et al., 2008	Multiple logistic regression	1		1				1			
Ladwig et al., 2008	Chi-squared test					0					
Mark et al., 2008	Mann-Whitney U test						1	1			
Pedersen et al., 2008a	Logistic regression									0	
Pedersen et al., 2008b	ANCOVA	1		1							
Van Den Broek et al., 2008	ANCOVA Multiple regression	1	0								
Jacq et al., 2009	Mann-Whitney U test Fisher's exact test Spearman correlation	1	1	1	0	1	1				
Noyes et al., 2009	Logistic and linear regressions (mediation models)						1	1			
Pedersen et al., 2009	ANCOVA	1		0							
Spindler et al., 2009	ANCOVA	1		0			0	0			1
Thomas et al., 2009	Linear mixed models	0		0							
Van Den Broek et al., 2009	Multiple regression		0					1			1
Kapa et al., 2010	MANOVA	1		0		1	0	0			
Pedersen et al., 2010a	Hierarchical, latent class regression models	1									
Redhead et al., 2010	Chi-squared test	1		0			1	0			
Suzuki et al., 2010	Chi-squared test			1							
Versteeg et al., 2010	Logistic regression					1					
Dickerson et al., 2010	ANOVA						0	0			
Habibovic et al., 2012	Multiple linear and logistic regression					0					
Pedersen et al., 2011	Multiple logistic regression	0									
Von Känel et al., 2011	Multiple linear and logistic regression					1					

1 means "significant effect," while 0 means "non-significant effect."

demonstrate any significant association between the methodological factors and the statistical significance of the shock effect on quality of life.

Post-Traumatic Stress Disorder (PTSD)

PTSD or PTSD symptoms were assessed as outcomes in five studies and were always measured with self-report questionnaires. A statistically significant effect of ICD shocks was found in 3 studies.

Psychiatric disorders

In four studies the effect of ICD shocks was assessed on psychiatric diagnosis of mental disorders and in 3 out of them the effect was statistically significant.

ICD acceptance and concerns

ICD acceptance was assessed as an outcome in 1 study but no significant effect of ICD shocks was found, while ICD concerns were measured in 3 studies and the effect of ICD shocks was statistically significant in all of them.

DISCUSSION

The critical appraisal of the mixed evidence concerning the relationship between ICD shocks and patient-centered outcomes (mainly QoL, anxiety and depression) is the main content of three recently published papers (Pedersen and Van Den Broek, 2008; Pedersen et al., 2010b; Sears and Kirian, 2010). Despite slightly different paradigmatic views on the relative importance of ICD shocks within the group of the numerous factors that may negatively influence the psychological adaptation and well-being of implanted patients, the authors agree that the heterogeneity of designs and methods across studies is most likely to account for the mixed findings.

The quasi-quantitative results of our review do not support this hypothesis. In particular, study design (cross-sectional vs. prospective studies), shock operationalization (the way ICD shocks were operationalized/quantified), shock analysis (the way the effect of ICD shocks was tested) and control for confounding (bivariate vs. multivariate analyses) were examined in vote-counting subgroup analysis, but statistical evidence was null for each of them.

As already noted by Pedersen et al. in a recent viewpoint (2010b), results are mixed even in the subgroup of RCTs. Hence, it seems that the statistical significance of the ICD shock effect on patients' QoL (anxiety and depression were not measured in RCTs) does not depend strictly on sample size. Furthermore, contrary to the hypothesis that a dose-response relationship may exist between the number of shocks and QoL, with only patients experiencing $\geq$5 shocks being at risk for impaired QoL (Irvine et al., 2002; Pedersen et al., 2010b), studies that categorized the shock variable in classes of increasing shock incidence (e.g., 0–4 vs. 5–9 vs. $\geq$10 shocks) did not show consistent significant results in any of the outcomes of interest.

However, such null evidence is far from being conclusive. This systematic review shows clearly that methods are very heterogeneous across studies and suggests that such methodological differences should be considered in a multivariate fashion rather than bivariately. However, subgrouping the included studies in a multivariate manner is unfeasible because it would parcel out studies in a number of cells that would be too small for valid statistical analysis.

Subgroup analyses were not performed on the few studies that evaluated the effect of ICD shock on PTSD development or PTSD symptoms, psychiatric disorders, ICD acceptance and ICD concerns. With the exception of the five studies that assessed PTSD and whose results are mixed as well, the evidences pertaining to the psychiatric diagnosis of mental disorders (4 studies) and to ICD concerns (3 studies) are consistently significant and support the hypothesis that one or more ICD shocks may cause the development of a psychiatric disorder and the hypothesis that shocked patients have significantly more concerns about the ICD. However, the strength of the former evidences is low because the very few studies that tested the effect of ICD shock on mental disorders used a cross-sectional approach. In none of them patients were actually administered the psychiatric interview before ICD implantation and the mental disorders that were diagnosed long after implantation might have been already present before or immediately after, even before the occurrence of the first shock. Despite the severe limitations of a vote-counting approach, the attempt to explore whether methodological differences across studies account for the mixed findings of the literature on the effect of ICD shocks on patients' QoL, anxiety and depression was not vain because it allowed the full discovery of the wide and multiple heterogeneities that exist across studies. Furthermore, it allowed the discovery of severe methodological flaws, the most important of which are undoubtedly the cross-sectional design that was applied by the great part of studies and the multiple wrong ways that were used to operationalize shocks.

Our description is not comprehensive inasmuch as other hypothetical accounting factors were intentionally overlooked. Some information on demographics (age and sex), ICD indication (primary or secondary prevention) and both inclusion and exclusion criteria was extracted from studies and tabulated (**Table 1**), but any explorative attempt to meta-correlate them with the significance of the shock effect failed. However, in many of the studies that were included in this review, a variety of patient characteristics (demographic, clinical, psychological, etc.) was considered for explaining why, in some patients, QoL and psychological health deteriorate after ICD implantation. Such variables were also entered in multivariate analyses together with ICD shocks, but their effects on patient-centered outcomes were mainly examined as competitors of ICD shocks. Surprisingly, only one study tested the moderating effect of a patient characteristic (i.e., Type-D personality) on the relationship between shocks and psychological distress (anxiety and depression) (Pedersen et al., 2004). A significant interaction (Type-D $\times$ Shocks $\geq$1) was found only for depression, i.e., ICD patients who received one or more shocks and had a type D personality (negative affectivity and social inhibition) reported an higher mean level of depression than ICD patients who received one or more shocks and had not a type D personality. However, this interesting result received no consideration in the discussion, probably because the authors were more concerned in looking beyond shocks toward other determinants such as the type-D personality.

CONCLUSIONS

Clinical practice suggests that ICD shocks have a detrimental effect on patients' QoL and account for the development of anxiety and depression disorders. However, results of studies that have investigated this issue are discordant. The heterogeneity of designs and methods has been ascribed as the main reason for the discrepancy but our findings do not support such hypothesis.

The attempt to solve the problem with a quasi-quantitative approach was daring due to its severe limitations but no other meta-analytic approach was feasible. Regardless of this, the systematic review allowed us to look more clearly at studies and to paint a partial picture of the current status of research on the impact of ICD shocks on patient-centered outcomes.

We think that drawing firm statements about the short, mid and long-term impact of ICD shocks on patients' QoL and psychological well-being is an important matter both for the optimal clinical management of patients and for the adoption of new ICD programming strategies that eliminate or reduce ICD shocks. It is thus imperative that research on the psychological effects of ICD shocks goes further. Future studies should avoid the methodological flaws described in this review and should also consider that the relationship between ICD shocks and patient-centered outcomes may not be as straightforward as expected. Some other putative variables such as personality traits (e.g., Type D personality), coping skills and social support play surely a role and their effects on ICD patients' psychological health should be investigated also in interaction with the occurrence of shocks in order to know the profile of patients who might respond badly and focus treatment resources on them.

REFERENCES

1. Anderson, J. L., Hallstrom, A. P., Epstein, A. E., Pinski, S. L., Rosenberg, Y., Nora, M. O., et al. (1999). Design and results of the antiarrhythmics vs implantable defib- rillators (AVID) registry. The AVID Investigators. *Circulation* 99, 1692–1699.
2. Bardy, G. H., Lee, K. L., Mark, D. B., Poole, J. E., Packer, D. L., Boineau, R., et al. (2005). Amiodarone or an implantable cardioverter-defibrillator for congestive heart failure. *N. Engl. J. Med.* 352, 225–237. doi: 10.1056/NEJMoa043399
3. Barnay, C., Taieb, J., and Morice, R. (2007). [Electrical storm]. *Ann. Cardiol. Angeiol.* 56, 183–187. doi: 10.1016/j.ancard.2007.08.003
4. Bilge, A. K., Ozben, B., Demircan, S., Cinar, M., Yilmaz, E., and Adalet, K. (2006). Depression and anxiety status of patients with implantable cardioverter defib- rillator and precipitating factors. *Pacing Clin. Electrophysiol.* 29, 619–626. doi: 10.1111/j.1540-8159.2006.00409.x
5. Burgess, E. S., Quigley, J. F., Moran, G., Sutton, F. J., and Goodman, M. (1997). Predictors of psychosocial adjustment in patients with implantable cardioverter defibrillators. *Pacing Clin. Electrophysiol.* 20, 1790–1795.
6. Burke, J. L., Hallas, C. N., Clark-Carter, D., White, D., and Connelly, D. (2003). The psychosocial impact of the implantable cardioverter defib- rillator: a meta-analytic review. *Br. J. Health Psychol.* 8, 165–178. doi: 10.1348/135910703321649141
7. Buxton, A. E., Lee, K. L., Fisher, J. D., Josephson, M. E., Prystowsky, E. N., and Hafley, G. (1999). A randomized study of the prevention of sud- den death in patients with coronary artery disease. Multicenter unsus- tained tachycardia trial investigators. *N. Engl. J. Med.* 341, 1882–1890. doi: 10.1056/NEJM199912163412503
8. Carroll, D. L., and Hamilton, G. A. (2005). Quality of life in implanted cardioverter defibrillator recipients: the impact of a device shock. *Heart Lung.* 34, 169–178. doi: 10.1016/j.hrtlng.2004.10.002
9. Chevalier, P., Verrier, P., Kirkorian, G., Touboul, P., and Cottraux, J. (1996). Improved appraisal of the quality of life in patients with automatic implantable cardioverter defibrillator: a psychometric study. *Psychother. Psychosom.* 65, 49–56.
10. Connolly, S. J., Gent, M., Roberts, R. S., Dorian, P., Roy, D., Sheldon, R. S., et al. (2000a). Canadian implantable defibrillator study (CIDS): a randomized trial of the implantable cardioverter defibrillator against amiodarone. *Circulation* 101, 1297–1302. doi: 10.1161/01.CIR.101.11.1297
11. Connolly, S. J., Hallstrom, A. P., Cappato, R., Schron, E. B., Kuck, K. H., Zipes, D. P., et al. (2000b). Meta-analysis of the implantable cardioverter defibrillator secondary prevention trials. AVID, CASH and CIDS studies. Antiarrhythmics vs Implantable Defibrillator study. Cardiac Arrest Study Hamburg. Canadian Implantable Defibrillator Study. *Eur. Heart J.* 21, 2071–2078. doi: 10.1053/euhj.2000.2476 S0195668X0092476X [pii]
12. Crossmann, A., Pauli, P., Dengler, W., Kuhlkamp, V., and Wiedemann, G. (2007). Stability and cause of anxiety in patients with an implantable cardioverter- defibrillator: a longitudinal two-year follow-up. *Heart Lung.* 36, 87–95. doi: 10.1016/j.hrtlng.2006.08.001
13. Cuculi, F., Herzig, W., Kobza, R., and Erne, P. (2006). Psychological distress in patients with ICD recall. *Pacing Clin. Electrophysiol.* 29, 1261–1265. doi: 10.1111/j.1540-8159.2006.00523.x
14. Dickerson, S. S., Kennedy, M., Wu, Y. W., Underhill, M., and Othman, A. (2010). Factors related to quality-of-life pattern changes in recipients of implantable defibrillators. *Heart Lung.* 39, 466–476. doi: 10.1016/j.hrtlng.2009.10.022
15. Dougherty, C. M. (1995). Psychological reactions and family adjustment in shock versus no shock groups after implantation of internal cardioverter defibrillator. *Heart Lung.* 24, 281–291.
16. Dunbar, S. B., Jenkins, L. S., Hawthorne, M., Kimble, L. P., Dudley, W. N., Slemmons, M., et al. (1999). Factors associated with outcomes 3 months after implantable cardioverter defibrillator insertion. *Heart Lung.* 28, 303–315. doi: 10.1053/hl.1999.v28.a101052
17. Duru, F., Buchi, S., Klaghofer, R., Mattmann, H., Sensky, T., Buddeberg, C., et al. (2001). How different from pacemaker patients are recipients of implantable cardioverter-defibrillators with respect to psychosocial adaptation, affective disorders, and quality of life? *Heart* 85, 375–379. doi: 10.1136/heart.85.4.375
18. Godemann, F., Ahrens, B., Behrens, S., Berthold, R., Gandor, C., Lampe, F., et al. (2001). Classic conditioning and dysfunctional cognitions in patients with panic disorder and agoraphobia treated with an implantable cardioverter/defibrillator. *Psychosom Med* 63, 231–238. doi: 10.1097/00006842-200103000-00006
19. Godemann, F., Butter, C., Lampe, F., Linden, M., Schlegl, M., Schultheiss, H. P., et al. (2004a). Panic disorders and agoraphobia: side effects of treatment with an implantable cardioverter/defibrillator. *Clin. Cardiol.* 27, 321–326. doi: 10.1002/clc.4960270604
20. Godemann, F., Butter, C., Lampe, F., Linden, M., Werner, S., and Behrens, S. (2004b). Determinants of the quality of life (QoL) in patients with an implantable cardioverter/defibrillator (ICD). *Qual. Life Res.* 13, 411–416.
21. Goodman, M., and Hess, B. (1999). Could implantable cardioverter defibrilla- tors provide a human model supporting the learned helplessness theory of depression? *Gen. Hosp. Psychiatry* 21, 382–385.
22. Habibovic, M., Van Den Broek, K. C., Alings, M., Van Der Voort, P. H., and Denollet, J. (2012). Posttraumatic stress 18 months following cardioverter defibrillator implantation: shocks, anxiety, and personality. *Health Psychol.* 31, 186–193. doi: 10.1037/a0024701
23. Heller, S. S., Ormont, M. A., Lidagoster, L., Sciacca, R. R., and Steinberg, S. (1998). Psychosocial outcome after ICD implantation: a current perspective. *Pacing Clin. Electrophysiol.* 21, 1207–1215.
24. Herbst, J. H., Goodman, M., Feldstein, S., and Reilly, J. M. (1999). Health-related quality-of-life assessment of patients with life-threatening ventricular arrhythmias. *Pacing Clin. Electrophysiol.* 22(6 Pt 1), 915–926.
25. Herrmann, C., Von Zur Muhen, F., Schaumann, A., Buss, U., Kemper, S., Wantzen, C., et al. (1997). Standardized assessment of psychological well-being and quality-of-life in patients with implanted defibrillators. *Pacing Clin. Electrophysiol.* 20, 95–103.
26. Irvine, J., Dorian, P., Baker, B., O'brien, B. J., Roberts, R., Gent, M., et al. (2002). Quality of life in the Canadian Implantable Defibrillator Study (CIDS). *Am. Heart J.* 144, 282–289. doi: 10.1067/mjh.2002.124049
27. Jacq, F., Foulldrin, G., Savoure, A., Anselme, F., Baguelin-Pinaud, A., Cribier, A., et al. (2009). A comparison of anxiety, depression and quality of life between device shock and nonshock groups in implantable car- dioverter defibrillator recipients. *Gen. Hosp. Psychiatry* 31, 266–273. doi: 10.1016/j.genhosppsych.2009.01.003
28. Johansen, J. B., Pedersen, S. S., Spindler, H., Andersen, K., Nielsen, J. C., and Mortensen, P. T. (2008). Symptomatic heart failure is the most important clinical correlate of impaired quality of life, anxiety, and depression in implantable cardioverter-defibrillator patients: a single-centre, cross-sectional study in 610 patients. *Europace* 10, 545–551. doi: 10.1093/europace/eun073

29. Kamphuis, H. C., De Leeuw, J. R., Derksen, R., Hauer, R., and Winnubst, J. A. (2002). A 12-month quality of life assessment of cardiac arrest survivors treated with or without an implantable cardioverter defibrillator. *Europace* 4, 417–425. doi: 10.1053/eupc.2002.0258
30. Kamphuis, H. C., De Leeuw, J. R., Derksen, R., Hauer, R. N., and Winnubst, J. A. (2003). Implantable cardioverter defibrillator recipients: quality of life in recip- ients with and without ICD shock delivery: a prospective study. *Europace* 5, 381–389. doi: 10.1016/S1099-5129(03)00078-3
31. Kapa, S., Rotondi-Trevisan, D., Mariano, Z., Aves, T., Irvine, J., Dorian, P., et al. (2010). Psychopathology in patients with ICDs over time: results of a prospective study. *Pacing Clin. Electrophysiol.* 33, 198–208. doi: 10.1111/j.1540-8159.2009.02599.x
32. Keren, A., Sears, S. F., Nery, P., Shaw, J., Green, M. S., Lemery, R., et al. (2011). Psychological adjustment in ICD patients living with advisory fidelis leads. *J. Cardiovasc. Electrophysiol.* 22, 57–63. doi: 10.1111/j.1540-8167.2010.01867.x
33. Keren, R., Aarons, D., and Veltri, E. P. (1991). Anxiety and depression in patients with life-threatening ventricular arrhythmias: impact of the implantable cardioverter-defibrillator. *Pacing Clin. Electrophysiol.* 14, 181–187.
34. Kuck, K. H., Cappato, R., Siebels, J., and Ruppel, R. (2000). Randomized compar- ison of antiarrhythmic drug therapy with implantable defibrillators in patients resuscitated from cardiac arrest: the Cardiac Arrest Study Hamburg (CASH). *Circulation* 102, 748–754. doi: 10.1161/01.CIR.102.7.748
35. Ladwig, K. H., Baumert, J., Marten-Mittag, B., Kolb, C., Zrenner, B., and Schmitt, C. (2008). Posttraumatic stress symptoms and predicted mortality in patients with implantable cardioverter-defibrillators: results from the prospective liv- ing with an implanted cardioverter-defibrillator study. *Arch. Gen. Psychiatry* 65, 1324–1330. doi: 10.1001/archpsyc.65.11.1324
36. Leosdottir, M., Sigurdsson, E., Reimarsdottir, G., Gottskalksson, G., Torfason, B., Vigfusdottir, M., et al. (2006). Health-related quality of life of patients with implantable cardioverter defibrillators compared with that of pacemaker recipients. *Europace* 8, 168–174. doi: 10.1093/europace/euj052
37. Liberati, A., Altman, D. G., Tetzlaff, J., Mulrow, C., Gotzsche, P. C., Ioannidis, J. P., et al. (2009). The PRISMA statement for reporting systematic reviews and meta-analyses of studies that evaluate health care interventions: explanation and elaboration. *Ann. Intern. Med.* 151, W65–W94. doi: 10.7326/0003-4819-151-4- 200908180-00136
38. Luderitz, B., Jung, W., Deister, A., Marneros, A., and Manz, M. (1993). Patient acceptance of the implantable cardioverter defibrillator in ventricular tach- yarrhythmias. *Pacing Clin. Electrophysiol.* 16, 1815–1821.
39. Luyster, F. S., Hughes, J. W., Waechter, D., and Josephson, R. (2006). Resource loss predicts depression and anxiety among patients treated with an implantable cardioverter defibrillator. *Psychosom. Med.* 68, 794–800. doi: 10.1097/01.psy. 0000227722.92307.35
40. Mark, D. B., Anstrom, K. J., Sun, J. L., Clapp-Channing, N. E., Tsiatis, A. A., Davidson-Ray, L., et al. (2008). Quality of life with defibrillator ther- apy or amiodarone in heart failure. *N. Engl. J. Med.* 359, 999–1008. doi: 10.1056/NEJMoa0706719
41. Mishkin, J. D., Saxonhouse, S. J., Woo, G. W., Burkart, T. A., Miles, W. M., Conti, J. B., et al. (2009). Appropriate evaluation and treatment of heart failure patients after implantable cardioverter-defibrillator discharge: time to go beyond the initial shock. *J. Am. Coll. Cardiol.* 54, 1993–2000. doi: 10.1016/j.jacc.2009. 07.039
42. Morris, P. L., Badger, J., Chmielewski, C., Berger, E., and Goldberg, R. J. (1991). Psychiatric morbidity following implantation of the automatic implantable cardioverter defibrillator. *Psychosomatics* 32, 58–64.
43. Moss, A. J., Zareba, W., Hall, W. J., Klein, H., Wilber, D. J., Cannom, D. S., et al. (2002). Prophylactic implantation of a defibrillator in patients with myocardial infarction and reduced ejection fraction. Multicenter Automatic Defibrillator Implantation Trial II Investigators. *N. Engl. J. Med.* 346, 877–883. doi: 10.1056/NEJMoa013474 NEJMoa013474 [pii]
44. Namerow, P. B., Firth, B. R., Heywood, G. M., Windle, J. R., and Parides, M. K. (1999). Quality-of-life six months after CABG surgery in patients randomized to ICD versus no ICD therapy: findings from the CABG Patch Trial. *Pacing Clin. Electrophysiol.* 22, 1305–1313.
45. Newman, D. M., Dorian, P., Paquette, M., Sulke, N., Gold, M. R., Schwartzman, D. S., et al. (2003). Effect of an implantable cardioverter defibrillator with atrial detection and shock therapies on patient-perceived, health-related quality of life. *Am. Heart J.* 145, 841–846. doi: 10.1016/S0002-8703(02)94817-9
46. Noyes, K., Corona, E., Veazie, P., Dick, A. W., Zhao, H., and Moss, A. J.
47. (2009). Examination of the effect of implantable cardioverter-defibrillators on health-related quality of life: based on results from the Multicenter Automatic Defibrillator Trial-II. *Am. J. Cardiovasc. Drugs* 9, 393–400. doi: 10.2165/11317980-000000000-00000
48. Passman, R., Subacius, H., Ruo, B., Schaechter, A., Howard, A., Sears, S. F., et al. (2007). Implantable cardioverter defibrillators and quality of life: results from the defibrillators in nonischemic cardiomyopathy treatment evaluation study. *Arch. Intern. Med.* 167, 2226–2232. doi: 10.1001/archinte.167.20.2226
49. Pauli, P., Wiedemann, G., Dengler, W., Blaumann-Benninghoff, G., and Kuhlkamp, V. (1999). Anxiety in patients with an automatic implantable cardioverter defib- rillator: what differentiates them from panic patients? *Psychosom. Med.* 61, 69–76.
50. Pedersen, S. S., den Broek, K. C., Theuns, D. A., Erdman, R. A., Alings, M., Meijer, A., et al. (2011). Risk of chronic anxiety in implantable defibrillator patients: a multi-center study. *Int. J. Cardiol.* 147, 420–423. doi: 10.1016/j.ijcard.2009. 09.549
51. Pedersen, S. S., Spindler, H., Johansen, J. B., and Mortensen, P. T. (2009). Clustering of poor device acceptance and Type D personality is associated with increased distress in Danish cardioverter-defibrillator patients. *Pacing Clin. Electrophysiol.* 32, 29–36. doi: 10.1111/j.1540-8159.2009.02173.x
52. Pedersen, S. S., Spindler, H., Johansen, J. B., Mortensen, P. T., and Sears, S. F. (2008a). Correlates of patient acceptance of the cardioverter defibrillator: cross- validation of the Florida patient acceptance survey in Danish patients. *Pacing Clin. Electrophysiol.* 31, 1168–1177. doi: 10.1111/j.1540-8159.2008.01158.x
53. Pedersen, S. S., Theuns, D. A., Erdman, R. A., and Jordaens, L. (2008b). Clustering of device-related concerns and type D personality predicts increased distress in ICD patients independent of shocks. *Pacing Clin. Electrophysiol.* 31, 20–27. doi: 10.1111/j.1540-8159.2007.00921.x
54. Pedersen, S. S., Theuns, D. A., Jordaens, L., and Kupper, N. (2010a). Course of anxiety and device-related concerns in implantable cardioverter defibrillator patients the first year post implantation. *Europace* 12, 1119–1126. doi: 10.1093/europace/euq154
55. Pedersen, S. S., Theuns, D. A., Muskens-Heemskerk, A., Erdman, R. A., and Jordaens, L. (2007). Type-D personality but not implantable cardioverter-defibrillator indication is associated with mpaired health- related quality of life 3 months post-implantation. *Europace* 9, 675–680. doi: 10.1093/europace/eum041
56. Pedersen, S. S., and Van Den Broek, K. C. (2008). Implantable cardioverter- defibrillator shocks and their adverse impact on patient-centered outcomes: fact or fiction? *J. Am. Coll. Cardiol.* 52, 1037–1038. doi: 10.1016/j.jacc.2008.04.066
57. Pedersen, S. S., Van Den Broek, K. C., Van Den Berg, M., and Theuns, D. A. (2010b). Shock as a determinant of poor patient-centered outcomes in implantable car- dioverter defibrillator patients: is there more to it than meets the eye? *Pacing Clin. Electrophysiol.* 33, 1430–1436. doi: 10.1111/j.1540-8159.2010.02845.x
58. Pedersen, S. S., Van Domburg, R. T., Theuns, D. A., Jordaens, L., and Erdman, R. A. (2004). Type D personality is associated with increased anxiety and depressive symptoms in patients with an implantable car- dioverter defibrillator and their partners. *Psychosom Med.* 66, 714–719. doi: 10.1097/01.psy.0000132874.52202.21 66/5/714 [pii]
59. Pedersen, S. S., Van Domburg, R. T., Theuns, D. A., Jordaens, L., and Erdman, R. A. (2005). Concerns about the implantable cardioverter defibrillator: a determi- nant of anxiety and depressive symptoms independent of experienced shocks. *Am. Heart J.* 149, 664–669. doi: 10.1016/j.ahj.2004.06.031
60. Piotrowicz, K., Noyes, K., Lyness, J. M., Mcnitt, S., Andrews, M. L., Dick, A., et al. (2007). Physical functioning and mental well-being in association with health outcome in patients enrolled in the multicenter automatic defibrilla- tor implantation Trial II. *Eur. Heart J.* 28, 601–607. doi: 10.1093/eurheartj/ ehl485
61. Redhead, A. P., Turkington, D., Rao, S., Tynan, M. M., and Bourke, J. P. (2010). Psychopathology in postinfarction patients implanted with cardioverter- defibrillators for secondary prevention. A cross-sectional, case-controlled study. *J. Psychosom. Res.* 69, 555–563. doi: 10.1016/j.jpsychores.2010.06.002
62. Schron, E. B., Exner, D. V., Yao, Q., Jenkins, L. S., Steinberg, J. S., Cook, J. R., et al. (2002). Quality of life in the antiarrhythmics versus implantable defibrillators trial: impact of therapy and influence of adverse symptoms and defibrillator shocks. *Circulation* 105, 589–594. doi: 10.1161/hc0502.103330
63. Sears, S. F., and Kirian, K. (2010). Shock and patient-centered outcomes research: is an ICD shock still a critical event? *Pacing Clin. Electrophysiol.* 33, 1437–1441. doi: 10.1111/j.1540-8159.2010.02872.x
64. Sears, S. F., Lewis, T. S., Kuhl, E. A., and Conti, J. B. (2005). Predictors of quality of life in patients with implantable cardioverter defibrillators. *Psychosomatics* 46, 451–457. doi: 10.1176/appi.psy.46.5.451

65. Sears, S. F., Sowell, L. V., Kuhl, E. A., Handberg, E. M., Kron, J., Aranda, J. M. Jr., et al. (2006). Quality of death: implantable cardioverter defibrillators and proactive care. *Pacing Clin. Electrophysiol.* 29, 637–642. doi: 10.1111/j.1540-8159.2006.00412.x
66. Sears, S. F. Jr., Todaro, J. F., Lewis, T. S., Sotile, W., and Conti, J. B. (1999). Examining the psychosocial impact of implantable cardioverter defibrillators: a literature review. *Clin. Cardiol.* 22, 481–489.
67. Sossong, A. (2007). Living with an implantable cardioverter defibrillator: patient outcomes and the nurse's role. *J. Cardiovasc. Nurs.* 22, 99–104.
68. Spindler, H., Johansen, J. B., Andersen, K., Mortensen, P., and Pedersen, S. S. (2009). Gender differences in anxiety and concerns about the cardioverter defibrillator. *Pacing Clin. Electrophysiol.* 32, 614–621. doi: 10.1111/j.1540-8159.2009.02334.x
69. Strickberger, S. A., Hummel, J. D., Bartlett, T. G., Frumin, H. I., Schuger, C. D., Beau, S. L., et al. (2003). Amiodarone versus implantable cardio-verter- defibrillator:randomized trial in patients with nonischemic dilated cardiomyopathy and asymptomatic nonsustained ventricular tachycardia– AMIOVIRT. *J. Am. Coll. Cardiol.* 41, 1707–1712. doi: 10.1016/S0735-1097(03) 00297-3
70. Suzuki, T., Shiga, T., Kuwahara, K., Kobayashi, S., Suzuki, S., Nishimura, K., et al. (2010). Prevalence and persistence of depression in patients with implantable cardioverter defibrillator: a 2-year longitudinal study. *Pacing Clin. Electrophysiol.* 33, 1455–1461. doi: 10.1111/j.1540-8159.2010.02887.x
71. Thomas, S. A., Friedmann, E., Gottlieb, S. S., Liu, F., Morton, P. G., Chapa, D. W., et al. (2009). Changes in psychosocial distress in outpatients with heart failure with implantable cardioverter defibrillators. *Heart and Lung: the J. Critical Care* 38, 109–120.
72. Van Den Broek, K. C., Nyklicek, I., and Denollet, J. (2009). Anxiety predicts poor perceived health in patients with an implantable defibrillator. *Psychosomatics* 50, 483–492. doi: 10.1176/appi.psy.50.5.483
73. Van Den Broek, K. C., Nyklicek, I., Van Der Voort, P. H., Alings, M., and Denollet, J. (2008). Shocks, personality, and anxiety in patients with an implantable defibrillator. *Pacing Clin. Electrophysiol.* 31, 850–857. doi: 10.1111/j.1540- 8159.2008.01099.x
74. Versteeg, H., Theuns, D. A., Erdman, R. A., Jordaens, L., and Pedersen, S. S. (2010). Posttraumatic stress in implantable cardioverter defibrillator patients: the role of pre-implantation distress and shocks. *Int. J. Cardiol.* 146, 438–439. doi: 10.1016/j.ijcard.2010.10.108
75. Von Känel, R., Baumert, J., Kolb, C., Cho, E.-Y. N., and Ladwig, K.-H. (2011). Chronic posttraumatic stress and its predictors in patients living with an implantable cardioverter defibrillator. *J. Affect. Disord.* 131, 344–352. doi: 10.1016/j.jad.2010.12.002
76. Wallace, R. L., Sears, S. F. Jr., Lewis, T. S., Griffis, J. T., Curtis, A., and Conti, J. B. (2002). Predictors of quality of life in long-term recipients of implantable cardioverter defibrillators. *J. Cardiopulm. Rehabil.* 22, 278–281.
77. Wathen, M. S., Degroot, P. J., Sweeney, M. O., Stark, A. J., Otterness, M. F., Adkisson, W. O., et al. (2004). Prospective randomized multicenter trial of empirical antitachycardia pacing versus shocks for spontaneous rapid ven- tricular tachycardia in patients with implantable cardioverter-defibrillators: pacing fast ventricular tachycardia reduces shock therapies (PainFREE Rx II) trial results. *Circulation* 110, 2591–2596. doi: 10.1161/01.CIR.0000145610. 64014.E4

4

A false-positive detection bias as a function of state and trait schizotypy in interaction with intelligence

Phillip Grant *, Mona Balser, Aisha Judith Leila Munk, Jens Linder and Juergen Hennig

Personality Psychology and Individual Differences, Department of Psychology, Justus-Liebig-University Giessen, Giessen, Germany

Edited by:
Caroline Gurvich, Monash University, Australia

Reviewed by:
Carmel Maree Loughland, University of Newcastle, Australia
Elias Tsakanikos, University of Roehampton, UK

***Correspondence:**
Phillip Grant, Personality Psychology and Individual Differences, Department of Psychology, Justus-Liebig-University Giessen, Otto-Behaghel-Str. 10F, Giessen D-35394, Hessen, Germany
e-mail: phillip.grant@psychol.uni-giessen.de

Hallucinatory experiences are by far not limited to patients with clinical psychosis. A number of internal and external factors may bring about such experiences in healthy individuals, whereby the personality trait of (positive) schizotypy is a major mediator of individual differences. Psychotic experiences are defined as associating abnormal meaning to real but objectively irrelevant perceptions. Especially, the ambiguity of a stimulus correlates positively with the likelihood of abnormal interpretation, and intelligence is believed to have an important influence and act as protective against clinical psychosis in highly schizotypic individuals. In this study, we presented 131 healthy participants with 216 15-letter strings containing either a word, a non-word, or only random letters and asked them to report, whether or not they believed to have seen a word. The aim was to replicate findings that participants with high values in positive schizotypy on the trait-level make more false-positive errors and assess the role of stimulus-ambiguity and verbal intelligence. Additionally, we wanted to examine whether the same effect could be shown for indices of state schizotypy. Our results support findings that both state and trait positive schizotypy explain significant variance in "seeing things that are not there" and that the properties of individual stimuli have additional strong effects on the false-positive hit rates. Finally, we found that verbal intelligence and positive schizotypy interact with stimulus-ambiguity in the production of false-positive perceptions.

Keywords: schizotypy, psychosis proneness, psychosis continuum, perception, intelligence

INTRODUCTION

Hallucinatory experiences, especially of an auditory nature, are sometimes erroneously believed to exist only as symptoms of psychosis and, by extension, schizophrenia. A number of studies have shown, however, that such phenomena are not exclusive to clinically psychotic patients, but can be found even in the healthy population; e.g., (1), reports a prevalence of hallucinations of any kind within a large tri-national sample ($n = 13{,}057$) of 38.7%, whereof no relation to specific pathology was found in more than half of the sample. Visual hallucinations were of considerably higher prevalence than auditory hallucinations (3.2 vs. 0.6%) in the entire sample.

Although a number of clinical and non-clinical factors exist that bring on individual hallucinatory experiences in non-psychotic patients [e.g., stress, caffeine, and the interaction of both; (2)], it has been repeatedly shown that the occurrence of such experiences is mediated by personality traits related to schizotypy [e.g., Ref. (3–5)].

On the phenomenological level, hallucinations have been shown not to actually be seeing or hearing, etc., "things that *are not there*," but rather – as proposed by Kurt Schneider – interpreting abnormal meaning(fulness) to truly existent but objectively meaningless stimuli [cited from Ref. (6)]. This definition translates well into the current biological model of psychosis and psychosis-proneness by Howes and Kapur (7), who plausibly argue that *abnormal meaning* comes from top-down cognitive explanations of *aberrant salience* attributed (as a function of a dysregulation of dopaminergic neurotransmission) to, essentially, irrelevant stimuli. The authors also clearly argue that individual differences in dopaminergic (dys)regulation in the healthy population also exist. Thus, these differences explain both the appearance of hallucinations in non-psychotic individuals, as well as a possible biological basis of the aforementioned personality trait of schizotypy/psychosis-proneness.

Within the schizotypy-framework as defined by Claridge (8), high levels in schizotypy are not necessarily pathological but potentially beneficial; a concept Claridge refers to as "benign schizotypy." Especially, when paired with above-average intelligence, which appears to protect high schizotypes against clinical psychosis (9), especially positive schizotypy is associated with creativity (10, 11) and can be found in higher levels in, e.g., artists, novelists, composers, philosophers, etc. [q.v., (9)]. In those cases, where eminent achievers exhibited biographical indices of clinical psychosis, it has to be noted that their major contributions usually preceded their first psychotic episode (12), or that their psychotic conditions had not caused serious disability or, alternatively, interrupted or ended their creative work (13). Thus, it seems that schizotypy (especially positive schizotypy) but not clinical psychosis is linked to benignly being able to see patterns where others see random noise. In the case of signals within noise, highly schizotypic persons have been shown to rely on less information in order to reach conclusions, whereby this *jumping-to-conclusions*-bias does not relate to the quality of conclusions (14–16).

A typical paradigm for the examination of hallucinatory experiences in healthy individuals is the "White Christmas"-paradigm, during which participants are primed with the eponymous Bing Crosby song and then listen to white noise, during which they are asked to press a button every time they believe to hear the song through the white noise. This paradigm has been used repeatedly by others [e.g., Ref. (3, 4, 17)] and has repeatedly shown the number of false-positive hits correlates positively with schizotypic traits. This paradigm is limited, however, as it allows for no modification of the signal-to-noise-ratio (i.e., difficulty), which has been shown to also be important for the occurrence of hallucinatory experiences (18).

Galdos et al. (19) also found a significant increase in the reporting of meaningful speech when, actually, random noise was presented in schizophrenia patients compared to controls. Within the control group, a similar effect was found as a function of positive but not negative schizotypy as well as of familial risk for schizophrenia. Relevant, in this context, are findings by Dubal and Viaud-Delmon (20) wherein self-reported auditory sensitivity was also positively associated with magical ideation.

Regarding other sensory modalities, Fyfe et al. (21) showed that persons high in schizotypic traits were more likely to interpret meaningfulness in the random movement of triangles, and Simmonds-Moore (22) found effects of schizotypic traits to be more pronounced in visual than auditory stimuli. Interestingly, however, in this publication, no main effect of schizotypy was discovered regarding the number of false-positive guesses in both modalities, but high schizotypes showed significantly greater confidence in their false-positive guesses. Similar results have been published by Corlett et al. (23) regarding the confidence in but not the number of false-positive memories. Contrary to these findings, however, Wilson and French (24) found that individuals significantly more often reporting false-positive memories, also had higher scores in schizotypic measures. Also of relevance is the often reported effect that highly schizotypic persons were more likely to display a tendency to say "yes" to ambiguous stimuli in forced-choice paradigms [e.g., Ref. (23, 25, 26)].

The group around Tsakanikos and Reed [e.g., Ref. (18, 27–30)], under the plausible assumption that the link between schizotypy and a false-positive detection bias was not limited to individual sensory modalities (27), thus, created a visual word-detection paradigm. Herein, participants were presented different moving words and non-words and asked to note (a) whether they had seen a "real" word and (b) which word they had seen. Through variations of the paradigm, the instructions or the difficulty of the task, they were able to link positive schizotypy [measured through the *Unusual Experiences*-scale of the O-LIFE (31)] to the tendency to significantly more often see (and also be able to write down) words when in fact non-words were presented. Furthermore, this link was significantly influenced through task-difficulty and instruction-induced expectancy; i.e., schizotypy had the highest influence in instances (a) where a higher rate of true-positive words was expected than was actually presented, (b) where the true-positive rate was actually high, and/or (c) when the task-difficulty was medium. These results suggest that too easy tasks have too high a signal-to-noise-ratio to make "jumping-to-conclusion" necessary and too difficult tasks lack a minimum of actual perceptual input to allow for the emergence of a false-positive detection bias as a function of schizotypy. A significant effect of stimulus-ambiguity was also reported by van Elk (26).

There are, however, some factors that were not examined so far: as briefly mentioned above, the role of intelligence (especially verbal intelligence or vocabulary) can be considered a relevant factor that may potentially moderate or mediate the effect of schizotypy on a false-positive detection bias in a word-detection task.

Furthermore, schizotypic features, although believed to be relatively stable (8), actually show a certain degree of intraindividual variation; although influenced by habitual (trait) schizotypy, the situational (state) proneness for psychotic-like experiences is dependent upon other internal and external factors. In other words, the probability of having a psychotic-like or hallucinatory experience may vary within the same individual; e.g., in response to environmental factors like perceived (social) stress [e.g., Ref. (32) or influences of recreational drugs (33)]. Therefore, the influences of state measures of schizotypy may prove better predictors of a false-positive detection bias than scores in trait questionnaires. Moreover, it can be expected that a combination of both aspects (trait and state), comparable to a diathesis – stress model, would explain the highest amount of variance in false-positive detection.

It was our aim in this paper to incorporate the aforementioned variables into a single experiment and to pose the following research-questions:

1. Can we replicate the findings of Tsakanikos; Reed and colleagues (q.v., above) that unusual experiences (UnEx) as an indicator of positive schizotypy is associated with a false-positive detection bias?
2. Is the false-positive detection bias additionally related to state indices of positive schizotypy and what is the role of perceived stress in this context?
3. What are the influences of signal-to-noise ratio, task-difficulty, and verbal intelligence/vocabulary on the false-positive detection bias?

MATERIALS AND METHODS

SAMPLE

The sample consisted of a total of 131 healthy participants (according to telephone and on-site self-report). Hereof, 27 were male and 104 female (aged between 17 and 73; $M = 27.43$; $MD = 24$; $SD = 10.63$). Participants were gathered through university adverts, personal communications, and newspaper adverts looking for individuals with telepathic or other extrasensory perceptive experiences. Participants were fully briefed during a telephone interview as well as immediately before the experiment; on both occasions, all participants stated not currently suffering or ever in the past having suffered from a psychological or relevant medical condition.

Research was approved by the ethics committee of the German Psychological Association (Deutsche Gesellschaft für Psychologie, DGPs).

SELF-REPORT MEASURES

Trait schizotypy was assessed using the German version of the Oxford-Liverpool Inventory of Feelings and Experiences [O-LIFE;

(34)]; the *Unusual Experiences* (UnEx) scale was used as a measure of positive schizotypy. The O-LIFE consists of 104 items in a yes/no-format. In order to use UnEx as a factor for a multifactorial ANOVA, participants were trichotomized according to the 33rd-percentiles.

State schizotypic or psychosis-like indices were assessed using a translation of the items used by Barrantes-Vidal et al. (32) for experience sampling methodology. These items are based on the Wisconsin Schizotypy Scales (WSS) and, thus, have a slightly different factor-structure than the O-LIFE [q.v., (35)]. We therefore combined items from the "psychotic-like index" with the "paranoid index" to assess state positive schizotypy. Items suited only for use in experience sampling methodology were omitted (e.g., "Since the last beep, I consumed: Food I Caffeine I Medication I Snuff I Alcohol I Cannabis or other drugs"). Additionally, the item "At the moment I am feeling stressed" was added. All state items were coded on a visual analog scale from 0 (not at all) to 100 (completely) and measured immediately before and after the word-detection paradigm. Verbal intelligence/vocabulary was measured using the Mehrfachwahl–Wortschatz–Intelligenz test [MWT-B; (36)]. The MWT-B consists of several sets of five-letter-combinations, whereof one is an actual word. The participant is tasked with identifying the word; the IQ can be extrapolated from the manual depending on the number of true identifications and the individual words that were (not) identified correctly. The MWT-B was specifically chosen, as it measures (verbal) intelligence in a fashion similar to the trials in our paradigm.

All self-report measures were programed as online-versions using the platform suscisurvey.de.

WORD-DETECTION PARADIGM

The paradigm was programed using Matlab (version 4.0.7 with Psychtoolbox 3.0.9). The paradigm consisted of 216 trials, each preceded by a fixation cross randomly shown between 1 and 2 s. Stimuli consisted of a 15-letter sequence presented in Arial (font size 24; white letters on black background) at a distance of 50 cm between the participant and the computer monitor. Testing was performed on two computers with identical monitors with equal settings; room illumination was kept at a constant level using window blackouts, and participants were alone in the room during the paradigm.

Stimuli were presented for 750 ms each, followed by the question "Did you see a word?" (with yes/no-format). If the participant answered "yes," a second question "Please type in the word you have seen" appeared. Thereafter, the participants were instructed to return to their upright-seated position and press the space-bar for the next trial to commence. Initially, four instruction trials were presented, the first containing a true word and the second not containing a true word (presented for 5 s), the third and fourth instruction trials again with a true word and no word, but presented for 2 s. These stimuli were not used during the main paradigm.

Since the words were German, they are not presented within the scope of this English manuscript. Interested researchers are, however, encouraged to contact the corresponding author.

Of the 216 experimental trials, 72 contained a true word (of five-letter length), 72 a non-word designed according to the corresponding true word using the non-word generator *Wuggy* (37) and the final 72 stimuli containing neither a true word nor a non-word. The true words were gathered from a list of 98 German five-letter words that fit certain criteria (i.e., they were singular-case common nouns that contained no umlaut). These 98 words were randomly embedded into 10 other nonsense letters and given to a sample of 242 unrelated students during a lecture at the University of Applied Science, Giessen, by the principal author. The student were asked to rate the word from "easy to detect" to "difficult to detect" (5-point Likert scale) without time limit. From this, average difficulties were calculated and the 12 "easiest" as well as the 12 "most difficult" words were chosen for the paradigm at hand. For each of these 24 words, a corresponding non-word was created. Words and non-words were each presented three times, namely once at the beginning, the middle, and the end of the 15-letter stimulus (e.g., **HEART**ZBKMLPTWFG, ZBKML**HEART**PTWFG, and ZBKMLPTWFG**HEART**; English word and bold print used just here for clarity). Presentation-order was randomized for each participant, but each participant was presented all 216 stimuli.

Responses were coded by hand (and double-checked by an independent persons) into either of four categories; namely, true-positive, true-negative, false-positive, and false-negative. With respect to the aim of these particular study questions, the categories other than false-positive as well as the reactions times shall not be used as dependent variables within this publication.

STATISTICAL ANALYSES

All statistical analyses were performed using SPSS (version 15). Due to reported effects of age and sex on UnEx [q.v., Ref. (31, 34)] respective variance was removed for between-subject analyses using the generalized linear model by saving standardized residuals and assigning these to the dependent variables. A similar approach was used for the false-positive hit rate in case of significant effects of factors not related to our research question (e.g., age, intelligence).

For within-subject analyses (i.e., influences of word difficulty and -position as well as signal-to-noide ratio), a dependent-samples GLM-analysis was performed with raw false-positive hits as dependent variables in a 2 × 3-design (two steps for difficulty; three steps for position). A second dependent-samples GLM-analysis was also performed for the analysis of effects of the signal-to-noise ratio on the false-positive hits. This was operationalized through the trial-condition (word, non-word, random letters); with increasingly fewer semantically interpretable entities (word > non-word > random letters) the signal-to-noise ratio was expected to decline.

For between-subject analyses (i.e., influences of schizotypy), an independent-sample GLM-analysis was performed with the standardized residuals of the false-positive hits (independently of difficulty or position) as dependent variables and the trichotomized UnEx-group as factor.

For the analyses of the effects of state schizotypic indices and stress, linear regressions were performed with the standardized residuals of the false-positive hits (again, independently of difficulty and position) as dependent variables and the positive schizotypy index and the stress-item as regressors.

In case of replication questions (i.e., the effects of trait or state positive schizotypy on the false-positive detection rate), one-tailed testing was called for Ref. (38); for all other analyses, two-tailed testing was performed.

Data were controlled for outliers, whereby for the effects of positive schizotypy on the false-positive detection rate one case was eliminated; for all other analyses, it was not necessary to remove this case.

RESULTS

Over the total of 216 trials, our 131 participants reported an average of 5.45 (SD = 4.93) false-positive hits. The range was from 0 (four participants) to 37 (one participant), whereby the latter was considered as the aforementioned outlier, as the next highest number of false-positive hits was 26, followed by 19, and then continuously from 16 through 0. The median was four and there were two modes (1 and 3, with 18 participants each); the second highest number of false-positive hits was four (14 participants). This appears to be substantially higher than in comparable studies by Tsakanikos and colleagues [e.g., Ref. (18)].

The first question was, whether state and trait positive schizotypy had significant influences on the false-positive detection rate. For these analyses, the age- and sex-corrected UnEx-scores were used as dependent variables (in the ANOVA, the sample was trichotomized as described above). Dependent variable was the false-positive detection rate, corrected (as described above) for confounding factors (i.e., intelligence, age, etc.).

We found a significant effect of UnEx (positive schizotypy) on the false-positive detection rate [$F_{2,127} = 3.01$; $p = 0.027$ (one-tailed)], whereby Bonferroni-corrected *post hoc* test showed that this effect was mainly explained by the highest scores in the high schizotypy group compared to the low schizotypy group [$p = 0.032$ (one-tailed)].

The regression of state positive schizotypy was also significant [$\beta = 0.254$; corrected $R^2 = 0.057$; $F_{1,128} = 8.85$; $p = 0.002$ (one-tailed)]. Perceived stress had no significant predictive power regarding the false-positive hits; the interaction with state positive schizotypy, however, was significant ($\beta = 0.231$; corrected $R^2 = 0.046$; $F_{1,128} = 4.72$; $p = 0.008$).

The effects of word-position and word difficulty were analyzed using a within-subjects model with Greenhouse-Geisser correction on the false-positive hits (uncorrected for between-subject confounders). Both main effects as well as their interaction were significant; i.e., word-position ($F_{1.8,243.46} = 9.16$; $p < 0.001$; partial $\eta^2 = 0.066$), word difficulty ($F_{1,130} = 20.01$; $p < 0.001$; partial $\eta^2 = 0.133$), and interaction ($F_{1.87,243.49} = 6.49$; $p = 0.002$; partial $\eta^2 = 0.048$). Descriptive statistics showed higher false-positive hits with difficult compared to easy words. Regarding word-position, with easy words the rate of false-positive hits was lower when the word was presented at the beginning of the 15-letter string compared to the middle or end. In the hard word category, false-positives were identical when the word was presented at the beginning or end, but higher when the word was presented in the middle. Over all, the highest and lowest false-positive hits were difficult words presented in the middle and easy words presented at the beginning, respectively.

Both main effects as well as the interaction were no longer significant when IQ was introduced into the model as a covariate; thus, suggesting that verbal intelligence moderates the effects of word-position and -difficulty. It has to be mentioned that an interaction between the within- and between-subject factors in one model could not be analyzed, since the within-subject design did not allow for correction of between-subject confounders, whereby the between-subject design necessitated a correction for between-subject confounders. Using between-subject factors as covariates and, apparently, "correcting" for these factors, is, in fact, not a probate method in this case (39).

When positive schizotypy was entered as a covariate, the main effect of difficulty and the interaction between position and difficulty remained significant, albeit with reduced effects sizes (difficulty: $F_{1,129} = 5.65$; $p = 0.019$; partial $\eta^2 = 0.042$; interaction: $F_{1.88,241.87} = 4.27$; $p = 0.017$; partial $\eta^2 = 0.032$). Additionally, although the main effect of position was no longer significant, there was a significant interaction between position and positive schizotypy ($F_{1.82,234.75} = 3.327$; $p = 0.042$; partial $\eta^2 = 0.025$). This effect was the only one that remained significant (with the same effect size), when both IQ and UnEx were simultaneously entered as covariates.

In case of the effect of the signal-to-noise-ratio (operationalized through "condition": word, non-word, random letters) the main effect was significant ($F_{1.68,217.84} = 102.81$; $p < 0.001$; partial $\eta^2 = 0.442$), showing similar false-positive hits in the conditions with the highest and lowest signal-to-noise ratio (word and random letters) but an increased detection bias in the non-word condition. The effect remained significant but of reduced size when UnEx, IQ, and both were entered as covariates into the model (respectively: $F_{1.69,218.1} = 22.67$; $p < 0.001$; partial $\eta^2 = 0.149$, $F_{1.68,216.63} = 4.34$; $p = 0.019$; partial $\eta^2 = 0.033$ and $F_{1.7,217.07} = 3.86$; $p = 0.029$; partial $\eta^2 = 0.029$). There were no significant interactions between condition and either positive schizotypy or IQ.

DISCUSSION

We found a significant effect of positive schizotypy on the false-positive detection rate, whereby especially highly schizotypic participants had more incidences of "seeing words that were not there" than low schizotypic individuals. This result is in complete agreement with the findings reported by Tsakanikos and Reed (27, 28). Due to the complexity of the other additionally analyzed factors in this study, we chose not to examine the effects of other schizotypy facets or other performance indices (i.e., true-positives and -negatives as well as false-negatives and reaction time) within the scope of this paper for reasons of brevity.

Additionally, we found that not only trait but also state schizotypy, as assessed through the items used in ESM-studies by Barrantes-Vidal et al. (32), significantly predicted the false-positive hits and interacts with self-reported stress. The latter, in and of itself, did not have predictive power regarding the detection bias in our paradigm. Thus, it would seem that the effects of stress moderate the influence of state schizotypy. This is in line with the supposition that stress (or stressful life events) not only act as facilitators of *inter*individual differences in schizotypy or psychotic-like experiences [e.g., Ref. (40)] and *intra*individual differences [e.g., Ref. 32)] but also that highly schizotypic persons are more susceptible to stress (41).

In within-subject designs, we found significant effects of the difficulty of the presented word and the position thereof as well as the interaction of both of these factors. Presenting words that had been rated as difficult to detect leads to higher false-positive errors than easy words. Furthermore, when words were presented in the middle of the 15-letter string, more false-positive errors were made, independently of word difficulty, than when words were presented at either the beginning or the end of the stimulus. In the interaction, easy words presented at the end of the string lead to the lowest and difficult words presented in the middle of the string to the highest rates of false-positive errors.

Regarding the signal-to-noise ratio, which was operationalized through the task condition (i.e., the relation of semantically interpretable unit to "letter jumble"), we found that the condition with middle signal-to-noise ratio (i.e., non-words) elicited higher false-positive hits than the high or low signal-to-noise ratios (i.e., word and random letters).

These results agree with the proposition by, i.a., Tsakanikos (18) that very easy tasks (e.g., high signal-to-noise ratio, easy words, words that began or ended the 15-letter string) usually require less cognitive "filling in the gaps" and, thus, incur less errors. In the highly difficult conditions, persons would make less false-positive errors as they would have more difficulty to identify potentially semantically relevant units and, thus, be more likely to answer that they had not seen a word. In this case, a follow-up question would be, whether these difficult conditions elicited significantly more false-negative errors. The finding most necessary to discuss, in our opinion, is that in case of the difficult words presented in the middle the high false-positive hits mean that participants made double-errors; i.e., an additional false-negative error, as they had, actually, not identified the presented word correctly. Extrapolated to clinical psychosis, this would be comparable to a situation where a patient, e.g., sees an unknown (but truly existent) face but erroneously interprets this as another person's face or even something else (e.g., the face of a demon). This would explain anecdotal evidence that hallucinations occur more often at night or in the early evening or morning [(42); q.v., patients' statements on schizophrenia.com]. Also in healthy individuals it is obviously more common to "see something" at night or during dusk and dawn.

The influence of IQ in this case is highly relevant and, to our knowledge, examined for the first time in research of this kind in healthy individuals. The introduction of verbal IQ as a covariate into the model completely eliminated the main effects of difficulty and position as well as their interaction and considerably reduced the effect size of condition. This can be interpreted along the same line of argumentation as before. The higher the intelligence, the more it is likely that difficulty and position will no longer influence the false- as well as the true-positive detection rates (especially considering that we specifically chose an intelligence test with the MWT-B that extrapolates IQ from a number of tasks inherently similar to our paradigm). In other words, the capability of identifying a word independently of its position or difficulty will increase with the aptitude for this kind of task (as measured through the MWT-B). Therefore, the main effects and the interaction will be most prominent in participants with (relatively) low verbal IQ and, thus, were to be expected to no longer be significant when IQ was entered as a covariate. Regarding the reduction of effect size of condition by IQ, the same explanation as above holds.

Going back to the supposition that intelligence may be protective in high schizotypes regarding their transition into clinical psychosis (9), our findings may help explain this. We chose an IQ-test that consisted of a task specifically measuring the aptitude to what we were also measuring in our paradigm. If one extrapolates to crystalline or g-factor intelligence in general, one would also expect that this will influence stimulus-processing on a broader range of levels. Thus, it should be expected that highly intelligent individuals experience less ambiguity in perceived stimuli and thus require less top-down cognitive "filling in" of gaps and are, therefore, less prone to (especially bizzare) psychotic experiences. Future studies will be necessary, in order to ascertain the verisimilitude of this supposition.

The effects of schizotypy are also of particular relevance, especially within the scope of this paper. In order to explore this further, we performed individual one-tailed *ex post facto* t-tests between the high and low schizotypy groups for each variety of word difficulty, word-position, and task condition in order to assess where the effect of schizotypy was strongest.

These analyses showed that differences were most pronounced in the non-word condition ($T_{82} = 2.55$; $p = 0.006$) with a trend in the word condition ($T_{82} = 1.5$; $p = 0.068$) and no difference in the random letters condition. Similarly, schizotypy did not explain significant differences when difficult words were presented, but there was a trend in the cases of presentation of easy words ($T_{72.74} = 1.53$; $p = 0.065$). With regards to position, words presented in the middle lead to the greatest schizotypy-dependent differences in false-positive hits ($T_{82} = 1.98$; $p = 0.025$), especially if these words were easy words ($T_{64.76} = 2.31$; $p = 0.012$). Interestingly, however, although there were not schizotypy-dependent differences in the false-positive hits when difficult words were presented or when words were presented at the beginning of the 15-letter strings, there was a trend in case these factors were combined; i.e., high schizotypes had tendentially higher false-positive hits in cases were difficult words were presented at the beginning of the stimulus ($T_{82} = 1.46$; $p = 0.074$). All effects were in the expected direction; i.e., highly schizotypic persons always had higher false-positive hits rates than low schizotypic persons.

These results, on the one hand, show that in the non-word condition, where most false-positive errors were made, these can be explained significantly by individual differences in trait positive schizotypy; this is, again, in agreement with Tsakanikos (18) that schizotypy-dependent differences are most pronounced in middle signal-to-noise ratios. The same goes for the differences explained by schizotypy regarding the false-positive reactions to word presented in the middle of a 15-letter string. Furthermore, although difficult words lead to a higher false-positive hit rate in general, highly schizotypic persons showed significantly, and borderline-significantly more errors in easy words compared to low schizotypic persons. It can, thus, be asserted that the effects of schizotypy (although significant) are less pronounced than those of the stimuli. This is in line with the repeated findings that (a) any person, independently of schizotypy, can experience psychotic-like experiences when presented with the "right conditions" and (b) that highly schizotypic persons will be more likely to experiences psychotic-like experiences not only in general but especially in situations were low schizotypic persons will not have a psychotic-like experience.

To summarize, we replicated findings that positive schizotypy leads to a "jumping-to-conclusions" bias and that this bias is most heavily pronounced in reaction to relatively highly ambiguous stimuli. Furthermore, we could show that the effects of schizotypy are considerably less strong than those of stimulus-quality and, thus, that schizotypy explains most variance in those conditions that are not of themselves ambiguous enough to lead to errors in judgment in most persons. In other words, ambiguity increases the amount of errors, but highly schizotypic persons require less ambiguity as a facilitator of a false-positive detection bias than low schizotypic individuals.

We extended upon previous findings by showing that (verbal) IQ significantly moderates both a general detection bias as well as the interactions between said bias and trait schizotypy. Furthermore, we showed that not only trait but also state schizotypy significantly predicted false-positive errors. Although both factors correlated significantly in our study [q.v., (32)], an interaction with stress shows that situational psychosis-like experiences in healthy individuals are not solely a factor of habitual schizotypy.

In conclusion, our results further the understanding that hallucinatory experiences in non-clinical individuals are not only a factor of healthy variations in schizotypy but also depend more heavily on the quality of stimulus-perception and cognition as well as (task-specific) cognitive abilities – as shown by the considerable effects explained through verbal IQ.

Over all, we believe that our study presents a significant add-on to other related findings. We replicate previous results and add relevant information regarding, especially, state schizotypy and intelligence. In the future, different variations of paradigms of this sort may be used and, additionally, combined with imaging and psychophysiological methods (e.g., fMRI and EEG). We are also currently in the process of examining the effects of genetic factors in this relation. It could be expected that specific polymorphisms as well as additive effects of different polymorphisms that are relevant to schizotypy may yield further insight. Preliminary results are highly promising, but we chose not to publish these as yet, due to the fact that the number of participants willing to provide a DNA-sample so far is not large enough to reach the statistical power needed for genetic association studies.

ACKNOWLEDGMENTS

The authors would like to thank Carina Damerau and Frieder Gabriel for their help in acquiring participants for this study as well as Anna Freier for her help in programing our paradigm.

REFERENCES

1. Ohayon MM. Prevalence of hallucinations and their pathological associations in the general population. *Psychiatry Res* (2000) **97**(2–3):153–64. doi:10.1016/S0165-1781(00)00227-4
2. Crowe SF, Barot J, Caldow S, D'Aspromonte J, Dell'Orso J, Di Clemente A, et al. The effect of caffeine and stress on auditory hallucinations in a non-clinical sample. *Pers Individ Dif* (2011) **50**(5):626–30. doi:10.1016/j.paid.2010.12.007
3. Bentall RP, Slade PD. Reality testing and auditory hallucinations: a signal detection analysis. *Br J Clin Psychol* (1985) **24**(Pt 3):159–69. doi:10.1111/j.2044-8260.1985.tb01331.x
4. Merckelbach H, van de Ven V. Another White Christmas: fantasy proneness and reports of 'hallucinatory experiences' in undergraduate students. *J Behav Ther Exp Psychiatry* (2001) **32**(3):137–44. doi:10.1016/S0005-7916(01)00029-5
5. Sommer IE, Daalman K, Rietkerk T, Diederen KM, Bakker S, Wijkstra J, et al. Healthy individuals with auditory verbal hallucinations; who are they? Psychiatric assessments of a selected sample of 103 subjects. *Schizophr Bull* (2010) **36**(3):633–41. doi:10.1093/schbul/sbn130
6. Weitbrecht HJ. *Psychiatrie Im Grundriss.* Berlin: Springer (1963).
7. Howes OD, Kapur S. The dopamine hypothesis of schizophrenia: version III the final common pathway. *Schizophr Bull* (2009) **35**(3):549–62. doi:10.1093/schbul/sbp006
8. Claridge G. Theoretical background and issues. 1st ed. In: Claridge G, editor. *Schizotypy – Implications for Illness and Health.* Oxford: Oxford University Press (1997). p. 3–18.
9. Brod JH. Creativity and schizotypy. 1 ed. In: Claridge G, editor. *Schizotypy – Implications for Illness and Health.* Oxford: Oxford University Press (1997). p. 274–98.
10. Poreh AM, Whitman DR, Ross TP. Creative thinking abilities and hemispheric asymmetry in schizotypal college student. *Curr Psychol* (1994) **12**:344–52. doi:10.1007/BF02686814
11. Batey M, Furnham A. The relationship between measures of creativity and schizotypy. *Pers Individ Dif* (2008) **45**(8):816–21. doi:10.1016/j.paid.2008.08.014
12. Lange-Eichbaum W. *The Problem of Genius (E. P. C. Paul, Trans.).* New York: Macmillan (1932).
13. Post F. Creativity and psychopathology. A study of 291 world-famous men. *Br J Psychiatry* (1994) **165**(1):22–34. doi:10.1192/bjp.165.1.22
14. Heilbrun AB Jr, Blum NA. Cognitive vulnerability to auditory hallucination. Impaired perception of meaning. *Br J Psychiatry* (1984) **144**:508–12. doi:10.1192/bjp.144.5.508
15. Garety PA, Hemsley DR, Wessely S. Reasoning in deluded schizophrenic and paranoid patients. Biases in performance on a probabilistic inference task. *J Nerv Ment Dis* (1991) **179**(4):194–201. doi:10.1097/00005053-199104000-00003
16. Dudley RE, John CH, Young AW, Over DE. Normal and abnormal reasoning in people with delusions. *Br J Clin Psychol* (1997) **36**(Pt 2):243–58. doi:10.1111/j.2044-8260.1997.tb01410.x
17. Rankin PM, O'Carroll PJ. Reality discrimination, reality monitoring and disposition towards hallucination. *Br J Clin Psychol* (1995) **34**(Pt 4):517–28. doi:10.1111/j.2044-8260.1995.tb01486.x
18. Tsakanikos E. Perceptual biases and positive schizotypy: the role of perceptual load. *Pers Individ Dif* (2006) **41**(5):951–8. doi:10.1016/j.paid.2006.04.004
19. Galdos M, Simons C, Fernandez-Rivas A, Wichers M, Peralta C, Lataster T, et al. Affectively salient meaning in random noise: a task sensitive to psychosis liability. *Schizophr Bull* (2010) **37**(6):1179–86. doi:10.1093/schbul/sbq029
20. Dubal S, Viaud-Delmon I. Magical ideation and hyperacusis. *Cortex* (2008) **44**(10):1379–86. doi:10.1016/j.cortex.2007.06.008
21. Fyfe S, Williams C, Mason OJ, Pickup GJ. Apophenia, theory of mind and schizotypy: perceiving meaning and intentionality in randomness. *Cortex* (2008) **44**(10):1316–25. doi:10.1016/j.cortex.2007.07.009
22. Simmonds-Moore C. Exploring the perceptual biases associated with believing and disbelieving in paranormal phenomena. *Conscious Cogn* (2014) **28**:30–46. doi:10.1016/j.concog.2014.06.004
23. Corlett PR, Simons JS, Pigott JS, Gardner JM, Murray GK, Krystal JH, et al. Illusions and delusions: relating experimentally-induced false memories to anomalous experiences and ideas. *Front Behav Neurosci* (2009) **3**:53. doi:10.3389/neuro.08.053.2009
24. Wilson K, French C. The relationship between susceptibility to false memories, dissociativity, and paranormal belief and experience. *Pers Individ Dif* (2006) **41**:1493–502. doi:10.1016/j.paid.2006.06.008
25. Krummenacher P, Mohr C, Haker H, Brugger P. Dopamine, paranormal belief, and the detection of meaningful stimuli. *J Cogn Neurosci* (2010) **22**(8):1670–81. doi:10.1162/jocn.2009.21313

26. van Elk M. Paranormal believers are more prone to illusory agency detection than skeptics. *Conscious Cogn* (2013) **22**(3):1041–6. doi:10.1016/j.concog.2013.07.004
27. Tsakanikos E, Reed P. Do positive schizotypal symptoms predict false perceptual experiences in nonclinical populations? *J Nerv Ment Dis* (2005) **193**(12):809–12. doi:10.1097/01.nmd.0000188974.44468.92
28. Tsakanikos E, Reed P. Seeing words that are not there: detection biases in schizotypy. *Br J Clin Psychol* (2005) **44**(Pt 2):295–9. doi:10.1348/014466505X28757
29. Cella M, Taylor K, Reed P. Violation of expectancies produces more false positive reports in a word detection task in people scoring high in unusual experiences scale. *Pers Individ Dif* (2007) **43**(1):59–70. doi:10.1016/j.paid.2006.11.007
30. Reed P, Wakefield D, Harris J, Parry J, Cella M, Tsakanikos E. Seeing non-existent events: effects of environmental conditions, schizotypal symptoms, and sub-clinical characteristics. *J Behav Ther Exp Psychiatry* (2008) **39**(3):276–91. doi:10.1016/j.jbtep.2007.07.005
31. Mason O, Claridge G. The Oxford-Liverpool inventory of feelings and experiences (O-LIFE): further description and extended norms. *Schizophr Res* (2006) **82**(2–3):203–11. doi:10.1016/j.schres.2005.12.845
32. Barrantes-Vidal N, Chun CA, Myin-Germeys I, Kwapil TR. Psychometric schizotypy predicts psychotic-like, paranoid, and negative symptoms in daily life. *J Abnorm Psychol* (2013) **122**(4):1077–87. doi:10.1037/a0034793
33. Mason OJ, Morgan CJ, Stefanovic A, Curran HV. The psychotomimetic states inventory (PSI): measuring psychotic-type experiences from ketamine and cannabis. *Schizophr Res* (2008) **103**(1–3):138–42. doi:10.1016/j.schres.2008.02.020
34. Grant P, Kuepper Y, Mueller E, Wielpuetz C, Mason O, Hennig J. Dopaminergic foundations of schizotypy as measured by the German version of the Oxford-Liverpool inventory of feelings and experiences (O-LIFE) – suitable endophenotype of schizophrenia. *Front Hum Neurosci* (2013) **7**(1). doi:10.3389/fnhum.2013.00001
35. Kwapil TR, Barrantes-Vidal N, Silvia PJ. The dimensional structure of the Wisconsin Schizotypy scales: factor identification and construct validity. *Schizophr Bull* (2008) **34**(3):444–57. doi:10.1093/schbul/sbm098
36. Lehrl S. *Mehrfachwahl-Wortschatz-Intelligenztest (MWT-B)*. Balingen: Spitta (2005).
37. Keuleers E, Brysbaert M. Wuggy: a multilingual pseudoword generator. *Behav Res Methods* (2010) **42**(3):627–33. doi:10.3758/BRM.42.3.627
38. Bland JM, Altman DG. Statistics notes – one-sided and 2-sided tests of significance.8. *Br Med J* (1994) **309**(6949):248. doi:10.1136/bmj.309.6949.248
39. Miller GA, Chapman JP. Misunderstanding analysis of covariance. *J Abnorm Psychol* (2001) **110**(1):40–8. doi:10.1037/0021-843X.110.1.40
40. Kocsis-Bogar K, Miklosi M, Forintos DP. Impact of adverse life events on individuals with low and high schizotypy in a nonpatient sample. *J Nerv Ment Dis* (2013) **201**(3):208–15. doi:10.1097/NMD.0b013e3182845cea
41. Smith NT, Lenzenweger MF. Increased stress responsivity in schizotypy leads to diminished spatial working memory performance. *Personal Disord* (2013) **4**(4):324–31. doi:10.1037/per0000014
42. Manford M, Andermann F. Complex visual hallucinations. Clinical and neurobiological insights. *Brain* (1998) **121**(Pt 10):1819–40. doi:10.1093/brain/121.10.1819

5

Factor analysis demonstrates a common schizoidal phenotype within autistic and schizotypal tendency: implications for neuroscientific studies

Talitha C. Ford* and David P. Crewther

Centre for Human Psychopharmacology, Faculty of Health, Arts and Design, School of Health Sciences, Swinburne University of Technology, Melbourne, VIC, Australia

Edited by:
Caroline Gurvich, Monash University, Australia

Reviewed by:
Linda Byrne, Deakin University, Australia
Suzanna Russell-Smith, The University of Western Australia, Australia

****Correspondence:***
Talitha C. Ford, Centre for Human Psychopharmacology, Faculty of Health, Arts and Design, School of Health Sciences, Swinburne University of Technology, 400B Burwood Road, Hawthorn, VIC 3122, Australia
e-mail: tcford@swin.edu.au

Behavioral and cognitive dysfunction, particularly social and communication impairments, are shared between autism and schizophrenia spectrum disorders, while evidence for a diametric autism-positive schizophrenia symptom profile is inconsistent. We investigated the shared phenotype at a personality trait level, particularly its resemblance to schizoid personality disorder, as well as differential aspects of the autism–schizophrenia model. Items of the autism spectrum quotient (AQ) and schizotypal personality questionnaire (SPQ) were pseudo-randomly combined, and were completed by 449 (162 male, 287 female) non-clinical participants aged 18–40. A factor analysis revealed three factors; the first represented a shared social disorganization phenotype, the second reflected perceptual oddities specific to schizotypy while the third reflected social rigidity specific to autism. The AQ and SPQ were strongly correlated with Factor 1 (AQ: $r = 0.75$, $p < 0.001$; SPQ: $r = 0.96$, $p < 0.001$), SPQ score was correlated with Factor 2 ($r = 0.51$, $p < 0.001$), particularly in cognitive–perceptual features ($r = 0.66$, $p < 0.001$), and AQ score was strongly correlated with Factor 3 ($r = 0.76$, $p < 0.001$). Furthermore, there was no relationship between Factor 1 and Factor 2. Thus, there is robust evidence for a shared social disorganization phenotype in autistic and schizotypal tendency, which reflects the schizoid phenotype. Discriminating and independent dimensions of schizotypal and autistic tendency exist in Factors 2 and 3, respectively. Current diagnostic protocols could result in different diagnoses depending on the instrument used, suggesting the need for neuromarkers that objectively differentiate autistic and schizotypal traits and resolve the question of commonality versus co-morbidity.

Keywords: autistic traits, schizotypal personality traits, schizoid personality disorder, factors analysis, autism, schizophrenia

INTRODUCTION

The phenotypic tangle of autism and schizophrenia spectrum symptomology has been hotly debated since Bleuler defined "autism" in 1911 as an exclusive psychiatric disorder (1, 2). Despite their obvious clinical differences in symptom onset and presentation, interpersonal and cognitive deficits, and disorganization are fundamental to both disorders (1, 3–9), yielding a potential confusion in diagnosis.

Autism and schizophrenia (the terms "autism" and "schizophrenia" refer to the full spectra of the respective disorders) are neurodevelopmental disorders with pervasive social impairments such as flattened facial and speech affect, reduced gesturing, eye contact and language, concrete and obsessional thinking, and unusual body movement (10). King and Lord (11) pointed to symptom similarity between schizotypal personality and autism in terms of unusual preoccupations, unusual perceptual experiences, odd thinking and speech, constricted affect, social anxiety, lack of close friends, and odd or eccentric speech and behavior. A clinical diagnosis of autism spectrum disorder (ASD) specifies early childhood presentation of social and communication dysfunction, in conjunction with restricted and repetitive behaviors (10). Schizophrenia is typically qualified with the onset of a psychotic episode, marked by hallucinations, delusions, disorganization, and/or catatonic behavior for up to 1 month, in late adolescence or early adulthood. Schizophrenia diagnoses can be established only if the psychosis is accompanied by enduring affective and interpersonal dysfunction, and disorganization in speech and behaviors (10).

The newly released Diagnostic and Statistical Manual of Psychiatric Disorders version five (DSM-5) (10) is naturally controversial due to its central role in clinical diagnosis, and the revision of symptom discrimination, differentiation, and co-morbidity. The new edition saw the removal of paranoid and schizoid personality disorder (PD), which may be detrimental to diagnostic specificity. Schizoid PD, as defined in DSM-IV-TR (12), describes pervasive social dysfunction and negative symptoms that are central to schizophrenia (including schizotypal PD). Such symptoms are also seen in autism. Core features of schizoid PD include: lack of interest in, and active avoidance of social situations both in occupation and daily life, restricted affect, odd communication, relationship detachment, and poor empathy. Mental rigidity and single-minded pursuit of interests are also characteristic (12–14).

These features can indirectly lead to positive-like symptoms such as fantasies, mania (13), and paranoid ideation (11). Schizoid PD, thought to be a milder form of schizotypal PD, has the potential to progress into more enduring schizophrenia spectrum disorders, with a genetic association to schizophrenia (14, 15). In fact, in a study of 32 children diagnosed with schizoid PD, 24 met the criteria for schizotypal PD, and two developed schizophrenia (14). Exclusion of schizoid PD was based on a lack of empirical evidence for the disorder. Schizoid PD was reported to have only 1% pathological prevalence (13), compared to 3% prevalence of schizotypal PD (12).

DSM-5, in similar vein, aligns Asperger's disorder with ASD resulting in the abolishment of key differential diagnostic criteria. Removing language delay and early onset symptom presentation criteria for ASD consequently reduces the discriminatory quality of diagnosis. Wolff et al. (14) suggest distinguishing between schizotypal PD, schizoid PD, and Asperger's disorder is not warranted. Thus, the relaxed exclusion criterion for ASD, and removal of schizoid PD, impacts the diagnosis, prognosis, and therapeutic techniques for autism and schizophrenia spectrum disorders. More accurate assessment of the schizoid phenotype may indeed reduce confusion between the apparent comorbid social dysfunction in the autism and schizophrenia spectra (13).

Social–cognitive dysfunction is evident in both autism (7, 16–19) and schizophrenia (7, 16–22). Social cognition is defined as the cognitive aspects of the social experience; including perceptions, processing, and interpreting social information (23) from basic facial affect recognition to theory of mind (22). Social anhedonia – social isolation and disinterest, is a prodromal, as well as an active and residual feature of schizophrenia (24, 25). Social anhedonia has also been found to predict severity in autism (26). However, it has been argued that social deficits in autism represent social anxiety and social skills, while negative schizotypy relates to social anhedonia and depression (27). The similarity between the two disorders in terms of social cognition and interpersonal deficit may lead to confusion in symptom interpretation, and consequently result in misdiagnosis (9, 22).

Due to the spectrum nature of both disorders, symptoms in the general population grade from clinical pathology to personality traits (1). Self-report measures such as the autism spectrum quotient (AQ) (28) and Schizotypal Personality Questionnaire (SPQ) (29) reliably identify autistic and schizotypal traits, respectively among clinical (3, 4, 6, 30–32) and non-clinical populations (5, 33–35). The AQ contains five subscales that reflect the DSM-IV criteria for autism: social skills, attention to detail, attention switching, communication, and imagination (36). The SPQ provides a measure of schizotypal tendency in accordance with the nine DSM-III-R criteria for schizotypal PD (37). Three superordinate dimensions encapsulate these nine subscales: Ideas of reference, odd beliefs, unusual perceptual experiences, and suspiciousness (cognitive–perceptual/positive); excessive social anxiety, no close friends and constricted affect (interpersonal/negative); odd behavior and odd speech (disorganized) (29, 38). A brief version of the SPQ (SPQ-B) was introduced in 1995 by Raine and Benishay (39) and then revised in 2010 by Cohen et al. (SPQ-BR) (40). Cohen et al. (40) reduced the SPQ to 32-items within seven subscales, uniting Ideas of Reference and Suspiciousness, and No Close Friends and Constricted Affect (40). Despite the obvious benefits of creating a briefer scale, the full-scale SPQ provides a comprehensive measure of schizotypy based on schizotypal PD, unlike the brief versions revised based on non-clinical student samples. Furthermore, in reducing the number of response opportunities, valuable information about the diversity of the schizotypal phenotype may well be missed. The SPQ-BR has only three or four items representing each of the nine criteria for schizotypal PD (40), compared with the seven to nine questions representing the same criteria in the full-scale SPQ (29). This relative paucity of assessment may result in noisier data, likely affecting diagnostic predictive power.

Autistic traits are particularly similar to disorganized (3–6) and interpersonal features of the SPQ (3, 5, 33, 34). Furthermore, Schizotypal tendency, quantified by the SPQ, is significantly higher in autism (3, 6) and Asperger's disorder (4, 5) than in controls, while AQ-measured autistic tendency is higher in schizophrenia (3, 31, 32). The common social–interpersonal dysfunction and communication–disorganization in schizotypal PD and Asperger's disorder may reflect true comorbid symptoms. Alternatively, the apparent co-morbidity could result from a lack of differentiation between distinct symptoms by measurement tools (5).

The diametric model argues that positive or cognitive–perceptual features are opposed to the social aspects of autism (3, 5, 33–35). The AQ's imagination subscale quantifies a rigidity of thought and convergent thinking, which is in contrast with the fluidity of thought characterizing schizophrenia (5, 41). Crespi and Badcock (2) suggested that social–cognitive dysfunction in autism is diametric to that in schizophrenia. Specifically, that social–cognitive dysfunction is under-developed in autism and over-developed in schizotypy (leading to hyper-developed theory of mind). Nevertheless, positive schizotypal features remain stronger in autism than controls (6, 35), and paranoid thinking in autism and schizophrenia may be a subsequent consequence of social–communication misperceptions (11). Furthermore, SPQ unusual perceptual experiences and Odd behavior's mimic AQ predictors of abnormal sensory responses and restrictive/repetitive behaviors, respectively (4). Altogether, the core social dysfunction, with evidence of broad trait similarities provides support for a shared schizoid phenotype in autism and schizophrenia spectrum disorders.

Dinsdale et al. (35) supported a shared social and communication dysfunction in autistic and schizotypal tendency, as well as supporting the diametric model of positive schizotypy and autism. The authors ran a principal component analysis (PCA) of combined AQ and SPQ-BR subscales revealing two components. The first component reflected social–communication disinterest, impairment, and abnormalities with predominant contributions from the AQ subscales social skills and communication, and SPQ-BR subscales constricted affect, social anxiety, odd behavior, and ideas of reference. The second component reflected a pattern of diametric social autism and positive schizotypy. Substantial contributions from SPQ-BR subscales Odd beliefs and unusual perceptions loaded positively and AQ subscales of social skills and imagination loaded negatively create an autism-positive schizotypy axis (35). The authors also carried out their own PCA analysis of Wakabayashi et al.'s (34) full-scale SPQ and AQ data (35).

The resulting two-component solution supported their own PCA results, however, differences in subscale contribution to the components suggests that the full-scale SPQ provides a more robust division of subscales than does the brief form. Specifically, attention switching was exclusive to the first component, odd behavior contributed equally to both components, and ideas of reference contributed more substantially to the second component (35). Put simply, in Wakabayashi et al.'s dataset, the first component appears to better represent a social behavioral dysfunction, while the second gives a stronger representation of cognitive–perceptual and disorganized subscales. Overall, the first component from both datasets supports a co-morbidity of traits within the broader social dysfunction phenotype in autistic and schizotypal tendencies, particularly those specific to Asperger's disorder and schizoid PD (35).

It is noteworthy that in these studies, the questionnaires were presented individually on different response scales (AQ: 4-point scale, SPQ-BR: 5-point scale, SPQ: 2-point scale), affecting response specificity and statistical analysis. Furthermore, the total contribution of the components to the total variance in their data was quite low in both datasets, at around 45%. PCA may not be the ideal analysis for this type of data, as it aims to simply reduce a large dataset to a smaller set of components exploring patterns in the data (42). All of the variables variance is included in the PCA, limiting the capacity to identify meaningful underlying constructs, thus, rendering it uninterpretable (43, 44). Factor analysis, on the other hand, can more accurately reveal the underlying constructs as only the variance that is shared among the variables is analyzed (42, 45). Factor analysis is recommended when there is a theoretical basis for a conceptual relationship between the variables (43), thus, this study will adopt factor analysis as the preferred method, and PCA simply to compare with Dinsdale et al. (35).

Co-morbidity between the disorders is seen at a clinical level. Solomon et al. (7) found that 20% of their high risk and first episode schizophrenia participants also met the criteria for autism. Waris et al. (8) identified pervasive developmental disorder (PDD – the diagnostic category in which ASD lies) in 10 of 18 adolescents with schizophrenia, and Rapoport et al. (46) found 20–30% of children with schizophrenia had prodromal and comorbid PDD, and expressive and receptive language deficits. Also, stress-induced behavior in autism can be additionally or misdiagnosed as schizophrenia (47, 48). These studies give evidence of the risk of incorrect behavioral assessment in autism and schizophrenia. Children with Asperger's were indistinguishable from "loner" (parent rated schizoid personality traits) children on a schizoid scale (49) suggesting potential misclassification of schizoid PD as Asperger's disorder due to comorbid schizoid trait in "loner" and Asperger's children. Schizoid PD, until its removal, was differentiated from schizotypal PD in its lacking positive symptom, identical to the distinction of autism from schizotypal PD (12). Misdiagnosis must be avoided in order to eliminate wrongly prescribed psychopharmacological medications, which may have limited success, instead exposing patients to potentially harmful side effects.

The argument for a shared phenotype is further reinforced by genetic and neuroimaging studies, providing an objective link between the disorders. Genome-wide association studies have found genetic overlap in copy number variants between schizophrenia and autism, suggesting similar processes in the development and regulation of synaptic transmission that influence common biological pathways in the two disorders (50). The heritability within and between autism (2, 50, 51) and schizophrenia (2, 10, 12, 50, 52) evidences a common biological foundation between the disorders (46, 50, 53, 54). Furthermore, schizoid traits are more likely in parents of children with autism (55), and parents of children with autism more likely to have a history of a mental disorder, particularly schizophrenia, than control parents (56). Similar social–cognitive neural dysfunction in conjunction with genetic associations further supports the schizoid phenotype as a link between autism and schizophrenia. Altogether, these studies underline adverse implications in the subjective nature of the DSM clinical classification process (50, 57).

Neuroimaging studies directly comparing autism and schizophrenia identify a neural network related to social cognition (18, 58) and other functional and structural similarities (19, 22, 58–62). Gray matter reduction around the STS and limbic-striato-thalamic network is associated with the degree of autistic tendency in schizophrenia and autism (31, 59, 61, 62). Metabolite similarities, such as glutamate, glutamine, gamma-aminobutyric acid (GABA), and *N*-acetylaspartylglutamic acid (NAAG) are related to negative symptoms of schizophrenia (63, 64) and autism (65), and have also been associated with social–cognitive dysfunction in both disorders [see Rossignol for a review (65, 66)]. On the other hand, reduced *N*-acetylaspartyl acid (NAA) has been associated with more severe symptoms in schizophrenia, particularly positive symptoms (64, 67) and reduced social functioning, but not negative symptoms alone (67). Reductions in NAA have also been identified in autism (65, 68), suggesting a common neurotransmitter link between the spectrum disorders and opposing the argument for diametric disorders.

To our knowledge, no previous study has explored the factor structure of a combined, pseudo-randomized version of the original SPQ and AQ (ASQ). Items were presented on a four-point Likert to reduce response bias and yield more reliable participant reports (69). The aim of this study was to extend Dinsdale et al.'s findings via a PCA of the complete ASQ followed by factor analysis in order to identify the underlying constructs (43–45). Furthermore, the study aimed to uncover a more robust phenotypic model for autism and schizophrenia spectrum disorders at a trait level, with particular interest in the schizoid phenotype. It was expected that, as with Dinsdale et al. (35), the ASQ PCA would reveal a factor specific to social AQ (social skills, communication, and attention switching) and Interpersonal SPQ (no close friends, constricted affect, and social anxiety), reflecting schizoid PD. In using only the shared variance in the model, and allowing the resulting factors to correlate, this research explored how cognitive–perceptual subscales (ideas of reference, odd beliefs, unusual perceptual experiences, and suspiciousness) contributed to the model. It was expected that the disorganization subscales would contribute across factors, as these traits are related to both social AQ and interpersonal and cognitive–perceptual dysfunction. In terms of the factor analysis, we expected that a similar model structure would emerge, but that this would provide a more robust model of the underling constructs within autistic and schizotypal traits. Furthermore, we predicted a strong relationship between the interpersonal dimension of the SPQ and AQ social subscales: social skills, attention switching, and communication.

MATERIALS AND METHODS

PARTICIPANTS

Participants were sourced through social media and advertisements targeting the general population. A total of 449 adults aged between 18 and 40 years, 162 males (mean = 24.20, SD = 4.92) and 287 female (mean = 23.08, SD = 5.01), volunteered for the study, accessing and completing a combined questionnaire online. On average males were older than females [one-way ANOVA, $F(1,448) = 5.22$, $p < 0.05$]. The Swinburne University Human Research Ethics Committee approved the collection of participant data; informed consent was obtained from each participant prior to completing the questionnaire.

MATERIALS

Autistic tendency was measured with Baron-Cohen et al.'s (28) AQ comprising 50 items within five subscales: social skills, attention switching, attention to detail, communication, and imagination. Schizotypal tendency was quantified using Raine's (29) 74-item SPQ. The SPQ has nine subscales in accordance with the DSM III-R diagnostic criteria of schizotypal PD, which represent the three core criteria of schizophrenia: cognitive–perceptual (ideas of reference, odd beliefs, unusual perceptual experiences, and suspiciousness), interpersonal (social anxiety, no close friends, and constricted affect), and disorganized (odd behavior and odd speech) (12, 29, 36, 38). Including the full-scale SPQ provided a richer schizotypal trait dataset, while also allowing the extraction of the 32-items that create the SPQ-BR. Subsequently, comparisons against both Dinsdale et al.'s and Wakabayashi et al.'s findings were made (35). Furthermore, we were able to identify any potential confounds of the SPQ-BR, as highlighted previously in relation to the PCA of Wakabayashi et al.'s data (34) conducted by Dinsdale et al. (35).

The original dichotomous "yes/no" response format of the SPQ raises concerns over trait insensitivity and social desirability response bias (70). A Likert scale design has been shown to improve internal reliability and convergence of the SPQ (70) and consequently this study employed a 4-point Likert scale to align with the AQ. Thus, creating a cohesive set of items that was not particularly associated with either questionnaire. The AQ and SPQ items were then combined, pseudo-randomized, and presented online with Opinio (71). Participant responses to combined AQ and SPQ (ASQ) items ranged from 1: "strongly agree," to 4: "strongly disagree." In broadening the response options from yes/no (2-point), and removing the "neutral" option in the 5-point scale, the opportunity for respondents to make a conservative response to potentially socially undesirable questions is reduced. There was acceptable internal consistency for SPQ total ($\alpha = 0.86$) and its superordinate subscales (cognitive–perceptual $\alpha = 0.77$; interpersonal $\alpha = 0.77$; disorganized $\alpha = 0.69$), AQ total ($\alpha = 0.66$), and ASQ total ($\alpha = 0.88$).

PROCEDURE

Participants volunteered to complete the online ASQ through the Opinio website (71). Raw ASQ item scores were converted to zero (0) for an unendorsed response ("strongly disagree" or "disagree") and one (1) for an endorsed response ("strongly agree" or "agree"). AQ and SPQ items were then extracted from the combined questionnaire to obtain conventional AQ (/50) and SPQ (/74) scores. Participants' individual subscale and total scores were entered into SPSS Version 20.0 for statistical analysis (72).

DATA ANALYSIS

An initial one-way analysis of variance (ANOVA) for gender differences in total AQ and SPQ score was performed. Pearson correlations were obtained within and between AQ and SPQ total and individual subscale scores.

As previously discussed, dimension reduction with PCA is not ideal for data that is interrelated. Therefore, factor analysis was the primary technique in this study. In order to directly compare these data with Dinsdale et al. (35), a PCA including all nine SPQ and five AQ subscales was also conducted. The 32-items of the SPQ-BR were then extracted and a PCA with the seven SPQ-BR and five AQ subscales was conducted (35, 40). Finally, the full-scale ASQ was subjected to a factor analysis with maximum likelihood estimation. Due to the well-reported relationship between AQ and SPQ subscales, there were reasonable theoretical grounds to conduct an oblique (direct oblimin) rotation, taking into account the relationship between the factors (43). The sampling adequacy (Kaiser–Meyer–Olkin measure – KMO) of the data was found to be suitable for each analysis (AQ: KMO = 0.670; SPQ: KMO = 0.887; ASQ: KMO = 0.894; ASBQ: KMO = 0.843). Correlations between the subscales were adequate for factor analysis with Bartlett's test of sphericity significant for AQ [$\chi(10) = 387.9$, $p < 0.001$], SPQ [$\chi(36) = 1610.1$, $p < 0.001$], ASQ [$\chi(91) = 2582.3$, $p < 0.001$], and ASBQ [$\chi(66) = 1417.6$, $p < 0.001$] (43). Factors/components with Eigenvalues >1.0 were retained as substantial representations of the variation in the model, and the Scree Plot was used as visual support for the retained factors. Subscale contributions to the model were referred to as "factor loadings" and reflected the strength of the relationship between the factor/component and the subscale. Factor loadings below 0.3 were suppressed in order to report only important factor contributions (43). Pearson correlations were obtained between on the resultant factor analysis factors, total AQ, total SPQ, cognitive–perceptual, interpersonal, and disorganized scores.

RESULTS

The mean AQ and SPQ scores for males and females are shown in **Table 1**. A one-way ANOVA revealed no significant gender effects on mean AQ score [$F(1,448) = 0.557$, $p = 0.456$], however, there was a significant difference in SPQ score [$F(1,448) = 4.71$, $p < 0.05$]. Participant age did not affect AQ ($r = 0.031$, $p = 0.507$) or SPQ ($r = -0.006$, $p = 0.904$) score.

AQ AND SPQ SUBSCALE CORRELATIONS

The correlation matrix in **Table 2**, consisting of total SPQ, total AQ, and all 14 subscales, showed strong correlations between total AQ and total SPQ scores. Each individual subscale was significantly correlated with AQ and SPQ total scores; however, there was only a weak relationship between total AQ and odd beliefs (SPQ), and between total SPQ and imagination (AQ).

Among the individual subscales, the strongest relationships were between social skills (AQ) and communication (AQ) and interpersonal subscales (SPQ): social anxiety, no close friends, and constricted affect. Communication (AQ) also had a robust relationship with the disorganized subscales (SPQ): odd behavior and odd speech. Notably, there were very weak to no relationship detected between imagination (AQ) and all SPQ subscales, and between odd beliefs (SPQ) and all AQ subscales.

COMPONENT AND FACTOR STRUCTURE OF COMBINED AQ AND SPQ (ASQ)

The PCA of the nine SPQ and five AQ subscales is presented in **Table 3** below. The comparison ASQ PCA resulted in a three-component solution. The unique contribution (component loading) of each ASQ subscale to the model was reported in the Pattern Matrix, summarized in **Table 3**. Scores below 0.3 are not shown.

Table 1 | Mean gender difference in AQ and SPQ.

N = 449	N	AQ M (SD)	Min	Max	SPQ M (SD)	Min	Max
Male	162	17.6(6.8)	1	36	24.6(12.6)	2	65
Female	287	17.1(6.6)	1	35	21.8(12.8)	2	61

AQ, autism spectrum quotient; SPQ, schizotypal personality questionnaire; M, mean; SD, standard deviation.

Table 3 illustrates clear overlap of AQ and SPQ subscales, particularly in component 1, which included disorganized (odd behavior and odd speech), interpersonal (no close friends, constricted affect, and social anxiety), cognitive–perceptual (suspiciousness ideas of reference and unusual perceptual experiences) and AQ (communication, social skills, and attention switching) subscales. Component 2 was loaded with imagination, attention to detail, and social skills of the AQ. Finally, component 3 comprised of cognitive–perceptual subscales odd beliefs, unusual perceptual experiences, and ideas of reference, as well as attention to detail from the AQ.

The factor analysis of the ASQ, with an oblimin rotation, resulted in a three-factor solution. The pattern and structure matrix are presented in **Table 4**. The pattern matrix reports the regression coefficient for each subscale on each factor, that is, the unique contribution that each subscale has to each factor. The structure matrix on the other hand, reports the correlation coefficient between the subscale and factor, thus the factor loading of each subscale takes into account the relationship between factors.

Table 4 illustrates the clear overlap found between AQ and SPQ subscales, particularly in Factor 1. AQ subscales (communication, social skills, and attention switching) and all SPQ subscales but odd beliefs (cognitive–perceptual) loaded on Factor 1. Factor 1 will be referred to as *Social Disorganization*. Factor 2 comprised cognitive-perceptual subscales odd beliefs, unusual perceptual experiences, and ideas of reference, as well as attention to detail from the AQ, with weak contributions from suspiciousness and odd speech. These factor loadings suggest intrinsic attributes that lead to unusual perceptions, speech and behaviors, and hereafter, Factor

Table 2 | Correlation matrix for total AQ, total SPQ, and individual subscales.

	1	2	3	4	5	6	7	8	9	10	11	12	13	14	15
Social skill															
Communication	0.501														
Attention switching	0.38**	0.41**													
Attention to detail	0.40**	0.12*	0.06												
Imagination	0.34**	0.19**	0.11**	0.29**											
AQ total	0.89**	0.67**	0.63**	0.58**	0.55**										
Ideas of ref	0.33**	0.41**	0.42**	0.16**	0.03	0.43**									
Odd beliefs	0.09	0.04	0.07	0.31**	0.03	0.17**	0.40**								
Unusual perceptual exp	0.21**	0.38**	0.34**	0.18**	−0.08	0.33**	0.56**	0.41**							
Suspiciousness	0.38**	0.42**	0.44**	0.21**	0.08	0.48**	0.63**	0.26**	0.47**						
Social anxiety	0.54**	0.50**	0.44**	0.23**	0.11*	0.57**	0.46**	0.13*	0.34**	0.45**					
No close friends	0.58**	0.48**	0.41**	0.23**	0.18*	0.58**	0.46**	0.07*	0.34**	0.51**	0.55**				
Constrict affect	0.52**	0.50**	0.32**	0.29**	0.22**	0.57**	0.38**	0.05	0.30**	0.42**	0.46**	0.62**			
Odd behavior	0.35**	0.52**	0.40**	0.08**	0.07	0.44**	0.47**	0.14*	0.42**	0.42**	0.36**	0.51**	0.45**		
Odd speech	0.31**	0.48**	0.32**	0.25**	0.10*	0.46**	0.52**	0.22**	0.50**	0.51**	0.36**	0.48**	0.50**	0.53**	
Total SPQ	0.54**	0.61**	0.52**	0.30**	0.12*	0.65**	0.79**	0.39**	0.69**	0.76**	0.68**	0.75**	0.70**	0.70**	0.75**

$^{*}p < 0.05$, $^{**}p < 0.001$.

Table 3 | Principal component analysis of combined AQ and SPQ subscales.

	Component 1	Component 2	Component 3
Communication	0.785		
No close friends	0.782		
Odd behavior	0.740		
Constricted affect	0.697		
Social anxiety	0.691		
Attention switching	0.683		
Suspiciousness	0.628		
Odd speech	0.625		
Ideas of reference	0.593		0.458
Social skill	0.592	0.512	
Attention to detail		0.744	0.446
Imagination		0.724	
Odd beliefs			0.884
Unusual perceptual experience	0.454		0.563
Eigenvalues	5.650	1.574	1.332
Variance explained	40.4%	11.2%	9.5%
Rotation sum of square	5.39	1.80	2.23
Total variance	61.1%		

Subscale: SPQ: *AQ:*

Table 4 | Factor analysis pattern and structure matrix of combined AQ and SPQ subscales.

	Pattern matrix			Structure matrix		
	F1	F2	F3	F1	F2	F3
No close friends	0.738			0.757		0.375
Communication	0.721			0.700		
Odd behavior	0.713			0.679		
Ideas of reference	0.648	0.376		0.701	0.528	
Suspiciousness	0.643			0.691	0.385	
Constricted affect	0.641			0.679		0.413
Odd speech	0.633			0.671	0.332	
Social anxiety	0.623			0.663		0.337
Attention switching	0.605			0.582		
Unusual perceptual experience	0.512	0.438		0.572	0.560	
Odd beliefs		0.721			0.716	
Attention to detail		0.361	0.664		0.330	0.642
Social skill	0.509		0.512	0.620		0.651
Imagination			0.458			0.473
Eigenvalues	5.181	1.091	0.828			
Variance explained	37.0%	7.8%	5.9%			
Rotation sum of square	5.005	1.527	1.605			
Rotation variance explained	30.0%	10.9%	9.8%			
Total variance	50.7%					

Subscale: SPQ: *AQ:* *F, factor.*

2 will be referred to as *Perceptual Oddities*. Factor 3 was loaded with imagination, attention to detail, and social skills of the AQ, with weaker contributions from constricted affect to social anxiety. Factor 3 will be referred to as *Social Rigidity*. In the subsequent discussions, the structure matrix is referred due to its representation of the relationship between the factors. It is important to note that the ASQ PCA component 2 and component 3 subscales in **Table 3** were opposite to ASQ factor analysis Factor 2 and Factor 3 subscales in **Table 4**.

The distribution of factor scores across 449 participants can be visualized easily via a RGB color additive model, where red represents Factor 1 (*Social Rigidity*), blue represents Factor 2 (*Perceptual Oddities*), and green represents Factor 3 (*Social Disorganization*) (see **Figure 1**). While individual differences in factor scores can be discerned, so can the general correlation between AQ and SPQ scores. Relative to the regression line, diametric tendencies are clearly observed with green/blue shadings to the bottom right and pink/purple/brown shades to the upper left.

Figure 1 is a visual representation of the relationship between SPQ and AQ scores for the 449 participants. The overall correlation between scores is evident through the main trend of the data points. The colors in the plot represent how each participant scored on the three factors of the Factor Analysis. It is clear that those with more *Social Rigidity* scored higher on total AQ and

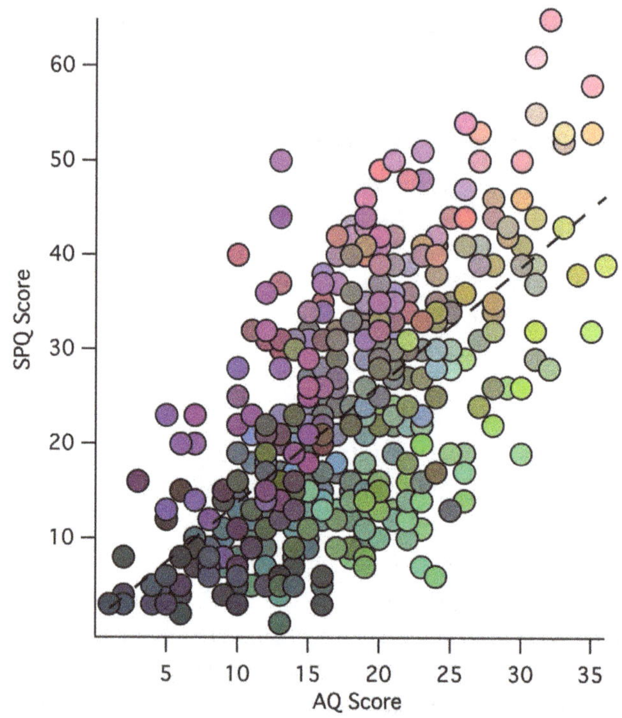

FIGURE 1 | Scatter plot of participant total SPQ vs. AQ scores: weightings of each participant's three-factor model scores is indicated by an RGB color model (scaled for each factor), where red represents Factor 1, blue represents Factor 2, and green represents Factor 3 (with the same scaling of factor values to color values for each factor). Thus, the low scores in both AQ and SPQ toward the origin tend to be shaded gray, while the extreme AQ and SPQ scores are more illuminant.

lower on total SPQ. Similarly, those with more *Perceptual Oddities* had higher total SPQ and lower total AQ. Shared *Social Disorganization* is seen along the line of best fit and into higher SPQ reflecting a relationship between the factors, and supporting the overall relationship between autism and schizophrenia spectrum disorders.

COMPARING THE PCA STRUCTURES OF THE ASQ AND ASBQ

To directly compare with Dinsdale et al. (35), we replicated the AQ and SPQ-BR subscales (ASBQ) and ran a PCA. A three-component solution was revealed, similar to our full-scale ASQ PCA, which explained 56.15% of the variance. However, there were some differences between the models (see Table S1 in Supplementary Material). The most significant change in the component structure from the ASQ to the ASBQ was the transfer of subscales no close friends and constricted affect from the ASQ component 1 to ASBQ component 2. In restricting these two subscales to one no close friends/constricted affect subscale, it fell in line with AQ subscales attention to detail, imagination, and social skills. Furthermore, social skills contributed more to component 2 than component 1 in the ASBQ compared to the ASQ PCA.

QUESTIONNAIRE AND FACTOR CORRELATIONS

Pearson correlations between participant scores on the three factors (*Social Desirability, Perceptual Oddities, and Social Rigidity*), total AQ, total SPQ, and the SPQ dimensions are shown in **Table 5**.

Strong correlations were evident between *Social Disorganization,* and AQ and all SPQ dimensions. There were strong correlations between *Perceptual Oddities,* and SPQ total and cognitive–perceptual subscales, this relationship was weak for total AQ. Finally, there was a strong correlation between *Social Rigidity* and total AQ, but weak for total SPQ. There was a weak positive relationship between *Social Disorganization,* and *Perceptual Oddities* and *Social Rigidity,* with no relationship present between *Perceptual Oddities* and *Social Rigidity.*

Table 5 | AQ and SPQ correlations with factor analysis factors.

	Social desirability	Perceptual oddities	Social rigidity
Total AQ	0.75**	0.15**	0.76**
Total SPQ	0.96**	0.51**	0.30**
Interpersonal	0.75**	0.08	0.42**
Cognitive–perceptual	0.66**	0.64**	0.08
Disorganized	0.62**	0.16*	0.07
Social desirability	–	0.3*	0.35*
Perceptual oddities	0.3*	–	−0.03
Social rigidity	0.35*	−0.03	–

*$p < 0.05$, **$p < 0.001$.

DISCUSSION

This study was the first to investigate the contributions of autistic and schizotypal traits through a combined, randomized autism schizotypal questionnaire (ASQ). We revealed a robust three-factor solution, as opposed to Dinsdale et al.'s (35) two-components, in the analysis of only shared variance between the subscales. The correlation and factor analyses provided face value support for a shared fundamental phenotype in autism and schizophrenia spectrum disorders; *Social Disorganization* (3, 5, 34, 35). Further, they exposed independent positive schizotypy and autistic rigidity phenotypes. This evidence brings to light an important question: does the relationship between autistic and schizotypal scores result from a common phenotype, or is it due simply to a lack of differentiation between distinct symptoms by measurement tools?

As expected, the first factor, *Social Disorganization,* supported a comorbid social–cognitive dysfunction central to autism and schizophrenia spectrum disorders (5, 16–19, 35). *Social Disorganization* included social AQ and all SPQ subscales but odd beliefs, explaining the majority of the variation in the subscale scores. The autism and schizophrenia spectra are presented in current diagnostic tools as completely separate disorders. Therefore, diagnosis relies on the subjective interpretation of symptoms that are specific to autism and schizophrenia spectrum disorders, excluding the shared phenotype. Clearly, relying on subjective symptom assessment risks confusion and misinterpretation, potentially leading to misdiagnosis and mistreatment of symptoms. The trait combination of the *Social Disorganization* factor is reminiscent of schizoid PD, defined by the DSM-IV-TR (12) as exclusively negative schizotypy (prior to its removal from the DSM-5). Core features of schizoid PD are fundamental to the pervasive social dysfunction in autism; lack of interest in, and active avoidance of social situations both in occupation and daily life, restricted affect and empathy, odd communication, and relationship detachment, as well as rigid pursuit of personal interests (12–14). Schizoid PD may be the conceptual or phenotypic link between autism and schizophrenia spectrum disorders, with impairments in empathy, communication oddities, social isolation, and mental rigidity some of the common central features (13, 14). Social anhedonia is another core feature of schizoid PD (24, 25, 73), the negative aspects of schizotypal PD (24, 25) and autism (26), which is characterized by atypical interpersonal behaviors. Collins et al. (24) found that social anhedonics have significantly higher scores on schizoid scales than controls; however, social anhedonics do not differ in level of schizotypy. This relationship suggests that the schizoid phenotype provides a more accurate representation of social anhedonia than does schizotypy (24). *Social Disorganization* appears to reflect the schizoid phenotype as a combination of social autistic and Interpersonal schizotypal tendencies. With the addition of disorganization in speech and behavior, *Social Disorganization* links the two spectrum disorders and raises cause for concern over the accuracy of current diagnostic processes.

Disorganized subscales of the SPQ were a substantial contributor to the *Social Disorganization* factor. Disorganization was not a specific criterion for schizoid PD; however, SPQ Disorganized subscales have explained a substantial amount of variance in the AQ, particularly in communication (5, 14) and motor behavior (14). Pervasive interpersonal dysfunction leads to disorganization in speech and behavior, which manifests in the social environment. This indirect effect provides an explanation for the role of disorganized subscales in the first factor. In addition to disorganization, cognitive–perceptual subscales contributed to the first factor, supporting broad shared traits between the disorders (3, 11, 33–35).

In both autism and schizophrenia, environmental interpretation plays an integral role in the individual's experience. Specifically, the misinterpretation of environmental stimuli is evident in both spectra and can be quantified with the SPQ subscale unusual perceptual experience, which has been found to mimic AQ predictors of abnormal sensory responses (4). Furthermore, schizoid individuals report more fantasy and heightened sensitivity experiences (14), explaining its role in the shared *Social Disorganization* factor.

The strength of the relationship between the AQ, and interpersonal and disorganized SPQ subscales, and weak relationship with cognitive–perceptual subscales, further support the underlying schizoid phenotype. These data suggest that the interpersonal and social AQ subscales scores are a reflection of each other, not differential measures of separate traits. Altogether, the correlations demonstrated a clear common *Social Disorganization* that links the two spectra, which can be defined in terms of schizoid PD.

The exclusion of schizoid PD from the DSM 5 was a consequence of little empirical research resulting in only 1% reported pathological prevalence of the disorder (13, 74). Although the diagnosis has been removed, the schizoid phenotype remains a distinct cluster of symptoms (75). The diagnostic exclusion criteria for schizoid PD; independence from schizophrenia, mood disorder with psychotic features, psychotic disorder, and pervasive developmental disorder, may have contributed to its removal from the DSM 5 (12). The very nature of the schizoid phenotype suggests that affected individuals may carry out a life that suits their social preference. Thus, seeking clinical intervention due to increasing symptom severity that is in line with more severe schizophrenia or autism spectrum pathology (13). Although schizoid PD tends to be more stable than schizotypal PD, schizoid symptoms can be prodromal to schizotypal PD, which in turn can be prodromal to more severe schizophrenia spectrum disorders (13, 14). A child presenting with profound negative symptoms (abnormal social interaction and interpersonal skills, lack of eye contact, impoverished language, and restricted range of thought and cognition) may be assigned a diagnosis of autism rather than child-onset schizoid PD, or alternate schizophrenia spectrum disorders. Furthermore, an additional schizophrenia diagnosis to pre-existing autism is possible should odd language and behavior be misinterpreted (47, 48). A diagnosis of autism relies on the individual's developmental history, and disclosure of this information could be difficult as it depends largely on the mental health of the parent (47). Relying on relatives to provide clinical information can be difficult due to the genetic association between the disorders. Schizoid, paranoid, and schizotypal PDs are more likely in relatives of schizophrenia and ASDs (12, 55). The mental health history of relatives may also lead to the symptoms classification that is in line with genetic predictions. The risk of misdiagnosis due to misinterpretation of social and communication dysfunction is accentuated by the removal of schizoid PD, incorporation of Asperger's disorder into autism, and removal of stringent age of onset and language development delay criteria in autism (10). These changes increase the variability and ambiguity in differentiating autism and schizophrenia spectrum disorders, thereby increasing diagnostic and therapeutic risks.

The second factor, *Perceptual Oddities*, separated the positive dimension of the schizophrenia spectrum from the shared *Social Disorganization* phenotype. After the relationship between the factors was taken into account, strongest contributions to this factor were from cognitive–perceptual SPQ subscales odd beliefs, unusual perceptions, ideas of reference, and weak suspiciousness. This factor provided some support for Dinsdale et al.'s (35) second component, however, with the absence of autistic subscales in the negative direction their autism-positive schizotypy axis was not supported. Disorganized odd speech loaded weakly also, adding weight to the argument of a differential schizotypal construct. Interestingly, attention to detail had a moderate contribution to *Perceptual Oddities*, as in Dinsdale et al. (35). Cognitive–perceptual features have been found to explain a substantial proportion of the variance in Attention to Detail (5), and those scoring highly may be particularly analytical of details leading to an over-interpretation of reality. Odd beliefs were the strongest contributor to *Perceptual Oddities*, and had no contribution to any other factor. Dinsdale et al. (35) found odd beliefs to be the most significant contributor to their second diametric component, suggesting that this trait may play a key role in the differentiation between autistic and schizotypal tendency. Suspiciousness, however, was not an influential predictor of *Perceptual Oddities*. Instead suspiciousness loaded substantially on the shared factor, *Social Disorganization*. The relationship between suspiciousness and *Social Disorganization* may be explained by the continual social distress, insecurities, and anxiety that lead to increased suspiciousness in children with autism, which remain to adulthood (4). The strength of the relationship between *Perceptual Oddities* and cognitive–perceptual subscales, but not total AQ, interpersonal and disorganized subscales, suggested this phenotype was specific to psychosis.

Together, the AQ subscales imagination, attention to detail, and social skills made up the third factor, *Social Rigidity*, which was exclusively autistic until the correlation between factors was taken into account. The factor correlations revealed a contribution, although weak, from all interpersonal subscales. *Social Rigidity* reflected the rigidity of thought, restricted, and repetitive behaviors, and social dysfunction that are key criteria for ASDs. This phenotypic construct was not found in Dinsdale et al.'s (35) restricted analysis. The AQ subscale imagination was only a moderate contributor to the *Social Rigidity* factor and had weak correlations across all subscales. This finding opposed the diametric model for rigidity of thought in autism and fluidity of thought in schizophrenia, as imagination was not diametric to AQ subscales (2, 5). Individuals with schizophrenia, as well as those with autism, report higher rigidity of thought as measured by imagination than controls (3, 32). This is perhaps a result of a deficit in the active control of imaginative thought in schizophrenia, while representing a lack of diversity in imagination in autism (3). Wolff et al. (14) reported high levels of fantasy in schizoid participants, but also rigidity of mental set, symptoms that are seen in schizophrenia and autism, respectively. Altogether, these imagination traits were highly reported across spectrum groups, but tap into differential thought processes, questions the specificity of the imagination subscale (32). Dinsdale et al.'s (35) data did not produce this autism-specific component, nor did their analysis of Wakabayashi et al.'s data. Instead, the autism-specific subscales loaded negatively against positive schizotypy subscales in a diametric second component, implications of which will be discussed below. *Social Rigidity* had a strong relationship with total AQ, but a weak relationship with total SPQ and its three dimensions, thus represented more classically autistic features.

Our restricted ASBQ PCA, conducted to contrast with Dinsdale et al. (35) and factor analysis as a data reduction technique, revealed some observable differences to the ASQ PCA. First, our PCA's second and third components are in reverse to those of our factor analysis. Second, the combined and restricted constricted affect/no close friends subscale shifted from component 1 in the ASQ PCA, to component 2 in the ASBQ PCA. This shift renders the subscale more "autistic" and thereby reduces its distinction between autistic tendency and negative schizotypy. Third, the ASBQ third component was almost exclusively loaded with odd beliefs, suggesting that odd beliefs are a separate phenotype of schizotypy in the restricted model. Odd beliefs are culturally and sample sensitive (5, 12), thus it is important to specify that these data were taken from an Australian population, while Dinsdale et al. (35) took their sample from Canadian Undergraduate students. Fourth, The AQ subscale attention to detail was strongly loaded on the second component for both ASQ and ASBQ models as a diagnostically specific autistic trait. However, Dinsdale et al. (35) suggested that attention to detail represents an independent dimension of autism, as the subscale did not contribute to either component in their restricted model. Finally, the ASBQ subscales explained less of the model variance than did the ASQ. This was particularly true of Component 1, providing further support that the full-scale questionnaire is a more comprehensive assessment of autistic and schizotypal traits. Due to the differences in dimension reduction process between PCA (using unique plus shared variance) and factor analysis (only shared variance), the factor analysis subscales explained slightly less of the total variation than the subscales in PCA extraction (42, 43, 45). While PCA is a suitable tool for analyzing datasets without *a priori* assumptions about the existence of underlying constructs, we argue that the use of factor analysis here was a superior method for this type of dataset, as it exposes underlying constructs in autistic and schizotypal tendency (42, 43, 45). Thus, the three-factor model was clearly a more accurate representation of shared and differential traits.

Dinsdale et al. (35) identified a shared social–communication disinterest, impairment, and abnormality despite their use of the SPQ-BR and PCA technique. This indicates that the common *Social Disorganization* phenotype is robust across instruments. However, we argue that the full-scale ASQ factor structure provides a more comprehensive representation of autistic and schizotypal tendency, as it more accurately reflects the underlying constructs that characterize the two spectra. Furthermore, the *Perceptual Oddities* and *Social Rigidity* phenotypes were somewhat unrelated, rather than diametric. Thus, these findings provide evidence against the diametric model of autism and schizophrenia (3, 5, 33, 34) and Dinsdale et al.'s (35) diametric autism-positive schizotypy axis. The underlying constructs identified in this study supported literature reporting positive schizophrenia symptoms in autism, and autistic symptoms in schizophrenia (4, 6, 11, 33, 34). The ASQ has shown a clear separation of disorder specific traits, thus may be a useful tool for distinguishing autistic and schizotypal tendency that could be validated in the clinical setting. However, the ASBQ also extracted three factors, suggesting that it is not merely the use of the full-scale instrument that exposes the differential factors.

The inclusion of a "neutral" response option in the SPQ-BR presented by Dinsdale et al. (35) creates noise in the data that may have resulted in their diametric second component. Forcing an affirmative or negative response, as in our 4-point scale, provided better discriminant value than a scale with a "neutral" response. Furthermore, it would expose those that tend to respond in a socially desirable manner despite possessing certain trait. Wakabayashi et al. (34) presented their questionnaires separately in their original form, with the SPQ in a "yes/no" forced choice format. With only two response options and the absence of reverse scored items in the SPQ, a bias to a socially desirable "no" response is possible. Moreover, a Likert scale design has been shown to improve internal reliability and convergence of the SPQ (70). In combining the AQ and SPQ, reverse scored items are included and all items are presented on a 4-point Likert scale with the neutral response option removed, thus response bias is reduced. Consequently, these data better represented the relationship between autistic and schizotypal tendency. The self-report nature of these results provided an individual's perspective of their own behavior and personal interests, but may be subjected to social desirability bias. The response quality does however reflect a very personal representation to an individual's thoughts, feelings, and behaviors, perhaps providing a richer response quality than clinically observed behaviors. However, it is possible that retaining 4-point scale in the scores may improve the item-by-item correlations and consequently the reliability and factor analysis (76).

Altogether, with the evident confusion in behavioral overlap between social AQ and interpersonal SPQ at a trait level, which reflects schizoid PD, there is a risk of misdiagnosis in clinical settings. These data highlight the need for care in diagnostic and research settings involving the two spectra, particularly in the recruitment of accurate and distinct sample groups to avoid unbiased conclusions. As imaging research continues to identify neuromarkers specific to social–cognitive function (2, 18, 31), the search for differential neuromarkers to separate social–cognitive dysfunction that distinguish autistic and schizophrenia spectrum disorders is imperative (2, 18, 22). However, in light of the similarity in behavioral phenotypes, researchers must be vigilant to ensure exclusion of possible co-morbidities and misdiagnoses within the participant sample (1, 8, 22). Ultimately, neuromarkers are likely to provide an efficient and effective means for intervention, diagnosis and treatment development (1).

In conclusion, we presented robust evidence for a shared *Social Disorganization* phenotype in autistic and schizotypal tendency that resembles schizoid PD. In addition, we revealed discriminating factors of *Social Rigidity* and *Perceptual Oddities* that represented a specific phenotype in autistic and schizotypal tendency, respectively. This is in contrast to Dinsdale et al.'s (35) diametric component. We suggest that these discriminating factors be validated and applied in neuroimaging studies to identify neuromarkers associated with these factors. The identification of neuromarkers that differentiate autistic and schizotypal traits may ultimately lead to an objective diagnostic tool. This in turn may prevent misdiagnosis arising from the misinterpretation of shared phenotypes.

ACKNOWLEDGMENTS

The researchers acknowledge project grant support (APP1004740) by the National Health and Medical Research Council of Australia.

REFERENCES

1. Nylander L, Lugnegard T, Hallerbačk MU. Autism spectrum disorders and schizophrenia spectrum disorders in adults – is there a connection? A literature review and some suggestions for future clinical research. *Clin Neuropsychiatry* (2008) **5**(1):43–54.
2. Crespi B, Badcock C. Psychosis and autism as diametrical disorders of the social brain. *Behav Brain Sci* (2008) **31**(3):241–61. doi:10.1017/S0140525X08004214
3. Spek AA, Wouters SGM. Autism and schizophrenia in high functioning adults: behavioral differences and overlap. *Res Autism Spectr Disord* (2010) **4**:709–17. doi:10.1016/j.rasd.2010.01.009
4. Kanai C, Iwanami A, Ota H, Yamasue H, Matsushima E, Yokoi H, et al. Clinical characteristics of adults with Asperger's syndrome assessed with self-report questionnaires. *Res Autism Spectr Disord* (2011) **5**(1):185–90. doi:10.1016/j.rasd.2010.03.008
5. Hurst RM, Nelson-Gray RO, Mitchell JT, Kwapil TR. The relationship of Asperger's characteristics and schizotypal personality traits in a non-clinical adult sample. *J Autism Dev Disord* (2007) **37**(9):1711–20. doi:10.1007/s10803-006-0302-z
6. Barneveld PS, Pieterse J, de Sonneville L, van Rijn S, Lahuis B, van Engeland H, et al. Overlap of autistic and schizotypal traits in adolescents with Autism Spectrum Disorders. *Schizophr Res* (2011) **126**(1–3):231–6. doi:10.1016/j.schres.2010.09.004
7. Solomon M, Olsen E, Niendam T, Ragland JD, Yoon J, Minzenberg M, et al. From lumping to splitting and back again: a typical social and language development in individuals with clinical-high-risk for psychosis, first episode schizophrenia, and autism spectrum disorders. *Schizophr Res* (2011) **131**(1–3):146–51. doi:10.1016/j.schres.2011.03.005
8. Waris P, Lindberg N, Kettunen K, Tani P. The relationship between Asperger's syndrome and schizophrenia in adolescence. *Eur Child Adolesc Psychiatry* (2013) **22**(4):217–23. doi:10.1007/s00787-012-0338-x
9. Sheitman B. Are the negative symptoms of schizophrenia consistent with an autistic spectrum illness? *Schizophr Res* (2004) **69**(1):119–20. doi:10.1016/s0920-9964(03)00177-4
10. American Psychological Association. *Diagnostic and Statistical Manual of Mental Disorders.* 5 ed. Washington, DC: American Psychological Association (2013).
11. King BH, Lord C. Is schizophrenia on the autism spectrum? *Brain Res* (2011) **1380**:34–41. doi:10.1016/j.brainres.2010.11.031
12. American Psychological Association. *Diagnostic and Statistical Manual of Mental Disorders.* 4 ed. Washington, DC: American Psychological Association (2000).
13. Esterberg ML, Goulding SM, Walker EF. Cluster A personality disorders: schizotypal, schizoid and paranoid personality disorders in childhood and adolescence. *J Psychopathol Behav* (2010) **32**:515–28. doi:10.1007/s10862-010-9183-8
14. Wolff S, Townshend R, McGuire RJ, Weeks DJ. 'Schizoid' personality in childhood and adult life. II: adult adjustment and the continuity with schizotypal personality disorder. *Br J Psychiatry* (1991) **159**:620–9. doi:10.1192/bjp.159.5.620
15. Kernberg OF. Overview and critique of the classification of personality disorders proposed for DSM-V. *Swiss Arch Neurol Psychiatr* (2012) **163**(7):234–8.
16. Eack SM, Bahorik AL, McKnight SA, Hogarty SS, Greenwald DP, Newhill CE, et al. Commonalities in social and non-social cognitive impairments in adults with autism spectrum disorder and schizophrenia. *Schizophr Res* (2013) **148**:24–48. doi:10.1016/j.schres.2013.05.013
17. Lugnegard T, Unenge Hallerback M, Hjarthag F, Gillberg C. Social cognition impairments in Asperger syndrome and schizophrenia. *Schizophr Res* (2013) **143**(2–3):277–84. doi:10.1016/j.schres.2012.12.001
18. Pinkham AE, Hopfinger JB, Pelphrey KA, Piven J, Penn DL. Neural bases for impaired social cognition in schizophrenia and autism spectrum disorders. *Schizophr Res* (2008) **99**(1–3):164–75. doi:10.1016/j.schres.2007.10.024
19. Sasson N, Tsuchiya N, Hurley R, Couture SM, Penn DL, Adolphs R, et al. Orienting to social stimuli differentiates social cognitive impairment in autism and schizophrenia. *Neuropsychologia* (2007) **45**(11):2580–8. doi:10.1016/j.neuropsychologia.2007.03.009
20. Fett AK, Maat A. Social cognitive impairments and psychotic symptoms: what is the nature of their association? *Schizophr Bull* (2013) **39**(1):77–85. doi:10.1093/schbul/sbr058
21. Derntl B, Habel U. Deficits in social cognition: a marker for psychiatric disorders? *Eur Arch Psychiatry Clin Neurosci* (2011) **261**(Suppl 2):8145–9. doi:10.1007/s00406-011-0244-0
22. Sasson NJ, Pinkham AE, Carpenter KL, Belger A. The benefit of directly comparing autism and schizophrenia for revealing mechanisms of social cognitive impairment. *J Neurodev Disord* (2011) **3**(2):87–100. doi:10.1007/s11689-010-9068-x
23. Brothers L. The social brain: a project for integrating primate behaviour and neurophysiology in a new domain. *Concepts Neurosci* (1990) **1**(1):27–51. doi:10.1093/schbul/sbq012
24. Collins LM, Blanchard JJ, Biondo KM. Behavioral signs of schizoidia and schizotypy in social anhedonics. *Schizophr Res* (2005) **78**(2–3):309–22. doi:10.1016/j.schres.2005.04.021
25. Kwapil TR. Social anhedonia as a predictor of the development of schizophrenia-spectrum disorders. *J Abnorm Psychol* (1998) **107**(4):558–65. doi:10.1037/0021-843X.107.4.558
26. Chevallier C, Grezes J, Molesworth C, Berthoz S, Happe F. Brief report: selective social anhedonia in high functioning autism. *J Autism Dev Disord* (2012) **42**(7):1504–9. doi:10.1007/s10803-011-1364-0
27. Russell-Smith SN, Bayliss DM, Maybery MT. Unique sets of social and mood characteristics differentiate autistic and negative schizotypy traits in a young adult non-clinical sample. *Pers Individ Dif* (2013) **55**:542–6. doi:10.1016/j.paid.2013.04.030
28. Baron-Cohen S, Wheelwright S, Skinner R, Martin J, Clubley E. The autism-spectrum quotient (AQ): evidence from Asperger syndrome/high-functioning autism, males and females, scientists and mathematicians. *J Autism Dev Disord* (2001) **31**(1):5–17. doi:10.1023/A:1005653411471
29. Raine A. The SPQ: a scale for the assessment of schizotypal personality based on DSM-III-R criteria. *Schizophr Bull* (1991) **17**(4):555–64. doi:10.1093/schbul/17.4.555
30. Naito K, Matsui Y, Maeda K, Tanaka K. Evaluation of the validity of the autism spectrum quotient (AQ) in differentiating high-functioning autistic spectrum disorder from schizophrenia. *Kobe J Med Sci* (2010) **56**(3):116–24.
31. Sasamoto A, Miyata J, Hirao K, Fujiwara H, Kawada R, Fujimoto S, et al. Social impairment in schizophrenia revealed by autism-spectrum quotient correlated with gray matter reduction. *Soc Neurosci* (2011) **6**(5–6):548–58. doi:10.1080/17470919.2011.575693
32. Wouters SGM, Spek AA. The use of the autism-spectrum quotient in differentiating high-functioning adults with autism, adults with schizophrenia and a neurotypical adult control group. *Res Autism Spectr Disord* (2011) **5**(3):1169–75. doi:10.1016/j.rasd.2011.01.002
33. Russell-Smith SN, Maybery MT, Bayliss DM. Relationships between autistic-like and schizotypy traits: an analysis using the autism spectrum quotient and Oxford-Liverpool Inventory of Feelings and Experiences. *Pers Individ Dif* (2011) **51**(2):128–32. doi:10.1016/j.paid.2011.03.027
34. Wakabayashi A, Baron-Cohen S, Ashwin C. Do the traits of autism-spectrum overlap with those of schizophrenia or obsessive-compulsive disorder in the general population? *Res Autism Spectr Disord* (2012) **6**(2):717–25. doi:10.1016/j.rasd.2011.09.008
35. Dinsdale NL, Hurd PL, Wakayabashi A, Elliot M, Crespi BJ. How are autism and schizotypy related? Evidence from a non-clinical population. *PLoS One* (2013) **8**(5):e63316. doi:10.1371/journal.pone.0063316
36. American Psychological Association. *Diagnostic and Statistical Manual of Mental Disorders.* 4 ed. Washington, DC: American Psychological Association (1994).
37. American Psychological Association. *Diagnostic and Statistical Manual of Mental Disorders.* 3 ed. Washington, DC: American Psychological Association (1987).
38. Raine A, Reynolds C, Lencz T, Scerbo A, Triphon N, Kim D. Cognitive-perceptual, interpersonal, and disorganized features of schizotypal personality. *Schizophr Bull* (1994) **20**(1):191–201. doi:10.1093/schbul/20.1.191
39. Raine A, Benishay D. The SPQ-B: a breif screening instrument for schizotypal personality disorder. *J Pers Disord* (1995) **9**(4):346–55. doi:10.1521/pedi.1995.9.4.346

40. Cohen AS, Matthews RA, Najolia GN, Brown LA. Toward a more psychometrically sound brief measure of schizotypal traits: introducing the SPQ-brief revised. *J Pers Disord* (2010) **24**(4):516–37. doi:10.1521/pedi.2010.24.4.516
41. Claridge G, McDonald A. An investigation into the relationships between convergent and divergent thinking, schizotypy, and autistic traits. *Pers Individ Dif* (2009) **46**(8):794–9. doi:10.1016/j.paid.2009.01.018
42. Brown JD. Principal components analysis and exploratory factor analysis – definitions, differences, and choices. *Shiken* (2009) **13**(1):26–30.
43. Tabachnick BG, Fidell LS. *Using Multivariate Statistics.* 6 ed. Boston: Allyn and Bacon (2013).
44. Fabrigar LR, Wengener DT, MacCallum RC, Strahan EJ. Evaluating the use of exploratory factor analysis in psychological research. *Psychol Methods* (1999) **4**(3):272–99. doi:10.1037/1082-989X.4.3.272
45. Kassim S, Hasan H, Ismon AM, Asri FM. Parameter estimation in factor analysis: maximum likelihood versus principal component. *AIP Conf Proc* (2013) **1522**:1293–9. doi:10.1063/1.4801279
46. Rapoport J, Chavez A, Greenstein D, Addington A, Gogtay N. Autism spectrum disorders and childhood-onset schizophrenia: clinical and biological contributions to a relation revisited. *J Am Acad Child Adolesc Psychiatry* (2009) **48**(1):10–8. doi:10.1097/CHI.0b013e31818b1c63
47. Crivelli B, Rocca P. Differential diagnosis between schizophrenia and autism in adulthood: a case report. *Neurocase* (2013) **19**(6):604–12. doi:10.1080/13554794.2012.713492
48. Konstantareas MM, Hewitt T. Autistic disorder and schizophrenia: diagnostic overlaps. *J Autism Dev Disord* (2001) **31**(1):19–28. doi:10.1023/A:1005605528309
49. Coolidge FL, Marle PD, Rhoades CS, Monaghan P, Segal DL. Psychometric properties of a new measure to assess autism spectrum disorder in DSM-5. *Am J Orthopsychiatry* (2013) **83**(1):126–30. doi:10.1111/ajop.12012
50. Carroll LS, Owen MJ. Genetic overlap between autism, schizophrenia and bipolar disorder. *Genome Med* (2009) **1**(102):1–7. doi:10.1186/gm102
51. Bishop DVM, Maybery M, Maley A, Wong D, Hill W, Hallmayer J. Using self-report to identify the broad phenotype in parents of children with autistic spectrum disorders: a study using the autism-spectrum quotient. *J Child Psychol Psychiatry* (2004) **45**(8):1431–6. doi:10.1111/j.1469-7610.2004.00325.x
52. Calkins ME, Curtis CE, Qrove WM, Iacono WQ. Multiple dimensions of schizotypy in first degree biological relatives of schizophrenia patients. *Schizophr Bull* (2004) **30**(2):317–25. doi:10.1093/oxfordjournals.schbul.a007081
53. Sporn AL, Addington AM, Gogtay N, Ordonez AE, Gornick M, Clasen L, et al. Pervasive developmental disorder and childhood-onset schizophrenia: comorbid disorder or a phenotypic variant of a very early onset illness? *Biol Psychiatry* (2004) **55**(10):989–94. doi:10.1016/j.biopsych.2004.01.019
54. Stone WS, Iguchi L. Do apparent overlaps between schizophrenia and autistic spectrum disorders reflect superficial similarities or etiological commonalities? *N Am J Med Sci* (2011) **4**(3):124–33. doi:10.7156/v4i3p124
55. Wolff S, Narayan S, Moyes B. Personality characteristics of parents of autistic children: a controlled study. *J Child Psychol Psychiatry* (1988) **29**(2):143–53. doi:10.1111/j.1469-7610.1988.tb00699.x
56. Daniels JL, Forssen U, Hultman CM, Cnattingius S, Savitz DA, Feychting M, et al. Parental psychiatric disorders associated with autism spectrum disorders in the offspring. *Pediatrics* (2008) **121**(5):1357–62. doi:10.1542/peds.2007-2296
57. Duan J, Sanders AR, Gejman PV. Genome-wide approaches to schizophrenia. *Brain Res Bull* (2010) **83**(3–4):93–102. doi:10.1016/j.brainresbull.2010.04.009
58. Sugranyes G, Kyriakopoulos M, Corrigall R, Taylor E, Frangou S. Autism spectrum disorders and schizophrenia: meta-analysis of the neural correlates of social cognition. *PLoS One* (2011) **6**(10):e25322. doi:10.1371/journal.pone.0025322
59. Cheung C, Yu K, Fung G, Leung M, Wong C, Li Q, et al. Autistic disorders and schizophrenia: related or remote? An anatomical likelihood estimation. *PLoS One* (2010) **5**(8):e12233. doi:10.1371/journal.pone.0012233
60. Fervaha G, Remington G. Neuroimaging findings in schizotypal personality disorder: a systematic review. *Prog Neuropsychopharmacol Biol Psychiatry* (2013) **43**:96–107. doi:10.1016/j.pnpbp.2012.11.014
61. Brieber S, Neufang S, Bruning N, Kamp-Becker I, Remschmidt H, Herpertz-Dahlmann B, et al. Structural brain abnormalities in adolescents with autism spectrum disorder and patients with attention deficit/hyperactivity disorder. *J Child Psychol Psychiatry* (2007) **48**(12):1251–8. doi:10.1111/j.1469-7610.2007.01799.x
62. Howard MA, Cowell PE, Boucher J, Broks P, Mayes A, Farrant A, et al. Convergent neuroanatomical and behavioural evidence of an amygdala hypothesis of autism. *Neuroreport* (2000) **11**(13):2931–5. doi:10.1097/00001756-200009110-00020
63. Rowland LM, Kontson K, West J, Edden RA, Zhu H, Wijtenburg SA, et al. In vivo measurements of glutamate, GABA, and NAAG in schizophrenia. *Schizophr Bull* (2013) **39**(5):1096–104. doi:10.1093/schbul/sbs092
64. Szulc A, Galinska B, Tarasow E, Dzienis W, Kubas B, Konarzewska J, et al. The effect of risperidone on metabolite measures in schizophrenic patients. A proton magnetic resonance spectroscopy (1H-MRS) study. *Pharmacopsychiatry* (2005) **38**:214–9. doi:10.1055/s-2005-873156
65. Horder J, Lavender T, Mendez MA, O'Gorman R, Daly E, Craig MC, et al. Reduced subcortical glutamate/glutamine in adults with autism spectrum disorders: a [(1)H]MRS study. *Transl Psychiatry* (2013) **3**:e279. Epub 2013/07/11. doi:10.1038/tp.2013.53
66. Rossignol E. Genetics and function of neocortical GABAergic interneurons in neurodevelopmental disorders. *Neural Plast* (2011) **2011**(649325):1–25. doi:10.1155/2011/649325
67. Sigmundsson T, Maier M, Toone BK, Williams SCR, Simmons A, Greenwood K, et al. Frontal lobe N-acetylaspartate correlates with psychopathology in schizophrenia: a proton magnetic resonance spectroscopy study. *Schizophr Res* (2003) **64**(1):63–71. doi:10.1016/s0920-9964(02)00533-9
68. Frieman SD, Shaw DW, Artru AA, Richards TL, Gardner J, Dawson G, et al. Regional brain chemical alterations in young children with autism spectrum disorder. *Neurology* (2003) **60**:100–7. doi:10.1212/WNL.60.1.100
69. Wuthrich VM, Bates TC. Confirmatory factor analysis of the three-factor structure of the schizotypal personality questionnaire and Chapman schizotypy scales. *J Pers Assess* (2006) **87**(3):292–304. doi:10.1207/s15327752jpa8703_10
70. Wuthrich V, Bates TC. Reliability and validity of two Likert versions of the Schizotypal Personality Questionnaire (SPQ). *Pers Individ Dif* (2005) **38**(7):1543–8. doi:10.1016/j.paid.2004.09.017
71. ObjectPlanet Inc. *Opinio Oslo Norway.* (1998–2013). Available from: http://www.objectplanet.com/Opinio/
72. IBM Corp. *IBM SPSS Statistics for Windows.* 20.0 ed. Armonk, NY: IBM Corp. (2011).
73. Cohen AS, Couture SM, Blanchard JJ. Neuropsychological functioning and social anhedonia: three-year follow-up data from a longitudinal community high risk study. *J Psychiatr Res* (2012) **46**(7):898–904. doi:10.1016/j.jpsychires.2012.03.020
74. Skodol AE. Personality disorders in DSM-5. *Annu Rev Clin Psychol* (2012) **8**:317–44. doi:10.1146/annurev-clinpsy-032511-143131
75. Blais MA, Malone JC. Structure of the DSM-IV personality disorders as revealed in clinician ratings. *Compr Psychiatry* (2013) **54**(4):326–33. doi:10.1016/j.comppsych.2012.10.014
76. Austin EJ. Personality correlates of the broader autism phenotype as assessed by the autism spectrum quotient (AQ). *Pers Individ Dif* (2005) **38**:451–60. doi:10.1016/j.paid.2004.04.022

6

The longitudinal course of gross motor activity in schizophrenia – within and between episodes

Sebastian Walther*, Katharina Stegmayer, Helge Horn, Luca Rampa, Nadja Razavi, Thomas J. Müller and Werner Strik

University Hospital of Psychiatry, University of Bern, Bern, Switzerland

Edited by:
Manuel Morrens, University of Antwerp, Belgium

Reviewed by:
Bernhard J. Mitterauer, Volitronics-Institute for Basic Research Psychopathology and Brain Philosophy, Austria
Assen Veniaminov Jablensky, The University of Western Australia, Australia

****Correspondence:***
Sebastian Walther, University Hospital of Psychiatry, University of Bern, Bolligenstrasse 111, Bern 60 3000, Switzerland
e-mail: walther@puk.unibe.ch

Schizophrenia is associated with heterogeneous course of positive and negative symptoms. In addition, reduced motor activity as measured by wrist actigraphy has been reported. However, longitudinal studies of spontaneous motor activity are missing. We aimed to explore whether activity levels were stable within and between psychotic episodes. Furthermore, we investigated the association with the course of negative symptoms. In 45 medicated patients, we investigated motor behavior within a psychotic episode. In addition, we followed 18 medicated patients across 2 episodes. Wrist actigraphy and psychopathological ratings were applied. Within an episode symptoms changed but activity levels did not vary systematically. Activity at baseline predicted the course of negative symptoms. Between two episodes activity recordings were much more stable. Again, activity at the index episode predicted the outcome of negative symptoms. In sum, spontaneous motor activity shares trait and state characteristics, the latter are associated with negative symptom course. Actigraphy may therefore become an important ambulatory instrument to monitor negative symptoms and treatment outcome in schizophrenia.

Keywords: actigraphy, psychosis, negative symptoms, PANSS, avolition

INTRODUCTION

Schizophrenia is characterized by positive symptoms, negative symptoms, and disorganization. Furthermore, cognitive and motor symptoms have been identified as relevant symptom clusters of schizophrenia. In fact, the current DSM5 concept of psychoses proposed eight dimensions of psychopathology to be assessed in subjects with schizophrenia, including motor symptoms (1). Schizophrenia is further associated with particular heterogeneity in course and outcome (2, 3). Generally, symptoms ameliorate during the course of a psychotic episode; however, negative symptoms do not respond as well to treatment as positive symptoms and disorganization too (4, 5). In longitudinal studies over years, negative symptoms generally tend to be stable (5, 6). However, findings of a recent meta-analysis suggest that negative symptoms may improve to a greater extent than what has previously been assumed (7).

Motor signs in schizophrenia include catatonia, neurological soft signs, psychomotor slowing, and extrapyramidal symptoms, i.e., abnormal involuntary movements, akathisia, and parkinsonism (8, 9). These motor symptoms are prevalent throughout the course of the disorder and may be affected by antipsychotic treatment. Particularly, gross motor behavior is important in schizophrenia; it is linked with medication, symptom dimensions, and relevant for physical health (10, 11). Spontaneous motor activity may be objectively assessed with continuous wrist actigraphy (12). A number of parameters can be calculated from actigraphy data, such as the activity level (AL; activity counts per hour), the movement index (MI; percentage of active periods), or the average duration of immobility periods (12). However, it was the AL that was associated with negative syndrome severity (13–15) and neuroimaging markers (16–18). In general, schizophrenia patients have reduced levels of daytime activity compared to healthy control subjects (15, 17, 19, 20). One study performed actigraphic recordings for seven consecutive days (19). Their graphs indicate rather stable measurements throughout a week, even though no statistical test had been applied to explore temporal fluctuations. Actigraphy has been used for cross-sectional comparisons of spontaneous motor behavior in schizophrenia; however, no study has addressed the longitudinal course within or even between psychotic episodes. Studies on motor abnormalities in first episode and chronic schizophrenia indicate that most motor symptoms including hypokinesia are attenuated by antipsychotic treatment within 4 weeks (21, 22). Therefore, we could assume that spontaneous motor activity is subject to changes within an episode. The longitudinal course of motor signs over more than a few weeks has only rarely been addressed. Few longitudinal studies included finger tapping and found no changes over time (23). Docx et al. report amelioration of catatonia and neurological soft signs in stable patients over 1 year (24). Likewise, neurological soft signs tend to decrease within the first year in schizophrenia (25).

The current study aimed at testing whether spontaneous motor activity would change during the course of a psychotic episode as well as during the course between two psychotic episodes. Furthermore, we wanted to investigate whether spontaneous motor activity at baseline would predict the course of symptoms in schizophrenia. The literature suggests wide distribution of activity levels between subjects with schizophrenia (15, 17). We hypothesized that a considerable proportion of the variance was stable over time (trait motor activity) and that some of the variable motor activity was state dependent and linked to negative symptoms of schizophrenia.

MATERIALS AND METHODS

PARTICIPANTS

Participants were recruited from the inpatient and outpatient department of the University Hospital of Psychiatry, Bern, Switzerland. This investigation includes data from three different studies that all used the same actigraphy procedures. Diagnoses were given after thorough clinical examination and review of all case files by board certified psychiatrists. The local mental health care system ensures that most of the patients are admitted to our clinic in every psychotic episode requiring inpatient treatment, allowing the collection of reliable diagnostic information. In a proportion of studies that contributed data to this analysis, the diagnoses were ascertained by structured clinical interviews (both SCID and MINI; 27% of cases). Patients were excluded in case of substance abuse other than nicotine, medical conditions affecting physical activity (e.g., injuries such as fractures or ligament ruptures and conditions such as idiopathic parkinsonism, arthrosis, or rheumatism) and epilepsy. Physical activity was recorded approximately 2 weeks after admission to the psychiatric department (24 h at each assessment time point). At the same time, psychopathology was assessed using the positive and negative syndrome scale (PANSS) (20). In the within-episode sample, actigraphy and PANSS assessments were repeated after the acute symptoms had been alleviated. In the between episodes sample, assessments were repeated within the first 2 weeks of the subsequent inpatient treatment due to a psychotic episode. Episode and inter-episode interval have been defined according the practice guidelines developed by the American Psychiatric Association codified a three-phase model of schizophrenia disease course, with the recognition that these phases "merge into one another without absolute, clear boundaries between them" (26). According to this model, the "acute phase," characterized by florid psychosis and severe positive and/or negative symptoms, which is followed by a "stabilization phase," during which symptoms recede and decrease in severity, and a subsequent "stable phase" with reduced symptom severity and relative symptom stability. In detail, the stable phase reflects the inter-episode interval while the acute phase including the stabilization phase has been defined as episode and within-episode interval (26, 27). Chlorpromazine equivalents (CPZ) of the current antipsychotic pharmacotherapy were calculated according to Woods (21). The protocols of the studies applying wrist actigraphy in schizophrenia spectrum disorders had been approved by the local ethics committee and participants provided written informed consent prior to study inclusion.

Within-episodes sample

In total, 45 patients (28 men and 15 women) were included with an average period between measurements of 42 days. Mean age was 36.9 ± 9.5 years, mean duration of illness 11.1 ± 10.7 years. Patients experienced 6.8 ± 6.6 episodes. The majority was treated with antipsychotics (94%; aripiprazole, clozapine, quetiapine, risperidone, olanzapine, haloperidol, amisulpride, zuclopenthixol, and flupenthixol), most of them atypical (91%).

Between episodes sample

In total, 18 patients (13 men and 5 women) were included with an average period between episodes of 639 days (4 subjects of the within-episode sample were also included in the between episode sample). Mean age was 34.7 ± 10.5 years, mean duration of illness 8.7 ± 8.0 years. Patients experienced 6.9 ± 7.2 episodes. All patients received antipsychotic treatment (aripiprazole, clozapine, quetiapine, risperidone, olanzapine, haloperidol, and amisulpride) with predominantly atypical antipsychotics (index episode 83%, later episode 94%).

ACTIGRAPHY

Participants wore an actigraph (Actiwatch, Cambridge Neurotechnology, Inc., Cambridge, UK) for 24 consecutive hours at the wrist of the non-dominant arm. The piezoelectronic sensor converts acceleration into movement counts. Data were sampled in 2 s intervals. Participants provided sleep log information and information on recording pauses (due to showering or bathing). Only the data collected during wakeful periods of the 24 h recording time were analyzed. Activity counts were averaged to provide the AL in counts/h.

STATISTICAL ANALYSES

Positive and negative syndrome scale scores were used to calculate two factors of negative symptoms as in previous studies (15, 28, 29): the expressivity factor including items N1 (blunted affect) and N6 (lack of spontaneity and flow of conversation) and the avolition factor including items N2 (emotional withdrawal) and N4 (passive/apathetic social withdrawal). Longitudinal comparisons of clinical and actigraphic parameters were calculated using paired T-tests. To test the explained variance, we entered AL baseline as predictor of a linear regression model of AL post. In both cohorts, we detected wide variability of AL changes. Using Pearson correlations, we explored associations between AL at baseline and clinical parameters at baseline and in the longitudinal course. Next, we aimed at testing groups according to their baseline AL values. In order to test the longitudinal course of PANSS scores according to baseline motor activity, we defined groups applying the 33rd and 66th percentile of the baseline AL in both cohorts. Group comparisons (low, medium, and high AL) were conducted using repeated measures ANOVAs. *Post hoc* analyses were Sidak corrected for multiple comparisons. All analyses were conducted with SPSS22.

RESULTS

WITHIN EPISODES

Within psychotic episodes longitudinal AL changes were wide-ranged. Paired T-tests of AL baseline and AL post indicated no change (see **Table 1**). However, only 28% of the patients had stable AL, i.e., AL changed by <20%. AL post ranged 35–272% of the AL at baseline. In contrast, PANSS positive and PANSS total scores were attenuated, a trend for improvement was detected in PANSS negative scores (see **Table 1**). Interestingly, baseline AL inversely correlated at trend level with% of change of activity ($r = -0.286$; $p = 0.063$), indicating that the less patients move at baseline the more likely AL changes within episodes. However, the magnitude of change from baseline AL was not predictive of the longitudinal course of PANSS scores (r-range: −0.17–0.10).

Table 1 | Paired *T*-tests within episode.

	Baseline	Post	*T*	df	*p*	*r*
AL (counts/h)	13735 ± 7274	13544 ± 8128	0.2	42	0.870	0.52
PANSS positive	17.1 ± 5.8	13.1 ± 4.8	4.3	42	<0.001	0.34
PANSS negative	18.4 ± 6.8	16.4 ± 6.2	1.7	42	0.099	0.30
PANSS avolition	5.3 ± 2.2	4.9 ± 2.4	0.8	42	0.406	0.10
PANSS expressivity	5.5 ± 3.0	5.0 ± 2.3	1.4	42	0.181	0.56
PANSS total	69.5 ± 16.6	59.0 ± 15.9	3.4	42	0.001	0.24
CPZ (mg)	543 ± 401	531 ± 435	0.2	42	0.807	0.69

Table 2 | Repeated measures ANOVAs within episode.

		AL baseline group			Time		Group		Time × group	
		Low	Medium	High	*F*	*p*	*F*	*p*	*F*	*p*
AL	Baseline	7742 ± 1178	11077 ± 1469	22577 ± 6016	0.3	0.863	47.2	<0.001	0.8	0.455
	Post	9096 ± 4684	11329 ± 4174	20366 ± 9781						
PANSS positive	Baseline	14.5 ± 4.9	19.5 ± 6.1	17.3 ± 5.7	17.7	<0.001	5.1	0.011	0.03	0.967
	Post	10.8 ± 3.6	15.3 ± 5.0	13.0 ± 4.8						
PANSS negative	Baseline	21.9 ± 6.9	19.3 ± 5.6	13.9 ± 5.7	3.3	0.078	4.1	0.025	3.5	0.039
	Post	15.8 ± 5.7	18.5 ± 7.4	14.8 ± 5.2						
PANSS avolition	Baseline	6.2 ± 2.6	5.6 ± 1.9	4.1 ± 1.6	0.9	0.357	1.5	0.230	4.5	0.017
	Post	4.0 ± 2.3	5.7 ± 2.4	5.0 ± 2.3						
PANSS expressivity	Baseline	7.5 ± 3.0	5.3 ± 2.8	3.7 ± 2.0	2.3	0.134	5.2	0.010	4.8	0.014
	Post	5.4 ± 2.2	5.5 ± 2.7	3.9 ± 1.9						
PANSS total	Baseline	69.8 ± 12.9	76.9 ± 20.5	61.4 ± 11.7	11.9	0.001	4.6	0.016	1.1	0.339
	Post	53.6 ± 15.4	66.2 ± 16.0	56.6 ± 14.3						

AL: high > low (p < 0.001) and high > medium (p < 0.001) post hoc Sidak tests.

Activity level at baseline predicted AL post ($R^2 = 0.26$, $F = 15.0$, $p < 0.001$). AL baseline correlated with PANSS negative baseline ($r = -0.53$, $p < 0.001$). Furthermore, AL post correlated with PANSS negative at both time points (PANSS negative baseline: $r = -0.39$, $p = 0.011$; PANSS negative post: $r = -0.35$, $p = 0.021$). Therefore, we explored whether AL baseline would indicate longitudinal changes in psychopathology. AL baseline was used to define three groups based on percentile rankings (33rd and 66th percentiles), i.e., low, medium, and high AL baseline. The three patient groups did not differ in terms of age ($F = 1.3$, df = 2, $p = 0.294$), duration of illness ($F = 1.4$, df = 2, $p = 0.258$), number of episodes ($F = 1.2$, df = 2, $p = 0.311$), CPZ ($F = 0.01$, df = 2, $p = 0.992$), and the time between measurements ($F = 0.5$, df = 2, $p = 0.609$). Time effects were strong for PANSS positive and total scores, indicating attenuation of symptoms during the episode (see **Table 2**; **Figure 1**). Significant group × time interactions were detected only for the measures of the negative syndrome: PANSS negative scores, avolition, and expressivity scores decreased significantly only in the group with low AL at baseline ($T = 3.4$, $p = 0.005$; $T = 2.7$, $p = 0.019$; $T = 3.2$, $p = 0.006$), while in the other groups negative syndrome scores remained stable.

BETWEEN EPISODES

Between episodes, AL was more stable than within episodes. In fact, 50% of the patients had AL changes of ±20%. AL at the later episode ranged 40–167% of AL at the index episode. Likewise, PANSS scores were similar between episodes (see **Table 3**), except a trend for deterioration in the PANSS avolition score. AL at index episode predicted AL at the later episode ($R^2 = 0.65$, $F = 30.0$, $p < 0.001$). Neither AL at index episode nor AL at a later episode correlated significantly with PANSS scores. Still, when the group was divided according to AL at index episode (low, medium, high AL), we detected a significant group effect on PANSS negative scores, as well as a trend to a time × group interaction (see **Table 4**; **Figure 2**). Negative syndrome scores increased between episodes in patients with high AL at index episode ($T = -2.6$, $p = 0.047$) and at trend level also in patients with low AL at index episode ($T = -2.1$, $p = 0.095$). Likewise, avolition scores increased at trend level in the group with high AL at index episode ($T = -2.7$, $p = 0.052$). In the group with low AL at index episode, we found single PANSS negative items to increase over time at trend level: N1 (blunted affect, $p = 0.076$) and N3 (poor rapport, $p = 0.076$). In the group with high AL at index episode, we found trends for changes of the items N2 (emotional withdrawal, $p = 0.070$) and N6 (lack of spontaneity, $p = 0.070$).

DISCUSSION

The present study explored the longitudinal course of spontaneous motor activity in schizophrenia. Results indicate considerable variance within psychotic episodes and stability of activity levels

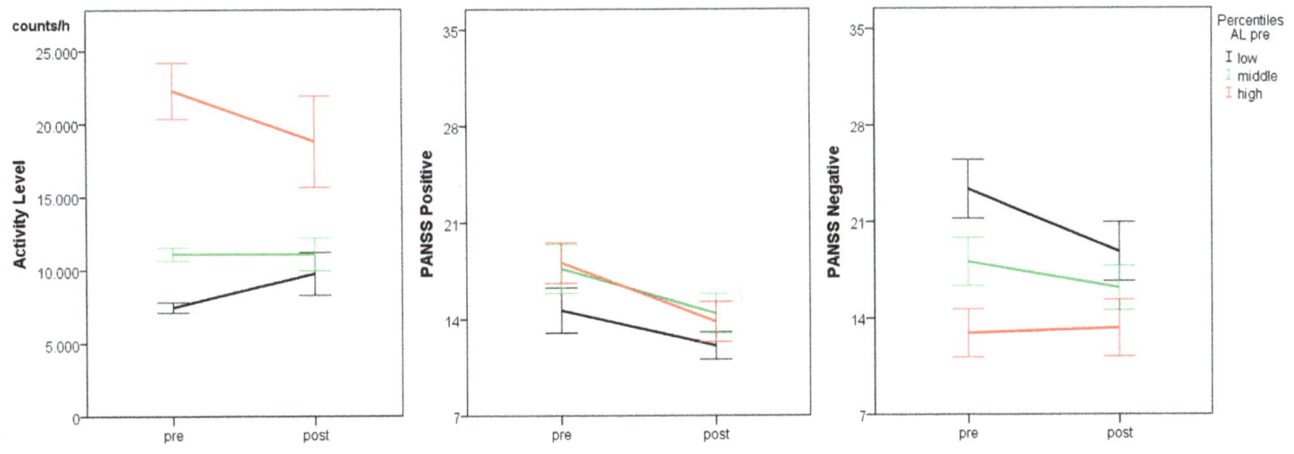

FIGURE 1 | Within-episode course of activity and psychopathology ($n = 45$) lines indicate mean ± SE.

Table 3 | Paired *T*-tests between episodes.

	Index episode	Later episode	*T*	df	*p*	*r*
AL (counts/h)	15472 ± 10152	13591 ± 7474	1.3	17	0.203	0.81
PANSS positive	13.3 ± 5.1	14.6 ± 6.0	−1.4	17	0.183	0.77
PANSS negative	17.7 ± 7.6	19.6 ± 7.7	−1.1	17	0.274	0.67
PANSS avolition	4.1 ± 2.0	5.5 ± 3.2	−2.1	17	0.051	0.53
PANSS expressivity	5.5 ± 3.1	6.1 ± 2.9	−1.0	17	0.351	0.69
PANSS total	60.0 ± 16.1	65.4 ± 16.1	−1.2	17	0.253	0.29
CPZ (mg)	440 ± 305	608 ± 387	−1.8	17	0.092	0.36

Table 4 | Repeated measures ANOVA between episodes ($n = 18$).

		AL index group			Time		Group		Time × group	
		Low	Medium	High	*F*	*p*	*F*	*p*	*F*	*p*
AL	Index	6870 ± 1669	13241 ± 2623	26305 ± 10256	2.4	0.143	13.0	0.001	4.1	0.038
	Later	7263 ± 3211	14016 ± 4016	19495 ± 8567						
PANSS positive	Index	15.5 ± 7.3	11.8 ± 3.8	12.7 ± 3.6	1.9	0.189	0.7	0.522	0.86	0.442
	Later	15.8 ± 5.4	12.3 ± 6.4	15.7 ± 6.7						
PANSS negative	Index	17.7 ± 7.9	17.2 ± 7.4	18.2 ± 8.9	1.6	0.231	4.1	0.025	2.9	0.088
	Later	22.0 ± 9.3	14.3 ± 2.3	21.7 ± 8.1						
PANSS avolition	Index	4.7 ± 2.7	4.0 ± 2.0	3.4 ± 0.9	4.8	0.047	0.6	0.539	1.7	0.217
	Later	6.3 ± 4.1	3.8 ± 2.0	6.2 ± 2.7						
PANSS expressivity	Index	5.5 ± 2.9	5.8 ± 3.0	5.2 ± 3.8	0.8	0.396	0.1	0.880	1.4	0.273
	Later	7.0 ± 3.6	5.0 ± 1.2	6.0 ± 3.4						
PANSS total	Index	62.3 ± 17.9	55.3 ± 17.5	62.3 ± 15.3	1.3	0.275	1.5	0.264	0.3	0.751
	Later	69.5 ± 15.4	55.7 ± 13.7	71.0 ± 16.9						

AL: high > low ($p < 0.001$) and high > medium ($p = 0.028$) post hoc Sidak tests.

between episodes. Furthermore, within-episodes baseline activity predicted the outcome of negative symptom severity. Therefore, our hypotheses were confirmed: spontaneous motor activity in schizophrenia has trait and state characteristics; the latter are associated with the negative syndrome.

WITHIN-EPISODE VARIANCE

Activity levels for the whole group demonstrated considerable variance, only 26% of the variance of AL post were predicted by AL at baseline. When we split the sample into three similar sized groups according to the baseline AL, we found no changes

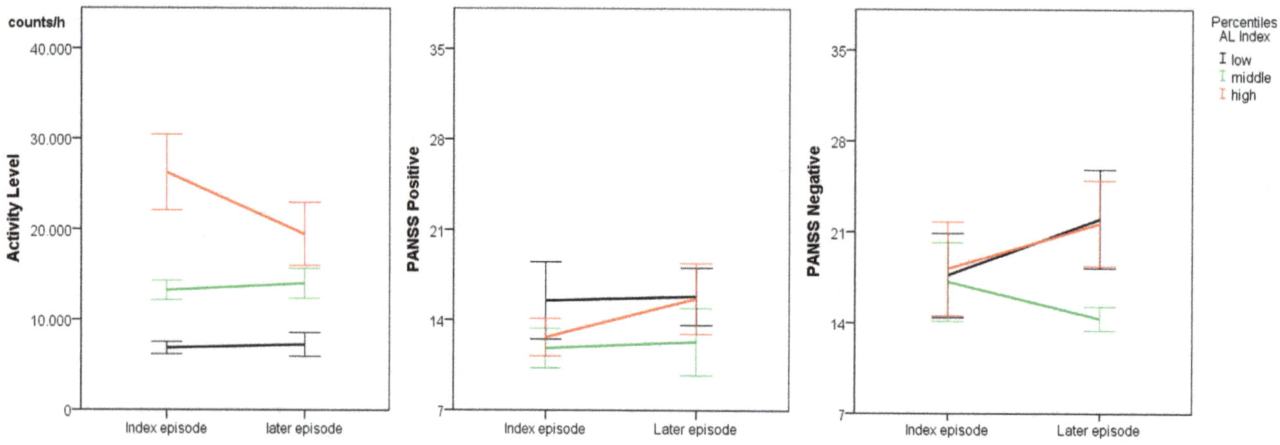

FIGURE 2 | Between episode course of activity and psychopathology ($n = 18$) lines indicate mean ± SE.

over time; instead, group differences remained throughout the episode. This stability of motor activity is congruent with the observations over 1 week (19). However, other motor signs in schizophrenia are attenuated by antipsychotic treatment. This is true for abnormal involuntary movements and neurological soft signs but also for hypokinesia, parkinsonism, and catatonia (21, 22, 25). Particularly, when hypokinetic movement disorders were ameliorated, we could expect an increase in AL within an episode. Our findings fail to support this notion. As noted above, there was considerable variance in the longitudinal course of AL within an episode. Peralta and Cuesta reported in their sample of 100 unmedicated first episode patients that 21% had parkinsonism and 18% catatonia at baseline (30). The two hypokinetic movement disorders demonstrated distinct courses with antipsychotic treatment; parkinsonism increased and catatonia declined within 4 weeks. Interestingly, for both syndromes, cases were identified who had drug emergent, drug responsive, and drug irresponsive courses (30). Therefore, patients can present with very different courses of movement disorders, which may explain our finding of stable AL in the paired T-test and only 26% of explained variance between assessments.

Activity level at baseline separated the groups according to negative syndrome severity. As in previous studies, lower AL was associated with increased negative syndrome scores (13–15). Furthermore, the groups differed in the course of negative syndrome. Patients in the low AL group experienced a pronounced decrease of negative syndrome scores within the episode, while the other groups did not. This finding was true for both, the avolition and the expressivity component of the PANSS negative syndrome score. Baseline AL may therefore predict who will have a higher probability of reduced negative symptoms with treatment. In line with the literature, within episodes in general PANSS positive and total scores decreased more than negative scores with antipsychotic treatment (4, 5, 31). In contrast, the avolition score remained stable (5, 32). Therefore, avolition may represent the invariant component of negative symptoms while other negative symptoms tend to improve (32). Interestingly, specifically deficits of "action-orientation" (slowing of the initiation of fine motor movements) have been associated with avolition (29). Likewise, problems of initiation of goal directed behavior might have led to psychomotor slowing in our study. Avolition is a critical component of the negative syndrome in schizophrenia, linked to impaired motivation and poor functional outcome (33). Measures of avolition are correlated with reduced AL in schizophrenia (15, 34). Because actigraphy is a well-accepted, ambulatory, and non-invasive way of obtaining objective data on spontaneous movement, it should be applied in larger pharmaceutical trials on negative symptoms in schizophrenia. At the very least, it could help to identify subjects at baseline with increased likelihood of responding to treatments for negative symptoms.

BETWEEN EPISODES STABILITY

Between two psychotic episodes AL was much more stable (65% explained variance) than within an episode. The time × group interaction indicated regression to the mean for AL in the longitudinal course. Our results argue for a trait component in AL in schizophrenia. Data on the long-term course of other motor phenomena are scarce and produced mixed results. Studies on neurological soft signs found subjects with increasing and subjects with decreasing symptoms (24, 25). The patients with increasing soft signs had poorer overall outcome (25). Catatonia was found to be reduced within 1 year even in chronic schizophrenia, but parkinsonism and motor retardation were unchanged (24). In contrast, cross-sectional reports of motor function in schizophrenia (chronic vs. first episode) noted generalized deterioration with ongoing course (35). Still, longitudinal studies of motor behavior during multiple episodes are missing.

Long-term studies starting in the first psychotic episodes indicate that considerable proportions of negative symptoms remain unchanged over several years (5, 6, 32). Again, avolition was most stable among the negative symptoms (5, 32). In our study, both positive and negative symptom scores displayed no time effect in the whole group, which may be accounted for by the small sample size. Still, correlations between index and later episode were strong for both syndromes. However, the avolition score indicated overall deterioration of this component of negative symptoms. In patients with high AL at baseline, single PANSS negative items emotional withdrawal (N2) and lack of spontaneity (N6) indicated deterioration at trend level in this group. Again, we noted an effect of AL on negative syndrome scores with a significant group effect and a group × time interaction at trend level. Here, patients with higher AL at index episode increased their negative syndrome scores between episodes. This is particularly interesting as the negative syndrome scores at baseline were similar between groups. Thus, only our measure of spontaneous motor activity had predictive value for negative syndrome scores. Again, results must be interpreted with caution due to the small groups.

LIMITATIONS

This was a truly naturalistic study design, which is not able to detect longitudinal changes associated with specific drug effects. There are various effects that may have contributed to the observed changes. Medication may have heterogeneous effects on motor activity (36). The observation period could not be standardized. In addition, the sample sizes were small, particularly for the inter-episode comparison. Thus, we may have missed effects due to type-II errors. In addition, diagnoses were given after thorough clinical psychiatric examination and chart review; however, structured clinical interviews (both SCID and MINI) were only applied in a proportion of (27% of cases) patients. We assessed negative symptoms with the PANSS negative syndrome scale and PANSS factors for avolition and expressivity. Additional negative scales such as the scale for the assessment of negative symptoms (SANS) (37) or the clinical assessment interview for negative symptoms (CAINS) (38) were not applied. Finally, future studies could include measures of motor syndromes such as catatonia, neurological soft signs, and parkinsonism to account for differential effects of medication on motor signs (30). In sum, we think our results are encouraging for large randomized controlled trials focusing on negative symptoms in schizophrenia.

CONCLUSION

Spontaneous gross motor behavior in schizophrenia shares trait and state characteristics. Within-episodes motor activity varies with negative syndrome scores, while between psychotic episodes motor activity remains stable. Wrist actigraphy should be considered as objective ambulatory non-invasive instrument to monitor the effects of treatment on negative symptoms.

AUTHOR CONTRIBUTIONS

SW and HH designed the study. SW wrote the protocol. LR, NR, KS, and SW recruited participants and performed assessments. SW performed the data analyses. All authors interpreted and discussed the findings. SW wrote the first draft of the manuscript. All authors contributed to the final version of the manuscript.

REFERENCES

1. Heckers S, Barch DM, Bustillo J, Gaebel W, Gur R, Malaspina D, et al. Structure of the psychotic disorders classification in DSM-5. *Schizophr Res* (2013) **150**(1):11–4. doi:10.1016/j.schres.2013.04.039
2. van Os J, Kapur S. Schizophrenia. *Lancet* (2009) **374**(9690):635–45. doi:10.1016/S0140-6736(09)60995-8
3. Insel TR. Rethinking schizophrenia. *Nature* (2010) **468**(7321):187–93. doi:10.1038/nature09552
4. Addington J, Addington D. Positive and negative symptoms of schizophrenia. Their course and relationship over time. *Schizophr Res* (1991) **5**(1):51–9. doi:10.1016/0920-9964(91)90039-T
5. Arndt S, Andreasen NC, Flaum M, Miller D, Nopoulos P. A longitudinal study of symptom dimensions in schizophrenia. Prediction and patterns of change. *Arch Gen Psychiatry* (1995) **52**(5):352–60. doi:10.1001/archpsyc.1995.03950170026004
6. Lang FU, Kosters M, Lang S, Becker T, Jager M. Psychopathological long-term outcome of schizophrenia – a review. *Acta Psychiatr Scand* (2013) **127**(3):173–82. doi:10.1111/acps.12030
7. Savill M, Banks C, Khanom H, Priebe S. Do negative symptoms of schizophrenia change over time? A meta-analysis of longitudinal data. *Psychol Med* (2014):1–15. doi:10.1017/S0033291714002712
8. Morrens M, Docx L, Walther S. Beyond boundaries: in search of an integrative view on motor symptoms in schizophrenia. *Front Psychiatry* (2014) **5**:145. doi:10.3389/fpsyt.2014.00145
9. Walther S, Strik W. Motor symptoms and schizophrenia. *Neuropsychobiology* (2012) **66**(2):77–92. doi:10.1159/000339456
10. Brown S, Birtwistle J, Roe L, Thompson C. The unhealthy lifestyle of people with schizophrenia. *Psychol Med* (1999) **29**(3):697–701. doi:10.1017/S0033291798008186
11. Vancampfort D, Probst M, Sweers K, Maurissen K, Knapen J, De Hert M. Relationships between obesity, functional exercise capacity, physical activity participation and physical self-perception in people with schizophrenia. *Acta Psychiatr Scand* (2011) **123**(6):423–30. doi:10.1111/j.1600-0447.2010.01666.x
12. Middelkoop HA, van Dam EM, Smilde-van den Doel DA, Van Dijk G. 45-hour continuous quintuple-site actimetry: relations between trunk and limb movements and effects of circadian sleep-wake rhythmicity. *Psychophysiology* (1997) **34**(2):199–203. doi:10.1111/j.1469-8986.1997.tb02132.x
13. Walther S, Koschorke P, Horn H, Strik W. Objectively measured motor activity in schizophrenia challenges the validity of expert ratings. *Psychiatry Res* (2009) **169**(3):187–90. doi:10.1016/j.psychres.2008.06.020
14. Walther S, Ramseyer F, Horn H, Strik W, Tschacher W. Less structured movement patterns predict severity of positive syndrome, excitement, and disorganization. *Schizophr Bull* (2014) **40**(3):585–91. doi:10.1093/schbul/sbt038
15. Docx L, Sabbe B, Provinciael P, Merckx N, Morrens M. Quantitative psychomotor dysfunction in schizophrenia: a loss of drive, impaired movement execution or both? *Neuropsychobiology* (2013) **68**(4):221–7. doi:10.1159/000355293
16. Walther S, Federspiel A, Horn H, Razavi N, Wiest R, Dierks T, et al. Resting state cerebral blood flow and objective motor activity reveal basal ganglia dysfunction in schizophrenia. *Psychiatry Res* (2011) **192**(2):117–24. doi:10.1016/j.pscychresns.2010.12.002
17. Walther S, Federspiel A, Horn H, Razavi N, Wiest R, Dierks T, et al. Alterations of white matter integrity related to motor activity in schizophrenia. *Neurobiol Dis* (2011) **42**(3):276–83. doi:10.1016/j.nbd.2011.01.017
18. Bracht T, Schnell S, Federspiel A, Razavi N, Horn H, Strik W, et al. Altered cortico-basal ganglia motor pathways reflect reduced volitional motor activity in schizophrenia. *Schizophr Res* (2013) **143**(2–3): 269–76. doi:10.1016/j.schres.2012.12.004
19. Wichniak A, Skowerska A, Chojnacka-Wojtowicz J, Taflinski T, Wierzbicka A, Jernajczyk W, et al. Actigraphic monitoring of activity and rest in schizophrenic patients treated with olanzapine or risperidone. *J Psychiatr Res* (2011) **45**(10):1381–6. doi:10.1016/j.jpsychires.2011.05.009
20. Berle JO, Hauge ER, Oedegaard KJ, Holsten F, Fasmer OB. Actigraphic registration of motor activity reveals a more structured behavioural pattern in schizophrenia than in major depression. *BMC Res Notes* (2010) **3**:149. doi:10.1186/1756-0500-3-149
21. Peralta V, Campos MS, De Jalon EG, Cuesta MJ. Motor behavior abnormalities in drug-naive patients with schizophrenia spectrum disorders. *Mov Disord* (2010) **25**(8):1068–76. doi:10.1002/mds.23050
22. Peralta V, Cuesta MJ. Motor features in psychotic disorders. I. Factor structure and clinical correlates. *Schizophr Res* (2001) **47**(2–3):107–16. doi:10.1016/S0920-9964(00)00035-9
23. Hoff AL, Svetina C, Shields G, Stewart J, DeLisi LE. Ten year longitudinal study of neuropsychological functioning subsequent to a first episode of schizophrenia. *Schizophr Res* (2005) **78**(1):27–34. doi:10.1016/j.schres.2005.05.010

24. Docx L, Sabbe B, Fransen E, Bervoets C, Hulstijn W, Van den Bossche B, et al. Longitudinal evaluation of the psychomotor syndrome in schizophrenia. *J Neuropsychiatry Clin Neurosci* (Forthcoming). doi:10.1111/j.1600-0447.2012.01846.x
25. Bachmann S, Bottmer C, Schroder J. Neurological soft signs in first-episode schizophrenia: a follow-up study. *Am J Psychiatry* (2005) **162**(12):2337–43. doi:10.1176/appi.ajp.162.12.2337
26. American Psychiatric Association. Practice guideline for the treatment of patients with schizophrenia. *Am J Psychiatry* (1997) **154**(4 Suppl):1–63. doi:10.1176/ajp.154.4.1
27. Andreasen NC, Carpenter WT Jr, Kane JM, Lasser RA, Marder SR, Weinberger DR. Remission in schizophrenia: proposed criteria and rationale for consensus. *Am J Psychiatry* (2005) **162**(3):441–9. doi:10.1176/appi.ajp.162.3.441
28. Van den Oord EJCG, Rujescu D, Robles JR, Giegling I, Birrell C, Bukszar J, et al. Factor structure and external validity of the PANSS revisited. *Schizophr Res* (2006) **82**(2–3):213–23. doi:10.1016/j.schres.2005.09.002
29. Bervoets C, Docx L, Sabbe B, Vermeylen S, Van Den Bossche MJ, Morsel A, et al. The nature of the relationship of psychomotor slowing with negative symptomatology in schizophrenia. *Cogn Neuropsychiatry* (2014) **19**(1):36–46. doi:10.1080/13546805.2013.779578
30. Peralta V, Cuesta MJ. The effect of antipsychotic medication on neuromotor abnormalities in neuroleptic-naive nonaffective psychotic patients: a naturalistic study with haloperidol, risperidone, or olanzapine. *Prim Care Companion J Clin Psychiatry* (2010) **12**(2). doi:10.4088/PCC.09m00799gry
31. Peralta V, Cuesta MJ, Martinez-Larrea A, Serrano JF. Patterns of symptoms in neuroleptic-naive patients with schizophrenia and related psychotic disorders before and after treatment. *Psychiatry Res* (2001) **105**(1–2):97–105. doi:10.1016/S0165-1781(01)00319-5
32. Ucok A, Ergul C. Persistent negative symptoms after first episode schizophrenia: a 2-year follow-up study. *Schizophr Res* (2014) **158**(1–3):241–6. doi:10.1016/j.schres.2014.07.021
33. Foussias G, Remington G. Negative symptoms in schizophrenia: avolition and Occam's razor. *Schizophr Bull* (2010) **36**(2):359–69. doi:10.1093/schbul/sbn094
34. Farrow TF, Hunter MD, Wilkinson ID, Green RD, Spence SA. Structural brain correlates of unconstrained motor activity in people with schizophrenia. *Br J Psychiatry* (2005) **187**:481–2. doi:10.1192/bjp.187.5.481
35. Sponheim SR, Jung RE, Seidman LJ, Mesholam-Gately RI, Manoach DS, O'Leary DS, et al. Cognitive deficits in recent-onset and chronic schizophrenia. *J Psychiatr Res* (2010) **44**(7):421–8. doi:10.1016/j.jpsychires.2009.09.010
36. Walther S, Horn H, Razavi N, Koschorke P, Wopfner A, Muller TJ, et al. Higher motor activity in schizophrenia patients treated with olanzapine versus risperidone. *J Clin Psychopharmacol* (2010) **30**(2):181–4. doi:10.1097/JCP.0b013e3181d2ef6f
37. Andreasen NC. The scale for the assessment of negative symptoms (SANS): conceptual and theoretical foundations. *Br J Psychiatry Suppl* (1989) (7):49–58.
38. Forbes C, Blanchard JJ, Bennett M, Horan WP, Kring A, Gur R. Initial development and preliminary validation of a new negative symptom measure: the clinical assessment interview for negative symptoms (CAINS). *Schizophr Res* (2010) **124**(1–3):36–42. doi:10.1016/j.schres.2010.08.039

7

Psychotic-like experiences and their cognitive appraisal under short-term sensory deprivation

Christina Daniel[1], Anna Lovatt[2] and Oliver John Mason[1]*

[1] *Research Department of Clinical, Educational and Health Psychology, University College London, London, UK*
[2] *Cheshire and Wirral Partnership NHS Foundation Trust, Chester, UK*

Edited by:
Caroline Gurvich, Monash University, Australia

Reviewed by:
Sabina Berretta, Harvard Medical School, USA
Bernhard J. Mitterauer, Volitronics-Institute for Basic Research Psychopathology and Brain Philosophy, Austria

****Correspondence:***
Oliver John Mason, Research Department of Clinical, Educational and Health Psychology, University College London, 1-19 Torrington Place, London WC1E 7HB, UK
e-mail: o.mason@ucl.ac.uk

Aims: This study aimed to establish and compare the effects of brief sensory deprivation on individuals differing in trait hallucination proneness.

Method: Eighteen participants selected for high hallucination proneness were compared against 18 participants rating low on this trait. The presence of psychotic-like experiences (PLEs), and participants' cognitive appraisals of these, was evaluated in three different settings: at baseline, in a "secluded office" environment, and in light-and-sound sensory deprivation.

Results: Psychotic-like experiences were experienced significantly more often in sensory deprivation for both groups. In particular, both experienced slight increases in perceptual distortions and anhedonia in seclusion, and these increased further during sensory deprivation. Highly hallucination prone individuals showed a significantly greater increase in perceptual distortions in sensory deprivation than did non-prone individuals suggesting a state-trait interaction. Their appraisals of these anomalous experiences were compared to both clinical and non-clinical individuals experiencing psychotic symptoms in everyday life.

Conclusion: Short-term sensory deprivation is a potentially useful paradigm to model psychotic experiences, as it is a non-pharmacological tool for temporarily inducing psychotic-like states and is entirely safe at short duration. Experiences occur more frequently, though not exclusively, in those at putative risk of a psychotic disorder. The appraisals of anomalous experiences arising are largely consistent with previous observations of non-clinical individuals though importantly lacked the general positivity of the latter.

Keywords: sensory deprivation, psychosis proneness, appraisals, anomalous body experiences, hallucinations

INTRODUCTION

Since around 2000 high risk research has increasingly investigated how psychotic-like experiences (PLEs) may be part of the risk trajectory for psychosis (1, 2). However, there is a long history of experimental paradigms attempting to induce such experiences in healthy individuals, much of it taking place back in the 1950s and 1960s. Many of these studies employed sensory deprivation of various kinds as the method for inducing anomalous experiences [e.g., Ref. (3)]. The findings were inconsistent, possibly due to an inadequate recognition of the complexity of the variables that enter into the situation of sensory restriction (4). Prolonged periods of deprivation were found to produce a range of psychotic-like phenomena in many, if not all participants. However, experiences at shorter durations varied depending on the nature of the deprivation, and the characteristics of the participants involved. Other studies (5, 6) concluded that PLEs occur in highly suggestible individuals who have a tendency to mistake "imaginary" events as veridical. Researchers lost interest in the field of inducing anomalous experiences, many dismissing the phenomena as more akin to fantasy or acts of imagination and not a true parallel of the hallucinations and other positive symptoms seen in psychosis.

While PLEs are interesting in their own right, we would propose that the theoretical construct of schizotypy conceived as a continuous dimension of risk is an important theoretical perspective from which to interpret individual differences in PLEs. Furthermore, the study of individuals with schizotypal characteristics has the advantage that results are not confounded by the contribution of variables such as hospitalization, medication effects, illness duration, and cognitive deficits. Within the theoretical framework of the continuum hypothesis, the study of a subclinical sample can lead the way toward understanding the perceptual–cognitive mechanisms underlying anomalous experiences both in and outside of psychosis.

With the potential utility for studying PLEs in the normal population now clearly re-established as part of the psychosis continuum (1) and schizotypy rubrics, researchers have taken a fresh look at methods to experimentally induce such experiences, with perhaps the most widely studied relating to the induction of auditory–verbal hallucinations. Many of these methods have been informed by recent theoretical accounts of "voice hearing" such as increased impact of top-down processing (7, 8), reality discrimination failure (9), and increased sensitivity to internally generated percepts (10). Overall, several studies suggest a tendency to erroneously allocate an external source to internally generated stimuli may underlie hallucination proneness in schizophrenia [for review see Ref. (11)]. These findings support a tentative hypothesis that in sensory deprivation, where external events are absent or minimal, highly schizotypal, or hallucination prone individuals are more likely to erroneously process inner thoughts as being external events, and hence experience PLEs. A more sophisticated Bayesian framework (12, 13) suggests that psychotic symptoms arise from a disturbance in error-dependent updating of inferences and beliefs about the world. Corlett et al. (12), in particular, point out how several psychotomimetic drugs may come to have their effects by temporarily disturbing this cognitive process. They go on to discuss how sensory deprivation "may share phenomenological and biological similarities with the serotonergic hallucinogens, both occur when the top-down system imposes structure on noisy, unpredictable bottom-up signals" (p. 524).

In the modern era, several studies have attempted to use a sensory deprivation paradigm to induce PLEs in the normal population (14–18). Using more modern techniques, all studies were successful in inducing hallucinations of varying complexity in many of the participants. What is more, PLEs have been shown to be successfully induced using such methods with as little as 15 min exposure to deprivation of sight and sound (17). Mason and Brady (17) used an anechoic chamber (an environment of total light-and-sound deprivation) to induce PLEs (perceptual disturbances, paranoia, and anhedonia) particularly in those prone to hallucinatory experiences. This pilot study had a number of methodological limitations, not least its sample size of only 19 in total. The study was also criticized for the fact that the procedure included a "panic" button (19) on the basis that a previous study (20) showed the group with just such a button reported many more perceptual aberrations, and cognitive and emotional disturbances, including heightened anxiety. Bell (19) also suggested that the increased PLEs in the high hallucination prone group might be accounted for by differential anxiety levels between high and low-prone groups. This is a serious potential confound, it has been demonstrated that hallucination proneness is linked to trait anxiety (21), and in individuals with psychosis, acute anxiety is clearly linked to an increase in hallucinatory experiences (22). Therefore, it is feasible that an increase in anxiety brought about by sensory deprivation acts to mediate the relationship between PLEs and hallucination proneness. Anxiety was not measured in the original study and this omission was a major limitation. Assessment at baseline was also an area for technical improvement. The pilot study assessed this prior to entering the anechoic chamber when preparatory anxiety may have been influential. The current study utilized a further "secluded office" environment condition as a potentially better matched control condition than standard "baseline."

Cognitive models of psychotic symptoms (23) place central emphasis on how anomalous experiences are appraised. Among the range of appraisals, those that are externalizing and personalizing are thought to play a significant role in determining the transition to clinical psychosis and so are considered of particular significance. Garety et al. (23) also suggested that some people who have anomalous experiences may reject external attributions and so be protected in some way from developing full-blown psychotic symptoms such as delusions. Appraisals and the continuum of psychotic experiences have been studied in depth by Brett et al. (24). Their measure, the appraisals of anomalous experiences interview (AANEX), assesses anomalous experiences and individuals' responses to them, including their appraisals. Individuals with schizophrenia spectrum disorders appraised their experiences as more negative, more dangerous, more likely to be external and personally caused, and made more paranoid/conspiracy interpretations than non-diagnosed controls. Several subsequent studies (25, 26) have further elucidated, which AANEX appraisals distinguish clinical from "at risk" and healthy samples, and which predict greater distress. Assessment of appraisal of PLEs during sensory deprivation has not been described and is novel to this study.

AIMS AND HYPOTHESES

The current study aimed to replicate the effects of brief sensory deprivation using an anechoic chamber in larger groups of low and high hallucination prone individuals. A one-way microphone was also used to monitor participants rather than using a panic-button in an attempt to reduce potential demand characteristics. In addition, state and trait anxiety were measured as potential confounds/covariates. A further aim was to characterize the cognitive appraisals of PLEs arising in sensory deprivation using the AANEX and compare these to existing data.

It was hypothesized that:

1. The high schizotypy group would exhibit a greater degree of PLEs than the low group under normal baseline conditions. This helps further validate the measure of PLEs.
2. Both high and low hallucination prone groups would experience a significant increase in psychotic-like symptoms from baseline in sensory deprivation.
3. The increase in psychotic-like symptoms in sensory deprivation would be significantly greater for the high schizotypy group than the low schizotypy group.
4. The above effects would remain after controlling for any state/trait anxiety differences between the groups.

MATERIALS AND METHODS

PARTICIPANTS

Participants between the ages of 18 and 65 years were recruited via a university psychology department website that advertises to both students and the general public. Exclusion criteria included a history of a major psychiatric or neurological disorder, or recreational or psychotropic drug use in the past 3 months. An advert was placed inviting participants to complete an online version of the revised hallucinations scale [RHS: (27)]. Three hundred seventeen participants from a wide range of ethnic backgrounds returned data. From this sample, 76 low scorers and 39 high scorers were invited to participate as these conformed to the upper and lower 20th percentiles, according to questionnaire norms. Of these, 18 low scorers (7 males, 11 females, mean age = 25.39 years, SD = 6.09, mean score = 26.22, SD = 1.77) and 18 high scorers (4 males, 14 females, mean age = 24.94 years, SD = 3.95, mean score = 54.94, SD = 5.25) gave informed consent, consistent with university ethical procedures.

POWER ANALYSIS

Very little is known about the effects of sensory deprivation on people who rate highly for hallucination proneness, and so it was challenging to accurately estimate effect sizes from existing literature. The most similar study to date (17) reported large effect sizes for increases in perceptual distortions (partial $\eta^2 = 0.56$) and anhedonia (partial $\eta^2 = 0.58$) measured using the psychotomimetic states inventory (PSI) (28) immediately after 15 min of sensory deprivation. The power calculation for the current study was based on the smaller of these effect sizes – partial $\eta^2 = 0.56$. This is a conservative estimate for current purposes since participants in the current study spent a longer length of time in sensory deprivation (25 min) presumably providing greater opportunity for perceptual distortions to arise. Power calculations suggested that a minimum total sample of 18 per group would provide statistical power for a between-within participants repeated measures ANOVA design that exceeded 80% ($\beta = 0.80$), with $\alpha = 0.05$.

MEASURES

Revised hallucinations scale

This is a 24-item questionnaire based on the Launay–Slade hallucination scale (29) measuring a predisposition to experience hallucinations. It uses a revised scoring method, which allows participants to respond on a 4-point scale (1 = never to 4 = almost always). The scale has been shown to have good reliability and predictive validity, and moderately stable internal consistency over a period of 4–6 weeks (27).

Psychotomimetic states inventory

This is a 48-item questionnaire measuring psychosis-like experiences. Items are rated on a 4-point scale (from 0 = never to 3 = strongly), with some items being reverse scored (28). The PSI has sub-scales of delusory thinking, perceptual distortions, cognitive disorganization, anhedonia, mania, and paranoia. Originally developed for use in drug studies, it has produced meaningful results in a previous preliminary study of sensory deprivation (17).

State-trait anxiety inventory

A pair of two 20-item questionnaires that measure the temporary condition of state anxiety, and the more longstanding quality of trait anxiety. Items are rated of a 4-point scale. The state-trait anxiety inventory (STAI) has been shown to have good construct validity with multiple other assessment tools. It has also been shown to have good test-retest reliability [0.54 correlation for state, and 0.86 correlation for trait anxiety (30)].

Appraisals of anomalous experiences interview

A multidimensional measure of psychological responses to anomalies associated with psychosis (24). The first section (the AANEX inventory) includes items reflecting schneiderian first-rank symptoms and anomalies of perception, cognition, affect, and "individuation" (sense of distinction between self and others), as well as some "paranormal" experiences. The inventory generates two sets of scores: "lifetime" (not used in this study) and "state." For state scores, items are rated between 0 and 2 (absent, marginal, and present). The present study assessed whether a particular experience could be used to generate a state score.

The second section (the AANEX-CAR) is a structured interview that assesses appraisals, context, and responses pertaining to any anomalous experiences endorsed from the inventory. It can also be used independently from the inventory to explore anomalies elicited with other clinical instruments (in this instance, the PSI). The format is flexible, and different sub-sections can be used to assess current anomalous experiences, lifetime anomalous experiences, and also changes in interpretation and response style over time. Assessing a person's current style of appraising and responding takes approximately 10–15 min. The AANEX has been shown to reliably differentiate between clinical and non-clinical groups (24, 25).

PROCEDURE

Baseline data were collected from participants a few weeks prior to attending the testing facility (in order to minimize any anticipatory anxiety this may have caused on the day of the experiment itself). The baseline data-set for both groups included AANEX inventory state scores; STAI (full version); PSI. All participants submitted their data via an online website. In order to minimize order effects, participants in both groups were randomly split into two counterbalanced halves. The first half completed the deprivation condition first, followed by the seclusion condition separated by a half-hour break. These were reversed for the remainder. Following completion of the experiment, participants were debriefed, and received a nominal fee (the standard one set for psychology experiments) for their time in taking part.

DEPRIVATION CONDITION

The anechoic chamber and associated procedure is described previously (17). The amendments were the absence of a panic-button and presence of a microphone so that participants could be heard externally by the experimenter should they become distressed. Participants were informed that if they wished to terminate the experiment at any point they should remain seated and tell the experimenter, who would immediately restore light and communication. No participants chose to terminate the experiment early. After a period of 25 min within the chamber, participants were moved to an ante-room where they were immediately asked to complete questionnaires referring to the time that they had spent in the anechoic chamber: the AANEX inventory (state items only); STAI (state items only); PSI. For participants who reported clear anomalous experiences, the AANEX-CAR interview was also administered to gather data on appraisal and responding styles.

SECLUDED OFFICE CONDITION

Participants were seated in an unoccupied office for same period of time as the sensory deprivation condition. They then completed the same questionnaires/interview: AANEX inventory (state items only); STAI (state items only); PSI. Once again, if participants reported clear anomalous experiences, the AANEX-CAR interview was administered to gather data on appraisal and responding styles.

RESULTS

PRELIMINARY STATISTICAL ANALYSES

All statistical analyses were conducted using SPSS 17.0. Data were checked for normality before analysis using descriptive statistics and histograms with normal distribution curves. Anxiety and PSI scores were normally distributed; however, AANEX scores violated parametric assumptions due to significant floor effects, and as a result were not submitted to analysis of variance. Since the AANEX and PSI were both used to measure the underlying construct of PLEs, a non-parametric test of correlation (Kendall's tau) was carried out to detect the strength of association between the two measures. There was a strong positive relationship between AANEX and PSI scores across all three conditions: baseline, $\tau = 0.54$, $p < 0.001$; seclusion, $\tau = 0.70$, $p < 0.001$; and deprivation, $\tau = 0.64$, $p < 0.001$. This supported the validity of using PSI scores as the measure of PLEs in the main analysis, despite this measure not having been formally validated for use in this experimental context. Age and sex were unrelated to PSI and anxiety scores and so were not considered further in analysis.

The order in which participants experienced seclusion and deprivation conditions was counterbalanced as part of the experimental procedure, however, a preliminary mixed between-within subjects repeated measures analysis of variance was carried out to test for any effect of order on anxiety or PSI scores. A significant main effect of order was found for both anxiety scores [$F(1,32) = 7.41$, $p < 0.01$] and PSI scores [$F(1,32) = 5.07$, $p < 0.05$], with participants who experienced seclusion first reporting higher anxiety and PSI scores throughout the experiment. There were no interactions between order and group, indicating that these order effects are not dependent on degree of hallucination proneness.

BASELINE GROUP COMPARISONS

It was hypothesized that the high scoring group would score significantly higher on measures of psychotic-like symptoms under normal baseline conditions. The high and low scoring groups did differ significantly in PSI scores at baseline [$F(1,34) = 6.145$, $p < 0.001$], with the high scoring group reporting a greater number of psychosis-like experiences (see **Table 1** for descriptives).

Baseline trait and state anxiety scores were significantly correlated ($r = 0.74$, $p < 0.001$). Significant differences in trait anxiety [$F(1,34) = 20.23$, $p < 0.001$] and state anxiety [$F(1,34) = 7.91$, $p < 0.01$] were found between the high and low hallucination prone groups at baseline, with the high hallucination prone group reporting higher levels of trait anxiety ($x = 47.78$, SD = 12.95 compared to 31.89, SD = 7.55) and state anxiety ($x = 42.28$, SD = 11.83 compared to 32.50, SE = 8.82). Although not specifically hypothesized all the above findings are in the expected direction.

PSYCHOSIS-LIKE EXPERIENCES ACROSS GROUPS AND CONDITIONS

It was hypothesized that while both groups would experience a significant increase in psychosis-like symptoms from baseline in near-total sensory deprivation, the increase would be significantly greater for the high scoring group. Results of a mixed between-within subjects repeated measures analysis of variance demonstrated a significant main effect of group for PSI scores [$F(1,34) = 31.31$, $p < 0.001$] (see **Table 1** for descriptives). This indicates that the high hallucination prone group experienced a significantly greater number of psychosis-like symptoms overall throughout the experiment, independent of condition (see **Figure 1**).

There was also a main effect of condition for PSI scores [$F(1,83) = 12.524$, $p < 0.001$] (see **Table 1** for descriptives). Planned contrasts revealed that PSI scores were significantly higher in deprivation than at baseline [$F(1,34) = 17.86$, $p < 0.001$] and PSI scores were significantly higher in deprivation than in seclusion [$F(1,34) = 14.05$, $p < 0.001$]. There was no significant difference in PSI scores between seclusion and baseline. There was no interaction effect detected between group and condition, suggesting that both high and low scoring groups responded in a similar way to the experimental conditions.

A further mixed between-within subjects repeated measures analysis of variance examining the PSI sub-scales of delusional thinking, perceptual distortion, cognitive disorganization, anhedonia, mania, and paranoia was conducted to investigate any difference in particular types of psychosis-like experiences reported across the different conditions. Consistent with hypotheses, there

Table 1 | Questionnaire mean scores for high and low hallucination-prone groups by condition.

Questionnaire scores	High scorers ($n = 18$)			Low scorers ($n = 18$)		
Revised hallucinations scale	54.94			26.22		
	Baseline	Seclusion	Deprivation	Baseline	Seclusion	Deprivation
Trait anxiety	47.78	–	–	31.89	–	–
State anxiety	42.78	36.33	38.89	32.50	33.17	36.17
AANEX	39.94	39.28	44.67	29.33	29.33	31.17
Psychotomimetic states inventory (sub-scales below)	37.00	36.83	49.28	13.83	19.89	27.11
Delusory thinking	4.83	4.94	5.50	2.17	1.78	2.22
Perceptual distortions	3.33	5.78	10.78	1.17	2.06	4.89
Cognitive disorganization	9.94	8.78	11.78	3.33	4.56	5.72
Anhedonia	9.17	8.06	10.56	3.67	6.83	8.72
Mania	5.89	6.17	7.28	2.78	3.89	4.50
Paranoia	3.83	3.11	3.39	0.72	0.78	1.06

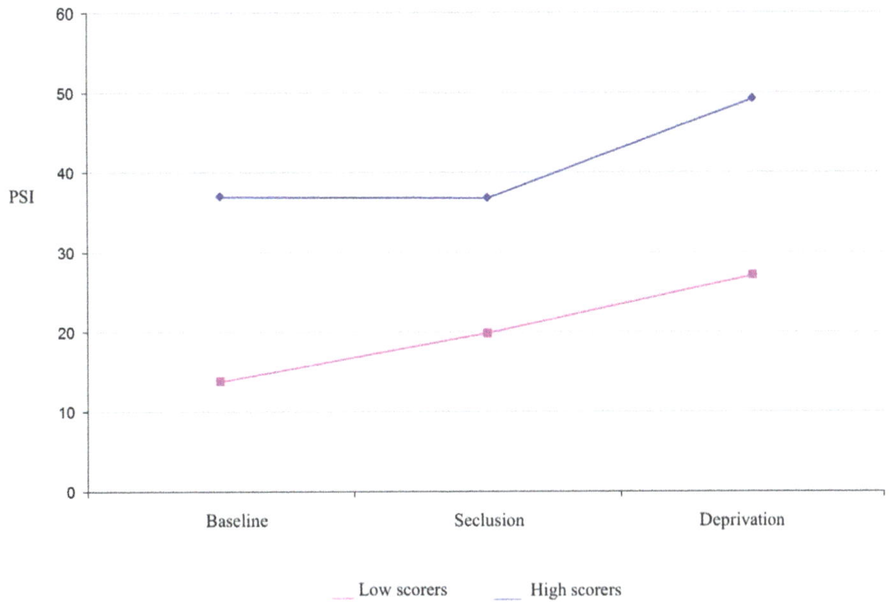

FIGURE 1 | Psychotomimetic states inventory scores in high and low hallucination-prone groups by condition.

was a significant main effect of condition for perceptual distortions [$F(2,68) = 34.15$, $p < 0.001$], anhedonia [$F(2,68) = 10.76$, $p < 0.001$], mania [$F(2,68) = 6.53$, $p < 0.01$], and cognitive disorganization [$F(2,68) = 3.22$, $p < 0.05$]. Planned contrasts indicated that perceptual distortions and anhedonia scores were significantly higher in seclusion than at baseline, and further increased during deprivation. Mania and cognitive disorganization were also significantly higher during deprivation than at baseline, but did not increase significantly in seclusion (see **Table 1**). A significant interaction between group and condition was found for the perceptual distortions subscale [$F(2,68) = 3.63$, $p < 0.05$], with high scorers showing a greater increase in these symptoms in deprivation than low scorers (a difference of around two SD, see **Table 1**). A significant interaction between group and condition was also found for the anhedonia subscale [$F(2,68) = 5.31$, $p < 0.01$], with low scorers showing a more marked increase in anhedonic symptoms in deprivation than high scorers (see **Table 1**).

STATE AND TRAIT ANXIETY ACROSS GROUPS AND CONDITIONS

Results of a mixed between-within subjects repeated measures analysis of variance demonstrated a significant main effect of group for state anxiety scores [$F(1,34) = 4.21$, $p < 0.05$] (see **Table 1** for descriptives). This indicates that the high hallucination prone group experienced higher state anxiety than the low hallucination prone group. There was no effect of condition for state anxiety, suggesting that anxiety did not differ between baseline, seclusion, and deprivation conditions (see **Figure 2**). Thus, state anxiety is unlikely to account for the differences in psychosis-like experiences between conditions. Trait anxiety differed between experimental groups, but did not correlate with PSI scores in any condition. Consequently, trait anxiety was not considered as a covariate for analysis of variance for PSI scores.

AANEX-CAR

AANEX-CAR semi-structured interviews were administered to all participants who reported clearly identifiable psychosis-like experiences in seclusion or deprivation. Interviews were indicated for 11 out of 18 participants in the high scoring group, and 4 out of 18 participants in the low scoring group. Consistent with PSI results, the hallucination prone group reported a greater number of psychosis-like experiences than the non-prone group ($\chi^2 = 4.11$, $p < 0.005$).

All interviews were indicated following experiences in deprivation. The types of experiences participants reported were varied, including hearing noises such as insects buzzing and whistling ($n = 2$); hearing music ($n = 2$); seeing shapes and colored lights ($n = 4$); visual hallucinations such as seeing faces and animals ($n = 2$); out-of-body experiences or the experience of watching events through another's eyes ($n = 3$); disorientation such as feelings of falling, the room spinning, and the walls closing in ($n = 2$). Interviews were scored according to the procedure described by Brett et al. (24), and ratings derived for appraisal dimensions, appraisal categories, emotional response, cognitive and behavioral response, perceived social understanding, and perceived controllability.

In order to establish whether AANEX-CAR scores reflected typical appraisal and cognitive/emotional response styles of people experiencing genuine symptoms that had not been experimentally "induced," the scores were compared with existing data from a clinical group (schizophrenia spectrum disorders) and a non-clinical group with anomalous experiences [Ref. (25), see **Table 2**]. Experiences under sensory deprivation were similar to those seen in the non-clinical group and differed from the clinical group in being appraised as less dangerous, less external, less due to others, and less anxiety provoking/negative emotionally; and as having a greater sense of agency, and more likely to have a psychological

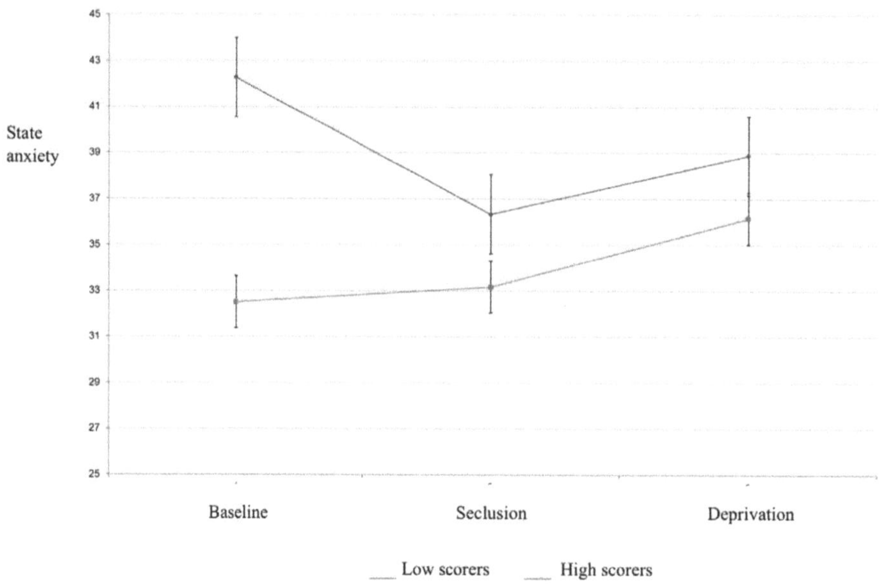

FIGURE 2 | State anxiety scores in high and low hallucination-prone groups by condition.

cause. However, the sensory deprivation group's appraisals differed from the non-clinical group in not being as positively valenced; not as spiritual in meaning; or positive emotionally. In these latter respects they did not differ significantly from the clinical group.

DISCUSSION

Consistent with hypotheses, hallucination proneness was associated with greater psychosis-like symptoms under all conditions. In addition, both high and low scoring groups experienced a significant increase in psychosis-like symptoms in sensory deprivation conditions. Sensory deprivation was found to produce a significant increase on four sub-scales of the PSI: perceptual distortions, anhedonia, mania, and cognitive disorganization. Findings with respect to perceptual distortions and anhedonia were highly marked and were consistent with the pilot study (17). However, unlike the previous study, paranoia did not appear to increase significantly. As the current study is larger and so better powered, and utilized a longer time period, it is likely to provide a more sensitive profile of the psychotic-like symptoms provoked by deprivation. In the current study, an interaction effect between condition and group was only seen for the perceptual distortion subscale clearly validating the RHS and suggesting a state-trait interaction. Consistent with this, the majority of hallucination prone individuals (11 of 19) reported clear anomalous experiences sufficient for AANEX-CAR interview, in contrast with a minority of non-prone (4 of 19). The potential role of state and trait anxiety was explored. Consistent with the previous literature (21), trait and state anxiety distinguished the high hallucination-prone from the low hallucination-prone groups at baseline. However, trait anxiety neither predicted changes in PSI scores nor differed across condition in either group. Therefore, the increase in psychosis-like symptoms seen in both groups during deprivation cannot be readily attributed to increased anxiety.

The considerable presence of anomalous perceptions that were experienced to some degree at least as autonomous, external, and "hallucination-like" are consistent with the "faulty source monitoring" hypothesis (9). It is also consistent with the framework offered by Fletcher and Frith (13) that unusual perceptions arise out of an abnormality in the brains' inferencing mechanism, so that new evidence (including sensations) is not properly integrated, leading to false prediction errors in psychotic and psychosis-prone individuals. In the absence of external stimuli, perceptual distortions are presumably internally generated by the individuals, but are misattributed as external in origin due to "top-down" processes (12). Overall, the range and frequency of psychotic-like symptoms are sufficient to endorse Corlett et al.'s (12) position that sensory deprivation offers a promising model of psychosis in psychiatrically healthy individuals. Future research should explore the underlying neurocognitive mechanisms of PLEs under sensory deprivation using neurobiological methods such as psychophysiological recording.

Also of interest, but not predicted, was that *low* scorers experienced a significantly greater increase in anhedonic symptoms during deprivation as compared to baseline measurement. Previously, this finding had only been seen in high scorers. This could be due to boredom effects in the low scoring group (related to the longer time duration), who otherwise reported few psychosis-like experiences during deprivation.

AANEX-CAR data showed the appraisal and cognitive/emotional response styles of participants were broadly consistent with those of non-clinical individuals with anomalous experiences. Participants strongly believed that the causes of their experiences were psychological in nature and that they had some agency within them. The unusual environmental context may have made them more likely to interpret their experiences in terms of internal mental processes. Anxiety, dangerousness, and

Table 2 | Appraisals under sensory deprivation compared with Lovatt et al. groups (25).

AANEX-CAR items	Sensory deprivation group ($n = 15$) mean (SD)	Clinical group ($n = 29$) mean (SD)	Non-clinical group ($n = 29$) mean (SD)	*F* test	*Post hoc* comparisons (Scheffe)
APPRAISAL: DIMENSIONS					
Valence	2.93 (1.24)	2.52 (1.25)	4.19 (1.04)	14.23**	NC > C = SD
Dangerousness	2.66 (1.74)	3.81 (1.18)	2.74 (1.10)	5.85**	C > NC = SD
Externality	2.00 (1.10)	3.44 (1.25)	2.33 (0.92)	10.61**	C > NC = SD
Agency	4.47 (0.72)	3.85 (1.2)	2.44 (1.15)	19.46**	C > NC = SD
APPRAISAL: CATEGORIES					
Biological	0.07 (0.25)	0.48 (0.80)	0.44 (0.80)	n.s	–
Psychological/normalizing	2.00 (0.00)	0.44 (0.75)	1.44 (0.75)	29.90**	C > NC = SD
Spiritual	0.33 (0.70)	0.67 (0.78)	1.33 (0.88)	8.54**	NC > C = SD
Other people	0.07 (0.25)	1.11 (0.93)	0.74 (0.26)	23.03**	C > NC = SD
EMOTIONAL RESPONSE					
Neutral arousal	2.33 (1.19)	2.59 (1.25)	2.70 (1.07)	n.s	–
Negative emotional response	2.12 (1.54)	3.70 (1.07)	2.00 (0.92)	17.09**	C > NC = SD
Positive emotional response	2.07 (1.24)	2.19 (0.92)	3.15 (1.13)	7.05**	NC > C = SD
Self-rated anxiety	2.53 (1.31)	3.96 (1.02)	1.96 (1.06)	22.69**	C > NC = SD
Self-rated excitement	2.27 (1.34)	2.48 (1.48)	3.03 (1.45)	n.s.	–

NC, non-clinical group; C, clinical group; SD, sensory deprivation group.
$^{**}p < 0.01$.

a negative emotional response were at the low levels seen in non-clinical individuals, and unlike the symptomatic experiences of those with psychotic disorders. However, non-clinical individuals with repeated anomalous experiences have often been shown to develop positively valenced appraisals with, for some, strong spiritual meanings. This did not prove the case, in general, for those in sensory deprivation. "Naturally" occurring – and reoccurring – anomalous experiences are plausibly more likely to develop idiosyncratic and personally highly meaningful appraisals than those "artificially" created by laboratory conditions.

LIMITATIONS

Despite attempting to address several potential confounds of the pilot study, other such as social desirability are suggestibility cannot be excluded and deserve further testing. Though the appraisal data go some way to detailing the similarities with clinical and non-clinical psychotic experiences there is some way to go before concluding the phenomena seen in sensory deprivation are equivalent as this is currently reliant on self-report. Biometric approaches such as psychophysiological or neurocognitive indices would clearly strengthen the argument.

The "secluded office" condition attempted to provide a closer analog to sensory deprivation (in duration at least) than the baseline but this was not highly successful. While, on many indices these two conditions appeared highly similar there were significant order effects across both groups, with participants who experienced seclusion first reporting more psychosis-like experiences throughout the experiment. It is possible that participants who experienced seclusion first responded to the perceived demand characteristics of the experiment, endorsing more items on the PSI and AANEX measures in this first condition. Counter-balancing was incorporated into the experimental design in an attempt to moderate any order effects, but demand characteristics may still have had some impact particularly on the seclusion data. As a consequence, the baseline condition is very probably the more stable one against which to compare the experimental deprivation condition.

CLINICAL IMPLICATIONS

The findings suggest that even during a quite brief period of sensory deprivation, perceptual distortions, and other psychosis-like experiences are common in the "normal" population. Although high hallucination prone individuals reported significantly greater levels of perceptual distortions, individuals not prone to experiencing hallucinations were also affected. In the current study, any psychosis-like symptoms were transient, and quickly resolved once participants were returned to normal conditions. Indeed, the distortions and other psychotic phenomena induced did not bring attendant anxiety as probably occurs with many early psychotic symptoms. Nevertheless, it is possible that a longer period of deprivation may have the potential to induce enduring symptoms of psychosis with consequent distress.

CONCLUSION

Overall, the study provides further support for use of sensory deprivation as a non-pharmacological tool for temporarily inducing psychotic-like states. Both high and low hallucination prone groups responded to sensory deprivation in a qualitatively similar manner, but with quantitative differences in the frequency of psychosis-like experiences reported. It appears possible to accurately predict individuals who are most likely to experience psychosis-like experiences in sensory deprivation based on the presence/absence of schizotypal traits (here as indexed by hallucination proneness). Sensory deprivation would seem a useful paradigm to model psychotic symptoms, to which we would add the important ethical principle of non-harm.

REFERENCES

1. Johns L, van Os J. The continuity of psychotic experiences in the general population. *Clin Psychol Rev* (2001) **21**(8):1123–41. doi:10.1016/S0272-7358(01)00103-9
2. Kelleher I, Cannon M. Psychotic-like experiences in the general population: characterizing a high-risk group for psychosis. *Psychol Med* (2011) **41**:1–6. doi:10.1017/S0033291710001005
3. Harris A. Sensory deprivation and schizophrenia. *J Mental Sci* (1959) **105**:235–7.
4. Ziskind E. A second look at sensory deprivation. *J Nerv Ment Dis* (1964) **138**:223–32. doi:10.1097/00005053-196403000-00002
5. Barber T, Calverley D. An experimental study of hypnotic (auditory and visual) hallucinations. *J Abn Soc Psychol* (1964) **68**:13–20. doi:10.1037/h0042175
6. Bowers K. The effects of demands for honesty on reports of visual and auditory hallucinations. *Int J Clin Exp Hypn* (1967) **15**:31–6. doi:10.1080/00207146708407503
7. Grossberg S. How hallucinations may arise from brain mechanisms of learning, attention, and volition. *J Int Neuropsychol Soc* (2000) **6**:583–92. doi:10.1017/S135561770065508X
8. Aleman A, Bocker K, Hijman R. Cognitive basis of hallucinations in schizophrenia: role of top-down information processing. *Schiz Res* (2003) **64**:175–85. doi:10.1016/S0920-9964(03)00060-4
9. Bentall RP. The illusion of reality: a review and integration of psychological research on hallucinations. *Psychol Bull* (1990) **107**:82–95. doi:10.1037/0033-2909.107.1.82
10. Blakemore SJ, Smith J, Steel R, Johnstone EC, Frith CD. The perception of self-produced sensory stimuli in patients with auditory hallucinations and passivity experiences: evidence for a breakdown in self-monitoring. *Psychol Med* (2000) **30**:1131–9. doi:10.1017/S0033291799002676
11. Ditman T, Kuperberg G. A source-monitoring account of auditory verbal hallucinations in patients with schizophrenia. *Harv Rev Psychiatry* (2005) **13**:280–99. doi:10.1080/10673220500326391
12. Corlett PR, Frith CD, Fletcher PC. From drugs to deprivation: a Bayesian framework for understanding models of psychosis. *Psychopharmacology (Berl)* (2009) **206**:515–30. doi:10.1007/s00213-009-1561-0
13. Fletcher PC, Frith CD. Perceiving is believing: a Bayesian approach to explaining the positive symptoms of schizophrenia. *Nat Rev Neurosci* (2008) **10**:48–58. doi:10.1038/nrn2536
14. Hayashi M, Morikawa T, Hori T. EEG alpha activity and hallucinatory experience during sensory deprivation. *Percept Mot Skills* (1992) **75**(2):403–412. doi:10.2466/pms.1992.75.2.403
15. McCreery C, Claridge G. A study of hallucinations in normal subjects – 1. Self report data. *Pers Indiv Diff* (1996) **21**:739–41. doi:10.1016/0191-8869(96)00115-8
16. Merabet L, Maguire D, Warde A. Visual hallucinations during prolonged blindfolding in sighted subjects. *J Neuroopthalmol* (2004) **24**(2):109–13. doi:10.1097/00041327-200406000-00003
17. Mason OJ, Brady F. The psychotomimetic effects of short-term sensory deprivation. *J Nerv Ment Dis* (2009) **97**:783–5. doi:10.1097/NMD.0b013e3181b9760b
18. Lloyd D, Lewis E, Payne J. A qualitative analysis of sensory phenomena induced by perceptual deprivation. *Phenomenol Cogn Sci* (2012) **11**:95–112. doi:10.1007/s11097-011-9233-z
19. Bell V. An alternative interpretation of "the psychotomimetic effects of short-term sensory deprivation". *J Nerv Ment Dis* (2010) **198**:166. doi:10.1097/NMD.0b013e3181cc0ba7
20. Orne M, Scheibe K. The contribution of nondeprivation factors in the production of sensory deprivation effects: the psychology of the "panic button". *J Abn Soc Psychol* (1964) **68**:3–12. doi:10.1037/h0048803
21. Allen P, Freeman D, McGuire P, Garety P, Kuipers E, Fowler D, et al. The prediction of hallucinatory predisposition in non-clinical individuals: examining the contribution of emotion and reasoning. *Br J Clin Psychol* (2005) **44**:127–32. doi:10.1348/014466504X20044
22. Delespaul P, deVries M, van Os J. Determinants of occurrence and recovery from hallucinations in daily life. *Soc Psychiatry Psychiatr Epidemiol* (2003) **37**:97–104. doi:10.1007/s001270200000
23. Garety PA, Kuipers E, Fowler D, Freeman D, Bebbington PE. A cognitive model of the positive symptoms of psychosis. *Psychol Med* (2001) **31**:189–95. doi:10.1017/S0033291701003312
24. Brett CMC, Peters EP, Johns LC, Tabraham PA, Valmaggia L, McGuire PK. The appraisals of anomalous experiences interview (AANEX): a multi-dimensional measure of psychological responses to anomalies associated with psychosis. *Br J Psychiatry Suppl* (2007) **51**:S23–30. doi:10.1192/bjp.191.51.s23
25. Lovatt A, Mason O, Brett C, Peters E. Psychotic-like experiences, appraisals, and trauma. *J Nerv Ment Dis* (2010) **198**:813–9. doi:10.1097/NMD.0b013e3181f97c3d
26. Brett CMC, Heriot-Maitland C, McGuire P, Peters EP. Predictors of distress associated with psychotic-like anomalous experiences in clinical and non-clinical populations. *Br J Clin Psychol* (2014) **53**:213–27. doi:10.1111/bjc.12036
27. Morrison AP, Wells A, Nothard S. Cognitive and emotional predictors of predisposition to hallucinations in non-patients. *Br J Clin Psychol* (2002) **41**:259–70. doi:10.1348/014466502760379127
28. Mason OJ, Morgan CJ, Stefanovic A, Curran HV. The psychotomimetic states inventory (PSI): measuring psychotic-type experiences from ketamine and cannabis. *Schiz Res* (2005) **103**:138–142. doi:10.1016/j.schres.2008.02.020
29. Launay G, Slade P. The measurement of hallucinatory predisposition in male and female prisoners. *Per Ind Diff* (1981) **2**:221–34. doi:10.1016/0191-8869(81)90027-1
30. Spielberger CD, Gorsuch RL, Lushene PR, Vagg PR, Jacobs AG. *Manual for the State-Trait Anxiety Inventory (Form Y)*. Palo Alto, CA: Consulting Psychologists Press, Inc (1983).

8

Preserved learning during the symbol–digit substitution test in patients with schizophrenia, age-matched controls, and elderly

Claudia Cornelis[1,2]*, Livia J. De Picker[1,2], Wouter Hulstijn[1,3], Glenn Dumont[1,2], Maarten Timmers[4], Luc Janssens[4], Bernard G. C. Sabbe[1,2] and Manuel Morrens[1,5]

[1] *Collaborative Antwerp Psychiatric Research Institute, University of Antwerp, Antwerp, Belgium*
[2] *University Psychiatric Center St. Norbertushuis, Duffel, Belgium*
[3] *Donders Institute for Brain, Cognition and Behaviour, Radboud University Nijmegen, Nijmegen, Netherlands*
[4] *Janssen Research and Development, Janssen Pharmaceutica N.V., Beerse, Belgium*
[5] *Psychiatric Hospital Broeders Alexianen, Boechout, Belgium*

Edited by:
Sebastian Walther, University Hospital of Psychiatry, Switzerland

Reviewed by:
Katharina Stegmayer, University Hospital of Psychiatry, Switzerland
Benny Liberg, Karolinska Institutet, Sweden

****Correspondence:***
Claudia Cornelis, Collaborative Antwerp Psychiatric Institute (CAPRI), University of Antwerp, Campus Drie Eiken, Universiteitsplein 1, Antwerp B-2610, Belgium
e-mail: claudia.cornelis@uantwerpen.be

Objective: Speed of processing, one of the main cognitive deficits in schizophrenia is most frequently measured with a digit–symbol-coding test. Performance on this test is additionally affected by writing speed and the rate at which symbol–digit relationships are learned, two factors that may be impaired in schizophrenia. This study aims to investigate the effects of sensorimotor speed, short-term learning, and long-term learning on task performance in schizophrenia. In addition, the study aims to explore differences in learning effects between patients with schizophrenia and elderly individuals.

Methods: Patients with schizophrenia ($N = 30$) were compared with age-matched healthy controls ($N = 30$) and healthy elderly volunteers ($N = 30$) during the Symbol–Digit Substitution Test (SDST). The task was administered on a digitizing tablet, allowing precise measurements of the time taken to write each digit (writing time) and the time to decode symbols into their corresponding digits (matching time). The SDST was administered on three separate days (day 1, day 2, day 7). Symbol–digit repetitions during the task represented short-term learning and repeating the task on different days represented long-term learning.

Results: The repetition of the same symbol–digit combinations within one test and the repetition of the test over days resulted in significant decreases in matching time. Interestingly, these short-term and long-term learning effects were about equal among the three groups. Individual participants showed a large variation in the rate of short-term learning. In general, patients with schizophrenia had the longest matching time whereas the elderly had the longest writing time. Writing time remained the same over repeated testing.

Conclusion: The rate of learning and sensorimotor speed was found to have a substantial influence on the SDST score. However, a large individual variation in learning rate should be taken into account in the interpretation of task scores for processing speed. Equal learning rates among the three groups suggest that unintentional learning in schizophrenia and in the elderly is preserved. These findings are important for the design of rehabilitation programs for schizophrenia.

Keywords: symbol–digit substitution test, coding task, processing speed, implicit learning, schizophrenia

INTRODUCTION

Schizophrenia is a psychiatric disorder, characterized by positive symptoms (e.g., hallucinations and delusions), negative symptoms (e.g., avolition and reduced emotional expressivity), and severe cognitive disabilities. Since cognitive deficits in schizophrenia are significantly correlated to poor functional outcomes (1) and quality of life (2), the development of pharmacological and remediation techniques addressing these impairments could be highly beneficial to the clinical outcome.

Cognition is not a single entity but can be divided into several domains. In schizophrenia research, the areas of primary interest are: processing speed, attention/vigilance, working memory, verbal learning, visual learning, executive functioning and social cognition (3). The combination of these domains may contribute differently to the overall clinical picture of cognitive decline in schizophrenia. Experimental tasks that focus on isolating the relative influence of these specific cognitive domains are needed to specify which deficits are most pronounced in order to provide a targeted treatment.

Processing speed has been shown to be a very distinguishing and reliable factor to characterize cognitive deficits in schizophrenia (4). This parameter reflects the speed with which different cognitive and sensorimotor functions are executed (5). Viewed from a traditional experimental psychology perspective, processing speed can be conceived as the total sum of three different stages of information processing, namely perceptual analysis, response selection, and response execution (6, 7).

Although there are several neuropsychological tests for measuring reduced processing speed, a recent meta-analysis (8) has demonstrated that a digit–symbol-coding task is the most sensitive test to apply to patients with schizophrenia. Moreover, this meta-analysis identified processing speed impairment as the largest single deficit in the cognitive abilities of schizophrenia (8, 9).

Digit–symbol-coding tasks have been carried out in two different ways. In one version, the Digit–Symbol Substitution Test (DSST), symbols have to be drawn under their corresponding digits according to a key of digit–symbol combinations, provided at the top of the sheet. The second version is the symbol-coding subtest of the Brief Assessment of Cognition in Schizophrenia included in the MATRICS Final Battery (7, 10). This task does not require the drawing of symbols but rather the numerals (1–9) have to be written as quickly as possible under the corresponding symbols, which are presented in rows on the response sheet. This version of the coding task has been called the Symbol–Digit Substitution Test (SDST). In the present study, as in our previous studies (5, 11), we have used the SDST in order to avoid drawing unfamiliar graphic symbols, which requires a time consuming process of motor planning.

In the measurement of processing speed using a digit–symbol-coding task, at least two factors might play a considerable role. First, digit–symbol-coding tasks have a strong sensorimotor component (i.e., fine motor writing skills of the symbols or the digits). A reduction in sensorimotor speed, characterized by a longer initiation and/or execution of graphic movements, might indeed contribute substantially to low coding task performance. Previous research by Morrens et al. has demonstrated that schizophrenia patients display both sensorimotor and cognitive slowing and that these two processes are unrelated to each other (11).

In addition to a possible sensorimotor component, a second possible factor, which may influence the measurement of processing speed is het effect of (implicit) learning of the specific symbol–digit combinations. Learning is a well-known impairment in schizophrenia (9, 12–14) in addition to processing speed. Once the symbol–digit relationships are learned, it is no longer necessary to rely on visual scanning of the key on top of the administration sheet, rather working or episodic memory can be used instead for the right response. This strategy might reduce the time in finding the right response, resulting in an increased score on the test. There may be large individual differences in the speed of learning these symbol–digit relations and in their memory capacity. Similarly, Bachman et al. (15) and Joy et al. (16) proposed that a reduced cognitive processing speed in schizophrenia might be partially due to a mnemonic deficit. Other studies on this topic concluded that the contribution of memory to symbol–digit coding performance might be relatively small but relevant (16).

However, many of these previous studies have used regression-based approaches in which coding performance was correlated with additional neuropsychological tests (15). In an older version of the Wechsler Adult Intelligence Scale (WAIS-III), the Digit–Symbol-coding test was even followed by an implicit learning test to assess the recall of the symbol–digit relations (17). Bachman et al. rightly argued for a complementary experimental approach in which the symbol-coding task is manipulated to determine the role that several sub-processes might play in coding tasks. However, a disadvantage of this latter approach is that changing the task might have consequences for the relative contribution of these sub-processes.

In this experimental study, the subjects' pen movements were recorded on a writing tablet under the test sheet in order to precisely measure the time taken to write each digit (writing time) as well as the preceding time necessary to decode a symbol into its corresponding digit (matching time). The task requires to write the digits as quickly as possible; therefore, the writing time provides an estimate of sensorimotor speed whereas matching time reflects the duration of the cognitive processes that are needed to find or recall the digit that corresponds to the stimulus symbol.

Because matching time and writing time were registered for every single digit, the decrease per symbol–digit combination offers an estimate of both the rate and the amount of learning within one (90 s) test administration. In addition, by administering the same test on three separate days, we were able to assess the amount of long-term learning of the symbol–digit relations.

Schizophrenia has been previously hypothesized as a generalized syndrome of accelerated aging (18). Since the earliest descriptions by Emil Kraepelin, schizophrenia has been referred to as "dementia praecox," literally meaning "a cognitive decline in young age." A number of studies have shown that processing speed as measured by the SDST is a fundamental mediator of age-related cognitive decline (19, 20). Therefore, comparing the performance of schizophrenia patients to elderly individuals could offer secondary, but valuable information as to what extent and in which domains the cognitive decline in schizophrenia resembles age-related cognitive impairment, referred to as "mild cognitive impairment." To our knowledge, a direct comparison of performance on the SDST between schizophrenic and elderly individuals has never been conducted.

In summary, the present study was set up to investigate the relative contribution of learning and sensorimotor speed during SDST performance. Patients with schizophrenia, age-matched healthy controls, and elderly volunteers were tested in order to assess different effects of these factors in the different groups. The first hypothesis was that overall test performance would be lower in schizophrenia patients compared with age-matched healthy controls. In addition, it was expected that this study would replicate the well-known findings of reduced writing speed in schizophrenia. As visual and verbal learning and memory have been frequently found to be impaired in patients with schizophrenia (7), it was further hypothesized that the rate and amount of the learning of the symbol–digit relations would be reduced in the schizophrenia patients. The comparison of schizophrenic and elderly individuals was exploratory.

MATERIALS AND METHODS

STUDY DESIGN

Our study group consisted of 30 patients with stable schizophrenia, 30 age- and sex-matched control participants, and 30 sex-matched elderly volunteers (aged 65–85 years). The SDST was administered three times on three separate assessment days. The test was conducted in accordance with the ethical principles that have their origin in the Declaration of Helsinki and that are consistent with Good Clinical Practices, applicable regulatory requirements, and in compliance with the study protocol. This study was held at the University Psychiatric Hospital Duffel, Belgium, and the study protocol was reviewed and approved by the institute's Ethics Committee.

PARTICIPANTS

The previously mentioned test subjects were recruited from the local community. Prior to the start of the study, they all provided a written informed consent and their eligibility for this study was assessed according to some inclusion and exclusion criteria. The inclusion criteria for patients were: (1) being an in- or outpatient with schizophrenia or schizoaffective disorder (DSM-IV), (2) having a known history of schizophrenia for at least 12 months, confirmed by the treating psychiatrist, and (3) receiving stable antipsychotic drug therapy (maximally 2) for at least 6 weeks prior to screening. The inclusion criteria for all participants were: (1) being a man or woman between 18 and 55 years old (schizophrenia patients and young controls) or between 65 and 85 years old (elderly volunteers) and (2) being medically stable.

The exclusion criteria applicable to all participants were (1) having a DSM-IV diagnosis of substance dependence or abuse within 3 months prior to screening evaluation (only caffeine dependence was not exclusionary), (2) use of benzodiazepines, tricyclic antidepressants, or anticholinergic medication, (3) having a positive urine screen for drug abuse or a positive alcohol breath test at screening on one of the test days, (4) having a clinically significant acute illness within 7 days prior to screening. Since the use of alcohol and drugs could potentially influence the study data, an alcohol breath test and a urine drug screen were performed before the start of each assessment day.

SYMBOL–DIGIT SUBSTITUTION TEST

The task was performed on two subsequent sessions (day 1 and day 2) and a third time (day 7). The SDST was the first task to be performed on every assessment day in a larger series of cognitive tests, which will be published elsewhere. In order to avoid influences of the circadian rhythm, also the time on which the test was administered was comparable for each subject.

The coding task required to translate 9 different symbols into the digits 1–9 on five rows each consisting of 25 symbols, according to a key of symbol–digit pairs, which was presented on top of the task sheet. The same symbol–digit combinations were repeated over the three session days. In line with our previous studies (5, 11, 21), we used the reversed version of the classical DSST where the digits had to be written under the symbols, denoted by SDST. We chose for this design in order to exclude the complication of processes of motor planning by the drawing of complex graphic symbols on SDST performance. The nine different symbols were presented in blocks. The sequence in which they were presented within each block was randomized.

A quiet environment was chosen to perform this task. The participants were asked to decode the list of symbols one by one as fast as possible within a preset 90s limit, based on the key above, writing the correct digit under the corresponding symbol on a sheet of paper placed on a digitizing tablet (WACOM1218RE) with a special pressure-sensitive normal-looking ballpoint pen. Pen position was recorded at 200 Hz and with 0.2 mm spatial accuracy, and stored on a standard personal computer. The signals were subsequently filtered by means of a fast-Fourier analysis. These digitized recordings allowed the computation of separate matching- and writing times.

Identical instructions were repeated each day, before the start of the task. Feedback was not provided at the end of the session. All subjects had to undergo a practice trial on the first assessment day, consisting of filling in the last 10 symbol–digit pairs, allowing them to get familiar with the experiment.

STATISTICAL ANALYSIS

All data were analyzed using a general linear model (GLM) repeated measures in IBM®SPSS® Version 22. First, we analyzed the Session effect (long-term learning) with Group (three levels) as the between-subjects variable and Session (or days, with three levels) as the within-subjects variable. A second analysis used Block (five levels; short-term learning) and Session (three levels) as the within-subject variables and Group (three levels) as the between-subject variable. We performed separate analyses for (1) the number of correct digits, (2) the mean matching time per digit, and (3) the mean writing time per digit. Wilk's Lambda was used in the tests of the within-variable effects. A p-value of <0.05 was considered significant.

The number of blocks that could be analyzed depended on the lowest test score (number correct) obtained by the participants. Matching and writing time were analyzed over five blocks (i.e., number correct is 45 or higher). This score was gained in all three sessions by 25 patients with schizophrenia, 28 elderly volunteers, and 28 controls. Including more participants in the analysis would result in too many missing values in the fourth and fifth block whereas analyzing more than five blocks would result in an unrepresentative low number of participants. Per block, the median matching time and median writing time were calculated. Only correct digits were analyzed and the first digit of a row was eliminated from analysis because the transport distance to this location was more than 20 cm instead of the normal 0.8 cm. In session 3, the data of one patient were missing.

RESULTS

The main objective of the present study was to evaluate the role of learning processes during SDST performance. Firstly, demographics will be prescribed (see Demographics) followed by their general test scores on the SDST [see Test score (Number of correct digits)]. Matching time and writing time of test scores were separately calculated (see Long-Term Learning Matching and Writing Time and Short-Term Learning Matching and Writing Time Over Blocks

Per session), and the added effects of long-term learning (section Long-Term Learning Matching and Writing Time) and short-term learning (see Short-Term Learning Matching and Writing Time Over Blocks Per session) were assessed. In a final section (see Estimating the Effect of Short-Term Learning on the SDST Score), the relative contribution of short-term learning on the overall SDST score was calculated.

DEMOGRAPHICS

The demographic features of the three study groups are shown in **Table 1**. All patients used antipsychotic medication at the time of testing. Sixteen schizophrenia patients were using more than one antipsychotic drug. The distribution of the different antipsychotic drugs and range of daily doses are summarized elsewhere (22). Seven young controls, two schizophrenia patients, and no elderly individuals were left-handed. A GLM repeated measures analysis was conducted on the performance of the SDST (number correct) for the young control group with "Session" as within-subject variable and "Handedness" as between-subject variable. "Handedness" did not have a significant influence on the overall test score. The schizophrenia group had a lower mean IQ, as measured by the Adult Reading Test/ART (Dutch version: Nederlandse Leestekst voor Volwassenen/NLV), than the control group ($t = 3.96, p = 0.0002$) and the elderly group ($t = 4.71, p < 0.0001$).

Table 1 | Demographics.

		Schizophrenia	Elderly	Control
N		**30**	**30**	**30**
Age	Mean (SD)	36.43 (7.83)	69.33 (3.89)	36.77 (8.55)
	Range	23–53	65–79	18–52
IQ (ART)	Mean (SD)	101.3 (10.30)	111.7 (6.43)	110.1 (6.39)
	Range	66–115	100–124	98–130
Sex	male: female	2:1	2:1	2:1
Race	Asian	0	0	1
	Maghreb	1	0	0
	White	29	30	29

TEST SCORE (NUMBER OF CORRECT DIGITS)

The mean number of correct digits per session is displayed in **Figure 1** for each group. This figure clearly shows an increase in task performance (long-term learning effect) over the three sessions, which was significant [$F(2,85) = 36.21$, $p < 0.001$]. This learning effect was about equal in the three groups (Session*Group interaction $p = 0.119$).

On average, the three groups differed significantly in their overall score [$F(2,86) = 21.69, p < 0.001$]. Both schizophrenia patients and the elderly volunteers achieved a lower test score than the controls ($p < 0.001$). **Figure 1** gives the impression that the schizophrenia group performed even worse than the elderly, but the difference between these groups was not significant ($p = 0.07$) but

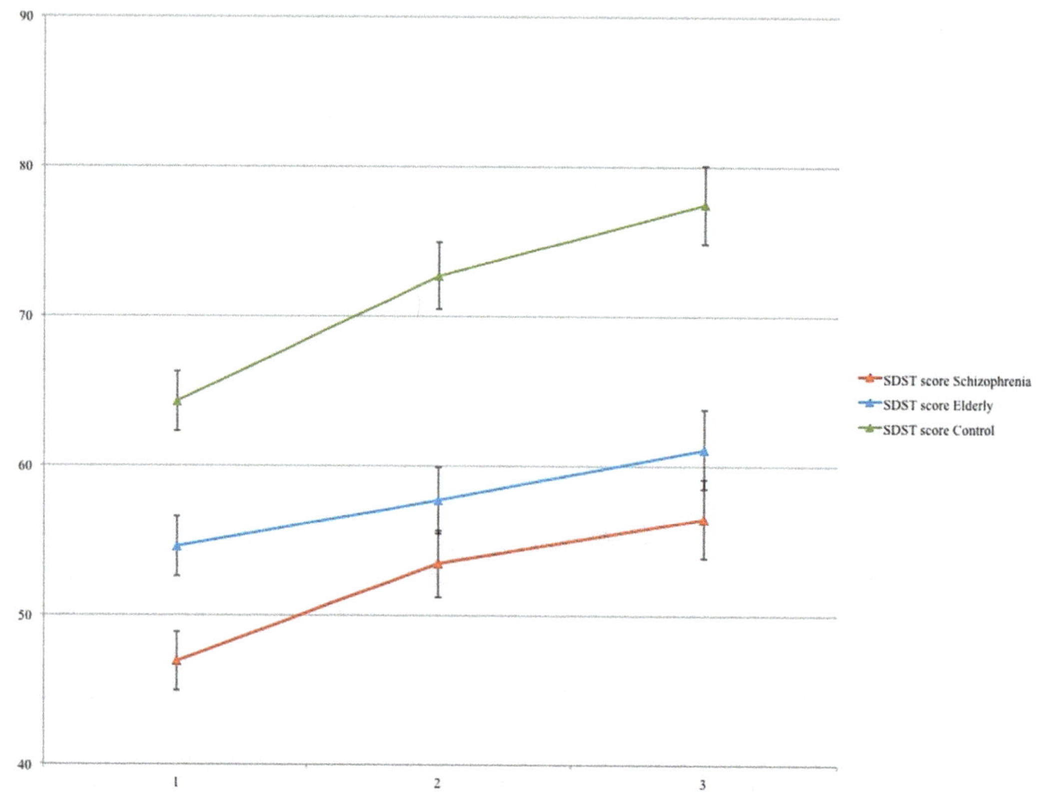

FIGURE 1 | Means and SE of the number of correct digits per session for schizophrenia patients, elderly volunteers, and young controls.

this was only true during the first session ($p = 0.028$). After incorporating IQ as a covariate in the analysis, the group difference between schizophrenia patients and controls remained significant [$F(1,56) = 23.61$, $p < 0.0001$], but the difference between schizophrenia and the elderly on session 1 was reduced to non-significance [$F(1,57) = 0.60$, $p = 0.443$].

LONG-TERM LEARNING MATCHING AND WRITING TIME

Mean matching time per digit and mean writing time per digit are presented in **Figure 2** for each session and each group.

Mean matching time per session

Figure 2 demonstrates that the matching times mirror the SDST performance of **Figure 1**. A clear learning effect over sessions was found [$F(2,85) = 32.46$, $p < 0.0001$], which was equal for the three groups [Group*Session interaction: $F(2,85) = 1.49$, $p = 0.206$]. Averaged over all sessions, the matching times in each group differed significantly from each other [$F(2,86) = 13.39$, $p < 0.001$]. Planned contrasts show a significant difference between patients and controls ($p < 0.0001$), between patients and elderly ($p = 0.002$ after Bonferroni correction), but not between the elderly and the controls ($p = 0.167$). IQ (ART) as a covariate was significant [$F(1,85) = 14.50$, $p = 0.0003$]. IQ did not influence the difference between patients and controls ($p = 0.001$) but reduced the difference between elderly and schizophrenic participants to non-significance ($p = 0.282$).

Mean writing time per session

The writing times as displayed in **Figure 2** do not show much variation over the test sessions, and the session effect was not significant [$F(2,85) = 1.36$, $p = 0.262$]. Therefore, we may conclude that there was no evident learning in the writing of the digits. Neither was the Group*Session interaction significant [$F(4,170) = 0.45$, $p = 0.771$]. On the other hand, the differences between the groups were relatively large and significant [$F(2,86) = 26.37$, $p < 0.0001$]. The elderly wrote significantly slower than the patients ($p = 0.0003$) and the patients wrote significantly slower than the controls ($p = 0.001$).

SHORT-TERM LEARNING MATCHING AND WRITING TIME OVER BLOCKS PER SESSION

Within-session learning effects are shown in **Figure 3**, which displays mean matching and writing times per digit for each of the five blocks in the three sessions.

Mean matching time per block

Figure 3 illustrates a decrease in matching time over the blocks and over sessions. A GLM repeated measures analysis confirmed that matching time decreased significantly over blocks [short-term learning; $F(4,75) = 21.66$, $p < 0.0001$] and over sessions [long-term learning; $F(4,75) = 21.66$, $p < 0.0001$]. The decrease over blocks was about equal in the three sessions [$F(8,71) = 1.74$, $p = 0.105$] and seemed to be similar in the three groups [$F(8,150) = 1.709$, $p = 0.101$], but the highest order interaction (session*block*group) was significant [$F(16,142) = 1.79$, $p = 0.038$]. Therefore, separate analyses were run per session. In these analyses, only the linear block effect was tested (i.e., a linear decrement of matching time over blocks; see the dashed lines in **Figure 3**). In session 1, this linear block effect was significant [$F(1,78) = 31.04$, $p < 0.0001$], denoting a significant short-term learning effect (decrement over blocks), but this learning effect was similar for the three groups [block*group Linear: $F(2,78) = 0.03$, $p = 0.597$]. In the second and third sessions, more participants reached the minimum criterion of 45

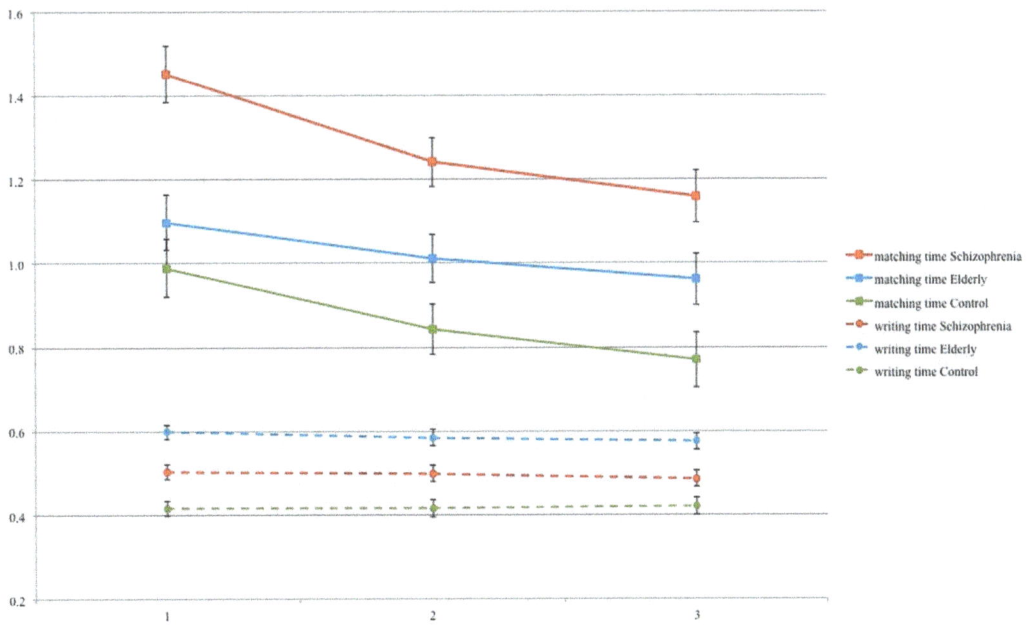

FIGURE 2 | Means and SE for matching and writing time per session for schizophrenia patients, elderly volunteers, and young controls.

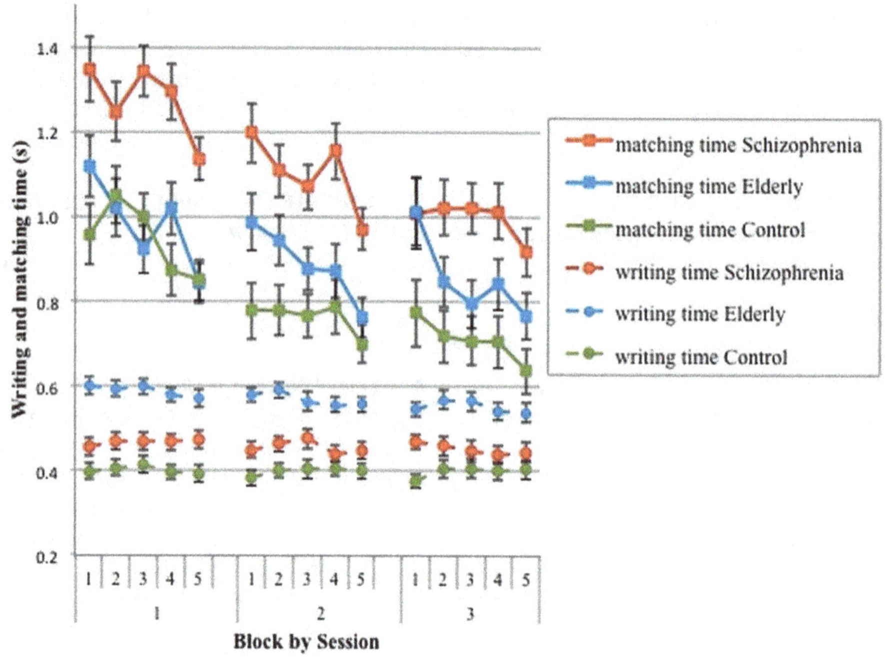

FIGURE 3 | Means and SE for writing and matching time per block and per session for schizophrenia patients, elderly volunteers, and young controls.

correct digits, but the analyses of the Linear trends yielded similar results [session 2: block: $F(1,83) = 29.08$, $p < 0.0001$; block*group Linear: $F(2,83) = 2.75$, $p = 0.070$; session 3: block: $F(1,83) = 25.20$, $p < 0.0001$; block*group Linear: $F(2,83) = 1.95$, $p = 0.148$]. Therefore, these results suggest that the rate and amount of short-term learning (repetition over blocks) was similar in the three sessions and about equal among the three groups.

Mean writing time per block

Writing time in **Figure 3** shows that there is not much variation over blocks and sessions. The only noteworthy result is the relatively long writing time of the elderly participants.

An analysis of writing time with session and block as the within-subject variables and group as the between-subject variable showed that the effect of session was not significant but the block effect was [$F(4,75) = 5.60$, $p = 0.0003$]. None of the interactions were significant either. In the first session, the linear block effect was not significant ($p = 0.216$), but the linear block*group interaction was significant [$F(2,78) = 3.55$, $p = 0.033$]. This is probably due to a slight decrement of writing time by the elderly but not by the other two groups. In the second and third session, the linear block effect and the linear block*group interactions were not significant, indicating that writing time remained stable in these sessions.

ESTIMATING THE EFFECT OF SHORT-TERM LEARNING ON THE SDST SCORE

To estimate the contribution of the linear decrease in matching time to the SDST score, we estimated the score that would have been obtained if the matching time (mt) and writing time (wt) of the first block (i.e., mt1 and wt1) had been maintained over all blocks in the 90 s of the test [i.e., estimated score = 90/(mt1 + wt1)]. We did the same for block five. The result of this estimation for session 1, i.e., for the standard test administration, was that the score of all participants had improved, more specifically from 50 to 56 for patients with schizophrenia, from 52 to 64 for the elderly and from 66 to 72 for the controls. These are increases of 12, 23, and 9%, respectively. It should, however, be stipulated that not all participants showed a decrease in matching time over blocks. Slopes ranged considerably, with the largest range found in the group of schizophrenia patients (from +78 ms/block to −301 ms/block; mean = −37 ms/block) compared to the ranges of the young controls (from + 50 ms/block to −284 ms/block; mean = −39 ms/block) and the elderly volunteers (from + 38 ms/block to −236 ms/block; mean = −55 ms/block).

DISCUSSION

SUMMARY OF RESULTS

The main purpose of this study was to assess to what extent differences in symbol–digit learning influence the performance on the SDST. The present findings demonstrate that the repetition of symbol–digit pairs during one test administration (short-term learning), and the repetition of the same test over several days (long-term learning), resulted in significant decreases of matching time. Interestingly, these learning effects on matching time were about equal for patients, age-matched controls, and elderly participants, while the overall test score differed among the groups. In contrast, writing time, reflecting sensorimotor speed, remained about equal over symbol–digit repetitions. Patients had the lowest overall score and the longest matching time; however, the difference between patients with schizophrenia and elderly was no longer significant after controlling for the lower IQ of the patients.

Sensorimotor speed had a smaller impact on the overall test performance, but there were significant differences between the three groups with the elderly clearly being the slowest writers.

RATIONALE FOR THE CHOSEN METHODOLOGICAL APPROACH

In an experimental approach of the coding task, like the one adopted by Bachman et al. (15), single symbol–digit pairs are presented trial by trial and on each trial the participant has to quickly decide whether the presented combination is identical to one of the digit–symbol pairs in the reference code that is simultaneously presented on the PC screen. In the more common paper-and-pencil version of the task, the participant can work at his own pace and might (learn to) combine the activities of both writing a digit and searching for the next digit that matches the next symbol in parallel. We opted to incorporate an experimental approach into the continuous paper-and-pencil version, because recording of the pen movements enables the separate measurement of reaction time (now denoted by "matching" time) and response execution time ("writing" time).

In addition, to allow an unbiased estimate of learning we adapted the presentation of the symbols that had to be coded. In standard symbol-coding tests, not all nine symbols are already shown in the first block but they are introduced gradually to promote the learning of the symbol–digit relations. For our SDST version, however, we preferred to present all nine symbols with the same frequency right from the start. As a result, a repetition of the same symbol–digit pair was separated by an average of eight other pairs. Yet, considerable learning did occur as evidenced by the linear decrease in matching time over nine-symbol blocks.

INFLUENCE OF LEARNING PROCESSES ON THE SDST TEST SCORE

Comparing the size of the learning effects with the SDST scores showed that the influence of learning processes on the SDST score in schizophrenia, the elderly and younger controls varies greatly from person to person. The average learning effects found in the present study of about 12% in the schizophrenia group and 23% in the elderly can be classified as rather substantial. This is in line with the conclusions drawn by Bachman et al. (15) and Joy (16). It deviates from Salthouse's (23) interpretation in which memory factors are assigned only "a very small role in contributing to the age decline in digit–symbol performance."

IDENTIFICATION OF LEARNING PROCESSES

Repetition of the same task results in learning. Therefore, the decrease in matching time over blocks within one session as well as over more sessions must be the result of a learning process. But what exactly is learned during the repetitions of symbol–digit pairs is less clear. Two critical processes are known to be involved in the search for the matching digit: visual scanning (24) and relational memory (16). First, visual scanning, refers to the early detection and identification of visual stimuli, either alone or in the presence of competing stimuli. The role of visual scanning is emphasized when participants consult the code key frequently during test administration. Possibly, visual scanning might improve by learning the position of the symbols in the key. Second, relational memory, refers in this context to the memory for associations in the SDST (10, 12). Learning the relations between symbols and digits will reduce the necessity for searching, which automatically results in a decreased matching time. A third process that might be involved in the reduction of matching time over repetitions is a change in the strategy to perform the task. An impairment in response selection (25, 26), i.e., the process of mapping stimuli to specific responses and decision making could possibly cause a considerable amount of the lower performance observed in schizophrenia. Most participants will start with performing matching and writing strictly after each other, while some participants might learn to do part of the writing and scanning in parallel. In that case, the search for the next digit has already started during the more or less automatic writing of the current number. Overall, various learning processes might contribute to a decreased matching time, but their relative contribution could not be deduced from the present study. To find more detailed answers, experimental changes of the task, like the manipulations tested by Bachman et al., are needed. For now, we can only conclude that these learning processes occurred unintentionally, and therefore, should be denoted by the term "implicit learning." An important outcome of this study is that the rate of this implicit learning was not significantly different among the three groups.

SENSORIMOTOR SPEED

The second aim of our investigation was to evaluate the effect of differences in writing speed on the SDST score. Group differences in writing speed were highly significant but smaller than the group differences in matching time. Schizophrenia patients wrote significantly slower than same-aged controls and the elderly had the lowest writing speed. The effects of reduced writing speed in schizophrenia and the elderly on the total test score were smaller than the estimated effects of learning (for schizophrenia, learning + 12%, writing speed + 4%; for the elderly, learning + 23%, writing speed + 13%). This leads us to the conclusion that the usual determination of the symbol-coding test score results in underestimation of the speed of information processing, particularly for the elderly.

SCHIZOPHRENIA AND THE ELDERLY COMPARED

Healthy elderly persons were included in this study in order to compare the reduction in the speed of information processing of the schizophrenia patients with normal, age-related cognitive decline. By correcting for sensorimotor speed and only taking the matching time as an index of processing speed, patients performed worse compared to the elderly volunteers (aged 65–85 years). However, when an estimate of premorbid intelligence (the Adult Reading Test) was taken into account, the differences in matching time were no longer statistically significant, while the difference between patients and same-aged controls still remained significant. Although the similarity between the elderly and the patients with schizophrenia on matching time is striking, we cannot deduce from these data whether schizophrenia should be seen as "dementia praecox." In addition, it should be acknowledged that the elderly had a small but significantly lower sensorimotor speed. Only sensorimotor speed differentiated all three groups.

STUDY LIMITATIONS

Due to patient selection, a bias might exist since only patients who were able to complete the test batteries were included in this study.

The neurocognitive abilities of the selected patients may therefore be higher than the group of schizophrenia at large. Thus, the results of this study may not be generalized to the whole population of patients with schizophrenia. However, the mean SANS score for schizophrenia patients of 25.7 (SD 17.39) that was measured on screening visit is comparable with the mean SANS score of 23.0 (SD 14.6) found in a large heterogeneous sample of schizophrenia patients (27). Additionally, only 4.2% of our study sample was excluded after screening visit, suggesting that the internal validity of our study is high.

IMPLICATIONS FOR FUTURE RESEARCH AND CLINICAL PRACTICE

There is a wide variation in the administration of symbol–digit coding tasks ranging from a classical pen-and-paper writing task to a purely computerized test, which simply requires pressing a button when the correct symbol–digit combination appears. These different methods may ask for different cognitive sub-processes in the total test score. As an example of this, the present study clearly showed that the time taken by the motor part of the test must be taken into account in interpreting symbol–digit coding test scores as measures of the speed of information processing. The large variation between individual participants in the rate of short-term learning could argue for the need of additional memory test information to assess to what extent the (possibly) low SDST score has been the result of a learning failure. Some healthy volunteers mentioned spontaneously at the end of a session that they had remembered the symbol–digit combinations but we did not give a questionnaire to draw further conclusions toward awareness differences among the groups. Therefore, we suggest that the addition of a self-rater or observer-rater questionnaire might be valuable to address the possibility of different explicit and implicit learning strategies.

Although schizophrenia is often characterized by a reduced speed of information processing, the present study showed a similarity with the control group and the elderly as far as the rate and amount of both short-term and long-term implicit learning was involved. This was found despite the general finding of impaired working memory and a lower rate of explicit verbal and visual learning in schizophrenia. Because we speculate that improving processing speed may be predictive for the functional outcome, we recommend that more attention should be paid to implicit learning in future schizophrenia research and in the design of specific rehabilitation programs.

CONCLUSION

We can conclude that the two factors that were studied both had an effect on the estimation of processing speed with the Symbol–Digit Substitution Test. The average effect of learning the symbol–digit relation on the SDST score was substantial and the large individual differences in the amount of learning deserves more attention. The effects of sensorimotor speed on the total test score were shown to be smaller than the learning effects, but cannot be neglected because they lead to an underestimation of the speed of information processing, particularly for the elderly.

The finding of equal unintentional learning effects in patients, their age-matched controls and elderly participants lead us to the conclusion that implicit learning might be preserved in schizophrenia. This finding has important consequences for the design of specific rehabilitation programs for schizophrenia patients.

AUTHOR CONTRIBUTIONS

All authors met ICMJE criteria and all those who fulfilled those criteria were listed as authors. All authors had access to the study data and made the final decision about where to present these data.

ACKNOWLEDGMENTS

The authors would like to thank Dr. Fransen (StatUA) for additional statistical guidance, Ms. Morsel for her guidance and refinement of the English writing style and Ms. Apers, Ms. Laureys and Ms. Vermeylen for their support in the testing of the study participants. The authors also thank the study participants, without whom the study would never have been accomplished.

REFERENCES

1. Weinberger DR, Gallhofer B. Cognitive function in schizophrenia. *Int Clin Psychopharmacol* (1997) **4**:29–36. doi:10.1097/00004850-199709004-00006
2. Nuechterlein KH, Ventura J, Subotnik KL, Bartzokis G. The early longitudinal course of cognitive deficits in schizophrenia. *J Clin Psychiatry* (2014) **75**:25–9. doi:10.4088/JCP.13065.su1.06
3. Nuechterlein KH, Barch DM, Gold JM, Goldberg TE, Green MF, Heaton RK. Identification of separable cognitive factors in schizophrenia. *Schizophr Res* (2004) **72**:29–39. doi:10.1016/j.schres.2004.09.007
4. Brébion G, Amador X, Smith MJ, Gorman JM. Memory impairment and schizophrenia: the role of processing speed. *Schizophr Res* (1998) **30**:31–9. doi:10.1016/S0920-9964(97)00123-0
5. Morrens M, Hulstijn W, Matton C, Madani Y, van BouwelL, Peuskens J, et al. Delineating psychomotor slowing from reduced processing speed in schizophrenia. *Cogn Neuropsychiatry* (2008) **13**:457–71. doi:10.1080/13546800802439312
6. Pashler H. Dual-task interference in simple tasks: data and theory. *Psychol Bull* (1994) **116**:220–44. doi:10.1037/0033-2909.116.2.220
7. Nuechterlein KH, Green MF, Kern RS, Baade LE, Barch DM, Cohen JD, et al. The MATRICS consensus cognitive battery, part 1: test selection, reliability, and validity. *Am J Psychiatry* (2008) **165**:203–13. doi:10.1176/appi.ajp.2007.07010042
8. Dickinson D, Ramsey ME, Gold JM. Overlooking the obvious: a meta-analytic comparison of digit symbol coding tasks and other cognitive measures in schizophrenia. *Arch Gen Psychiatry* (2007) **64**:532–42. doi:10.1001/archpsyc.64.5.532
9. Knowles EEM, David AS, Reichenberg A. Processing speed deficits in schizophrenia: reexamining the evidence. *Am J Psychiatry* (2010) **167**:828–35. doi:10.1176/appi.ajp.2010.09070937
10. Green MF, Nuechterlein KH, Gold JM, Barch DM, Cohen J, Essock S, et al. Approaching a consensus cognitive battery for clinical trials in schizophrenia: the NIMH-MATRICS conference to select cognitive domains and test criteria. *Biol Psychiatry* (2004) **56**:301–7. doi:10.1016/j.biopsych.2004.06.023
11. Morrens M, Hulstijn W, Van Hecke J, Peuskens J, Sabbe BGC. Sensorimotor and cognitive slowing in schizophrenia as measured by the symbol digit substitution test. *J Psychiatr Res* (2006) **40**:200–6. doi:10.1016/j.jpsychires.2005.04.014
12. Horan WP, Green MF, Knowlton BJ, Wynn JK, Mintz J, Nuechterlein KH. Impaired implicit learning in schizophrenia. *Neuropsychology* (2008) **22**:606–17. doi:10.1037/a0012602
13. McDowd J, Tang T-C, Tsai P-C, Wang S-Y, Su C-Y. The association between verbal memory, processing speed, negative symptoms and functional capacity in schizophrenia. *Psychiatry Res* (2011) **187**:329–34. doi:10.1016/j.psychres.2011.01.017
14. Morrens M, Hulstijn W, Sabbe B. Psychomotor slowing in schizophrenia. *Schizophr Bull* (2007) **33**:1038–53. doi:10.1093/schbul/sbl051
15. Bachman P, Reichenberg A, Rice P, Woolsey M, Chaves O, Martinez D, et al. Deconstructing processing speed deficits in schizophrenia: application of a parametric digit symbol coding test. *Schizophr Res* (2010) **118**:6–11. doi:10.1016/j.schres.2010.02.1029
16. Joy S, Fein D, Kaplan E. Decoding digit symbol: speed, memory, and visual scanning. *Assessment* (2003) **10**:56–65. doi:10.1177/0095399702250335

17. Lezak MD, Howieson DB, Loring DW. *Neuropsychological Assessment. Fourth Edition*. New York: Oxford University Press (2004).
18. Kirkpatrick B, Messias E, Harvey PD, Fernandez-Egea E, Bowie CR. Is schizophrenia a syndrome of accelerated aging? *Schizophr Bull* (2008) **34**:1024–32. doi:10.1093/schbul/sbm140
19. Crawford JR, Bryan J, Luszcz MA. The executive decline hypothesis of cognitive aging: do executive deficits qualify as differential deficits and do they mediate age-related memory decline? *Aging Neuropsychol Cogn* (2000) **7**:9–31. doi:10.1076/anec.7.1.9.806
20. Baudouin A, Clarys D, Vanneste S, Isingrini M. Executive functioning and processing speed in age-related differences in memory: contribution of a coding task. *Brain Cogn* (2009) **71**:240–5. doi:10.1016/j.bandc.2009.08.007
21. Morrens M, Hulstijn W, Sabbe B. The effects of atypical and conventional antipsychotics on reduced processing speed and psychomotor slowing in schizophrenia: a cross-sectional exploratory study. *Clin Ther* (2008) **30**:684–92. doi:10.1016/j.clinthera.2008.04.012
22. De Picker L, Cornelis C, Hulstijn W, Dumont G, Fransen E, Morrens M. Preserved sensorimotor learning in stable schizophrenia patients but not in elderly participants compared to young controls in two variations of the Rotary Pursuit. *Front Psychiatry* (2014) **5**:165. doi:10.3389/fpsyt.2014.00165
23. Salthouse TA. The role of memory in the age decline in digit-symbol substitution performance. *J Gerontol* (1978) **33**:232–8. doi:10.1093/geronj/33.2.232
24. Mahurin RK, Velligan DI, Miller AL. Executive-frontal lobe cognitive dysfunction in schizophrenia: a symptom subtype analysis. *Psychiatry Res* (1998) **79**:139–49. doi:10.1016/S0165-1781(98)00031-6
25. Woodward ND, Duffy B, Karbasforoushan H. Prefrontal cortex activity during response selection predicts processing speed impairment in schizophrenia. *J Int Neuropsychol Soc* (2013) **19**:782–91. doi:10.1017/S1355617713000532
26. Krieger S, Lis S, Janik H, Cetin T, Gallhofer B, Meyer-Lindenberg A. Executive function and cognitive subprocesses in first-episode, drug-naive schizophrenia: an analysis of N-back performance. *Am J Psychiatry* (2005) **162**:1206–8. doi:10.1176/appi.ajp.162.6.1206
27. van Erp TG, Preda A, Nguyen D, Faziola L, Turner J, Bustillo J, et al. Converting positive and negative symptom scores between PANSS and SAPS/SANS. *Schizophr Res* (2014) **152**:289–94. doi:10.1016/j.schres.2013.11.013

9

Neurological soft signs in aging, mild cognitive impairment, and Alzheimer's disease – the impact of cognitive decline and cognitive reserve

Nadja Urbanowitsch[1]*, Christina Degen[1], Pablo Toro[3] and Johannes Schröder[1,2]

[1] *Section of Geriatric Psychiatry, University of Heidelberg, Heidelberg, Germany*
[2] *Institute of Gerontology, University of Heidelberg, Heidelberg, Germany*
[3] *Department of Psychiatry, Centro Interdisciplinario de Neurociencias, School of Medicine, Pontificia Universidad Católica de Chile, Santiago, Chile*

Edited by:
Sebastian Walther, University Hospital of Psychiatry, Switzerland

Reviewed by:
Katharina Stegmayer, University Hospital of Psychiatry, Switzerland
Lise Docx, University of Antwerp, Belgium

****Correspondence:***
Nadja Urbanowitsch, Section of Geriatric Psychiatry, University of Heidelberg, Voßstraße 4, 69115 Heidelberg, Germany
e-mail: nadja.urbanowitsch@med.uni-heidelberg.de

Objectives: Neurological soft signs (NSS), i.e., minor motor and sensory changes, are a common feature in severe psychiatric disorders. We sought to establish the frequency of NSS in patients with mild cognitive impairment (MCI) and Alzheimer's disease (AD) on basis of a large population-based sample and to identify their neuropsychological correlates including cognitive reserve.

Methods: Neurological soft signs were examined using an abbreviated version of the Heidelberg NSS Scale in 221 "old" participants born between 1930 and 1932 (63 with MCI, 15 with AD, 143 healthy old controls) and 256 healthy "young" participants (born between 1950 and 1952) of the population-based interdisciplinary longitudinal study of aging. Subjects received thorough neuropsychological testing; years of school education were used as a proxy for cognitive reserve.

Results: Neurological soft signs scores were significantly ($p < 0.001$) higher in the AD patients (5.6 ± 3.11) than in the healthy old controls (2.8 ± 1.90) and in the MCI patients (3.0 ± 1.96). This result was confirmed after years of school education, which were inversely correlated ($r = -0.25$; $p < 0.001$) with NSS were entered as a covariate. In the patients, but not in the controls, NSS were significantly correlated with deficits in executive functioning and visuospatial functioning. Comparison of NSS scores between "old" (2.84 ± 1.9) and "young" (2.46 ± 1.97) controls yielded only minor, non-significant differences after education (13.86 ± 3.0 vs. 14.61 ± 2.48 years, respectively) was controlled for.

Conclusion: Our results demonstrate that NSS are frequently found in mild AD, but not in MCI. NSS refer to frontal-executive deficits and visuospatial dysfunction rather than age *per se* and can be partly compensated for by cognitive reserve.

Keywords: NSS, MCI, AD, cognitive reserve, ILSE

INTRODUCTION

Recent studies (1, 2) demonstrate that neurological soft signs (NSS) – i.e., minor motor and sensory deficits – are frequently found in Alzheimer's disease (AD) and mild cognitive impairment (MCI) as they were consistently described in other major psychiatric conditions such as bipolar disorder or especially schizophrenia (3, 4). Corresponding to the significant association found between NSS and negative symptoms in schizophrenia (5) and Seidl et al. (2) reported a significant correlation between NSS and apathy in a large group of nursing home residents ($n = 120$) with mild to severe AD. Similar to earlier reports in schizophrenia [reviewed in Ref. (6)], Seidl et al. (2) did not find NSS to be associated with neuroleptic treatment. However, other important aspects of NSS known from studies in schizophrenia – in particular, the associations of NSS with neuropsychological deficits (7–10) – were not yet tested in AD. This question is of particular importance as positive effects of physical activity on cognitive performance are generally accepted (11).

It is generally accepted that high levels of physical activity are associated with a reduced risk for developing AD potentially by facilitating the brain and cognitive reserve. Another study of our group (11) investigated muscular strength as measured by a vigorimeter and motor coordination, which was operationalized by means of the one-foot-standing test, with respect to the risk of developing MCI or AD in the interdisciplinary longitudinal study of aging (ILSE). In the framework of this prospective population-based study, subjects (born 1930–1932) were examined at three examination waves (t_1:1993/1994; t_2: 1997/1998; t_3: 2005/2007). The study demonstrated that motor coordination evaluated at t_1 but not muscular strength was a significant predictor of cognitive impairment at t_3.

Another important question refers to the nature of NSS as signs of generalized rather than discrete cerebral changes. Along with this, neuroimaging studies in schizophrenia identified a number of dispersed cerebral sites associated with NSS (12–15). Hence, one may expect to find increased NSS scores in manifest AD where cerebral changes involve large parts of the brain rather than in MCI where cerebral changes still remain localized in the medial temporal lobe. Accordingly, NSS scores should be rather stable in the process of healthy aging since the latter does not involve major cerebral changes.

We therefore thought to investigate NSS with respect to neuropsychological deficits and school education, as a proxy of cognitive reserve and to compare NSS scores between patients with MCI or AD and healthy old controls. In addition, NSS scores obtained in the latter were compared with scores measured in young controls to identify age-related changes.

MATERIALS AND METHODS

PARTICIPANTS

The ILSE-study is based on two birth cohorts born during 1930–1932 and 1950–1952 who were randomly recruited according to community registers in the urban regions of Leipzig (Saxony) and Heidelberg/Mannheim (Palatine). The study was approved by the ethical committee of the University of Heidelberg and written informed consent after complete description of the study to the subjects was obtained. The first examinations took place between December 1993 and January 1996. Data of the present study correspond to the third examination wave, which were performed between 2005 and 2008, i.e., more than 12 years after the initiation of the study. At this time, 381 participants of the 1930–1932 cohort and 408 participants of the 1950–1952 – corresponding to more than 75 and 80%, respectively, of the original cohorts – could be reinvestigated. Participants with a current episode of major depression, substance abuse, anxiety disorder, bipolar disorder, schizophrenia, or meeting ICD 10 criteria for a cognitive disorder due to a general medical condition were excluded from the analysis since these conditions usually course with both neurological signs and cognitive deficits and may overlap with dementia. Hence, a sample of 477 participants was available for analyses comprising 256 participants of the 1950–1952 cohort and 221 participants of the 1930–1932 cohort.

Sixty-three participants out of 221 (28.51%) were diagnosed with MCI and 15 with AD (6.79%) in the 1930–1932 cohort. Because we were interested in investigating the effects of age on NSS performance 256 otherwise healthy participants from the young cohort were also included. Hence, three groups were constituted: healthy young controls, ($n = 256$), healthy old controls ($n = 143$) old-aged with MCI (MCI; $n = 63$), and old-aged with AD (AD; $n = 15$). All participants selected for the present study had complete core data sets (socio-demographic variables, diagnoses, NSS), while the thorough neuropsychological test battery could be completed in the whole group. The mini-mental state examination [MMSE, (16)] was not applied in the young cohort.

SURVEY MEASURES

All participants were carefully screened for physical and mental health by extensive clinical interviews, physical examinations, laboratory tests, and a thorough assessment of neuropsychological functioning. Cognitive assessment included the MMSE and subtests of the Nürnberger-Alters-Inventar [NAI, (17)] and the Leistungsprüfsystem (18), both of which are well-established and commonly used test batteries in Germany [for more details, see Ref. (19)]. Subjective cognitive complaints were assessed by interviewing and applying the respective items of the Nürnberger Selbsteinschätzungsliste [NSL; (20)].

Neurological soft signs were examined by using the modified version (2) of the Heidelberg Neurological Soft Signs Scale (4), which included five items, named – (a) finger-to-nose movement, (b) diadochokinesia, (c) pronation and supination, (d) finger-thumb opposition, and (e) mirror movements. The scores of the items were scaled from 0 (no prevalence) to 3 (marked prevalence), with a total score of maximum 18. The subtests were selected from the original scale based upon clinical and research experience collected with demented patients. Examination subtest had to be easy to understand by AD patients.

PSYCHIATRIC DIAGNOSES

Clinical axis I diagnoses were obtained by using the German version of the Structured Clinical Interview for the DSM-III-R [SKID I, (21)]. MCI was defined by using the aging-associated cognitive decline (AACD) criteria, which were already applied in the first two examination waves (19, 22). Diagnostic criteria for AACD have been proposed by the international psychogeriatric association (23) and include (1) subjective impairment: a report by the individual (or a reliable informant) that cognitive function has declined and (2) objective impairment in any of the following cognitive domains, as indicated by a neuropsychological test performance of at least 1 SD below normal age and educational levels: memory and learning, attention and concentration, abstract thinking (problem solving, abstraction), language, and visuospatial functioning. AD was diagnosed according to the NINCDS–ADRA (24). All diagnoses were confirmed by both specialists in old age psychiatry involved.

STATISTICAL ANALYSES

Clinical variables, NSS, and neuropsychological performances were compared between groups by calculating separate analyses of covariance (ANCOVA) with group (healthy young controls vs. healthy old controls vs. MCI vs. AD) as predictor variable and years of education as covariate. *Post hoc* comparison analyses were based on Duncan's test. The potential relations between NSS, clinical variables, and neuropsychological findings were addressed by calculating Pearson product-moment correlation coefficients, which were controlled for years of education. All computations were performed by using the 9.2 version of the SAS Software.

RESULTS

The clinical characteristics, neuropsychological performance, and total NSS scores obtained in the diagnostic groups are summarized in **Table 1**. Diagnostic groups differed significantly with respect to age and years of school education but showed no significant differences in sex distribution. As expected, AD patients scored significantly lower than MCI patients, followed by healthy old controls, on the MMSE. With respect to neuropsychological test performance, three patterns of group differences arose: performance on verbal memory, digit symbol, D2, and visuospatial thinking tests conformed to the expected order with the highest scores achieved by healthy young controls, followed by healthy old controls and MCI, and the lowest scores obtained by AD.

Table 1 | Demographic and neuropsychological characteristics by subgroup with the results of a Duncan test at the 5%-level.

	Healthy young controls ($n=256$)	Healthy old controls ($n=143$)	MCI ($n=63$)	AD ($n=15$)	F (df)	p	Duncan/Chi Square
DEMOGRAPHICS							
Age	55.15 (0.97)	73.94 (0.99)	74.21 (1.03)	74.73 (1.03)	14525 (3, 473)	<0.001	HY < HO = OMCI = OAD
Sex (women/men)	126/130	75/68	32/31	7/8	n.a.	n.s.	Chi-Sq: 0.469
Education	14.61 (2.48)	13.86 (2.99)	12.22 (2.41)	11.20 (1.78)	20.07 (3, 473)	<0.001	HY = HO > OMCI = OAD
MMSE ($n=218$)	n.a.	28.91 (1.12)	28.07 (1.41)	24.13 (2.39)	90.02 (2, 215)	<0.001	HO > OMCI > OAD
NEUROPSYCHOLOGY							
Verbal memory: immediate recall ($n=438$)	14.59 (3.16)	12.36 (3.47)	10.35 (3.46)	7.5 (3.50)	31.7 (3, 434)	<0.001	HY > HO > OMCI > OAD
Verbal memory: delayed recognition ($n=438$)	7.93 (2.27)	6.91 (2.35)	5.81 (2.50)	4.0 (2.63)	14.5 (3, 434)	<0.001	HY = HO > OMCI > OAD
DST ($n=438$)	53.94 (9.33)	44.15 (9.51)	36.11 (8.73)	25.8 (8.94)	72.4 (3, 434)	<0.001	HY > HO > OMCI > OAD
D2 ($n=432$)	164.45 (32.06)	136.79 (33.08)	105.67 (33.93)	76.67 (43.37)	50.1 (3, 428)	<0.001	HY > HO > OMCI > OAD
Finding similarities ($n=439$)	26.64 (4.17)	26.77 (4.07)	22.6 (6.27)	16.0 (6.62)	18.1 (3, 435)	<0.001	HY = HO > OMCI > OAD
Verbal fluency ($n=439$)	32.38 (9.36)	32.15 (8.23)	24.47 (8.48)	18.8 (8.9)	11.0 (3, 435)	<0.001	HY = HO > OMCI > OAD
Visuospatial thinking ($n=437$)	25.41 (6.04)	21.79 (5.72)	17.53 (7.41)	11.56 (6.93)	24.2 (3, 433)	<0.001	HY > HO > OMCI > OAD
NSS	2.46 (1.97)	2.84 (1.91)	3.0 (1.96)	5.6 (3.11)	8.0 (3, 473)	<0.001	HY = HO = OMCI < OAD

MCI, mild cognitive impairment; AD, Alzheimer's disease; MMSE, mini-mental state examination; DST, digit symbol test; D2, D2-test; NSS, neurological soft signs; n.a., not applicable; n.s., not significant.

In the subtests, verbal memory recognition, verbal fluency, and finding similarities, significant group differences were found only between MCI and AD, while healthy young controls and healthy old controls showed similar results. AD patients demonstrated significantly more NSS compared to the other three subgroups. As demonstrated in **Figure 1** across all diagnostic groups, NSS scores were inversely correlated with years of school education ($r=-0.25$; $p<0.001$). The ANCOVA with years of school education as a covariate [$F(4,472)=15.78$, $p<0.0001$] yielded a significant main effect (type III ss) of diagnostic group on NSS scores [$F(3,473)=7.95$, $p<0.0001$].

To further analyze the correlations between NSS and neuropsychology deficits, the subgroups of patients with MCI and AD were collapsed. Within this joint group of cognitively impaired, NSS scores were significantly inversely correlated with scores on the MMSE, on the DST, and on the tests for visuospatial functioning and verbal fluency, processing speed, and cognitive flexibility, respectively (**Table 2**).

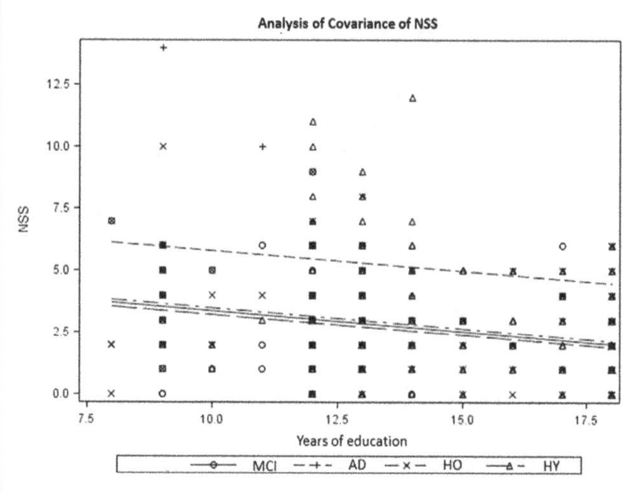

FIGURE 1 | NSS and years of education across diagnostic subgroups. NSS, neurological soft signs; HO, healthy old controls; HY, healthy young controls; MCI, patients with MCI; AD, patients with Alzheimer's disease.

DISCUSSION

The main findings of the present study can be summarized as follows: significantly increased NSS scores (i) were found in patients with AD but not in patients with MCI or healthy old controls compared to healthy young controls, (ii) correspond to deficient executive functioning and visuospatial apraxia and can be partially compensated for by cognitive reserve, and (iii), are not the sequelae of aging *per se*.

The present study confirmed increased NSS scores in patients with mild AD as previously described by a number of studies (2, 25, 26), which also examined patients in more advanced stages of the disease. This increase was not observed patients with MCI. In contrast, Li et al. (1) reported significantly increased NSS scores – which particularly involved motor coordination signs – in 29 MCI patients who were compared with 28 healthy controls. This discrepancy might refer to methodological differences, such as sample size and mode of recruitment, as well as the relatively greater severity of cognitive deficits in their MCI group, in particular (mean MMSE scores: 26.07 ± 2.33 vs. 28.07 ± 1.41, respectively).

Similar to the study of Chan et al. (27), NSS scores were significantly correlated with neuropsychological deficits involving executive functioning (verbal fluency, digit symbol test) and

Table 2 | Neuropsychological correlates of NSS in patients with MCI or AD.

NP-test	MMSE	Verbal memory (immediate recall)	Verbal memory (delayed recognition)	DST	D2-test	Finding similarities	Verbal fluency	Visuospatial thinking
NSS								
r uncorrected	***r* = −0.45****	*r* = −0.08	*r* = −0.03	***r* = −0.37***	*r* = −0.13	*r* = −0.21	***r* = −0.37***	***r* = −0.41****
(corrected)		(*r* = −0.04)	(*r* = −0.03)	**(*r* = −0.39*)**	(*r* = −0.15)	(*r* = −0.18)	**(*r* = −0.37*)**	**(*r* = −0.36*)**

Values corrected for education in brackets. Bold font indicates significant correlations.

NP, neuropsychology; MCI, mild cognitive impairment; AD, Alzheimer's disease; MMSE, mini-mental state examination; DST, digit symbol test; D2, D2-test; NSS, neurological soft signs.

$^*p < 0,005$; $^{**}p < 0.001$.

visuospatial thinking. Verbal memory was not associated with NSS. In the light of these findings, the significant correlation of NSS and logical memory reported by Chan et al. (27) may refer to the fact that the latter also involves some aspects of executive functioning in the sense of mnestic strategies. It is notable that similar associations between NSS and executive deficits were also reported in schizophrenia [for review see Ref. (7)] and in HIV associated neurocognitive disorders (28). That motor performance in AD is related to executive functioning is further supported by the results of dual-task studies, which even yielded interactions between fall risk and executive dysfunctions (29–32).

In all subgroups under investigation, NSS were inversely related with years of school education as a marker of cognitive reserve. This association corresponded to a wealth of studies [for review see Ref. (11)], which identified motor abilities to be a protective factor for cognitive decline and could be mediated by the beneficial effects of aerobic exercise on the hippocampus (33) and the frontal cortices (34).

Despite the large sample size, a comparison of NSS scores between healthy young controls and healthy old controls yielded only minor, non-significant differences. In contrast, Chan et al. (27) who examined 180 subjects aged 60–96 suggested that NSS were very common among the elderly. Their study, however, differs with respect to a variety of important methodological details from the present investigation, among them the definition of cognitively intact controls by a MMSE score of >24. This definition may well have led to the inclusion of patients with mild AD who often showed MMSE scores up to 26. Along with this, educational levels were in the range of 6.8 ± 4.4 years and do not compare with the respective value found in our sample. Similarly, Kodama et al. (35) found deficits in diadochokinesis, finger-to-nose test, and tandem gate to increase with age in 348 subjects aged 60–89. However, educational level and MMSE scores were considerably lower than in our birth cohorts rendering a direct comparison of the results difficult. Therefore, our finding only applies to the rather "young" old investigated here and needs to be confirmed in the further course of the ILSE when subjects have reached a higher age.

Another important methodological limitation of our study involves the fact that only motor NSS were examined. Motor NSS are generally considered to be of particular importance (5) and can be easily applied (2). Likewise, Kodama et al. (35) demonstrated significant age effects only for the motor NSS cited above and vibration sense of the lower limbs but not for other sensory NSS.

As hypothesized, our investigation of two large birth cohorts confirmed increased NSS scores in patients with mild AD but not patients with MCI. According to our findings, NSS do not appear to be the sequelae of healthy aging since the two birth cohorts examined showed only minor, non-significant differences with respect to NSS. That NSS were found to be significantly associated with executive dysfunction corresponds to earlier studies in patients with schizophrenia. However, NSS are not only a marker of brain damage in AD but also reflect aspects of cognitive reserve. Longitudinal studies are necessary to establish the stability of NSS in aging, their prognostic value in MCI and – ultimately – to determine norm values for NSS. From a clinical standpoint, NSS should be considered as a reliable and easy to administer tool in the routine examination of patients with cognitive decline.

ACKNOWLEDGMENTS

The ILSE was supported in part by the Dietmar-Hopp-Foundation/St. Leon-Rot, Germany. PT was supported by Comisión Nacional de Investigación Científica y Tecnológica de Chile (CONICYT) through Fondo Nacional de Desarrollo Científico y Tecnológico (FONDECYT) project no. 11121301. We acknowledge the financial support of the Deutsche Forschungsgemeinschaft and Ruprecht-Karls-Universität Heidelberg within the funding programme Open Access Publishing. We are grateful to Dr. Phil. Franz-Josef Geider for statistical consulting.

REFERENCES

1. Li HJ, Wang PY, Jiang Y, Chan RCK, Wang HL, Li J. Neurological soft signs in persons with amnestic mild cognitive impairment and the relationships to neuropsychological functions. *Behav Brain Funct* (2012) **8**:29. doi:10.1186/1744-9081-8-29
2. Seidl U, Thomann PA, Schröder J. Neurological soft signs in nursing home residents with Alzheimers' disease. *J Alzheimers Dis* (2009) **18**:525–30. doi:10.3233/JAD-2009-1159
3. Bombin I, Arango C, Buchanan RC. Significance and meaning of neurological signs in schizophrenia: two decades later. *Schizophr Bull* (2005) **31**(4):962–77. doi:10.1093/schbul/sbi028
4. Schröder J, Niethammer R, Geider FJ, Reitz C, Binkert M, Jauss M, et al. Neurological soft signs in schizophrenia. *Schizophr Res* (1992) **6**:25–30. doi:10.1016/0920-9964(91)90017-L
5. Jahn T, Hubmann W, Karr M, Mohr F, Schlenker R, Heidenreich T. Motoric neurological soft signs and psychopathological symptoms in schizophrenic psychoses. *Psychiatry Res* (2006) **142**:191–9. doi:10.1016/j.psychres.2002.12.003
6. Schröder J. Soft signs, neuroleptic side effects, and schizophrenia. *Psychiatr Ann* (2003) **33**(3):214–20. doi:10.3928/0048-5713-20030301-10
7. Chan RCK, Wang Y, Wang L, Chen EYH, Manschreck TC, Li Z, et al. Neurological soft signs and their relationships to neurocognitive functions: a re-visit

with the structural equation modeling design. *PLoS One* (2009) **4**(12):e8469. doi:10.1371/journal.pone.0008469

8. Chan RCK, Xu T, Heinrichs RW, Yu Y, Wang Y. Neurological soft signs in schizophrenia: a meta-analysis. *Schizophr Bull* (2010) **36**(6):1089–104. doi:10.1093/schbul/sbp011
9. Mohr F, Hubmann W, Albus M, Franz U, Hecht S, Scherer J, et al. Neurological soft signs and neuropsychological performance in patients with first episode schizophrenia. *Psychiatry Res* (2003) **121**(1):21–30. doi:10.1016/S0165-1781(03)00203-8
10. Schröder J. Subsyndrome der chronischen schizophrenie. *Untersuchungen mit bildgebenden Verfahren zur Heterogenität schizophrener Psychosen*. Berlin: Springer-Verlag (1998). p. 43–9.
11. Sattler C, Erickson KI, Toro P, Schröder J. Physical fitness as a protective factor for cognitive impairment in a prospective population-based study in Germany. *J Alzheimers Dis* (2011) **26**(4):709–18. doi:10.3233/JAD-2011-110548
12. Dazzan P, Morgan KD, Orr KG, Hutchinson G, Chitnis X, Suckling J, et al. The structural brain correlates of neurological soft signs in AeSOP first-episode psychoses study. *Brain* (2004) **127**:143–53. doi:10.1093/brain/awh015
13. Thomann PA, Roebel M, Dos Santos V, Bachmann S, Essig M, Schröder J. Cerebellar substructures and neurological soft signs in first-episode schizophrenia. *Psychiatry Res* (2009) **173**:83–7. doi:10.1016/j.pscychresns.2008.07.006
14. Heuser M, Thomann PA, Essig M, Bachmann S, Schröder J. Neurological signs and morphological cerebral changes in schizophrenia: an analysis of NSS subscales in patients with first episode psychosis. *Psychiatry Res* (2011) **192**(2):69–76. doi:10.1016/j.pscychresns.2010.11.009
15. Zhao Q, Li Z, Huang J, Yan C, Dazzan P, Pantelis C, et al. Neurological soft signs are not "soft" in brain structure and functional networks: evidence from ALE meta-analysis. *Schizophr Bull* (2014) **40**(3):626–41. doi:10.1093/schbul/sbt063
16. Folstein MF, Folstein SE, McHugh PR. "Mini-mental state". A practical method for grading the cognitive state of patients for the clinician. *J Psychiatr Res* (1975) **12**(3):189–98. doi:10.1016/0022-3956(75)90026-6
17. Oswald WD, Fleischmann VM. *Nürnberger-Alters-Inventar*. Erlangen-Nürnberg: Universität Erlangen-Nürnberg (1991).
18. Horn WC. *Leistungsprüfsystem*. Göttingen: Hogrefe (1983).
19. Schönknecht P, Pantel J, Kruse A, Schröder J. Prevalence and natural course of aging-associated cognitive decline in a population-based sample of young-old subjects. *Am J Psychiatry* (2005) **162**(11):2071–7. doi:10.1176/appi.ajp.162.11.2071
20. Oswald WD, Fleischmann VM. *Nürnberger Selbsteinschätzungsliste (NSL)*. Erlangen-Nürnberg: Universität Erlangen-Nürnberg (1986).
21. Wittchen HU, Zaudig M, Schramm E, Spengler P, Mombour W, Klug J, et al. *SKID: Strukturiertes Klinisches Interview für DSM-III-R*. Göttingen: Beltz-Test (1991).
22. Schröder J, Kratz B, Pantel J, Minnemann E, Lehr U, Sauer H. Prevalence of mild cognitive impairment in an elderly community sample. *J Neural Transm Suppl* (1998) **54**:51–9. doi:10.1007/978-3-7091-7508-8_5
23. Levy R. Aging-associated cognitive decline. *Int Psychogeriatr* (1994) **6**(1):63–8. doi:10.1017/S1041610294001626
24. McKhann G, Drachmann D, Folstein M, Katzmann R, Price D, Stadlan EM. Clinical diagnosis of Alzheimer's disease: report of the NINCDS-ADRDA work group under the auspices of the department of health and human services task force on Alzheimer's disease. *Neurology* (1984) **34**:939–65. doi:10.1212/WNL.34.7.939
25. Lam LL, Lui VWC, Chiu HFK. Associations between neurological soft signs and clinical progression Alzheimer's disease. *Hong Kong J Psychiatry* (2005) **15**:43–9.
26. Lautenschläger NT, Wu JS, Laws SM, Almeida OP, Clarnette RM, Joesbury K, et al. Neurological soft signs are associated with APOE genotype, age and cognitive performance. *J Alzheimers Dis* (2005) **7**(4):325–30.
27. Chan RCK, Xu T, Li HJ, Zhao Q, Liu HH, Wang Y, et al. Neurological abnormalities and neurocognitive functions in healthy elderly people: a structural equation modeling analysis. *Behav Brain Funct* (2011) **7**:32. doi:10.1186/1744-9081-7-32
28. Inostroza F, Valenzuela D, Schröder J, Toro P. [Neurological soft signs in HIV-infection and healthy controls – a clinical marker of cerebral damage]. *Revista chilena de neuropsiquiatria* (2014) **52**(2):121.
29. Beauchet O, Dubost V, Herrmann F, Rabilloud M, Gonthier R, Kressig RW. Relationship between dual-task related gait changes and intrinsic risk factors for falls among transitional frail older adults. *Aging Clin Exp Res* (2005) **17**(4):270–5. doi:10.1007/BF03324609
30. Lundin-Olsson L, Nyberg L, Gustafson Y. "Stops walking when talking" as a predictor of falls in elderly people. *Lancet* (1997) **349**:617. doi:10.1016/S0140-6736(97)24009-2
31. Lundin-Olsson L, Nyberg L, Gustafson Y. Attention, frailty, and falls: the effect of a manual task on basic mobility. *J Am Geriatr Soc* (1998) **46**:758–61.
32. Bloem BR, Steijns JAG, Smits-Engelsman BC. An update on falls. *Curr Opin Neurol* (2003) **16**:15–26. doi:10.1097/00019052-200302000-00003
33. Erickson KI, Voss MW, Prakash RS, Basak C, Szabo A, Chaddock L, et al. Exercise training increases size of hippocampus and improves memory. *Proc Natl Acad Sci U S A* (2011) **108**(7):3017–22. doi:10.1073/pnas.1015950108
34. Colcombe SJ, Erickson KI, Scalf PE, Kim JS, Prakash R, McAuley E, et al. Aerobic exercise training increases brain volume in aging humans. *J Gerontol A Biol Sci Med Sci* (2006) **61**(11):1166–70. doi:10.1093/gerona/61.11.1166
35. Kodama T, Nakagawa M, Arimura K, Koriyama C, Akiba S, Osame M. Cross-sectional analysis of neurological findings among healthy elderly: study in a remote island in Kagoshima, Japan. *Neuroepidemiology* (2002) **21**:36–43. doi:10.1159/000048612

10

An overview of the association between schizotypy and dopamine

Christine Mohr[1]* and Ulrich Ettinger[2]*

[1] Institute of Psychology, University of Lausanne, Lausanne, Switzerland
[2] Department of Psychology, University of Bonn, Bonn, Germany

Edited by:
Caroline Gurvich, Monash University, Australia

Reviewed by:
Ahmed A. Moustafa, University of Western Sydney, Australia
Maria R. Dauvermann, Massachusetts Institute of Technology, USA
Colin G. DeYoung, University of Minnesota, Twin Cities, USA

***Correspondence:**
Christine Mohr, Institute of Psychology, University of Lausanne, Quartier Mouline, Bâtiment Géopolis, Lausanne 1015, Switzerland
e-mail: christine.mohr@unil.ch;
Ulrich Ettinger, Department of Psychology, University of Bonn, Kaiser-Karl-Ring 9, Bonn 53111, Germany
e-mail: ulrich.ettinger@uni-bonn.de

Schizotypy refers to a constellation of personality traits that are believed to mirror the subclinical expression of schizophrenia in the general population. Evidence from pharmacological studies indicates that dopamine (DA) is involved in the etiology of schizophrenia. Based on the assumption of a continuum between schizophrenia and schizotypy, researchers have begun investigating the association between DA and schizotypy using a wide range of methods. In this article, we review published studies on this association from the following areas of work: (1) experimental investigations of the interactive effects of dopaminergic challenges and schizotypy on cognition, motor control, and behavior (2), dopaminergically supported cognitive functions (3), studies of associations between schizotypy and polymorphisms in genes involved in dopaminergic neurotransmission, and (4) molecular imaging studies of the association between schizotypy and markers of the DA system. Together, data from these lines of evidence suggest that DA is important to the expression and experience of schizotypy and associated behavioral biases. An important observation is that the experimental designs, methods, and manipulations used in this research are highly heterogeneous. Future studies are required to replicate individual observations, to enlighten the link between DA and different schizotypy dimensions (positive, negative, cognitive disorganization), and to guide the search for solid DA-sensitive behavioral markers. Such studies are important in order to clarify inconsistencies between studies. More work is also needed to identify differences between dopaminergic alterations in schizotypy compared to the dysfunctions observed in schizophrenia.

Keywords: schizotypy, personality, dopamine, cognition, psychopharmacology, neuroimaging, genetics

INTRODUCTION

Schizotypy, first coined by Rado (1), is a set of personality traits thought to mirror the subclinical expression of schizophrenia in the general population. Schizotypy encompasses behaviors, cognitions, and emotions resembling the signs and symptoms of schizophrenia. It is typically assessed in the general population using psychometric self-report questionnaires including, among others, the Schizotypal Personality Questionnaire (SPQ) (2), the Oxford–Liverpool Inventory of Feelings and Experiences (O-LIFE) (3), the Chapman scales (4), and the Rust Inventory of Schizotypal Cognitions (RISC) (5). Factor analytic studies have shown that schizotypy consists broadly of three subdimensions (3, 6). The *positive* schizotypy dimension describes perceptual aberrations resembling the hallucinations of schizophrenia as well as unusual views and ideas resembling the delusions of schizophrenia. The *negative* schizotypy dimension describes a loss of normal emotional, physical, and social functions such as the experience of pleasure or interest in social contacts. Finally, the *disorganized* dimension encompasses eccentric behavior and odd speech. Overall, the symptomatic phenomenology of schizotypy thus resembles the factor structure of symptoms reported in schizophrenia (7).

The literature tends to draw upon two scientific approaches toward the study of schizotypy, i.e., the quasi-dimensional and fully dimensional approaches. The quasi-dimensional, psychiatrically oriented approach, proposed by Meehl (8, 9), regards schizotypy as the subclinical expression of the symptoms of schizophrenia (10, 11). In that approach, schizotypal individuals are hypothesized to carry the genetic risk for schizophrenia. Evidence for this approach stems from some (12), but not all (13), taxometric studies. The fully dimensional approach (14), championed by Eysenck and Claridge (13, 15–18), regards schizotypy as a personality trait which is continuously distributed. It is assumed that schizotypal symptoms in the healthy population are qualitatively similar though quantitatively milder than those observed in schizophrenia. Evidence for the fully dimensional approach stems from taxometric studies that consider positive skewness of sample distribution (13). The high prevalence of psychotic-like experiences in the general population is also in accordance with the fully dimensional approach (19, 20). Importantly, both approaches emphasize the observation of variation in schizotypal features in the population. More work is, however, needed on the exact nature of the distribution and the boundary between non-clinical schizotypy and clinical schizophrenia (12, 13, 21, 22).

Irrespective of these open psychometric questions, biopsychological research on schizotypy is also based on the continuum assumption. There is considerable evidence that behavioral and brain correlates of schizophrenia are also related to schizotypy [for review, see, e.g., Ref. (11, 23, 24)]. By and large, the focus of these schizotypy studies has been on behavioral, cognitive, brain structural, and brain functional measures. Neuronal information transfer is, however, only possible with functional neurochemical transmissions at synapses. Therefore, neurochemical studies involving pharmacological challenges or molecular imaging methods are of utmost importance for our understanding of schizotypy. Most prominent so far are studies that link schizotypy to dopamine (DA). Comparable to above mentioned study domains, this link originates in the continuum assumption because schizophrenia has been linked to DA (25, 26), schizotypy might be associated with DA as well. In the following, we will explore this possible link. We will describe a selection of relevant psychopharmacological studies in patients with schizophrenia before referring to schizotypy studies that test the possible link to DA. First, however, we briefly introduce the structure and function of the DA system.

At this point, it should be mentioned that the schizophrenia spectrum also of course includes individuals with schizotypal personality disorder (SPD) and those at increased genetic or clinical risk for the illness. However, in the interest of focus, we restrict this overview to psychometrically identified schizotypy. Of course, it should be acknowledged that some, but not all, individuals with high levels of schizotypy also qualify for a diagnosis of SPD. For example, Raine (2) observed SPD in 55% of participants with SPQ scores in the top 10% of the distribution.

THE STRUCTURE AND FUNCTION OF HUMAN DOPAMINE SYSTEMS

Neurotransmitters exert different actions throughout the brain; the type of action depends on the neurotransmitter, action site, and/or neuronal circuit (27). For instance, the amino acids GABA (inhibitory) and glutamate (excitatory) are found throughout the brain. Acetylcholine and monoamines (DA, norepinephrine, serotonin), on the other hand, are organized in systems. Systems imply that cell bodies producing these substances are located subcortically in anatomically circumscribed regions (27). In the case of DA, the nigrostriatal (important to motor control), mesolimbic (important to reward and motivation), and mesocortical (important to prefrontal functions) pathways have been distinguished on the basis of where their cell bodies are located and where their axons project. Moreover, two major DA receptor families have been identified, viz. the D1-like (D1 and D5) and D2-like (D2, D3, D4) receptors that are widely distributed throughout the brain. Because of the importance of the DA system to various mental health conditions, its complexity and functioning remain intensively investigated (28).

Of course, complex mental health disorders cannot be explained by single changes to complex neurotransmitter systems. Instead, subsystems are likely contributors to different psychopathologies. DA has indeed been associated with diverse neurological and psychiatric conditions such as Parkinson's disease, schizophrenia, addiction, and attention deficit hyperactivity disorder [e.g., Ref. (29, 30)]. Also, neurotransmitter systems are not modular, i.e., they do not exert their actions in isolation. A given neurotransmitter system is in constant interaction with other systems. In schizophrenia, interactions between the DA and glutamate systems are intensively debated (31). Accordingly, pharmacological compounds can enhance DA release while also enhancing the release of the other two monoamines (norepinephrine, serotonin). The latter release might happen directly or indirectly through metabolism of DA into norepinephrine and the latter into serotonin (32, 33). This overall complexity in neurotransmitter systems highlights the fact that individual psychopharmacological studies have inherent limitations in investigating the link between schizotypy and DA. As exemplified in the following sections, we depend on findings from a multitude of studies using different but complementary approaches.

DOPAMINERGIC EFFECTS IN PATIENTS WITH SCHIZOPHRENIA

Neuroleptics were first discovered in the early 1950s (34). Since their discovery, it has been shown that these DA antagonists ameliorate acute psychotic symptoms [e.g., Ref. (35, 36)]. It is still accepted that DA is key in the treatment and pathophysiology of schizophrenia (37–39). For example, patients with schizophrenia profit from DA antagonistic treatment (38) and show symptom worsening after DA agonistic treatment (40, 41). In healthy populations, DA agonists can trigger psychotic or psychosis-like symptoms (42, 43). Such findings led to the suggestion that a hyperactive DA system results in acute psychotic symptoms (25, 38). Davis et al. (25) further elaborated on this suggestion by proposing DA abnormalities to depend on the brain region, i.e., D1 receptors being predominantly found cortically and D2 receptors subcortically. They specified that frontal hypodopaminergia would result in striatal hyperdopaminergia. Regarding symptoms, they related negative symptoms to frontal hypodopaminergia and positive symptoms to striatal hyperdopaminergia.

Howes and Kapur (44) refined this previous DA theory by suggesting that multiple "hits" (e.g., social, environmental, and cultural stressors) result in DA dysregulation at the pre-synaptic level. Such DA dysregulation is hypothesized to lead to changes in how events are appraised, potentially because events become overly salient (i.e., attract increased allocation of meaning). According to these authors, an alteration in pre-synaptic DA is the final common pathway to psychosis and psychosis-proneness (45). Yet, other evidence points to the role of post-synaptic processes (46). Very recently, Seeman (39) outlined how dynamic changes of post-synaptic D2 receptors might contribute to symptoms experienced in schizophrenia. Mainly based on animal studies, Seeman reports on D2 receptors that can either take a high affinity state for DA (D2High) or a low affinity state for DA (D2Low). Reviewing the literature, he suggests that psychosis is associated with the more active and normally less common D2High state.

Overall, despite various suggestions on the involvement of alternative neurotransmitter systems in psychosis and, by inference, schizophrenia (31, 47), recent notions highlight that DA is the likely final common pathway to psychosis. The precise mechanisms and sites of action remain inconclusive, and continued research reveals ever more complex synaptic dynamics such as the ones described for the D2High and D2Low affinity states. It remains to be clarified whether such alterations of the DA system are specific to overt clinical psychosis or are also evident, though less pronounced, along the schizophrenia spectrum including healthy schizotypy. Howes and Kapur (44) previously reviewed a number of studies showing an involvement of DA in the prodromal state, in ultra-high risk populations, in relatives of schizophrenia patients and in schizotypy. Because these populations lie on the psychosis continuum, part of these and additional studies will be discussed in more detail.

In an 18F-dopa positron emission tomography (PET) study, Howes et al. (48) observed that patients with prodromal psychotic symptoms showed enhanced striatal 18F-dopa uptake, intermediate to that of patients with schizophrenia and healthy controls. This enhanced uptake correlated positively with prodromal symptomatology and neuropsychological impairments [but see in Ref. (49)]. In a 3-year follow-up study, Howes et al. (50) observed that greater striatal DA synthesis capacity was observed in a psychosis transition group as compared to a group that did not transit into psychosis. Moreover, this capacity in the transition group correlated positively with symptom severity. In another study, elevated pre-synaptic striatal uptake was comparable between patients with SPD and remitted patients with schizophrenia (51). It was also elevated for individuals at ultra-high risk for psychosis, i.e., those who show impaired socio-occupational functions and attenuated psychotic symptoms (e.g., perceptual abnormalities, paranoia) (52). An increase of striatal pre-synaptic DA synthesis has also been observed in first-degree relatives of patients with schizophrenia (53). Relatives additionally showed an altered stress response, demonstrated by increased levels of plasma DA metabolites when compared to healthy controls (54). This increase was associated with psychotic-like symptoms subsequent to daily stressors (experience sampling methodology) (55). In yet another study, psychotic patients and unaffected relatives released significantly more DA in striatal regions subsequent to the inhalation of delta-9-tetrahydrocannabinol (the main psychoactive ingredient of cannabis) than healthy controls (56). In sum, these studies show that DA abnormalities are not restricted to individuals with a clinical diagnosis of schizophrenia, but are also evident in the extended phenotype. Findings specific to schizotypy are presented further below.

METHODS IN THE STUDY OF DOPAMINE AND ITS RELATION TO SCHIZOTYPY AND COGNITION

Various methods are available to measure aspects of the DA system in healthy humans. The most promising to study the link between schizotypy and DA include (1) experimental pharmacological challenges of the DA system, (2) neurobiologically informed, DA-sensitive cognitive and behavioral measures, (3) molecular studies of genes involved in DA neurotransmission, and (4) molecular neuroimaging of the DA system. Here, we briefly outline these methods. In the next section, we discuss how they have been used in work on schizotypy.

The first methodological approach directly tests the link between schizotypy and DA. For instance, one could test DA agonistic and antagonistic treatment effects on the experience of schizotypy as well as related correlates in healthy populations. This approach corresponds to tests of medication effects in patients. In patients, however, pharmacological treatment consists of the daily administration of medication over many weeks, given that the clinical antipsychotic effects of such compounds take several weeks to emerge (57). When testing healthy populations, such long-term drug administration would be unethical and potentially dangerous. For instance, antipsychotic treatment causes severe side effects [e.g., Ref. (58) for a meta-analysis]. These and other (e.g., economic and clinical) factors explain why the investigation of long-term medication effects is common in clinical studies while single (or limited) short-term drug effects are frequently investigated in healthy volunteers.

Importantly, short-term dopaminergic drug applications directly modulate the DA system, thereby allowing the evaluation of dopaminergic effects on domains of cognition, emotion, motor control and their neural correlates. Such studies tend to take place in well-controlled laboratory settings using tight methodological controls, such as double-blind procedures and placebo conditions [e.g., Ref. (59–61)]. Such paradigms inform on acute drug effects and their interaction with schizotypy. They also allow addressing clinical questions hard to implement in patients (40–43). As outlined above, however, it should be borne in mind that the DA system does not work in isolation but instead interacts with other neurotransmitter systems; therefore, the specificity of any pharmacological effect on behavior and cognition remains to be characterized further.

The second methodological approach involves the assessment of DA-mediated cognitive and behavioral performance measures and their covariance with schizotypal personality traits. This approach is indirect in comparison to the first approach. Yet, the use of DA-mediated performance measures is popular. Various paradigms have been drawn upon (62–67). Of importance, previous studies have shown that these performance measures are sensitive to modulations of the DA system. In particular, such measures are affected by dopaminergic drugs in humans [e.g., Ref. (61, 68, 69)], human mental health conditions in which the DA system is affected [e.g., Ref. (64, 65)] and by experimental dopaminergic interventions in animals [e.g., Ref. (64, 69)].

The third methodological approach involves molecular imaging methods. As indicated above, methods such as PET and single photon emission computed tomography (SPECT) can provide *in vivo* data on markers of the DA system (such as DA synthesis or receptor and transporter availability) in the human brain (45). These markers can be quantified and related directly to schizotypy scores. As will be detailed below, PET and SPECT methods have recently been applied to study the DA system as a function of schizotypy.

The fourth methodological approach involves the exploration of the role of DA in schizotypy by studying statistical associations of schizotypy scores with variants in genes whose protein products are known to be involved in the DA system (70, 71). Such genes may include those coding for receptors, transporters or enzymes involved in DA synthesis, release, reuptake, degradation or any other aspect of DA transmission. The effects on DA transmission of such genetic variants, when known, allow drawing conclusions about differences in DA transmission in relation to individual differences in schizotypy.

DOPAMINE AND SCHIZOTYPY: EMPIRICAL EVIDENCE

A role of DA in schizophrenia and schizotypy has long been postulated (67, 72–74). Empirical evidence on the nature of the association between DA and schizotypy has been scarce and the association has rarely been investigated directly (68, 75). However, studies have accumulated over the last 15 years. Here, we give an overview on the outcome of these studies, irrespective of which methodological approach has been applied. In case that DA was investigated indirectly (the second methodological approach mentioned above), we distinguish between studies that assessed more basic behavioral functions and those that assessed higher cognitive functions. Often these studies added a direct manipulation of the DA system using the first methodological approach outlined above. Therefore, we discuss these together with the purely behavioral data on simple or complex behavioral functions. In the case of molecular genetic and molecular imaging studies, many findings are based on associations with questionnaire scores. We discuss these studies separately.

BASIC BEHAVIORAL FUNCTIONS

Turning behavior is a behavioral marker of a relatively hyperactive DA system in one over the other hemisphere. Animal studies [Ref. (76) for overview] and a study testing patients with asymmetrical Parkinson's disease (77) showed that whole-body turning occurs away from the hemisphere with the more active DA system. Acutely psychotic patients (65) and individuals with elevated positive schizotypal features (74) yielded a preference for left- over right-sided turns pointing to a relative hyperactive right-hemispheric DA system along the schizophrenia spectrum. In a study that directly tested the influence of DA on turning behavior, half of the participants received a placebo and the other half a non-specific DA agonist (levodopa) (78). Turning biases were investigated as a function of participants' positive and negative schizotypal features. The authors found that elevated positive schizotypy associated with a left- over right-sided turning preference in the placebo group. In this same group, negative schizotypy associated with a right- over left-sided turning preference. In the levodopa group, these relationships were not strengthened, but actually reversed. The authors argued that a higher than normal DA availability might have balanced out pre-existing DA asymmetries. In another experiment on the same participants, schizotypy and levodopa treatments were unrelated to lateral turning biases in a computer-based object-rotation task (66).

Spontaneous eye blink rate (SBR) is indicative of cerebral DA activity. Eye blinks occur spontaneously, frequently, and mostly without awareness. They are primarily important for the health of the eye surface and clarity of vision. Decades ago, SBR has been suggested to be a sensitive marker of striatal DA activity (64). SBR has been associated with changes in concurrent cognitive processes, perceptual load, and level of arousal (79, 80). It is enhanced in schizophrenia, in particular in the unmedicated or drug-naïve state (64, 81, 82), and decreases with antipsychotic treatment (64, 82, 83). In line with Davis et al.'s (25) notion of a link between negative symptoms and hypodopaminergia on the one hand and positive symptoms and hyperdopaminergia on the other hand, negative symptoms were associated with a decreased SBR (83) and positive symptoms with an increased SBR (82, 83). Additionally, SBR increased with a DA agonistic treatment in healthy individuals (84, 85).

In a dopaminergic challenge study, half of the participants received a placebo while the others received an unspecific DA agonist (levodopa) (86). SBR did not differ between substance groups, but correlated positively with negative (but not positive) schizotypy scores after levodopa intake. The authors conjectured that this effect occurred because negative schizotypy is *a priori* related to hypodopaminergia. In another study, however, SBR correlated positively with participants' psychoticism scores, a subdimension of the Eysenck Personality Questionnaire (87). Some authors argued that psychoticism forms part of the schizotypy spectrum (88). Other authors linked psychoticism to impulsiveness, lack of cooperation, rigidity, low superego control, low social sensitivity, low persistence, lack of anxiety, and lack of feelings of inferiority (89) – features associated with borderline and antisocial personality disorder rather than with the schizophrenia spectrum (90, 91). The psychoticism dimension seems indeed the least clear-cut dimension of the three Eysenckian dimensions (90, 91). Whatever the psychoticism dimension is measuring, the latter SBR finding suggests that psychoticism is probably more sensitive to the DA system subserving SBR than is schizotypy (or negative schizotypy) as such.

Stereotyped behavior is thought to be sensitive to DA. It is observable in schizophrenia (92, 93) and after amphetamine consumption in healthy individuals (69). In schizophrenia, stereotyped behavior occurs on the motor (e.g., walking backwards and forwards, repetitive jaw movements) (94) and higher cognitive level. For instance, perseverative errors in the Wisconsin Card Sorting Test are elevated in schizophrenia [Ref. (95) for overview], SPD (96, 97) and as a function of both high positive and negative schizotypy (98, 99). Random number generation tasks show that patients with schizophrenia (100, 101), healthy participants after amphetamine administration (69), and healthy positive schizotypal participants (102, 103) yield stereotypical response biases when compared to respective controls. Finally, when rotating figures into advantageous target positions on a computer screen, left or right turns had to be applied dynamically to obtain maximal scores (66). Sticking stereotypically to one or the other direction would be disadvantageous. The latter study reported on two experiments with one being a between-subject levodopa placebo-controlled experiment. The authors observed that individuals with relatively high as compared to low positive schizotypy were behaving more stereotypically. Yet, in the levodopa group, high positive schizotypal individuals performed less stereotypically than the low positive schizotypal individuals. Comparable to the findings on turning behavior, results seem to suggest that a higher than normal DA availability in positive schizotypes balances out pre-existing DA-mediated behavioral abnormalities.

Prepulse inhibition (PPI) is another DA-sensitive measure that has been studied in relation to schizotypy. PPI is a cross-species phenomenon that refers to a reduction in the amplitude of the startle response to a strong sensory stimulus, the pulse, if this stimulus is preceded by 30–500 ms by a weak stimulus, the prepulse (104). The weak prestimulus is thought to evoke inhibitory mechanisms, which limit further stimulation until the processing of the prepulse has been completed, resulting in a reduced impact of the pulse. PPI is thought to reflect an early sensory gating process to avoid interference from simultaneous processing of several stimuli. It is, thus, a largely automatic measure of inhibitory function. Experimental studies in animals have shown that a cortico-striato-pallido-thalamic circuitry underlies PPI (105).

Patients with schizophrenia (106) and SPD (107) show reproducible reductions in the magnitude of PPI, which is thought to lead to sensory overstimulation causing cognitive and behavioral confusion. Also, PPI deficits are induced in numerous experimental models of schizophrenia through, e.g., isolation rearing (108), ketamine (109), sleep deprivation (110, 111), and phencyclidine (112). The robust and reliable PPI reduction in schizophrenia can be restored, at least partially, with antipsychotic treatment, with some advantage of atypical compounds over first-generation, typical antipsychotics (113–119).

Importantly, reduced PPI has been observed in relation to elevated SPQ total, cognitive-perceptual and interpersonal scores (120), Minnesota Multiphasic Personality Inventory (MMPI) psychosis-proneness scores (121) and Eysenckian psychoticism scores (122). Evidence from a functional magnetic resonance imaging (fMRI) study of PPI points to reduced activation in the insula, putamen, thalamus, inferior parietal cortex, hippocampal gyrus, and fusiform gyrus in relation to higher levels of Eysenckian psychoticism scores (122). These BOLD patterns show some resemblance with the data obtained from samples of patients with schizophrenia (123). Of relevance to the present discussion, areas such as the putamen are rich in DA receptors, consistent with the hypothesis that PPI is at least in part dopaminergically mediated (124–126).

A final basic DA-mediated paradigm is latent inhibition (LI) (62, 127, 128). Comparable to PPI, LI is a cross-species phenomenon, which is sensitive to pro- and antidopaminergic challenges (62). LI refers to the finding that non-reinforced pre-exposure to a stimulus, that is later to be conditioned, causes less efficient conditioning when the same stimulus is subsequently reinforced. This phenomenon has been observed in both humans and animals. LI has also been investigated in relation to schizophrenia and schizotypy. A recent review showed reduced LI in the acute phase of patients with schizophrenia and preserved LI in chronic schizophrenia (129). That review also found a modest but relatively consistent relationship between schizotypy and LI, particularly of positive schizotypy (130). In particular, higher levels of positive schizotypy seem to be associated with less LI in healthy participants. These studies, together, suggest an involvement of dopaminergic alterations in the LI deficits in schizophrenia and positive schizotypy.

HIGHER COGNITIVE FUNCTIONS

Dopamine is thought to modulate the signal-to-noise ratio in semantic networks (131, 132). The reduction of prefrontal tonic dopaminergic modulation (hypofrontality) in schizophrenia is assumed to decrease the contrast between a signal and noise. This decreased contrast leads to a disinhibited spreading activation within semantic networks [see in Ref. (132) for an overview]. This increased spreading activation would result in remote associations (psychotic symptom) and enhanced semantic priming effects (laboratory measures) in schizophrenia (132). In healthy populations, on the other hand, an experimentally enhanced DA availability (levodopa consumption) focused such priming effects (133). Yet, this dopaminergic modulation of semantic networks differed for the two cerebral hemispheres with a hyperdopaminergia being more prominent in the right than left hemisphere (see previous section). This hyperdopaminergia (potentially resulting from a frontal hypodopaminergia) has been considered to explain the observation that enhanced spreading activation was more relevant for the right than left hemisphere in schizophrenia (134) and healthy individuals high in positive schizotypy (60, 135). Independent studies suggested that these DA-mediated functions explain both these lateralized priming effects and enhanced remote associative processing more generally (136, 137) as well as right-hemisphere shifts of functions in a broader sense. Indeed, the left hemisphere seems compromised in patients with schizophrenia with DA antagonists restoring if not reversing such altered hemispheric asymmetries (138–143).

Studies showed that lateralized lexical decision performance is relatively biased toward the right hemisphere in high as compared to low scorers on a positive but not negative schizotypy questionnaire (144, 145). In a pharmacological challenge study, superior left hemisphere language dominance was associated with elevated negative schizotypy scores in a levodopa (but not placebo) group (145). Thus, levodopa might restore left hemisphere language dominance in healthy individuals through (i) the attenuation of the contribution of the right hemisphere to language as a function of positive schizotypy and (ii) an increased contribution of the left hemisphere as a function of negative schizotypy. In an independent sample, but using the same task, the authors calculated signal detection theory measures of sensitivity (d-prime) and response tendency (criterion) (146). Results showed lower d-prime in the levodopa than in the placebo group in individuals low in positive schizotypy. For the response criterion, individuals in the placebo group showed a loosened versus conservative response criterion when being high versus low in positive schizotypy. In the levodopa group, these response tendencies were attenuated. This study suggests that a higher than normal DA availability (i) reduces d-prime in low positive schizotypy individuals and (ii) turns low positive schizotypy individuals less conservative and high positive schizotypy individuals more conservative in their response behavior.

Higher cognitive functions such as working memory and cognitive control have also been studied using experimental psychopharmacological designs. Using a between-subjects, double-blind, placebo-controlled design with groups of high and medium total SPQ scores, amisulpride, a clinically effective antipsychotic with strong D2/D3 receptor antagonistic action, improved working memory and verbal fluency performance in the schizotypy group but impaired it in the medium schizotypy control group (59). The same multi-center study investigated the effects of risperidone, a clinically effective atypical antipsychotic with action on D2 as well as 5-HT receptors, on performance on the antisaccade task, a prominent measure of response inhibition (147, 148). It was found that risperidone impaired antisaccade performance in the medium schizotypy group, whereas performance in the high schizotypy group showed a non-significant tendency toward improvement (149). These findings are in agreement with previous evidence of risperidone impairing antisaccade performance in healthy controls (150) but improving it in patients with schizophrenia (151, 152).

To summarize, findings of this section suggest that individuals with high levels of schizotypy may benefit from DA agonists in terms of cognitive performance. In contrast, individuals with low levels of schizotypy may deteriorate in cognition with DA agonists. Concerning DA antagonists, people with high levels of (particularly positive) schizotypy may benefit in cognitive function from DA antagonistic compounds similar to patients with schizophrenia, or at least tolerate them. People with low or medium levels in (particularly positive) schizotypy may become impaired in these functions. Overall, given the role of DA in the effects of clinically effective antipsychotics (153), the presented data indicate that DA impacts some of the cognitive deficits observed in high (mainly positive) schizotypy (24, 78, 154). However, antipsychotics such as risperidone do not act only on the DA system, thereby limiting the implications for a dopaminergic basis of schizotypy (149).

SCHIZOTYPY AND DOPAMINE SYSTEM GENES

Twin studies have established that individual differences in the various subdimensions of schizotypy in the general population are to a significant part explained by additive genetic factors. Heritability estimates are in the range of 30–50% [see, e.g., Ref. (155–157)], although not all studies have found significant heritabilities (158). These behavioral genetic studies, thus, provide a basis for molecular genetic investigations such as those specifically targeting candidate genes related to the DA system.

The most frequently studied gene in the context of schizotypy is the gene coding for catechol-*O*-methyltransferase, the *COMT* gene (159–161). These studies were originally informed by significant associations of a single nucleotide polymorphism (SNP) in the *COMT* gene with schizophrenia (162); however, later meta-analyses have suggested that this association is not significant (163, 164). The COMT enzyme degrades catecholamines including DA in the synaptic cleft. Due to the paucity of the DA transporter in the prefrontal cortex, COMT plays a particularly prominent role in degrading pre-synaptic DA in that part of the brain. The *COMT* gene (located in chromosome 22q11.1-q11.2) contains a G to A missense mutation, resulting in a substitution of methionine (met) for valine (val) at codon 158 of the membrane-bound isoform of the protein (reference sequence identification code rs4680). This allelic variation (val158met) is a functional polymorphism: The met158 allele has about one third to one fourth of the activity of the val158 allele, resulting in less efficient catecholamine catabolism and, therefore, higher DA levels.

A number of published studies have reported associations between schizotypy and the *COMT* val158met polymorphism in healthy subjects. A series of publications from a large-scale study of apparently healthy young men, the ASPIS study, has provided evidence that the high-activity Val allele may be associated with schizotypy. In particular, the Val allele was found to be associated with elevated total SPQ and Perceptual Aberration Scale scores in a first analysis of 379 subjects (165). In a subsequent study using an extended sample of 543 individuals and a factor analysis of SPQ into four factors (cognitive-perceptual, negative, disorganization and paranoia) the Val loading was associated with increased total SPQ and increased negative and disorganized factor scores (71). In a further extension of 908 subjects where the analysis was also performed for individual SPQ dimensions, an association of Val with increased total SPQ, negative disorganized, and paranoia factors was observed. Additionally, there were specific relations of Val loading with increased scores in magical thinking, constricted affect, and odd speech subscales of the SPQ (166).

Broadly confirming this evidence, Grant et al. (167) observed in an independent sample of 280 healthy volunteers that Val/Val homozygotes had significantly higher positive schizotypy scores (O-LIFE unusual experiences) than Met carriers.

Other studies obtained evidence of an association between the Val allele and increased schizotypy in samples of relatives of psychiatric patients. One study (168) observed that among 81 first-degree relatives of schizophrenia patients the Val allele was associated with high negative schizotypy (social and physical anhedonia), while no association was found in 38 relatives of patients with bipolar disorder or in 30 healthy controls. Schürhoff et al. (70) studied *COMT* rs4680 and schizotypy in a combined sample of relatives of schizophrenic patients, relatives of bipolar patients and healthy controls (total $N = 106$). The authors observed higher total, positive and negative SPQ schizotypy (but not disorganization) scores in association with an increasing number of Val alleles.

Overall, these studies suggest that the Val allele is associated with higher levels of various schizotypy subdimensions. However, evidence to the contrary as well as failures to replicate have also been published. For example, Sheldrick and colleagues (169) reported higher SPQ-B Disorganization scores in the *COMT* Met/Met group than in the Val/Val group ($N = 522$ volunteers). Also, no significant association of overall schizotypy with rs4680 genotype was observed in individuals with velo-cardio-facial syndrome (170) or in a mixed sample of members from families with bipolar disorder as well as unaffected controls (total $N = 222$) (171). Ma and colleagues (172) similarly reported a lack of significant associations between rs4680 and SPQ total and subscale scores in 465 Chinese participants. Finally, Ettinger et al. (173) found no statistically significant association of positive schizotypy (RISC) with rs4680 in a small sample of healthy males ($N = 31$).

These inconsistencies remain to be resolved, both through additional original studies and a comprehensive meta-analysis that also addresses potential moderator variables. A number of factors may play a role, including the choice of schizotypy questionnaire (174) as well as the ethnic and sociodemographic composition of the sample (175). Other moderating variables may also be important. For example, the above mentioned study by Savitz and colleagues (171) observed, in the absence of an overall association of rs4680 with STA schizotypy, that there was an interaction between childhood trauma (as measured with the Childhood Trauma Questionnaire) and rs4680 on STA: The genotype was associated with STA only in individuals with higher trauma scores, such that Val/Val individuals showed increasing STA with increasing trauma, whereas other genotype groups did not. The possibility of interactive effects of genes and the environment is intriguing and needs to be examined in more detail.

In addition to *COMT*, a number of other DA-related genes have been investigated in relation to schizotypy. Ettinger et al. (173) obtained no evidence of significant associations of positive schizotypy (RISC) with polymorphisms in the *DRD3, DRD4,* and *SLC6A3* genes in a sample of 31 healthy subjects. Grant et al. (167), however, reported significant associations of different O-LIFE subscales with *DRD2 Taq1A*, *MAOA*-uVNTR and *SLC6A3* in 288 participants. Finally, a recent study by Taurisano et al. (176) observed an association between SPQ total score and *DRD2* rs1076560 in 67 subjects, with GT heterozygotes showing higher scores than G allele homozygotes.

Overall, the discussed molecular genetic findings are promising but must be considered preliminary; they require replication and further investigation in larger samples. Genetic research has the possibility of informing the molecular basis of inter-individual variation in schizotypy and as such makes a unique, non-invasive contribution to the neuroscientific method arsenal available to schizotypy researchers. An additional appeal of this method is the possibility of combining genetic data with other neuroscience methods, such as functional and structural neuroimaging (177).

MOLECULAR IMAGING OF THE DOPAMINE SYSTEM IN RELATION TO SCHIZOTYPY

Measures of the DA system in humans can also be obtained *in vivo* using molecular imaging techniques such as PET and SPECT. These methods have been applied successfully to the study of the dopaminergic basis of schizophrenia (45). In contrast, relatively few PET or SPECT studies have investigated the relationship between DA system markers and schizotypy.

An early ^{123}I-IBZM single photon emission tomography investigation (178) reported a significant *negative* relationship between Eysenckian psychoticism scores and D2 receptor binding in the basal ganglia (relative to frontal cortex) in a small sample of healthy volunteers. Extending this first evidence, a [^{11}C]raclopride PET study (179) found lower D2 receptor density in putamen to be associated with higher scores on the Karolinska Scales of Personality detachment scale, a measure tapping aspects of negative schizotypy. Breier and colleagues replicated this finding, reporting a negative association between the Karolinska detachment scale and striatal D2 receptor binding using [^{11}C]raclopride PET in an independent sample of healthy volunteers (180).

In contrast, a more recent SPECT study observed a positive relationship between the disorganization score of the SPQ and D2/3 receptor binding in the right striatum (relative to occipital cortex) (181). Most recently, Taurisano et al. (176) used SPECT and found a positive correlation between D2 receptor binding in the right putamen and total SPQ score in individuals heterozygous for the *DRD2* rs1076560 genotype but not in individuals homozygous for the G allele, suggesting interactive effects of genotype and D2 availability on schizotypal personality. No association between whole striatum DA synthesis capacity and total SPQ score was observed in a PET study of subjects with persistent auditory verbal hallucinations (182).

A different line of molecular imaging studies has focused on dopaminergic challenges in relation to schizotypy. It has previously been shown that patients with schizophrenia, both in the acute phase and in remission, exhibit amphetamine-induced reductions in D2 and D3 DA receptor binding potential in the striatum (40, 183). This result suggests increased striatal DA release in schizophrenia and complements the evidence of heightened pre-synaptic DA function in this disorder (45). Interestingly, a similar pattern of increased striatal amphetamine-induced DA release has been observed in SPD (51). Further evidence confirming and extending this pattern across the schizophrenia spectrum comes from a [^{18}F]fallypride PET study (184). That study showed significant correlations between striatal DA release after a single administration of amphetamine and SPQ total and disorganized dimension scores in healthy volunteers (184). Together, these studies provide evidence for a common striatal dopaminergic dysregulation in both schizotypy and schizophrenia.

Finally, based on evidence of stress as a possible risk factor for schizophrenia (185), molecular imaging methods have been employed to investigate the effects of experimentally induced stress on DA turnover as a function of schizotypy. Using [^{11}C]raclopride PET, it was shown that participants with high levels of negative schizotypy – but not controls or participants with high levels of positive schizotypy – showed a significant stress-induced striatal reduction in binding potential (186).

Overall, studies using molecular imaging methods such as PET or SPECT are able to provide relatively direct markers of the DA system *in vivo* and, as such, can be used profitably to investigate its relationship not only to schizophrenia but also to schizotypy. However, evidence of associations between DA markers and levels of schizotypy in healthy participants is still scarce. To summarize, while there are associations between lower D2 receptor availability and higher psychoticism and detachment, there is also a report of an association between lower D2/3 receptor binding and lower disorganized dimension schizotypy. This pattern may imply differential associations of DA levels with different dimensions of schizotypy. Finally, there is evidence of increased striatal DA release following amphetamine administration or stress induction in schizotypy.

CONCLUSIONS

In this overview, we discussed studies linking DA and schizotypy. We first introduced the neurotransmitter DA and sketched some *in vivo* methods of its study in patients with schizophrenia and healthy controls. We presented evidence from the behavioral literature showing that high levels of schizotypy (in particular positive schizotypy) are associated with DA-sensitive functions, in line with behavioral tendencies previously reported in schizophrenia. In addition, we presented evidence that both increased (DA agonists) and decreased (DA antagonists) DA availability seems to be beneficial to behavioral deficits in high schizotypes (mainly positive schizotypy). Those low in schizotypy, however, seemed to deteriorate in their behavioral performance following antipsychotic treatment. While only a careful conjecture, it seems that an increase as well as a decrease of DA may restore function in high schizotypes but deteriorate it in low schizotypes. Overall, we conclude that variance in schizotypy may be explained in part by alterations to the DA system. Of course, as noted, the DA system does not act in isolation but in constant and complex interactions with other neurotransmitter systems.

An underdeveloped theoretical point not only here, but also in schizotypy research more generally, is a well-recognized framework integrating empirical evidence on links between DA and schizotypy from various levels of analysis (not only concerning DA) into a coherent theory. Important theoretical contributions by Meehl (8, 9) and others (16, 187) have influenced our current thinking on schizotypy. A significant body of new data has been amassed that needs to be theoretically linked. In particular, we think of the psychopharmacological, imaging and genetic findings that are based on techniques that had not been available before. To achieve this aim, it may be instructive to turn in two directions for inspiration, viz. in the direction of (i) personality theory in individual differences research and (ii) clinical schizophrenia research.

Regarding individual differences, DeYoung (188) recently integrated previous assumptions into a theoretical framework that is relevant to our discussion of the role of DA in schizotypy. Particularly relevant is his discussion of "apophenia," i.e., individuals' tendency for overinclusive thinking and perception. Conrad (189) termed apophenia as the "unmotivated seeing of connections" accompanied by a "specific experience of an abnormal meaningfulness" (p. 46). For instance, one can refer to apophenia when individuals see and create pattern in random noise, whether this noise is perceptual (190, 191), semantic (136), or probabilistic (192). The suggestion of a link between apophenia and positive schizotypy in particular (136, 193) including its modulation by DA (60, 194) is not new. However, DeYoung (188) links apophenia not only with positive schizotypy and the positive symptoms of psychosis but adds another link, namely that apophenia can be predicted by openness, one of the personality traits of the five factor model of personality (195). Accordingly, apophenia can be called "openness to implausible patterns" [Ref. (188); p. 13]. This openness and its link to apophenia are hypothesized to stem from high-activity levels in the dopaminergic salience system. As mentioned above (44), recent theories on the role of DA in schizophrenia suggest that stressors dysregulate DA at the pre-synaptic control level. This is hypothesized to lead to changes in the appraisal of events, making them more salient (i.e., causing apophenia). Thus, DeYoung's (188) DA theory of personality is of interest as it ties schizotypy in with other personality traits and establishes parallels with schizophrenia at the cognitive (overinclusive pattern detection) and neurophysiological (DA) level.

These parallels link directly to the second direction of inspiration, i.e., clinical schizophrenia research. Here, aberrant salience has become a predominant topic. Current theorizing has provided promising explanations as to how DA links with the symptomatic expression of the clinical condition (153, 196). Specifically, these theories start to fill the explanatory gap between an apparent neurochemical disturbance in the brain and the formation of complex delusions and hallucinations. The argument is that delusions arise as a result of individuals' explanations of experienced aberrant salience. This argument is based on the role of DA in mediating both the presence or absence of reward and the salience, such as novelty, of stimuli. Increased DA neurotransmission is thought to lead to aberrant salience, that is, the direction of attention to objectively irrelevant internal or external stimuli. Delusions are by this account thought to arise through individuals' attempts to explain this distressing experience, likely in interaction with prior experiences and beliefs, both personal and socio-cultural. While it is not clear yet which aspect of salience is particularly disturbed in schizophrenia, this work provides a promising model for understanding an important symptom of schizophrenia. Additionally, it remains unclear from this work how other symptoms of schizophrenia, such as hallucinations, thought disorder and negative symptoms arise. Because we know of numerous established similarities between high schizotypy and schizophrenia [see in Ref. (24) for a recent overview], such theories may be drawn upon for our understanding of schizotypy as well.

In sum, we conclude that there is some evidence of an association between altered DA neurotransmission and schizotypy, particularly positive schizotypy. Such work informs not only neurobiological, but also cognitive models of the schizophrenia spectrum (196) and potential neuropharmacological treatments (197).

FUTURE WORK

The current overview illustrates the numerous and varied ways in which researchers have aimed to investigate the link between schizotypy and DA. The heterogeneity in the approaches and the sometimes conflicting results make it difficult to arrive at a clear-cut conclusion. Most of the time, we cannot directly compare results across study domains. This heterogeneity is of course frustrating but may also be constructive in providing directions as to where more work needs to be done.

Specific suggestions for future work include (1) the need to continue working on the development of an overarching theory of schizotypy (2), the assessment of the direction of effects of increasing and decreasing DA availability in high and low schizotypy of different dimensions (3), the role of concomitant illegal and legal drug use (4), the role of individuals' genetic makeup, and (5) the identification of schizotypal markers that are truly unfavorable concerning high-risk states and those that are potentially of little psychopathological impact.

In our view, the field needs both carefully controlled laboratory experiments and studies that account for the spontaneous self-administration of psychoactive ingredients that frequently act on the DA system. For instance, there is insufficient knowledge as to why schizotypal individuals and patients with schizophrenia consume DA-sensitive drugs to a higher degree than controls (198–200). It remains to be investigated whether this drug consumption is a potential trigger for psychosis or whether such individuals medicate themselves by altering their DA systems.

Also, inconsistencies in the literature remain regarding the molecular genetics of schizotypy. Future studies are needed to provide firmer answers on the important question of the molecular genetic makeup of schizotypy. Given the advance in sample sizes in the genetics of schizophrenia and the likely small sizes of genetic effects on schizophrenia spectrum phenotypes (201), it will be important to substantially increase sample sizes in the study of molecular genetic correlates of schizotypy. A promising way to achieve appropriate sample sizes is the establishment of multi-site collaborations under the guidance of consortia.

An additional avenue for future work concerns the direct comparison between individuals with high levels of schizotypy and patients with schizophrenia. While differences between individuals with high and low schizotypy scores have been shown on numerous occasions, much less is known about differences between highly schizotypal individuals and schizophrenia patients. Such a comparison would allow the identification of factors that perhaps protect schizotypes from developing the full-blown clinical condition (24).

Finally, it should be pointed out as a limitation that this overview provides merely a qualitative discussion of the evidence of an association between DA and schizotypy. An important future contribution to this literature would be a formal meta-analysis of the size and significance of this association across different studies and methods.

REFERENCES

1. Rado S. Dynamics and classification of disordered behaviour. *Am J Psychiatry* (1953) **110**:406–16.
2. Raine A. The SPQ: a scale for the assessment of schizotypal personality based on DSM-III-R criteria. *Schizophr Bull* (1991) **17**:555–64. doi:10.1093/schbul/17.4.555
3. Mason O, Claridge G. The Oxford–Liverpool Inventory of Feelings and Experiences (O-LIFE): further description and extended norms. *Schizophr Res* (2006) **82**:203–11. doi:10.1016/j.schres.2005.12.845
4. Chapman LJ, Kwapil TR. Scales for the measurement of schizotypy. In: Raine A, Lencz T, Mednick SA, editors. *Schizotypal Personality*. Cambridge: Cambridge University Press (1995). p. 79–106.
5. Rust J. The Rust Inventory of Schizotypal Cognitions (RISC). *Schizophr Bull* (1988) **14**:317–22. doi:10.1093/schbul/14.2.317
6. Raine A. Schizotypal personality: neurodevelopmental and psychosocial trajectories. *Annu Rev Clin Psychol* (2006) **2**:291–326. doi:10.1146/annurev.clinpsy.2.022305.095318
7. Liddle PF. The symptoms of chronic schizophrenia. A re-examination of the positive-negative dichotomy. *Br J Psychiatry* (1987) **151**:145–51. doi:10.1192/bjp.151.2.145
8. Meehl PE. Toward an integrated theory of schizotaxia. *J Pers Disord* (1990) **4**:1–99. doi:10.1521/pedi.1990.4.1.1
9. Meehl PE. Schizotaxia, schizotypy, schizophrenia. *Arch Gen Psychiatry* (1962) **46**:935–44. doi:10.1001/archpsyc.1989.01810100077015
10. Meehl PE. Schizotaxia revisited. *Arch Gen Psychiatry* (1989) **46**:935–44. doi:10.1001/archpsyc.1989.01810100077015
11. Lenzenweger MF. *Schizotypy and Schizophrenia: The View from Experimental Psychopathology*. New York, NY: Guilford Press (2010).
12. Haslam N, Holland E, Kuppens P. Categories versus dimensions in personality and psychopathology: a quantitative review of taxometric research. *Psychol Med* (2012) **42**:903–20. doi:10.1017/S0033291711001966
13. Rawlings D, Williams B, Haslam N, Claridge G. Taxometric analysis supports a dimensional latent trait structure for schizotypy. *Pers Indiv Differ* (2008) **44**:1640–51. doi:10.1016/j.paid.2007.06.005
14. Claridge G. *Schizotypy: Implications for Illness and Health*. Oxford: Oxford University Press (1997).
15. Claridge G. The schizophrenias as nervous types. *Br J Psychiatry* (1972) **121**:1–17. doi:10.1192/bjp.121.1.1
16. Claridge G. 'The schizophrenias as nervous types' revisited. *Br J Psychiatry* (1987) **151**:735–43. doi:10.1192/bjp.151.6.735
17. Eysenck HJ. *The Biological Basis of Personality*. Springfield: Thomas (1967).
18. Eysenck SB, Eysenck HJ. The measurement of psychoticism: a study of factor stability and reliability. *Br J Soc Clin Psychol* (1968) **7**:286–94. doi:10.1111/j.2044-8260.1968.tb00571.x
19. Barrett TR, Etheridge JB. Verbal hallucinations in normals, I: people who hear "voices.". *Appl Cogn Psychol* (1992) **6**:379–87. doi:10.1002/acp.2350060503
20. Lincoln TM. Relevant dimensions of delusions: continuing the continuum versus category debate. *Schizophr Res* (2007) **93**:211–20. doi:10.1016/j.schres.2007.02.013
21. Johns LC, van Os J. The continuity of psychotic experiences in the general population. *Clin Psychol Rev* (2001) **21**:1125–41. doi:10.1016/S0272-7358(01)00103-9
22. Barrantes-Vidal N, Gross GM, Sheinbaum T, Mitjavila M, Ballespí S, Kwapil TR. Positive and negative schizotypy are associated with prodromal and schizophrenia-spectrum symptoms. *Schizophr Res* (2013) **145**:50–5. doi:10.1016/j.schres.2013.01.007
23. Nelson MT, Seal ML, Pantelis C, Phillips LJ. Evidence of a dimensional relationship between schizotypy and schizophrenia: a systematic review. *Neurosci Biobehav Rev* (2013) **37**:317–27. doi:10.1016/j.neubiorev.2013.01.004
24. Ettinger U, Meyhöfer I, Steffens M, Wagner M, Koutsouleris N. Genetics, cognition, and neurobiology of schizotypal personality: a review of the overlap with schizophrenia. *Front Psychiatry* (2014) **5**:18. doi:10.3389/fpsyt.2014.00018
25. Davis KL, Kahn RS, Ko G, Davidson M. Dopamine in schizophrenia: a review and reconceptualization. *Am J Psychiatry* (1991) **148**:1474–86.
26. Laruelle M, Abi-Dargham A, van Dyck CH, Gil R, D'Souza CD, Erdos J, et al. Single photon emission computerized tomography imaging of amphetamine-induced dopamine release in drug-free schizophrenic subjects. *Proc Natl Acad Sci U S A* (1996) **93**:9235–40. doi:10.1073/pnas.93.17.9235
27. Banich MT. *Banich, Cognitive Neuroscience and Neuropsychology*. Boston: Houghton Mifflin Company (2004).
28. Tritsch NX, Sabatini BL. Dopaminergic modulation of synaptic transmission in cortex and striatum. *Neuron* (2012) **76**:33–50. doi:10.1016/j.neuron.2012.09.023
29. Mehler-Wex C, Riederer P, Gerlach M. Dopaminergic dysbalance in distinct basal ganglia neurocircuits: implications for the pathophysiology of Parkinson's disease, schizophrenia and attention deficit hyperactivity disorder. *Neurotox Res* (2006) **10**:167–79. doi:10.1007/BF03033354
30. Montgomery AJ, Lingford-Hughes AR, Egerton A, Nutt DJ, Grasby PM. The effect of nicotine on striatal dopamine release in man: a [11C]raclopride PET study. *Synapse* (2007) **61**:637–45. doi:10.1002/syn.20419
31. Javitt DC. Glutamate and schizophrenia: phencyclidine, *N*-methyl-D-aspartate receptors, and dopamine-glutamate interactions. *Int Rev Neurobiol* (2007) **78**:69–108. doi:10.1016/S0074-7742(06)78003-5
32. Kuczenski R, Segal DS. Exposure of adolescent rats to oral methylphenidate: preferential effects on extracellular norepinephrine and absence of sensitization and cross-sensitization to methamphetamine. *J Neurosci* (2002) **22**:7264–71.
33. Rothman RB, Baumann MH, Dersch CM, Romero DV, Rice KC, Carroll FI, et al. Amphetamine-type central nervous system stimulants release norepinephrine more potently than they release dopamine and serotonin. *Synapse* (2001) **39**:32–41. doi:10.1002/1098-2396(20010101)39:1<32::AID-SYN5>3.0.CO;2-3
34. Stip E. Happy birthday neuroleptics! 50 years later: la folie du doute. *Eur Psychiatry* (2002) **17**:115–9. doi:10.1016/S0924-9338(02)00639-9
35. Klein D, Davis J. *Diagnosis and Drug Treatment of Psychiatric Disorders*. Baltimore: Williams & Wilkins (1969).
36. Matthysse S. Antipsychotic drug actions: a clue to the neuropathology of schizophrenia? *Fed Proc* (1973) **32**:200–5.
37. Kapur S, Mamo D. Half a century of antipsychotics and still a central role for dopamine D2 receptors. *Prog Neuropsychopharmacol Biol Psychiatry* (2003) **27**:1081–90. doi:10.1016/j.pnpbp.2003.09.004
38. Laruelle M, Abi-Dargham A. Dopamine as the wind of the psychotic fire: new evidence from brain imaging studies. *J Psychopharmacol* (1999) **13**:358–71. doi:10.1177/026988119901300405
39. Seeman P. Schizophrenia and dopamine receptors. *Eur Neuropsychopharmacol* (2013) **23**:999–1009. doi:10.1016/j.euroneuro.2013.06.005
40. Abi-Dargham A, Gil R, Krystal J, Baldwin RM, Seibyl JP, Bowers M, et al. Increased striatal dopamine transmission in schizophrenia: confirmation in a second cohort. *Am J Psychiatry* (1998) **155**:761–7.
41. Davidson M, Keefe RS, Mohs RC, Siever LJ, Losonczy MF, Horvath TB, et al. L-Dopa challenge and relapse in schizophrenia. *Am J Psychiatry* (1987) **144**:934–8.
42. Janowsky DS, Risch C. Amphetamine psychosis and psychotic symptoms. *Psychopharmacology (Berl)* (1979) **65**:73–7. doi:10.1007/BF00491982
43. Sekine Y, Iyo M, Ouchi Y, Matsunaga T, Tsukada H, Okada H, et al. Methamphetamine-related psychiatric symptoms and reduced brain dopamine transporters studied with PET. *Am J Psychiatry* (2001) **158**:1206–14. doi:10.1176/appi.ajp.158.8.1206
44. Howes OD, Kapur S. The dopamine hypothesis of schizophrenia: version III – the final common pathway. *Schizophr Bull* (2009) **35**:549–62. doi:10.1093/schbul/sbp006
45. Howes OD, Kambeitz J, Kim E, Stahl D, Slifstein M, Abi-Dargham A, et al. The nature of dopamine dysfunction in schizophrenia and what this means for treatment. *Arch Gen Psychiatry* (2012) **69**:776–86. doi:10.1001/archgenpsychiatry.2012.169
46. Thompson JL, Urban N, Slifstein M, Xu X, Kegeles LS, Girgis RR, et al. Striatal dopamine release in schizophrenia comorbid with substance dependence. *Mol Psychiatry* (2013) **18**:909–15. doi:10.1038/mp.2012.109

47. Papanastasiou E, Stone JM, Shergill S. When the drugs don't work: the potential of glutamatergic antipsychotics in schizophrenia. *Br J Psychiatry* (2013) **202**:91–3. doi:10.1192/bjp.bp.112.110999
48. Howes OD, Montgomery AJ, Asselin MC, Murray RM, Valli I, Tabraham P, et al. Elevated striatal dopamine function linked to prodromal signs of schizophrenia. *Arch Gen Psychiatry* (2009) **66**:13–20. doi:10.1001/archgenpsychiatry.2008.514
49. Allen P, Modinos G, Hubl D, Shields G, Cachia A, Jardri R, et al. Neuroimaging auditory hallucinations in schizophrenia: from neuroanatomy to neurochemistry and beyond. *Schizophr Bull* (2012) **38**:695–703. doi:10.1093/schbul/sbs066
50. Howes O, Bose S, Turkheimer F, Valli I, Egerton A, Stahl D, et al. Progressive increase in striatal dopamine synthesis capacity as patients develop psychosis: a PET study. *Mol Psychiatry* (2011) **16**:885–6. doi:10.1038/mp.2011.20
51. Abi-Dargham A, Kegeles LS, Zea-Ponce Y, Mawlawi O, Martinez D, Mitropoulou V, et al. Striatal amphetamine-induced dopamine release in patients with schizotypal personality disorder studied with single photon emission computed tomography and [123I]iodobenzamide. *Biol Psychiatry* (2004) **55**:1001–6. doi:10.1016/j.biopsych.2004.01.018
52. Egerton A, Chaddock CA, Winton-Brown TT, Bloomfield MA, Bhattacharyya S, Allen P, et al. Presynaptic striatal dopamine dysfunction in people at ultra-high risk for psychosis: findings in a second cohort. *Biol Psychiatry* (2013) **74**:106–12. doi:10.1016/j.biopsych.2012.11.017
53. Huttunen J, Heinimaa M, Svirskis T, Nyman M, Kajander J, Forsback S, et al. Striatal dopamine synthesis in first-degree relatives of patients with schizophrenia. *Biol Psychiatry* (2008) **63**:114–7. doi:10.1016/j.biopsych.2007.04.017
54. Brunelin J, d'Amato T, van Os J, Cochet A, Suaud-Chagny MF, Saoud M. Effects of acute metabolic stress on the dopaminergic and pituitary-adrenal axis activity in patients with schizophrenia, their unaffected siblings and controls. *Schizophr Res* (2008) **100**:206–11. doi:10.1016/j.schres.2007.11.009
55. Myin-Germeys I, Marcelis M, Krabbendam L, Delespaul P, van Os J. Subtle fluctuations in psychotic phenomena as functional states of abnormal dopamine reactivity in individuals at risk. *Biol Psychiatry* (2005) **58**:105–10. doi:10.1016/j.biopsych.2005.02.012
56. Kuepper R, Ceccarini J, Lataster J, van Os J, van Kroonenburgh M, van Gerven JM, et al. Delta-9-tetrahydrocannabinol-induced dopamine release as a function of psychosis risk: 18F-fallypride positron emission tomography study. *PLoS One* (2013) **8**:e70378. doi:10.1371/journal.pone.0070378
57. Nordstrom AL, Farde L, Halldin C. Time course of D2-dopamine receptor occupancy examined by PET after single oral doses of haloperidol. *Psychopharmacology (Berl)* (1992) **106**:433–8. doi:10.1007/BF02244811
58. Leucht S, Cipriani A, Spineli L, Mavridis D, Orey D, Richter F, et al. Comparative efficacy and tolerability of 15 antipsychotic drugs in schizophrenia: a multiple-treatments meta-analysis. *Lancet* (2013) **382**:951–62. doi:10.1016/S0140-6736(13)60733-3
59. Koychev I, McMullen K, Lees J, Dadhiwala R, Grayson L, Perry C, et al. A validation of cognitive biomarkers for the early identification of cognitive enhancing agents in schizotypy: a three-center double-blind placebo-controlled study. *Eur Neuropsychopharmacol* (2012) **22**:469–81. doi:10.1016/j.euroneuro.2011.10.005
60. Mohr C, Landis T, Brugger P. Lateralized semantic priming: modulation by levodopa, semantic distance, and participants' magical beliefs. *Neuropsychiatr Dis Treat* (2006) **2**:71–84.
61. Schmechtig A, Lees J, Perkins A, Altavilla A, Craig KJ, Dawson GR, et al. The effects of ketamine and risperidone on eye movement control in healthy volunteers. *Transl Psychiatry* (2013) **3**:e334. doi:10.1038/tp.2013.109
62. Weiner I, Arad M. Using the pharmacology of latent inhibition to model domains of pathology in schizophrenia and their treatment. *Behav Brain Res* (2009) **204**:369–86. doi:10.1016/j.bbr.2009.05.004
63. Braff DL. Prepulse inhibition of the startle reflex: a window on the brain in schizophrenia. *Curr Top Behav Neurosci* (2010) **4**:349–71. doi:10.1007/7854_2010_61
64. Karson CN. Spontaneous eye-blink rates and dopaminergic systems. *Brain* (1983) **106**(Pt 3):643–53. doi:10.1093/brain/106.3.643
65. Bracha HS, Livingston RL, Clothier J, Linington BB, Karson CN. Correlation of severity of psychiatric patients' delusions with right hemispatial inattention (left-turning behavior). *Am J Psychiatry* (1993) **150**:330–2.
66. Mohr C, Landis T, Sandor PS, Fathi M, Brugger P. Nonstereotyped responding in positive schizotypy after a single dose of levodopa. *Neuropsychopharmacology* (2004) **29**:1741–51. doi:10.1038/sj.npp.1300500
67. Kopp B, Wolff M, Hruska C, Reischies FM. Brain mechanisms of visual encoding and working memory in psychometrically identified schizotypal individuals and after acute administration of haloperidol. *Psychophysiology* (2002) **39**:459–72. doi:10.1111/1469-8986.3940459
68. Kumari V, Cotter PA, Mulligan OF, Checkley SA, Gray NS, Hemsley DR, et al. Effects of D-amphetamine and haloperidol on latent inhibition in healthy male volunteers. *J Psychopharmacol* (1999) **13**:398–405. doi:10.1177/026988119901300411
69. Ridley RM, Baker HF, Frith CD, Dowdy J, Crow TJ. Stereotyped responding on a two-choice guessing task by marmosets and humans treated with amphetamine. *Psychopharmacology (Berl)* (1988) **95**:560–4. doi:10.1007/BF00172977
70. Schürhoff F, Szöke A, Chevalier F, Roy I, Méary A, Bellivier F, et al. Schizotypal dimensions: an intermediate phenotype associated with the COMT high activity allele. *Am J Med Genet B Neuropsychiatr Genet* (2007) **144**:64–8. doi:10.1002/ajmg.b.30395
71. Stefanis NC, Van Os J, Avramopoulos D, Smyrnis N, Evdokimidis I, Hantoumi I, et al. Variation in catechol-o-methyltransferase val158 met genotype associated with schizotypy but not cognition: a population study in 543 young men. *Biol Psychiatry* (2004) **56**:510–5. doi:10.1016/j.biopsych.2004.06.038
72. Brugger P, Graves RE. Right hemispatial inattention and magical ideation. *Eur Arch Psychiatry Clin Neurosci* (1997) **247**:55–7. doi:10.1007/BF02916254
73. Gray NS, Pickering AD, Snowden RJ, Hemsley DR, Gray JA. The partial reinforcement extinction effect in humans: effects of schizophrenia, schizotypy and low doses of amphetamine. *Behav Brain Res* (2002) **133**:333–42. doi:10.1016/S0166-4328(02)00019-0
74. Mohr C, Bracha HS, Brugger P. Magical ideation modulates spatial behavior. *J Neuropsychiatry Clin Neurosci* (2003) **15**:168–74. doi:10.1176/appi.neuropsych.15.2.168
75. Williams JH, Wellman NA, Geaney DP, Feldon J, Cowen PJ, Rawlins JN. Haloperidol enhances latent inhibition in visual tasks in healthy people. *Psychopharmacology (Berl)* (1997) **133**:262–8. doi:10.1007/s002130050400
76. Pycock CJ. Experimental model of hemi-parkinsonism. In: Myslobodsky MS, editor. *Hemisyndromes: Psychobiology, Neurology, Psychiatry*. New York, NY: Academic Press (1983). p. 69–90.
77. Bracha HS, Shults C, Glick SD, Kleinman JE. Spontaneous asymmetric circling behavior in hemi-parkinsonism; a human equivalent of the lesioned-circling rodent behavior. *Life Sci* (1987) **40**:1127–30. doi:10.1016/0024-3205(87)90576-5
78. Mohr C, Landis T, Bracha HS, Fathi M, Brugger P. Levodopa reverses gait asymmetries related to anhedonia and magical ideation. *Eur Arch Psychiatry Clin Neurosci* (2005) **255**:33–9. doi:10.1007/s00406-004-0531-0
79. Chermahini SA, Hommel B. The (b)link between creativity and dopamine: spontaneous eye blink rates predict and dissociate divergent and convergent thinking. *Cognition* (2010) **115**:458–65. doi:10.1016/j.cognition.2010.03.007
80. Ettinger U, Klein C. Eye movements. In: Reuter M, Montag C, editors. *Neuroeconomics*. Berlin: Springer Verlag (in press).
81. Jacobsen LK, Hommer DW, Hong WL, Castellanos FX, Frazier JA, Giedd JN, et al. Blink rate in childhood-onset schizophrenia: comparison with normal and attention-deficit hyperactivity disorder controls. *Biol Psychiatry* (1996) **40**:1222–9. doi:10.1016/S0006-3223(95)00630-3
82. Mackert A, Woyth C, Flechtner KM, Volz HP. Increased blink rate in drug-naive acute schizophrenic patients. *Biol Psychiatry* (1990) **27**:1197–202. doi:10.1016/0006-3223(90)90417-Z
83. Chen EY, Lam LC, Chen RY, Nguyen DG. Blink rate, neurocognitive impairments, and symptoms in schizophrenia. *Biol Psychiatry* (1996) **40**:597–603. doi:10.1016/0006-3223(95)00482-3
84. Blin O, Masson G, Azulay JP, Fondarai J, Serratrice G. Apomorphine-induced blinking and yawning in healthy volunteers. *Br J Clin Pharmacol* (1990) **30**:769–73. doi:10.1111/j.1365-2125.1990.tb03848.x
85. Strakowski SM, Sax KW, Setters MJ, Keck PE Jr. Enhanced response to repeated D-amphetamine challenge: evidence for behavioral sensitization in humans. *Biol Psychiatry* (1996) **40**:872–80. doi:10.1016/0006-3223(95)00497-1
86. Mohr C, Sándor PS, Landis T, Fathi M, Brugger P. Blinking and schizotypal thinking. *J Psychopharmacol* (2005) **19**:513–20. doi:10.1177/0269881105056538

87. Colzato LS, Slagter HA, van den Wildenberg WPM, Hommel B. Closing one's eyes to reality: evidence for a dopaminergic basis of Psychoticism from spontaneous eye blink rates. *Pers Indiv Differ* (2009) **46**:377–80. doi:10.1016/j.paid.2008.10.017
88. Ettinger U, Corr PJ, Mofidi A, Williams SC, Kumari V. Dopaminergic basis of the psychosis-prone personality investigated with functional magnetic resonance imaging of procedural learning. *Front Hum Neurosci* (2013) **7**:130. doi:10.3389/fnhum.2013.00130
89. Corr PJ. Psychoticism. In: Kazdin AE, editor. *Encyclopedia of Psychology*. Washington, DC: Oxford University Press/APA (2000). p. 469–70.
90. Howarth E. What does Eysenck's psychoticism scale really measure? *Br J Psychol* (1986) **77**(Pt 2):223–7. doi:10.1111/j.2044-8295.1986.tb01996.x
91. Farmer A, Redman K, Harris T, Webb R, Mahmood A, Sadler S, et al. A sib-pair study of psychoticism, life events and depression. *Pers Indiv Differ* (2003) **34**:613–23. doi:10.1016/S0191-8869(02)00036-3
92. Kraepelin E. *Dementia Praecox and Paraphrenia*. New York, NY: RE Krieger (1919).
93. Peralta V, Cuesta MJ. Motor features in psychotic disorders. I. Factor structure and clinical correlates. *Schizophr Res* (2001) **47**:107–16. doi:10.1016/S0920-9964(00)00035-9
94. Jones IH. Observations on schizophrenic stereotypies. *Compr Psychiatry* (1965) **6**:323–35. doi:10.1016/S0010-440X(65)80026-8
95. Perry W, Braff DL. A multimethod approach to assessing perseverations in schizophrenia patients. *Schizophr Res* (1998) **33**:69–77. doi:10.1016/S0920-9964(98)00061-9
96. Cadenhead KS, Perry W, Shafer K, Braff DL. Cognitive functions in schizotypal personality disorder. *Schizophr Res* (1999) **37**:123–32. doi:10.1016/S0920-9964(98)00147-9
97. Raine A, Sheard C, Reynolds GP, Lencz T. Pre-frontal structural and functional deficits associated with individual differences in schizotypal personality. *Schizophr Res* (1992) **7**:237–47. doi:10.1016/0920-9964(92)90018-Z
98. Gooding DC, Kwapil TR, Tallent KA. Wisconsin card sorting test deficits in schizotypic individuals. *Schizophr Res* (1999) **40**:201–9. doi:10.1016/S0920-9964(99)00124-3
99. Lenzenweger MF, Jensen ST, Rubin DB. Finding the "genuine" schizotype: a model and method for resolving heterogeneity in performance on laboratory measures in experimental psychopathology research. *J Abnorm Psychol* (2003) **112**:457–68. doi:10.1037/0021-843X.112.3.457
100. Brugger P. Variables that influence the generation of random sequences: an update. *Percept Mot Skills* (1997) **84**:627–61. doi:10.2466/pms.1997.84.2.627
101. Salame P, Danion JM, Peretti S, Cuervo C. The state of functioning of working memory in schizophrenia. *Schizophr Res* (1998) **30**:11–29. doi:10.1016/S0920-9964(97)00107-2
102. Avons SE, Nunn JA, Chan L, Armstrong H. Executive function assessed by memory updating and random generation in schizotypal individuals. *Psychiatry Res* (2003) **120**:145–54. doi:10.1016/S0165-1781(03)00174-4
103. Brugger P, Landis T, Regard M. A sheep goat effect in repetition avoidance – extra-sensory perception as an effect of subjective-probability. *Br J Psychol* (1990) **81**:455–68. doi:10.1111/j.2044-8295.1990.tb02372.x
104. Graham FK. Presidential Address, 1974. The more or less startling effects of weak prestimulation. *Psychophysiology* (1975) **12**:238–48. doi:10.1111/j.1469-8986.1975.tb01284.x
105. Swerdlow NR, Geyer MA, Braff DL. Neural circuit regulation of prepulse inhibition of startle in the rat: current knowledge and future challenges. *Psychopharmacology (Berl)* (2001) **156**:194–215. doi:10.1007/s002130100799
106. Braff DL. Information processing and attention dysfunctions in schizophrenia. *Schizophr Bull* (1993) **19**:233–59. doi:10.1093/schbul/19.2.233
107. Cadenhead KS, Swerdlow NR, Shafer KM, Diaz M, Braff DL. Modulation of the startle response and startle laterality in relatives of schizophrenic patients and in subjects with schizotypal personality disorder: evidence of inhibitory deficits. *Am J Psychiatry* (2000) **157**:1660–8. doi:10.1176/appi.ajp.157.10.1660
108. Varty GB, Higgins GA. Examination of drug-induced and isolation-induced disruptions of prepulse inhibition as models to screen antipsychotic drugs. *Psychopharmacology (Berl)* (1995) **122**:15–26. doi:10.1007/BF02246437
109. Swerdlow NR, Bakshi V, Waikar M, Taaid N, Geyer MA. Seroquel, clozapine and chlorpromazine restore sensorimotor gating in ketamine-treated rats. *Psychopharmacology (Berl)* (1998) **140**:75–80. doi:10.1007/s002130050741
110. Frau R, Orrù M, Puligheddu M, Gessa GL, Mereu G, Marrosu F, et al. Sleep deprivation disrupts prepulse inhibition of the startle reflex: reversal by antipsychotic drugs. *Int J Neuropsychopharmacol* (2008) **11**:947–55. doi:10.1017/S1461145708008900
111. Petrovsky N, Ettinger U, Hill A, Frenzel L, Meyhöfer I, Wagner M, et al. Sleep deprivation disrupts prepulse inhibition and induces psychosis-like symptoms in healthy humans. *J Neurosci* (2014) **34**:9134–40. doi:10.1523/JNEUROSCI.0904-14.2014
112. Li M, He E, Volf N. Time course of the attenuation effect of repeated antipsychotic treatment on prepulse inhibition disruption induced by repeated phencyclidine treatment. *Pharmacol Biochem Behav* (2011) **98**:559–69. doi:10.1016/j.pbb.2011.03.007
113. Kumari V, Soni W, Sharma T. Normalization of information processing deficits in schizophrenia with clozapine. *Am J Psychiatry* (1999) **156**:1046–51.
114. Kumari V, Sharma T. Effects of typical and atypical antipsychotics on prepulse inhibition in schizophrenia: a critical evaluation of current evidence and directions for future research. *Psychopharmacology (Berl)* (2002) **162**:97–101. doi:10.1007/s00213-002-1099-x
115. Oranje B, Van Oel CJ, Gispen-De Wied CC, Verbaten MN, Kahn RS. Effects of typical and atypical antipsychotics on the prepulse inhibition of the startle reflex in patients with schizophrenia. *J Clin Psychopharmacol* (2002) **22**:359–65. doi:10.1097/00004714-200208000-00005
116. Leumann L, Feldon J, Vollenweider FX, Ludewig K. Effects of typical and atypical antipsychotics on prepulse inhibition and latent inhibition in chronic schizophrenia. *Biol Psychiatry* (2002) **52**:729–39. doi:10.1016/S0006-3223(02)01344-6
117. Quednow BB, Wagner M, Westheide J, Beckmann K, Bliesener N, Maier W, et al. Sensorimotor gating and habituation of the startle response in schizophrenic patients randomly treated with amisulpride or olanzapine. *Biol Psychiatry* (2006) **59**:536–45. doi:10.1016/j.biopsych.2005.07.012
118. Swerdlow NR, Light GA, Cadenhead KS, Sprock J, Hsieh MH, Braff DL. Startle gating deficits in a large cohort of patients with schizophrenia: relationship to medications, symptoms, neurocognition, and level of function. *Arch Gen Psychiatry* (2006) **63**:1325–35. doi:10.1001/archpsyc.63.12.1325
119. Swerdlow NR, Light GA, Sprock J, Calkins ME, Green MF, Greenwood TA, et al. Deficient prepulse inhibition in schizophrenia detected by the multi-site COGS. *Schizophr Res* (2014) **152**:503–12. doi:10.1016/j.schres.2013.12.004
120. Takahashi H, Iwase M, Canuet L, Yasuda Y, Ohi K, Fukumoto M, et al. Relationship between prepulse inhibition of acoustic startle response and schizotypy in healthy Japanese subjects. *Psychophysiology* (2010) **47**:831–7. doi:10.1111/j.1469-8986.2010.01000.x
121. Swerdlow NR, Filion D, Geyer MA, Braff DL. "Normal" personality correlates of sensorimotor, cognitive, and visuospatial gating. *Biol Psychiatry* (1995) **37**:286–99. doi:10.1016/0006-3223(94)00138-S
122. Kumari V, Antonova E, Geyer MA. Prepulse inhibition and "psychosis-proneness" in healthy individuals: an fMRI study. *Eur Psychiatry* (2008) **23**:274–80. doi:10.1016/j.eurpsy.2007.11.006
123. Kumari V, Gray JA, Geyer MA, ffytche D, Soni W, Mitterschiffthaler MT, et al. Neural correlates of tactile prepulse inhibition: a functional MRI study in normal and schizophrenic subjects. *Psychiatry Res* (2003) **122**:99–113. doi:10.1016/S0925-4927(02)00123-3
124. Braff DL, Geyer MA, Swerdlow NR. Human studies of prepulse inhibition of startle: normal subjects, patient groups, and pharmacological studies. *Psychopharmacology (Berl)* (2001) **156**:234–58. doi:10.1007/s002130100810
125. Kumari V, Ettinger U. Prepulse inhibition deficits in schizophrenia: static or amenable to treatment? In: Lang MV, editor. *Progress in Schizophrenia Research*. New York, NY: Nova Publishers (2004). p. 95–117.
126. Völter C, Riedel M, Wöstmann N, Aichert DS, Lobo S, Costa A, et al. Sensorimotor gating and D2 receptor signalling: evidence from a molecular genetic approach. *Int J Neuropsychopharmacol* (2012) **15**:1427–40. doi:10.1017/S1461145711001787
127. Weiner I. The "two-headed" latent inhibition model of schizophrenia: modeling positive and negative symptoms and their treatment. *Psychopharmacology (Berl)* (2003) **169**:257–97. doi:10.1007/s00213-002-1313-x
128. Lubow RE, Gewirtz JC. Latent inhibition in humans: data, theory, and implications for schizophrenia. *Psychol Bull* (1995) **117**:87–103. doi:10.1037/0033-2909.117.1.87
129. Kumari V, Ettinger U. Latent inhibition in schizophrenia and schizotypy: a review of the empirical literature. In: Lubow RE, editor. *Latent Inhibition*. Cambridge: Cambridge University Press (2010). p. 419–47.

130. Evans LH, Gray NS, Snowden RJ. A new continuous within-participants latent inhibition task: examining associations with schizotypy dimensions, smoking status and gender. *Biol Psychol* (2007) **74**:365–73. doi:10.1016/j.biopsycho.2006.09.007
131. Servan-Schreiber D, Printz H, Cohen JD. A network model of catecholamine effects: gain, signal-to-noise ratio, and behavior. *Science* (1990) **249**:892–5. doi:10.1126/science.2392679
132. Spitzer M. A cognitive neuroscience view of schizophrenic thought disorder. *Schizophr Bull* (1997) **23**:29–50. doi:10.1093/schbul/23.1.29
133. Kischka U, Kammer T, Maier S, Weisbrod M, Thimm M, Spitzer M. Dopaminergic modulation of semantic network activation. *Neuropsychologia* (1996) **34**:1107–13. doi:10.1016/0028-3932(96)00024-3
134. Weisbrod M, Maier S, Harig S, Himmelsbach U, Spitzer M. Lateralised semantic and indirect semantic priming effects in people with schizophrenia. *Br J Psychiatry* (1998) **172**:142–6. doi:10.1192/bjp.172.2.142
135. Pizzagalli D, Lehmann D, Brugger P. Lateralized direct and indirect semantic priming effects in subjects with paranormal experiences and beliefs. *Psychopathology* (2001) **34**:75–80. doi:10.1159/000049284
136. Gianotti LR, Mohr C, Pizzagalli D, Lehmann D, Brugger P. Associative processing and paranormal belief. *Psychiatry Clin Neurosci* (2001) **55**:595–603. doi:10.1046/j.1440-1819.2001.00911.x
137. Mohr C, Graves RE, Gianotti LR, Pizzagalli D, Brugger P. Loose but normal: a semantic association study. *J Psycholinguist Res* (2001) **30**:475–83. doi:10.1023/A:1010461429079
138. Levine J, Martine T, Feraro R, Kimhi R, Bracha HS. Medicated chronic schizophrenic patients do not demonstrate left turning asymmetry. *Neuropsychobiology* (1997) **36**:22–4. doi:10.1159/000119355
139. Maruff P, Hay D, Malone V, Currie J. Asymmetries in the covert orienting of visual spatial attention in schizophrenia. *Neuropsychologia* (1995) **33**:1205–23. doi:10.1016/0028-3932(95)00037-4
140. Purdon SE, Flor-Henry P. Asymmetrical olfactory acuity and neuroleptic treatment in schizophrenia. *Schizophr Res* (2000) **44**:221–32. doi:10.1016/S0920-9964(99)00212-1
141. Purdon SE, Woodward ND, Flor-Henry P. Asymmetrical hand force persistence and neuroleptic treatment in schizophrenia. *J Int Neuropsychol Soc* (2001) **7**:606–14. doi:10.1017/S1355617701755087
142. Schröder J, Bubeck B, Silvestri S, Demisch S, Sauer H. Gender differences in D2 dopamine receptor binding in drug-naive patients with schizophrenia: an [123I]iodobenzamide single photon emission computed tomography study. *Psychiatry Res* (1997) **75**:115–23. doi:10.1016/S0925-4927(97)00046-2
143. Tomer R, Flor-Henry P. Neuroleptics reverse attention asymmetries in schizophrenic patients. *Biol Psychiatry* (1989) **25**:852–60. doi:10.1016/0006-3223(89)90264-3
144. Brugger P, Gamma A, Muri R, Schäfer M, Taylor KI. Functional hemispheric asymmetry and belief in ESP: towards a "neuropsychology of belief". *Percept Mot Skills* (1993) **77**:1299–308. doi:10.2466/pms.1993.77.3f.1299
145. Mohr C, Krummenacher P, Landis T, Sandor PS, Fathi M, Brugger P. Psychometric schizotypy modulates levodopa effects on lateralized lexical decision performance. *J Psychiatr Res* (2005) **39**:241–50. doi:10.1016/j.jpsychires.2004.08.006
146. Krummenacher P, Mohr C, Haker H, Brugger P. Dopamine, paranormal belief, and the detection of meaningful stimuli. *J Cogn Neurosci* (2010) **22**:1670–81. doi:10.1162/jocn.2009.21313
147. Hutton SB, Ettinger U. The antisaccade task as a research tool in psychopathology: a critical review. *Psychophysiology* (2006) **43**:302–13. doi:10.1111/j.1469-8986.2006.00403.x
148. Miyake A, Friedman NP, Emerson MJ, Witzki AH, Howerter A, Wager TD. The unity and diversity of executive functions and their contributions to complex "Frontal Lobe" tasks: a latent variable analysis. *Cogn Psychol* (2000) **41**:49–100. doi:10.1006/cogp.1999.0734
149. Schmechtig A, Lees J, Grayson L, Craig KJ, Dadhiwala R, Dawson GR, et al. Effects of risperidone, amisulpride and nicotine on eye movement control and their modulation by schizotypy. *Psychopharmacology (Berl)* (2013) **227**:331–45. doi:10.1007/s00213-013-2973-4
150. Barrett SL, Bell R, Watson D, King DJ. Effects of amisulpride, risperidone and chlorpromazine on auditory and visual latent inhibition, prepulse inhibition, executive function and eye movements in healthy volunteers. *J Psychopharmacol* (2004) **18**:156–72. doi:10.1177/0269881104042614
151. Burke JG, Reveley MA. Improved antisaccade performance with risperidone in schizophrenia. *J Neurol Neurosurg Psychiatry* (2002) **72**:449–54. doi:10.1136/jnnp.72.4.449
152. Harris MS, Reilly JL, Keshavan MS, Sweeney JA. Longitudinal studies of antisaccades in antipsychotic-naive first-episode schizophrenia. *Psychol Med* (2006) **36**:485–94. doi:10.1017/S0033291705006756
153. Kapur S. Psychosis as a state of aberrant salience: a framework linking biology, phenomenology, and pharmacology in schizophrenia. *Am J Psychiatry* (2003) **160**:13–23. doi:10.1176/appi.ajp.160.1.13
154. Giakoumaki SG. Cognitive and prepulse inhibition deficits in psychometrically high schizotypal subjects in the general population: relevance to schizophrenia research. *J Int Neuropsychol Soc* (2012) **18**:643–56. doi:10.1017/S135561771200029X
155. Claridge G, Hewitt J. A biometrical study of schizotypy in a normal population. *Pers Indiv Differ* (1987) **8**:303–12. doi:10.1016/0191-8869(87)90030-4
156. Linney YM, Murray RM, Peters ER, MacDonald AM, Rijsdijk F, Sham PC. A quantitative genetic analysis of schizotypal personality traits. *Psychol Med* (2003) **33**:803–16. doi:10.1017/S0033291703007906
157. Macare C, Bates TC, Heath AC, Martin NG, Ettinger U. Substantial genetic overlap between schizotypy and neuroticism: a twin study. *Behav Genet* (2012) **42**:732–42. doi:10.1007/s10519-012-9558-6
158. MacDonald AW, Pogue-Geile MF, Debski TT, Manuck S. Genetic and environmental influences on schizotypy: a community-based twin study. *Schizophr Bull* (2001) **27**:47–58. doi:10.1093/oxfordjournals.schbul.a006859
159. Lachman HM, Papolos DF, Saito T, Yu YM, Szumlanski CL, Weinshilboum RM. Human catechol-O-methyltransferase pharmacogenetics: description of a functional polymorphism and its potential application to neuropsychiatric disorders. *Pharmacogenetics* (1996) **6**:243–50. doi:10.1097/00008571-199606000-00007
160. Weinshilboum RM, Otterness DM, Szumlanski CL. Methylation pharmacogenetics: catechol O-methyltransferase, thiopurine methyltransferase, and histamine N-methyltransferase. *Annu Rev Pharmacol Toxicol* (1999) **39**:19–52. doi:10.1146/annurev.pharmtox.39.1.19
161. Montag C, Jurkiewicz M, Reuter M. The role of the catechol-O-methyltransferase (COMT) gene in personality and related psychopathological disorders. *CNS Neurol Disord Drug Targets* (2012) **11**:236–50. doi:10.2174/187152712800672382
162. Egan MF, Goldberg TE, Kolachana BS, Callicott JH, Mazzanti CM, Straub RE, et al. Effect of COMT Val108/158 Met genotype on frontal lobe function and risk for schizophrenia. *Proc Natl Acad Sci U S A* (2001) **98**:6917–22. doi:10.1073/pnas.111134598
163. Munafo MR, Bowes L, Clark TG, Flint J. Lack of association of the COMT (Val158/108 Met) gene and schizophrenia: a meta-analysis of case-control studies. *Mol Psychiatry* (2005) **10**:765–70. doi:10.1038/sj.mp.4001664
164. Okochi T, Ikeda M, Kishi T, Kawashima K, Kinoshita Y, Kitajima T, et al. Meta-analysis of association between genetic variants in COMT and schizophrenia: an update. *Schizophr Res* (2009) **110**:140–8. doi:10.1016/j.schres.2009.02.019
165. Avramopoulos D, Stefanis NC, Hantoumi I, Smyrnis N, Evdokimidis I, Stefanis CN. Higher scores of self reported schizotypy in healthy young males carrying the COMT high activity allele. *Mol Psychiatry* (2002) **7**:706–11. doi:10.1038/sj.mp.4001070
166. Smyrnis N, Avramopoulos D, Evdokimidis I, Stefanis CN, Tsekou H, Stefanis NC. Effect of schizotypy on cognitive performance and its tuning by COMT val158 met genotype variations in a large population of young men. *Biol Psychiatry* (2007) **61**:845–53. doi:10.1016/j.biopsych.2006.07.019
167. Grant P, Kuepper Y, Mueller EA, Wielpuetz C, Mason O, Hennig J. Dopaminergic foundations of schizotypy as measured by the German version of the Oxford-Liverpool Inventory of Feelings and Experiences (O-LIFE)-a suitable endophenotype of schizophrenia. *Front Hum Neurosci* (2013) **7**:1. doi:10.3389/fnhum.2013.00001
168. Docherty AR, Sponheim SR. Anhedonia as a phenotype for the Val158Met COMT polymorphism in relatives of patients with schizophrenia. *J Abnorm Psychol* (2008) **117**:788–98. doi:10.1037/a0013745
169. Sheldrick AJ, Krug A, Markov V, Leube D, Michel TM, Zerres K, et al. Effect of COMT val158met genotype on cognition and personality. *Eur Psychiatry* (2008) **23**:385–9. doi:10.1016/j.eurpsy.2008.05.002
170. Murphy KC, Jones LA, Owen MJ. High rates of schizophrenia in adults with velo-cardio-facial syndrome. *Arch Gen Psychiatry* (1999) **56**:940–5. doi:10.1001/archpsyc.56.10.940

171. Savitz J, van der Merwe L, Newman TK, Stein DJ, Ramesar R. Catechol-o-methyltransferase genotype and childhood trauma may interact to impact schizotypal personality traits. *Behav Genet* (2010) **40**:415–23. doi:10.1007/s10519-009-9323-7
172. Ma X, Sun J, Yao J, Wang Q, Hu X, Deng W, et al. A quantitative association study between schizotypal traits and COMT, PRODH and BDNF genes in a healthy Chinese population. *Psychiatry Res* (2007) **153**:7–15. doi:10.1016/j.psychres.2007.02.003
173. Ettinger U, Joober R, DeGuzman R, O'Driscoll GA. Schizotypy, attention deficit hyperactivity disorder, and dopamine genes. *Psychiatry Clin Neurosci* (2006) **60**:764–7. doi:10.1111/j.1440-1819.2006.01594.x
174. Schofield K, Mohr C. Schizotypy and hemispheric asymmetry: results from two Chapman scales, the O-LIFE questionnaire, and two laterality measures. *Laterality* (2014) **19**:178–200. doi:10.1080/1357650X.2013.789883
175. Mohr C, Hubener F, Laska M. Deviant olfactory experiences, magical ideation, and olfactory sensitivity: a study with healthy German and Japanese subjects. *Psychiatry Res* (2002) **111**:21–33. doi:10.1016/S0165-1781(02)00132-4
176. Taurisano P, Romano R, Mancini M, Giorgio AD, Antonucci LA, Fazio L, et al. Prefronto-striatal physiology is associated with schizotypy and is modulated by a functional variant of DRD2. *Front Behav Neurosci* (2014) **8**:235. doi:10.3389/fnbeh.2014.00235
177. Meyer-Lindenberg A, Weinberger DR. Intermediate phenotypes and genetic mechanisms of psychiatric disorders. *Nat Rev Neurosci* (2006) **7**:818–27. doi:10.1038/nrn1993
178. Gray NS, Pickering AD, Gray JA. Psychoticism and dopamine D2 binding in the basal ganlia using single photon emission tomography. *Pers Indiv Differ* (1994) **17**:431–4. doi:10.1016/0191-8869(94)90289-5
179. Farde L, Gustavsson JP, Jonsson E. D2 dopamine receptors and personality traits. *Nature* (1997) **385**:590. doi:10.1038/385590a0
180. Breier A, Kestler L, Adler C, Elman I, Wiesenfeld N, Malhotra A, et al. Dopamine D2 receptor density and personal detachment in healthy subjects. *Am J Psychiatry* (1998) **155**:1440–2.
181. Chen KC, Lee IH, Yeh TL, Chiu NT, Chen PS, Yang YK, et al. Schizotypy trait and striatal dopamine receptors in healthy volunteers. *Psychiatry Res* (2012) **201**:218–21. doi:10.1016/j.pscychresns.2011.07.003
182. Howes OD, Shotbolt P, Bloomfield M, Daalman K, Demjaha A, Diederen KM, et al. Dopaminergic function in the psychosis spectrum: an [18F]-DOPA imaging study in healthy individuals with auditory hallucinations. *Schizophr Bull* (2013) **39**:807–14. doi:10.1093/schbul/sbr195
183. Breier A, Su TP, Saunders R, Carson RE, Kolachana BS, Bartolomeis A, et al. Schizophrenia is associated with elevated amphetamine-induced synaptic dopamine concentrations: evidence from a novel positron emission tomography method. *Proc Natl Acad Sci U S A* (1997) **94**:2569–74. doi:10.1073/pnas.94.6.2569
184. Woodward ND, Cowan RL, Park S, Ansari MS, Baldwin RM, Li R, et al. Correlation of individual differences in schizotypal personality traits with amphetamine-induced dopamine release in striatal and extrastriatal brain regions. *Am J Psychiatry* (2011) **168**:418–26. doi:10.1176/appi.ajp.2010.10020165
185. van OJ, Kenis G, Rutten BP. The environment and schizophrenia. *Nature* (2010) **468**:203–12. doi:10.1038/nature09563
186. Soliman A, O'Driscoll GA, Pruessner J, Holahan AL, Boileau I, Gagnon D, et al. Stress-induced dopamine release in humans at risk of psychosis: a [11C]raclopride PET study. *Neuropsychopharmacology* (2008) **33**:2033–41. doi:10.1038/sj.npp.1301597
187. Gruzelier J. A Janusian perspective on the nature, development and structure of schizophrenia and schizotypy. *Schizophr Res* (2002) **54**:95–103. doi:10.1016/S0920-9964(01)00356-5
188. Deyoung CG. The neuromodulator of exploration: a unifying theory of the role of dopamine in personality. *Front Hum Neurosci* (2013) **7**:762. doi:10.3389/fnhum.2013.00762
189. Conrad K. *Die Beginnende Schizophrenie. Versuch Einer Gestaltanalyse Des Wahns.* Stuttgart: Thieme (1958).
190. Brugger P, Regard M, Landis T, Cook N, Krebs D, Niederberger J. 'Meaningful' patterns in visual noise: effects of lateral stimulation and the observer's belief in ESP. *Psychopathology* (1993) **26**:261–5. doi:10.1159/000284831
191. van Elk M. Paranormal and religious believers are more prone to illusory face perception than skeptics and non-believers. *Appl Cogn Psychol* (2013) **27**:150–5. doi:10.1016/j.concog.2013.07.004
192. Bressan P. The connection between random sequences, everyday coincidences, and belief in the paranormal. *Appl Cogn Psychol* (2002) **16**:17–34. doi:10.1002/acp.754
193. Brugger P. From haunted brain to haunted science: a cognitive neuroscience view of paranormal and pseudoscientific thought. In: Houran J, Lange R, editors. *Hauntings and Poltergeists: Multidisciplinary Perspectives.* McFarland (2001). p. 195–213.
194. Shaner A. Delusions, superstitious conditioning and chaotic dopamine neurodynamics. *Med Hypotheses* (1999) **52**:119–23. doi:10.1054/mehy.1997.0656
195. McCrae RR, John OP. An introduction to the five-factor model and its applications. *J Pers* (1992) **60**:175–215. doi:10.1111/j.1467-6494.1992.tb00970.x
196. Winton-Brown TT, Fusar-Poli P, Ungless MA, Howes OD. Dopaminergic basis of salience dysregulation in psychosis. *Trends Neurosci* (2014) **37**:85–94. doi:10.1016/j.tins.2013.11.003
197. Carpenter WT, Koenig JI. The evolution of drug development in schizophrenia: past issues and future opportunities. *Neuropsychopharmacology* (2008) **33**:2061–79. doi:10.1038/sj.npp.1301639
198. Skosnik PD, Spatz-Glenn L, Park S. Cannabis use is associated with schizotypy and attentional disinhibition. *Schizophr Res* (2001) **48**:83–92. doi:10.1016/S0920-9964(00)00132-8
199. Larrison AL, Briand KA, Sereno AB. Nicotine, caffeine, alcohol and schizotypy. *Pers Indiv Differ* (1999) **27**:101–8. doi:10.1016/S0191-8869(98)00217-7
200. Williams JH, Wellman NA, Rawlins JN. Tobacco smoking correlates with schizotypal and borderline personality traits. *Pers Indiv Differ* (1996) **20**:267–70. doi:10.1016/0191-8869(95)00179-4
201. Ripke S, O'Dushlaine C, Chambert K, Moran JL, Kähler AK, Akterin S, et al. Genome-wide association analysis identifies 13 new risk loci for schizophrenia. *Nat Genet* (2013) **45**:1150–9. doi:10.1038/ng.2742

11

Stable schizophrenia patients learn equally well as age-matched controls and better than elderly controls in two sensorimotor rotary pursuit tasks

Livia J. De Picker[1,2]*, Claudia Cornelis[1,2], Wouter Hulstijn[1,3], Glenn Dumont[1,2], Erik Fransen[4], Maarten Timmers[5], Luc Janssens[5], Manuel Morrens[1] and Bernard G. C. Sabbe[1,2]

[1] *Collaborative Antwerp Psychiatric Research Initiative (CAPRI), University of Antwerp, Antwerp, Belgium*
[2] *University Psychiatric Hospital St. Norbertushuis, Duffel, Belgium*
[3] *Donders Institute for Brain, Cognition and Behaviour, Radboud University Nijmegen, Nijmegen, The Netherlands*
[4] *StatUA, University of Antwerp, Antwerp, Belgium*
[5] *Janssen Research and Development, Janssen Pharmaceutica N.V., Beerse, Belgium*

Edited by:
Sebastian Walther, University Hospital of Psychiatry, Switzerland

Reviewed by:
Dusan Hirjak, University of Heidelberg, Germany
Valentin Johannes Benzing, University Hospital of Psychiatry, Switzerland

****Correspondence:***
Livia J. De Picker, Collaborative Antwerp Psychiatric Research Institute (CAPRI), University of Antwerp, Campus Drie Eiken R.321, Universiteitsplein 1, 2610 Wilrijk, Belgium
e-mail: livia.depicker@uantwerp.be

Objective: To compare sensorimotor performance and learning in stable schizophrenia patients, healthy age- and sex-matched controls and elderly controls on two variations of the rotary pursuit: circle pursuit (true motor learning) and figure pursuit (motor and sequence learning).

Method: In the circle pursuit, a target circle, rotating with increasing speed along a predictable circular path on the computer screen, must be followed by a cursor controlled by a pen on a writing tablet. In the eight-trial figure pursuit, subjects learn to draw a complex figure by pursuing the target circle that moves along an invisible trajectory between and around several goals. Tasks were administered thrice (day 1, day 2, day 7) to 30 patients with stable schizophrenia (S), 30 healthy age- and sex-matched controls (C), and 30 elderly participants (>65 years; E) and recorded with a digitizing tablet and pressure-sensitive pen. The outcome measure accuracy (% of time that cursor is within the target) was used to assess performance.

Results: We observed significant group differences in accuracy, both in circle and figure pursuit tasks ($E < S < C$, $p < 0.01$). Strong learning effects were found in each group. Learning curves were similar in circle pursuit but differed between groups in figure pursuit. When corrected for group differences in starting level, the learning gains over the three sessions of schizophrenia patients and age-matched controls were equal and both were larger than those of the elderly controls.

Conclusion: Despite the reduced sensorimotor performance that was found in the schizophrenia patients, their sensorimotor learning seems to be preserved. The relevance of this finding for the evaluation of procedural learning in schizophrenia is discussed. The better performance and learning rate of the patients compared to the elderly controls was unexpected and deserves further study.

Keywords: rotor pursuit, schizophrenia, motor skills, learning curve, aging and cognitive function, procedural learning, motor learning

INTRODUCTION

The functional outcome of schizophrenia patients is highly impacted by the severity of their cognitive symptoms and their capacity to learn new skills (1). Two variants of learning are generally distinguished: declarative and procedural learning, the latter referring to skill, habit, or knowledge acquisition that occurs in an implicit manner, i.e., automatically and outside of conscious awareness (2). Sensorimotor learning, the incremental spatial and temporal accuracy of movements with repetition, represents a form of procedural learning involving different corticostriatal circuits from those in other forms, such as probabilistic classification (3).

Designed as a tool to evaluate motor learning, the rotor pursuit task has been first used in 1947 (4). It measures the ability to keep a stylus on a rotating target, requiring motor control over the proximal upper limb (including shoulder–elbow control and postural control), as well as the ability to continuously process and adapt to sensory (visual and proprioceptive) feedback. Rotor pursuit

---

Abbreviations: CPR, circle pursuit rotor; E group, elderly participants; FPR, figure pursuit rotor; GLM, general linear model; LCT, line-copying task; MT, movement time; NLV, *Nederlandse Leestest voor Volwassenen;* PR, pursuit rotor/rotary pursuit; RPM, rotations per minute; S group, schizophrenia patients; WCST, Wisconsin card sorting test; Y group, young controls.

performance is known to be altered in several pathologies involving the basal ganglia; impaired performance has been demonstrated in Huntington's and Parkinson's disease and enhanced performance in the early trials of the task is seen in patients with obsessive–compulsive disorder (5). The key substrate of the basal ganglia's involvement in sensorimotor performance and learning is represented by their extensive reciprocal connections to motor and premotor areas of the frontal lobe, implicated in planning and execution of movements (6). Besides the role of the striatal–cortical circuitry, which is considered particularly important in learning operated through the implicit mode, tracts involving the (pre)motor cortex, the supplementary motor area, and the cerebellum are also implicated in the generation of precise forces and spatial knowledge required for learning new motor skills (7).

In contrast to declarative tasks, in which schizophrenia patients have consistently shown impaired performance and learning compared to healthy controls, procedural learning has been less well studied. Both corticofrontal and striatal involvement are presumed in the pathophysiology of schizophrenia, and abnormal dopamine regulation within the basal ganglia is thought to contribute to the psychotic symptoms of the disease. However, studies examining patients with schizophrenia on the pursuit rotor motor-skill learning task have so far produced mixed results when comparing both general performance and learning rate of patients to healthy controls (see **Table 1**) (8–15). Reasons for the conflicting results may reflect methodological differences including in instrumentation, in equating for initial performance, in number of trials administered, or influences of intrinsic moderating variables, such as

Table 1 | Summary of sensorimotor skill studies with Pursuit rotor task in schizophrenia patients.

Author (year)	Huston and Shakow (1949)[8]	Goldberg et al. (1993)[9]	Granholm et al. (1993)[10]	Clare et al. (1993)[11]	Schwartz et al. (1996)[12]	Kern et al. (1997)[13]	Weickert et al. (2002)[14]	Gomar et al. (2011)[15]
Version	Contact	Contact	Photoelectric	Not specified	Contact	Photoelectric	Not specified	Digital
Design	2 blocks × 5 trials × 10 s	3 blocks × 5 trials × 20 s	6 blocks × 4 trials × 20 s	5 blocks × 6 trials × 20 s	6 blocks × 4 trials × 20 s	6 blocks × 4 trials × 20 s	6 blocks	6 blocks × 4 trials × 20 s
Days	d1	d1	d1	d1–d8	d1	d1	d1	d1–d8
N	SZ 122, C 60	24 discordant and 7 normal MZ twin pairs	SZ 11, C 11	SZ 11, C 12	SZ 40, C 40 (each 20 elderly, 20 young)	SZ 18, C 15	SZ 35, C 35	SZ 43, C 22
SZ age; mean (range)		31 (17–44)	38.4	42.7 (21–70)	YSZ 33.1 (26–40), ESZ 63.2 (55–70)	36.7	Not specified	46.9 (24–64)
SZ sex M:F		14:10	11:0	7:5	38:2	18:0	Not specified	34:9
RPM	60	30 and 60	45	30	ESZ 40.50, EC 48.75, YSZ 47.25, YC 56.25	SZ 37.2, C 62.7	Not specified	Not specified
Trial 1 matched?	No	No	No	No	Yes	Yes	Not specified	Yes
IQ matched?	No	No	No	No	No	No	Yes (subsample *n* = 14)	Yes (subsample *n* = 22)
Absolute performance difference	SZ < C	SZ = C	SZ = C	SZ < C	SZ < C	SZ = C	SZ < C; IQ matched SZ = C	SZ < C; IQ matched SZ = C
Learning rate difference	Not specified	Not specified	SZ = C	SZ = C	SZ < C	SZ = C	SZ = C	SZ = C

SZ, schizophrenia patients; C, controls; ESZ, elderly schizophrenia patients; EC, elderly controls; YSZ, young schizophrenia patients; YC, young controls; RPM, rotations per minute.

general intellectual capacity and declarative memory, as well as the effect of psychotropic drugs. It is also debated whether any impaired performance on the rotor pursuit may be related more to underlying psychomotor deficits or to general cognitive decline, both features of schizophrenia (16).

Considering the outcomes of previous studies using the rotor pursuit task in schizophrenia, we hypothesized that true sensorimotor learning would be preserved in schizophrenia patients (10, 11, 13–15). However, many tasks that measure procedural learning also include a cognitive aspect, e.g., in the form of an implicit sequence to be learned. It has been postulated that motor and cognitive aspects of procedural tasks are governed by different brain processes; motor or skill learning aspects have been associated with a corticostriatal motor circuit involving the putamen, whereas aspects of cognitive or habit learning are suggested to operate the dorsolateral prefrontal cortex circuit involving the caudate (14). Previous studies that have tried to compare performance on these two aspects have been using combinations of methodologically distinct tasks (e.g., rotor pursuit and a probabilistic classification task, such as the weather prediction task), complicating the direct comparison of their relative outcomes (14).

In this study, we aim to assess the cognitive and motor aspects involved in sensorimotor skill learning in the same pursuit task set up, by using two separate task variations, one of which incorporates also a sequence component.

Furthermore, a longitudinal set up with repeated sessions over several days offers the added value of distinguishing between early (encoding and acquisition) and late (retention/consolidation) phases of sensorimotor learning, as distinguished in literature (7).

An age-related decline in sensorimotor performance and learning on the rotor pursuit has been described (17). Besides the schizophrenia patients and age-matched controls, we, therefore, also included a group of elderly healthy participants to investigate whether the sensorimotor deficits in schizophrenia patients are comparable to those associated with advanced age. We expected both schizophrenia subjects and elderly participants to perform poorer than young control subjects in the sensorimotor rotary pursuit tasks.

MATERIALS AND METHODS

STUDY DESIGN

For all subjects enrolled, the study consisted of an eligibility screening examination (up to 21 days prior) and three cognitive assessment days. The screening examination included baseline assessments of executive functioning (Wisconsin Card Sorting Test; WCST), premorbid IQ (Dutch Adult Reading Test/*Nederlandse Leestest voor Volwassenen*; NLV), and psychomotor speed (measured with a line-copying task on a digitizing tablet; LCT).

Cognitive assessments were made in two subsequent sessions (days 1 and 2), which were separated by overnight sleep. An additional third session was performed on day 7. The pursuit task was part of a cognitive test battery of approximately 90 min that was administered to all subjects in the same way and will be reported elsewhere. The time of day for completion of the cognitive test batteries was comparable on all test days for each subject, but not identical for all subjects.

The study was conducted in accordance with the ethical principles that have their origin in the Declaration of Helsinki and that are consistent with Good Clinical Practices, applicable regulatory requirements, and in compliance with the study protocol. The study protocol was reviewed and approved by the Institutional Ethics Committee.

PARTICIPANTS

After giving written informed consent, subjects were screened to ascertain their eligibility for the study according to the in- and exclusion criteria specific for the population enrolled. The patient sample consisted of 30 outpatients aged 18–55 with a known history of schizophrenia or schizo-affective disorder (based on DSM-IV criteria) of at least 12 months, as confirmed by the referring psychiatrist. Exclusion criteria were current use of drugs with anticholinergic properties (including tricyclic antidepressants) and benzodiazepines, or comorbid DSM-IV diagnosis of substance dependence within 3 months prior to screening evaluation (except for caffeine and nicotine dependence); patients with a positive drug screen at screening could be included provided they did not meet DSM-IV diagnosis of substance dependence and consented to abstain from illegal drugs at any time during the study. An alcohol breath test and urine drug screening were performed at each of the cognitive assay days. All patients were stably treated with antipsychotic medication for at least 6 weeks, with no more than two different antipsychotic drugs used concurrently. Patients were judged to be in stable clinical condition at the time of testing through subject interview and medical history review by a trained clinician. Symptom severity of patients was rated at screening by a trained psychology assistant using the scale for the assessment of negative symptoms and positive symptoms (SANS-SAPS) (18, 19).

Thirty age- and gender-matched control participants, as well as 30 gender-matched elderly participants (>65 years of age) were recruited from the local community. They met the same exclusion criteria as the patients. They were also interviewed by a clinician to verify that they had no personal history of psychiatric disorders nor first-degree relatives with psychotic disorders and that they were not using any psychotropic medication.

PURSUIT TASK SET UP

Based on the classical rotary pursuit task (20), our pursuit rotor (PR) continuous sensorimotor tasks required subjects to follow the movements of a target circle (12 mm in diameter) on the computer screen with a cursor they could control by manipulating a pressure-sensitive pen on a digitizing writing tablet (WACOM1218RE), recording at 200 Hz frequency and 0.2 mm spatial accuracy.

In the circle pursuit (CPR) task, the target circle rotates along a predictable circular path with a radius of 7.5 cm (see **Figure 1**). This task consisted of two trials of 30 s duration with six rotations each. The speed of the target was gradually increased from 10 s per 360° rotation (6 RPM) to 3 s per full rotation (20 RPM).

The CPR was directly followed by the figure pursuit (FPR) task in which subjects had to follow a trajectory between and around several on-screen goals (see **Figure 2**). This task can be perceived as learning to draw a complex figure in a so-called "pursuit" condition in which a person is asked to keep the pen cursor on a target

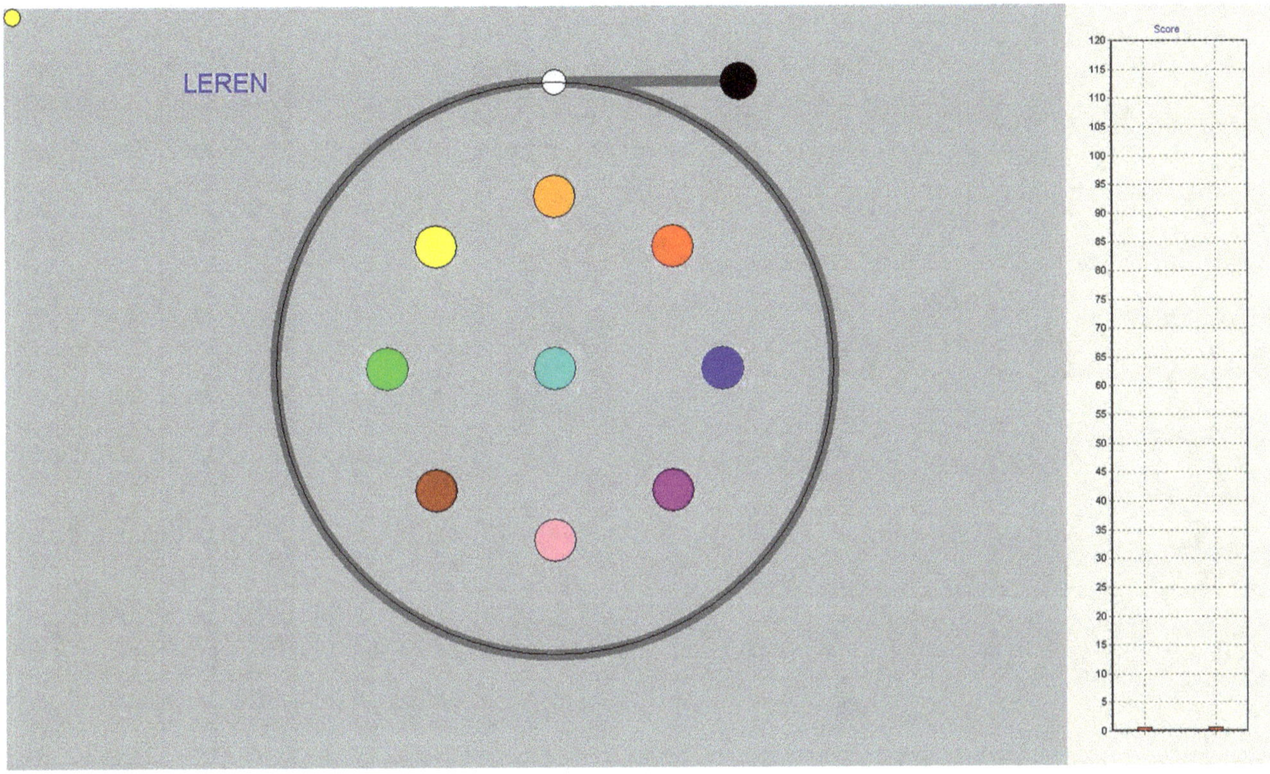

FIGURE 1 | Circle pursuit task on-screen, gray line indicating pursuit trajectory, not seen by participants. On the right-hand side, performance bars appeared as feedback after each trial.

circle that moves along the (invisible) trajectory that has to be learned. The start and end positions of the sequence are marked by white and black circles, signaling with a high and low beep, respectively, when the cursor reaches them. This task consisted of eight identical trials of 10 s duration.

Both during circle and figure pursuit, subjects were able to follow their level of performance throughout the task, with vertical score bars appearing on the right side of the screen after each trial, indicating their relative level of target contact (see **Figures 1** and **2**).

The dependent variable in both task variations was accuracy (% of time that the cursor is within the target circle, higher numbers indicating better performance). The total time of the PR tasks was approximately 3 min.

STATISTICAL ANALYSIS

We performed all statistical analyses in IBM SPSS Statistics for Windows, Version 22.0 (Armonk, NY, USA). Demographic features and baseline assessment results were analyzed using independent samples T-tests to evaluate significant group differences. There were some missing data for the Y group on the LCT ($n = 3$) and for the E group on the WCST ($n = 2$) and the LNS ($n = 1$). WCST outcome was defined as the number of categories completed. The movement time (MT) on the LCT was chosen as the relevant outcome measure for psychomotor speed.

The PR performance was quantified by the variable accuracy, and measured in three groups (schizophrenia patients = S, young controls = C, elderly participants = E). We tested each individual repeatedly in three sessions (day 1, day 2, day 7). Within each session, several identical trials were performed (two trials in CPR, eight trials in FPR). There were no missing data on the PR tasks. To provide a measure for the amount of learning over sessions, we computed two learning measures for each session: the mean and the cumulative learning gain, the latter correcting for the participant's starting level (performance on the first trial in the first session). In the figure pursuit, the cumulative learning gain was calculated as (T1 + T2 + T3 + T4 + T5 + T6 + T7 + T8)/8-S1T1. In circle pursuit, this was (T1 + T2)/2-S1T1.

We analyzed the PR data using a general linear model (GLM) with repeated measures. Because the time variable is accounted for by two separate variables in our study design, we first conducted an overall analysis with two within-subjects factors (SessionNumber, TrialNumber) and one between-subjects factor (Group, three levels). A *post hoc* analysis was used to contrast the three study groups, using Bonferroni correction to adjust for multiple comparisons (Analyses 1 and 2).

In the second step, we applied separate GLM repeated measures analyses to compare the learning over trials of groups Y–S and Y–E within the first session, which we expected to express the greatest learning effect. Subsequently, we compared the between-subjects effects of group in this analysis to the effects of group in a second analysis accounting for a covariate variable that was expected to influence the between-group differences (Analyses 3 and 4).

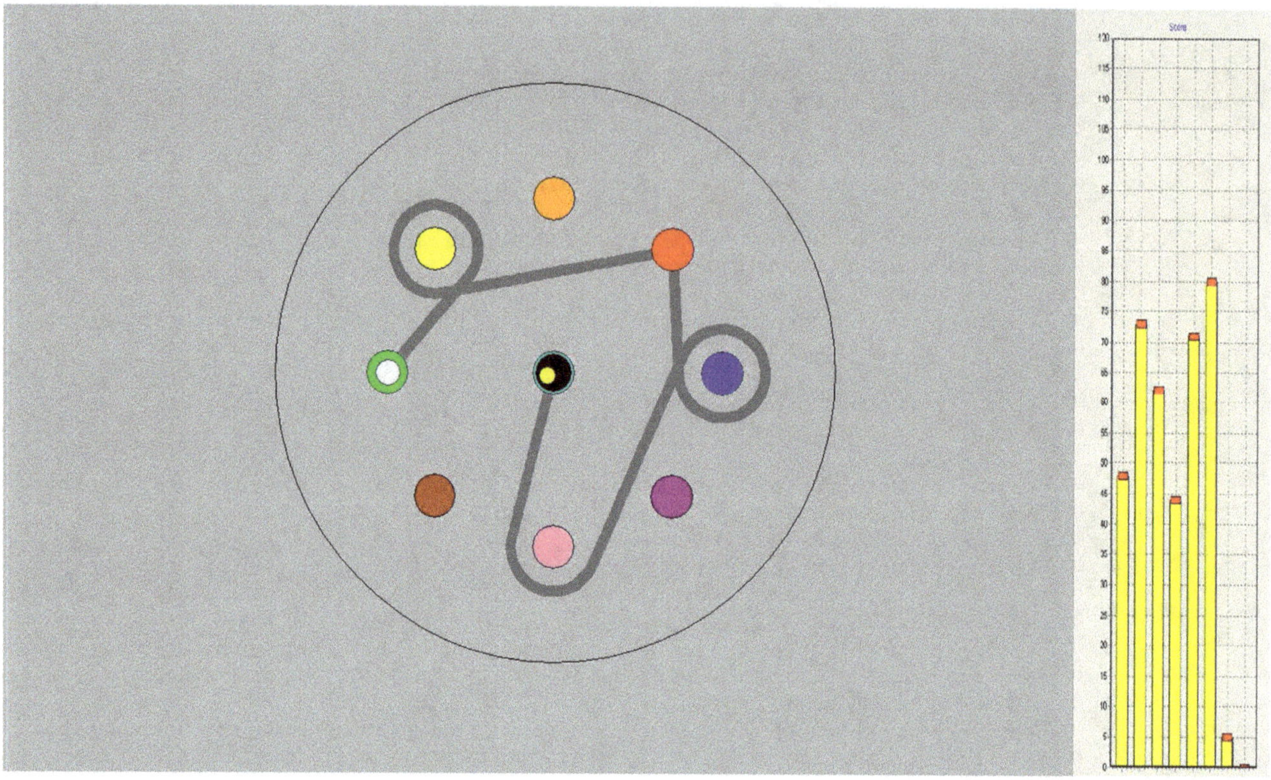

FIGURE 2 | Figure pursuit task on-screen, gray line indicating pursuit trajectory, not seen by participants. On the right-hand side, performance bars appeared as feedback after each trial.

Table 2 | Demographic and baseline assessment results.

	Schizophrenia patients (S)	Young controls (Y)	Elderly participants (E)	*T*-test S–Y	*T*-test E–Y
N	30	30	30	Matched	Matched
Age; mean (range)	36.4 (23–53)	37.3 (18–52)	69.2 (65–79)	$t(58) = 0.16$; $p = 0.875$	$t(58) = 18.99$; $p < 0.001$**
Sex M:F	20:10	20:10	20:10	Matched	Matched
Education years; mean (SD)	12.2 (±2.4)	15.1 (±2.6)	14.5 (±3.4)	$t(58) = 4.50$; $p < 0.001$**	$t(58) = 0.74$; $p = 0.465$
NLV Premorbid IQ; mean (SD)	101.30 (±10.29)	110.07 (±6.39)	111.73 (±6.43)	$t(58) = 3.96$; $p < 0.001$**	$t(58) = 1.01$; $p = 0.318$
LCT movement time; mean (SD)	0.36 (±0.15)	0.27 (±0.12)	0.40 (±0.13)	$t(55) = 2.40$; $p = 0.020$*	$t(55) = 3.65$; $p = 0.001$**
WCST categories completed; median (range)	3 (0–5)	5 (0–5)	3 (0–6)	$t(58) = 2.60$; $p = 0.012$*	$t(56) = 3.35$; $p = 0.001$**

NLV, Dutch adult reading test/Nederlandse Leestest voor Volwassenen; LCT, line-copying task); WCST, Wisconsin card sorting test.
*T-test differences are reported as t(df) and p-values (*significant at the 0.05 level; **significant at the 0.01 level).*

This procedure was repeated for three different covariates: LCT movement time (LCT_MT, an estimate of motor speed), WCST categories completed (WCST_cat, a measure of executive functioning), and education years.

In the third step, we used the computed learning measures (mean and cumulative learning gain) in separate GLM repeated measures analyses to evaluate the learning across sessions between groups Y–S and Y–E (Analyses 5 and 6).

RESULTS

DEMOGRAPHICS AND BASELINE ASSESSMENTS

Demographic features, baseline assessment results and group differences are summarized in **Table 2**. Schizophrenia patients (S) had a significantly lower level of education and premorbid IQ compared to the young controls (Y), whereas the young controls and elderly participants (E) did not differ significantly for this parameter. The Y group significantly outperformed both E and S

Table 3 | Antipsychotic drug prescriptions in schizophrenia patients.

Antipsychotic drug name	Number of prescriptions	Dose range
Clozapine	8	50–700 mg/day
Amisulpiride	7	200–800 mg/day
Haloperidol decanoate	7	75–200 mg/month
Quetiapine	6	50–600 mg/day
Olanzapine	3	5–20 mg/day
Paliperidone	3	3–6 mg/day
Paliperidone depot	3	75–200 mg/month
Aripiprazole	2	10–30 mg/day
Olanzapine depot	2	210–405 mg/month
Risperidone depot	2	50 mg/month
Clotiapine	1	40 mg/day
Flupentixol	1	1 mg/day
Bromperidol decanoate	1	125 mg/month
Zuclopentixol depot	1	200 mg/month
Risperidone	1	4 mg/day

groups on the LCT and WCST measures (see **Table 2**). Composite symptom scores for schizophrenia patients were 25.67 ± 17.39 on the SANS scale and 14.24 ± 19.68 on the SAPS scale. A summary of the use of antipsychotic drugs in schizophrenia patients included in the study is provided in **Table 3**.

ANALYSES OF CIRCLE AND FIGURE PURSUIT

Learning the PR tasks over all trials and sessions

In Analysis 1, independent of groups, learning effects were demonstrated by significant main effects of TrialNumber and SessionNumber and a significant interaction TrialNumber*SessionNumber both in the CPR task and the FPR task, indicating that the learning curves over trials for each session were different [see **Table 4A**].

Upon addition of Group as between-subjects factor in analysis 2, in both PR tasks, a significant main effect of Group was found [see **Table 4A**]. *Post hoc* analysis with Bonferroni correction demonstrated that the performance of schizophrenia patients and elderly participants was significantly poorer than the young control subjects at all stages of the task ($p < 0.001$), and that the elderly participants were the worst performing group (E-S CPR mean difference −13.62, SE 3.11, $p < 0.001$; E-S FPR mean difference −14.42, SE 2.97, $p < 0.001$).

In contrast, the interaction of TrialNumber*SessionNumber*Group was only significant in FPR, indicating that the learning curves of the groups also followed different slopes (with significant linear, quadratic, and cubic components). In CPR, the slopes were similar for the three groups [see **Table 4A; Figures 3** and **4**].

Learning the PR tasks over trials within session 1

In Analysis 3, comparisons of groups Y–S and Y–E on the FPR session 1 showed both a difference in performance, indicated by the significant between-subjects effect of the Group variable, as well as a different learning slope over trials, indicated by the significant TrialNumber*Group interaction. However, the significant Y–S group effect was reduced to a non-significant value when accounting for significant covariates: LCT_MT, WCST_cat, and education years in Analysis 4 [see **Table 4B**]. Combination of two individually significant covariates (LCT_MT plus WCST_cat and LCT_MT plus education years) further reduced the FPR Group effect.

In CPR session 1, again there was only a significant between-subjects effect of Group without TrialNumber*Group interaction. Furthermore, only the WCST_cat covariate reached a level of significance in the between-groups effect in this task, reducing also the Group difference between Y and S to a non-significant level [see **Table 4B**].

Interestingly, when these same covariates were added to the Y–E comparison, in both PR tasks the between-subjects Group effect remained significant [see **Table 4B**].

None of the analyses with covariates demonstrated a significant TrialNumber*Covariate or Group*Covariate interaction, suggesting the main effects of the covariates on the Accuracy variable can be interpreted independently of Group or Trialnumber.

Learning the PR tasks over sessions

The mean accuracy over trials was compared across sessions 1–3 in Analysis 5. In both PR tasks, a difference in performance between Y–S and Y–E groups was observed (i.e., significant main between-subjects effect of Group), but the SessionNumber*Group interaction was only significant for Y–E comparison, suggesting that schizophrenia patients showed a similar learning pattern across sessions as did young controls, but elderly participants did not [see **Table 4C; Figures 5** and **6**].

In Analysis 6, the same analyses were repeated with the learning measure cumulative learning gain, which corrects the mean for the participant's starting level performance on the first trial in session 1. Here, when Y and S groups were compared, neither the SessionNumber*Group interaction nor the between-subjects effect of Group was significant in either of the PR tasks. In the comparison of Y and E groups, a significant interaction of SessionNumber*Group was maintained for both PR tasks, but the main effect of Group was only significant for FPR [see **Table 4C; Figures 3** and **4**].

DISCUSSION

KEY RESULTS

General performance

Our results demonstrate poorer performance both in schizophrenia patients and in elderly participants compared to young controls, thereby matching findings of previous rotary pursuit studies (8, 11, 12, 14, 15, 17). This finding was observed in both pursuit tasks, and both on a within- and across-session level.

In FPR session 1, the poorer performance in patients was found to be attributable to differences in other functional parameters, such as psychomotor speed (LCT_MT), executive functioning (WCST categories completed), and years of education, with an additive effect. This implies that patients performing worse than healthy controls on the FPR task also perform worse on one or several of these baseline measures. One could thus hypothesize that the impaired FPR performance of patients is caused by reduced psychomotor speed and/or executive functioning or a lower level of education. Alternatively, it could also point out the existence of

Table 4 | Results of the GLM repeated measures analyses.

		Figure pursuit		Circle pursuit	
		F (hypothesis df, error df)[a]	p	F (hypothesis df, error df)[a]	p
(A) Y, S, AND E GROUPS					
SessionNumber[b]		285.76 (2, 88)	<0.001**	173.36 (2, 88)	<0.001**
TrialNumber[b]		179.77 (7, 83)	<0.001**	140.82 (1, 89)	<0.001**
SessionNumber*TrialNumber[b]		4.17 (14, 76)	<0.001**	13.34 (2, 88)	<0.001**
Group[c]		31.59	<0.001**	30.80	<0.001**
SessionNumber*TrialNumber*Group[c]		1.97 (28, 148)	0.005**	0.54 (4, 172)	0.710
(B) SESSION 1, Y GROUP – S GROUP					
TrialNumber*Group[d]		2.80 (7, 52)	0.015*	0.07 (1, 58)	0.799
Group[d]		7.80	0.007**	6.51	0.013*
WITH COVARIATE					
WCST_cat	Covariate[e]	19.42	<0.001**	9.35	0.003**
	Group[e]	4.57	0.114	2.54	0.117
LCT_MT	Covariate[e]	7.32	0.009**	3.15	0.082
	Group[e]	2.98	0.090	3.03	0.087
Education years	Covariate[e]	4.97	0.030*	2.18	0.146
	Group[e]	1.82	0.183	1.84	0.181
WCST(1) + LCT_MT(2)	Covariate1[e]	16.33	<0.001**		
	Covariate2[e]	5.84	0.010**		
	Group[e]	0.67	0.418		
Education years (1) + LCT_MT(2)	Covariate1[e]	5.48	0.023*		
	Covariate2[e]	8.86	0.004**		
	Group[e]	0.17	0.685		
SESSION 1, Y GROUP – E GROUP					
	TrialNumber*Group[d]	3.42 (7, 52)	0.004**	0.08 (1, 58)	0.775
	Group[d]	85.77	<0.001**	43.63	<0.001**
WITH COVARIATE					
WCST_cat	Covariate[e]	9.01	0.004**	6.84	0.011*
	Group[e]	61.35	<0.001**	27.38	<0.001**
LCT_MT	Covariate[e]	5.24	0.024*	0.61	0.439
	Group[e]	52.51	<0.001**	27.55	<0.001**
(C) LEARNING MEASURE OVER SESSIONS					
Mean	Y, S, and E groups				
	SessionNumber*Group[f]	2.51 (4, 172)	0.043*	1.59 (4, 172)	0.179
	Group[f]	31.59	<0.001**	30.80	<0.001**
	Y group – S group				
	SessionNumber*Group[f]	0.10 (2, 57)	0.905	0.87 (2, 57)	0.424
	Group[f]	9.16	0.004**	11.74	0.001**
	Y group – E group				
	SessionNumber*Group[f]	3.42 (2, 57)	0.039*	3.19 (2, 57)	0.049*
	Group[f]	83.78	<0.001**	70.26	<0.001**

(Continued)

Table 4 | Continued

		Figure pursuit		Circle pursuit	
		F (hypothesis df, error df)[a]	*p*	*F* (hypothesis df, error df)[a]	*p*
Cumulative learning gain	Y, S, and E groups				
	SessionNumber*Group[g]	2.51 (4, 172)	0.043*	1.59 (4, 172)	0.179
	Group[g]	7.81	0.001**	1.54	0.220
	Y group – S group				
	SessionNumber*Group[g]	0.10 (2, 57)	0.905	0.87 (2, 57)	0.424
	Group[g]	1.04	0.312	1.50	0.225
	Y group – E group				
	SessionNumber*Group[g]	3.42 (2, 57)	0.039*	3.19 (2, 57)	0.049*
	Group[g]	16.23	<0.001**	0.269	0.107

[a]*Wilk's Lambda F for multivariate analysis results.*
[b]*Analysis 1: within-subjects factors SessionNumber(3) and TrialNumber (8 FPR; 2 CPR).*
[c]*Analysis 2: within-subjects factors SessionNumber(3) and TrialNumber (8 FPR; 2 CPR) and between-subjects factor Group (3).*
[d]*Analysis 3: within-subjects factor TrialNumber (8 FPR; 2 CPR) and between-subjects factor Group (2).*
[e]*Analysis 4: within-subjects factor TrialNumber (8 FPR; 2 CPR), between-subjects factor Group (2) and covariate.*
[f]*Analysis 5: within-subjects factor SessionNumber(3), between-subjects factor Group (3 or 2), variable mean.*
[g]*Analysis 6: within-subjects factor SessionNumber(3), between-subjects factor Group (3 or 2), variable cumulative learning gain.*
**Significant at the 0.05 level; **significant at the 0.01 level.*

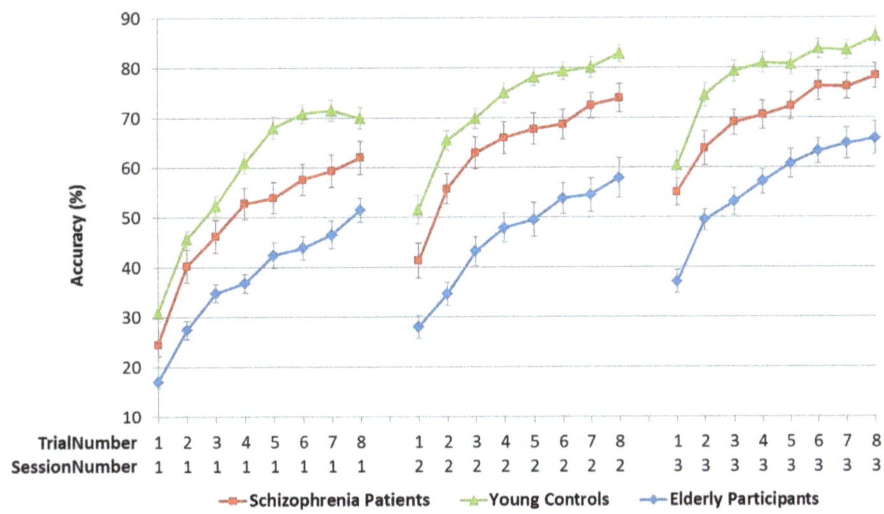

FIGURE 3 | Figure pursuit accuracy over three sessions and eight trials.

a separate subgroup of schizophrenia patients exhibiting impairments on all of these domains. In contrast, the difference in FPR performance between elderly participants and young controls could not be accounted for by differences in psychomotor speed nor executive functioning, indicating a performance gap between these groups that is independent of other functional parameters.

In CPR, contrasting to what was expected, psychomotor speed did not have a significant effect on the performance in session 1. Only executive functioning level appeared to account significantly for the difference between schizophrenia patients and controls in this task.

After the mean performance per session was corrected for the initial starting level, there was no longer a significant difference in performance across sessions between patients and controls. This finding suggests that the lower mean performance of patients is caused by a significantly lower starting level, which is not recovered by additional practice. However, in two other recent PR studies, an individual equation of the target speed was applied to account for participants' starting level performance; yet, the general performance in schizophrenia patients was found to be impaired nonetheless (12, 15). Thus, adjusting the difficulty of the task does not seem to solve the performance gap. Further study is needed to understand these seemingly contradictory findings. Regarding the elderly participants, their poorer mean level of performance was amended in the CPR, but remained in the FPR after correction for their significantly lower starting level by the cumulative learning gain measure.

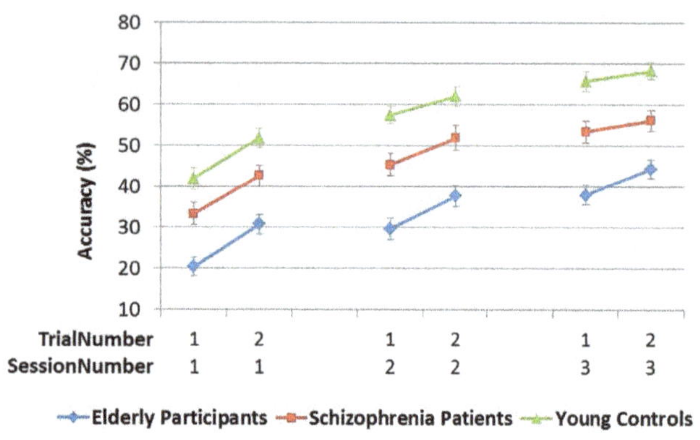

FIGURE 4 | Circle pursuit accuracy over three sessions and two trials.

Skill learning rate

We have established that all groups learned the new FPR and CPR sensorimotor skills over trials and sessions, but whereas the overall learning rate of schizophrenia patients and elderly participants was preserved in CPR, it differed between the three groups in FPR.

The early phase of learning the FPR skill was characterized by a significantly different learning curve of the schizophrenia patients and the elderly participants compared to young controls, who reached their peak performance earlier, as illustrated in **Figure 3**. The CPR consisted of only two trials in the first session, and therefore by definition the learning rate was marked by a linear increase, of which the slopes did not differ between the three groups (see **Figure 4**). In the later phase of learning of both PR tasks, schizophrenia patients and control subjects showed comparable learning gains over sessions, but elderly participants learned significantly less.

STUDY LIMITATIONS

By using two variations of the PR task, we have attempted to distinguish motor and sequence learning components, yet it remains difficult to single out and evaluate separately the processes involved in sensorimotor learning and performance. We cannot rule out the impact of declarative and spatial memory, attention capacity, and motor coordination on our PR skill performance and learning results. Also, while our CPR task was similar to the classical rotary pursuit task, we used a different methodology regarding the number of trials and rotation speed (see **Table 1**), which complicates the comparison of our results in the CPR to

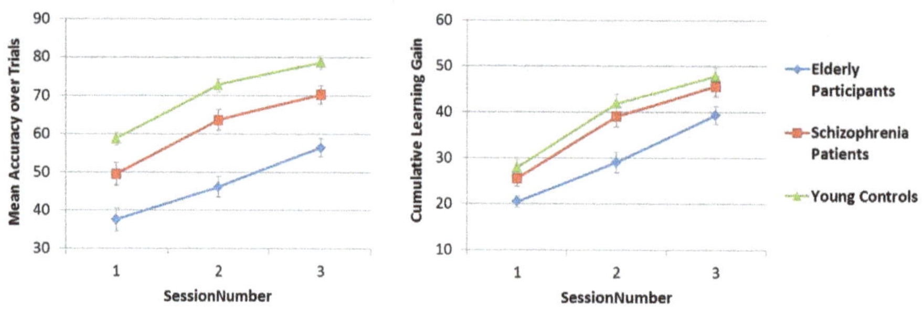

FIGURE 5 | Figure pursuit mean accuracy and cumulative learning gain over three sessions.

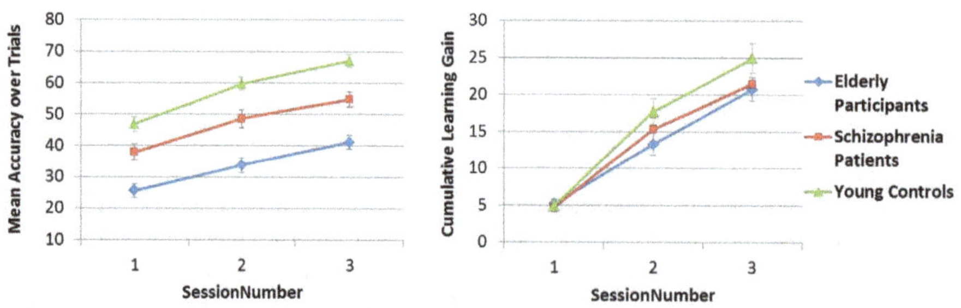

FIGURE 6 | Circle pursuit mean accuracy and cumulative learning gain over three sessions.

those of previous PR studies. It is possible that the number of trials per session in our CPR was too limited to establish within-session learning differences, which were found in FPR but not in CPR.

This study included only schizophrenia outpatients who were able to complete the test batteries and results can, therefore, not necessarily be generalized to the whole population of patients with schizophrenia. However, the mean SAPS and SANS composite scores in our sample concurred with scores found by van Erp et al. in a sample of 205 schizophrenia patients: mean composite SAPS 16.8 ± 14.2 compared to 14.2 ± 19.7 in our sample, and mean composite SANS 23.0 ± 14.6 compared to 25.7 ± 17.4 in our sample (21). Our patient population can, therefore, not be presumed to differ significantly in terms of symptom severity from other schizophrenia patient samples.

A large within-group heterogeneity in performance existed, particularly in the starting performance level of schizophrenia patients and the final performance level of elderly subjects. The relatively higher performance heterogeneity of the patients and elderly participants compared to the young controls may imply performance on the PR tasks in these groups was influenced by other variables than those accounted for in our study design. Problems with the evaluation of cognition of schizophrenia patients include lack of motivation and attention problems caused by negative symptomatology. Patients were instructed to complete the tasks to the best of their ability and our experience during test procedures was that being able to follow the feedback of their performance live on-screen provided an additional stimulus for performance optimization to subjects in all groups.

Other variables that may affect task performance include general cognitive functioning and medication use. We did not evaluate the study groups for their current IQ scores, and the schizophrenia patients had a significantly lower premorbid IQ score compared to young and elderly controls. In previous studies, comparing IQ-matched subgroups reduced or abolished differences in the overall level of performance between schizophrenic patients and control subjects on the rotor pursuit and other tasks of procedural learning (14, 15). However, IQ matching may also introduce a bias, considering research of general intelligence in schizophrenia has shown that only about a quarter of schizophrenia patients have a preserved IQ compared to the general population (22). Moreover, correlations between motor and cognitive functioning in schizophrenia patients have been repeatedly demonstrated (23, 24), and matching for cognitive parameters in studies of motor learning may, therefore, greatly influence the primary outcome measure. It is often argued that cognitive impairments in schizophrenia, and specifically psychomotor ones, are caused by psychotropic substances in general and antipsychotic medication in particular. All patients in our study had been stably treated with antipsychotic medication at the time of testing, and 16 patients were using more than one antipsychotic drug concomitantly (see **Table 3**). The reduced performance on PR tasks combined with a normal learning rate in patients may be hypothesized to be due to the use of antipsychotic drugs, known to affect psychomotor functioning (25).

IMPLICATIONS FOR FUTURE RESEARCH AND CLINICAL PERSPECTIVES

Our study provides important caveats toward future research on procedural learning in schizophrenia. Researchers should be aware that motor tasks including a sequence component should be distinguished from true motor learning tasks. As shown in this study, small variations applied to commonly used procedural tasks may allow to distinguish between operationally different components that may be important to further elucidate the nature of the deficits in schizophrenia. Particularly, the combination of different sensorimotor learning tasks with imaging techniques can be valuable to evaluate structural and functional brain alterations in the motor system. Furthermore, a longitudinal design should be a key feature of any study design interested in aspects of learning and memory, with differentiation of early and late learning phases.

Cognitive functioning, and specifically also executive functioning as measured with the Wisconsin card sorting test, has been shown to be a major predictor of functional outcome in schizophrenia (1). Motor learning in schizophrenia has been less studied, and its relation to functional outcome is currently unknown. However, evidence that motor performance is not only related to cognitive and executive functioning but also a predictor of cognitive deficits in schizophrenia patients at 1-year follow-up (23) suggests an association between motor performance or learning capacity, and functional outcome may exist that merits further investigation.

An age-related decline in sensorimotor learning has been previously recognized (17, 26), and in our study indeed the elderly participants demonstrated both poorer performance and lower learning gains in both PR tasks. Unexpectedly, the schizophrenia patients even outperformed the elderly healthy participants. Although this finding needs to be confirmed, it governs a more optimistic message about the functioning of patients than has hitherto been assumed. However, it is uncertain whether this pattern is maintained throughout different cognitive domains. Findings of our research group, as reported elsewhere in this journal (Cornelis et al., in press), suggest that in other cognitive domains, elderly participants may outperform schizophrenia patients. It might be interesting for future studies to include both elderly and non-elderly schizophrenia and control participants to differentiate between the mechanisms of cognitive impairment related to aging and schizophrenia.

A generally lower level of performance in schizophrenia (starting and ending the learning phase at a lower level than control subjects) has been a frequent finding in PR studies (11, 12, 14). Some authors have interpreted this phenomenon as reflecting impaired procedural learning in schizophrenia patients. However, since this reduced overall level of performance is usually accompanied with a normal learning rate, the mechanisms that underlie these two aspects of task performance are likely to differ to some extent. Because of this difficulty to differentiate between y-intercept (absolute performance) and slope (learning rate), and because of the high degree of within-group heterogeneity on performance level, many studies have not been able to conclude as to the actual capacity for sensorimotor skill learning of schizophrenia patients. Based on our results, it seems that schizophrenia patients have a mostly preserved capacity to learn sensorimotor skills, with any deficit related more to the early learning phase of sequence-holding skills and depending largely on the starting level performance of patients. This knowledge may prove important to the development and evaluation of therapies to improve such deficits in schizophrenia, in which the rotary pursuit, a well-established, easy and quick to administer task, may be used for the initial and follow-up evaluation of motor learning capacity and performance in patients. Because the late-phase learning of patients was preserved, it can be suspected that with an extended number of trials, the patients could eventually reach the same performance level as the final level in young controls. Thus, schizophrenia patients maintain the ability to acquire new skills, of vital importance to everyday functioning, given extra room for rehearsal. On the other hand, since more complex skills often also require additional cognitive components related to planning and organization, it is unclear whether this finding may be translated to all real-life skills.

CONCLUSION

Both in circle pursuit (motor task) and figure pursuit (motor plus sequence task), learning was evident in all groups, with equal learning gains of schizophrenia patients compared to age-matched controls, but reduced learning in elderly participants. In terms of general performance, the schizophrenia patients fell between the young controls and the elderly participants, differing significantly from both. Our results suggest that the lower performance of schizophrenia patients compared to age-matched controls can be accounted for by impaired speed of movement and executive functioning.

AUTHOR CONTRIBUTIONS

All the authors met ICMJE criteria and all those who fulfilled those criteria were listed as authors. All the authors had access to the study data and made the final decision about where to present these data.

ACKNOWLEDGMENTS

This clinical trial was sponsored by Janssen Research and Development, Janssen Pharmaceutica N.V. (Beerse, Belgium). The authors would like to thank Ms. Apers, Ms. Laureys, and Ms. Vermeylen for their support in the testing of the study participants. The authors also thank the study participants, without whom the studies would never have been accomplished. The study is registered at ClinicalTrials.gov: NCT01788436.

REFERENCES

1. Green MF, Kern RS, Heaton RK. Longitudinal studies of cognition and functional outcome in schizophrenia: implications for MATRICS. *Schizophr Res* (2004) **72**:41–51. doi:10.1016/j.schres.2004.09.009
2. Squire LR. Declarative and nondeclarative memory: multiple brain systems supporting learning and memory. *J Cogn Neurosci* (1992) **4**:232–43. doi:10.1162/jocn.1992.4.3.232
3. Marsh R, Alexander GM, Packard MG, Zhu H, Peterson BS. Perceptual-motor skill learning in Gilles de la Tourette syndrome. Evidence for multiple procedural learning and memory systems. *Neuropsychologia* (2005) **43**:1456–65. doi:10.1016/j.neuropsychologia.2004.12.012
4. Ammons RB. Acquisition of motor skill; rotary pursuit performance with continuous practice before and after a single rest. *J Exp Psychol* (1947) **37**:393–411. doi:10.1037/h0054334
5. Roth RM, Baribeau J, Milovan D, O'Connor K, Todorov C. Procedural and declarative memory in obsessive-compulsive disorder. *J Int Neuropsychol Soc* (2004) **10**:647–54. doi:10.1017/S1355617704105018
6. Graybiel AM, Aosaki T, Flaherty AW, Kimura M. The basal ganglia and adaptive motor control. *Science* (1994) **265**:1826–31. doi:10.1126/science.8091209
7. Doyon J, Bellec P, Amsel R, Penhune V, Monchi O, Carrier J, et al. Contributions of the basal ganglia and functionally related brain structures to motor learning. *Behav Brain Res* (2009) **199**:61–75. doi:10.1016/j.bbr.2008.11.012
8. Huston P, Shakow D. Learning capacity in schizophrenia. *Am J Psychiatry* (1949) **105**:881–8.
9. Goldberg TE, Torrey EF, Gold JM, Ragland JD, Bigelow LB, Weinberger DR. Learning and memory in monozygotic twins discordant for schizophrenia. *Psychol Med* (1993) **23**:71–85. doi:10.1017/S0033291700038861
10. Granholm E, Bartzokis G, Asarnow RF, Marder SR. Preliminary associations between motor procedural learning, basal ganglia T2 relaxation times, and tardive dyskinesia in schizophrenia. *Psychiatry Res* (1993) **50**:33–44. doi:10.1016/0925-4927(93)90022-A
11. Clare L, McKenna PJ, Mortimer AM, Baddeley AD. Memory in schizophrenia: what is impaired and what is preserved? *Neuropsychologia* (1993) **31**:1225–41. doi:10.1016/0028-3932(93)90070-G
12. Schwartz BL, Rosse RB, Veazey C, Deutsch SI. Impaired motor skill learning in schizophrenia: implications for corticostriatal dysfunction. *Biol Psychiatry* (1996) **39**:241–8. doi:10.1016/0006-3223(95)00130-1
13. Kern R, Green M, Wallace C. Declarative and procedural learning in schizophrenia: a test of the integrity of divergent memory systems. *Cogn Neuropsychol* (1997) **2**:39–50. doi:10.1080/135468097396405
14. Weickert TW, Terrazas A, Bigelow LB, Malley JD, Hyde T, Egan MF, et al. Habit and skill learning in schizophrenia: evidence of normal striatal processing with abnormal cortical input. *Learn Mem* (2002) **9**:430–42. doi:10.1101/lm.49102
15. Gomar JJ, Pomarol-Clotet E, Sarro S, Salvador R, Myers CE, McKenna PJ. Procedural learning in schizophrenia: reconciling the discrepant findings. *Biol Psychiatry* (2011) **69**:49–54. doi:10.1016/j.biopsych.2010.07.013
16. Gold JM, Hahn B, Strauss GP, Waltz JA. Turning it upside down: areas of preserved cognitive function in schizophrenia. *Neuropsychol Rev* (2009) **19**:294–311. doi:10.1007/s11065-009-9098-x
17. Kennedy KM, Partridge T, Raz N. Age-related differences in acquisition of perceptual-motor skills: working memory as a mediator. *Neuropsychol Dev Cogn B Aging Neuropsychol Cogn* (2008) **15**:165–83. doi:10.1080/13825580601186650
18. Andreasen N. *The Scale for the Assessment of Negative Symptoms (SANS)*. Iowa City, Iowa: University of Iowa (1983).
19. Andreasen N. *The Scale for the Assessment of Positive Symptoms (SAPS)*. Iowa City, Iowa: University of Iowa (1984).
20. Siegel D. A multivariate study of pursuit rotor skill development. *Res Q Exerc Sport* (1990) **61**:201–5. doi:10.1080/02701367.1990.10608676
21. van Erp TG, Preda A, Nguyen D, Faziola L, Turner J, Bustillo J, et al. Converting positive and negative symptom scores between PANSS and SAPS/SANS. *Schizophr Res* (2014) **152**:289–94. doi:10.1016/j.schres.2013.11.013
22. Weickert TW, Goldberg TE, Gold JM, Bigelow LB, Egan MF, Weinberger DR. Cognitive impairments in patients with schizophrenia displaying preserved and compromised intellect. *Arch Gen Psychiatry* (2000) **57**:907–13. doi:10.1001/archpsyc.57.9.907
23. Salazar-Fraile J, Balanza-Martinez V, Selva-Vera G, Martinez-Aran A, Sanchez-Moreno J, Rubio C, et al. Motor speed predicts stability of cognitive deficits in both schizophrenic and bipolar I patients at one-year follow-up. *Eur J Psychiatry* (2009) **23**:184–97. doi:10.4321/S0213-61632009000300007
24. Cuesta MJ, Sanchez-Torres AM, de Jalon EG, Campos MS, Ibanez B, Moreno-Izco L, et al. Spontaneous parkinsonism is associated with cognitive impairment in antipsychotic-naive patients with first-episode psychosis: a 6-month follow-up study. *Schizophr Bull* (2014) **40**:1164–73. doi:10.1093/schbul/sbt125
25. Morrens M, Hulstijn W, Sabbe B. The effects of atypical and conventional antipsychotics on reduced processing speed and psychomotor slowing in schizophrenia: a cross-sectional exploratory study. *Clin Ther* (2008) **30**:684–92. doi:10.1016/j.clinthera.2008.04.012
26. Ghisletta P, Kennedy KM, Rodrigue KM, Lindenberger U, Raz N. Adult age differences and the role of cognitive resources in perceptual-motor skill acquisition: application of a multilevel negative exponential model. *J Gerontol B Psychol Sci Soc Sci* (2010) **65B**:163–73. doi:10.1093/geronb/gbp126

12

Deficits in agency in schizophrenia, and additional deficits in body image, body schema, and internal timing, in passivity symptoms

Kyran T. Graham*[1,2], *Mathew T. Martin-Iverson*[1,2], *Nicholas P. Holmes*[3], *Assen Jablensky*[4] and *Flavie Waters*[2,4]

[1] *Pharmacology, Pharmacy and Anaesthesiology Unit, School of Medicine and Pharmacology, Faculty of Medicine, Dentistry and Health Sciences, The University of Western Australia, Perth, WA, Australia*
[2] *Statewide Department of Neurophysiology and Clinical Research Centre, Graylands Hospital, North Metropolitan Health Services – Mental Health, Perth, WA, Australia*
[3] *Centre for Integrative Neuroscience and Neurodynamics, School of Psychology and Clinical Language Sciences, University of Reading, Reading, UK*
[4] *Centre for Clinical Research in Neuropsychiatry, School of Psychiatry and Clinical Neurosciences, The University of Western Australia, Perth, WA, Australia*

Edited by:
Susan L. Rossell, Swinburne University of Technology, Australia

Reviewed by:
Jakob Hohwy, Monash University, Australia
Ryan Kaplan, Monash University, Australia

****Correspondence:***
Flavie Waters, Clinical Research Centre, Graylands Hospital, Private Bag No 1, Claremont, WA 6910, Australia
e-mail: flavie.waters@health.wa.gov.au

Individuals with schizophrenia, particularly those with passivity symptoms, may not feel in control of their actions, believing them to be controlled by external agents. Cognitive operations that contribute to these symptoms may include abnormal processing in agency as well as body representations that deal with body schema and body image. However, these operations in schizophrenia are not fully understood, and the questions of general versus specific deficits in individuals with different symptom profiles remain unanswered. Using the projected-hand illusion (a digital video version of the rubber-hand illusion) with *synchronous* and *asynchronous* stroking (500 ms delay), and a hand laterality judgment task, we assessed sense of agency, body image, and body schema in 53 people with clinically stable schizophrenia (with a current, past, and no history of passivity symptoms) and 48 healthy controls. The results revealed a stable trait in schizophrenia with no difference between clinical subgroups (sense of agency) and some quantitative (specific) differences depending on the passivity symptom profile (body image and body schema). Specifically, a reduced sense of self-agency was a common feature of all clinical subgroups. However, subgroup comparisons showed that individuals with passivity symptoms (both current and past) had significantly greater deficits on tasks assessing body image and body schema, relative to the other groups. In addition, patients with current passivity symptoms failed to demonstrate the normal reduction in body illusion typically seen with a 500 ms delay in visual feedback (*asynchronous* condition), suggesting internal timing problems. Altogether, the results underscore self-abnormalities in schizophrenia, provide evidence for both trait abnormalities and state changes specific to passivity symptoms, and point to a role for internal timing deficits as a mechanistic explanation for external cues becoming a possible source of self-body input.

Keywords: schizophrenia, passivity symptoms, first-rank symptoms, rubber-hand illusion, hand laterality, agency, body schema, body image

INTRODUCTION

In the field of cognitive neuroscience, the "sense of self" refers to a complex framework, which is derived from cognitive, sensory, and motor systems. In this context, a subjective experience of "self" is drawn, at least in part, from information gained from body and motor senses. Self-abnormalities in schizophrenia have long been documented in the clinical literature. Kurt Schneider noted that symptoms described "a loss of the very contours of the self" (1), and Bleuler (2) described the tearing apart or splitting of psychic functions. Such self-abnormalities appear to be characteristic of schizophrenia (3, 4), and are particularly pronounced in passivity symptoms (experience of alien control), where individuals do not feel in control of their movements and believe that their actions and intentions are controlled by an external agent. In passivity symptoms, the primary experience is that of a perceptual change regarding how the self is experienced alongside the subjective experience of an external locus of control for internally generated events.

A contemporary model suggests that such abnormalities arise from a failure in the mental operations responsible for predicting the sensory consequences of intended motor commands (the forward model), where the brain "anticipates" an action taking place (5–7). Cognitive self-monitoring models, by contrast, have explained the observed self-distortions as a failure of higher order cognitive processes involving source-monitoring, biases, and *post hoc* inferences that enable coherent self-referencing over time (8, 9). It is becoming clear, however, that these proposals are not adequate or sufficient as theoretical frameworks for motor passivity symptoms (10, 11). Criticisms include that motor commands are neither necessary nor sufficient to engender a sense of agency, and that *post hoc* inferences and biases cannot fully account for pervasive changes in self-experience and self-awareness reported by people with schizophrenia. In support, structured clinical interviews using a clinical–phenomenological approach demonstrate fundamental changes in embodied self-presence, self-experience, and self-judgment in individuals with schizophrenia (12) and in those at high risk of psychosis (13). In addition, disruptions in the forward model should precipitate gross motor problems in people with schizophrenia, for which there is contrary evidence (14, 15).

BODY REPRESENTATION DISTORTIONS AS AN ALTERNATIVE FRAMEWORK FOR EXPLAINING SELF-ABNORMALITIES IN SCHIZOPHRENIA

A focus on purely motor or cognitive mechanisms fails to consider other somatic and psychological processes that are necessary prerequisites for a coherent sense of self. It was recently suggested that self-deficits in schizophrenia may be better described as broad deficits in body representations that extend beyond self-agency (16). This proposal was drawn from evidence showing that the self emerges from the concurrent activation of multiple body representations, which are derived from multimodal sensory input as well as motor monitoring sources, and that are based on anatomical and neural networks, which play a critical role in one's sense of self. Body representations are intrinsically linked to one's sense of awareness, identity, self-concept, and sense of uniqueness. They are needed for the differentiation of body parts and for the accurate performance of purposeful actions.

A general framework for conceptualizing body representations includes at least two important representations: body image and body schema. *Body image* refers to a top-down cognitive representation that integrates the conscious perceptual experiences of one's body and contributes to one's belief and attitude about one's body (17–21). *Body schema* is typically defined as an unconscious dynamic sensory representation that reflects the position and movement of the body and limbs in space (17–20). The validity of these body representations is supported by studies of neurological patients, where localized lesions can selectively impair one or more representations (22–26), and from brain imaging studies pointing to differential activation of neural networks on tasks selective for each body representation (27–31). Finally, for the purposes of the current study, the *sense of agency* is defined as the experience that one is the initiator and in control of one's actions. The sense of agency is different from body representations as it is critically dependent on actions and intentions (32–34).

BODY REPRESENTATION DISTORTIONS IN PEOPLE WITH SCHIZOPHRENIA

As detailed previously, people with schizophrenia have difficulty in correctly attributing agency to self-made movements (35, 36), indicating distortions in agency. There is also emerging evidence for disturbances of these multiple body representations in schizophrenia. For example, empirical findings point to difficulties in imagining movements (37) pointing to deficits in body schema. People with schizophrenia also have abnormal body image, as assessed using a body distortion questionnaire (38). From these findings, it would appear that the internal modeling of the self is weakened or more malleable in people with schizophrenia.

The question of general versus specific deficits in individuals with different symptom profiles, however, has not yet been addressed. Specifically, are these body representation-deficits present in all individuals with schizophrenia or only those with passivity symptoms? According to the philosophical–theoretical tradition of self-disturbances in schizophrenia (3), passivity symptoms represent the more severe and elaborated form of self-disturbances in a continuum from non-psychotic experiences through intermediate phenomena into the manifest psychotic symptoms. Individuals then transit back and forth between manifest psychosis and the intermediary forms as their clinical condition changes over time. According to this view, there should be quantitative differences between people with passivity symptoms compared to individuals with a history of these symptoms and individuals with no lifetime history of passivity. The performance of individuals with schizophrenia with different symptom profile was therefore of interest in the current study.

ASSESSING BODY REPRESENTATIONS IN THE CURRENT STUDY

Body illusions, such as the rubber-hand illusion, are frequently used to examine processes underlying self-recognition. In the rubber-hand illusion, participants watch a fake hand being stroked, while their own hand is synchronously stroked out of view. This produces an illusory sensation of ownership of the rubber hand and a shift in perceived hand location toward the fake hand. A key requirement of the illusion is that of synchronous input between sensory modalities (tactile and vision). In the asynchronous condition, the illusion can be abolished or diminished by introducing a temporal delay between brush strokes and visual feedback (39). This condition allows an examination of the effects of a timing delay on each type of body representation.

People with schizophrenia tend to experience the rubber-hand illusion more strongly (40, 41) and faster (42) compared to healthy controls. Additionally, the relocation of the perceived position of one's own hand toward the image ("proprioceptive drift") has been shown to be greater in schizophrenia than controls, indicating stronger visual capture of proprioceptive information (40). The *projected*-hand illusion, however, has not yet been reported in the schizophrenia literature. The projected-hand illusion uses a live video image of the participant's own hand projected onto a video screen, allowing a more realistic image of the hand than the traditional "rubber-hand" methodology, more precise control over the timing of brush strokes, as well as enhanced merging of reality into the illusion.

This task assesses two aspects of the sense of self in one experimental set-up. Using a post-performance questionnaire, body image can be assessed on domains of "embodiment (of the 'other' projected hand)" and "disembodiment (of one's own hand)," and the sense of agency with the subjective sensation of motor control (over both the "other" and own hand). Psychometric studies show that illusory sensations over the "other" hand are simultaneously associated with a reduction of the same sensations in the real hand (43). For example, embodiment of the "other" hand is proportionally related to disembodiment of one's real hand, with the total embodiment of both being equal to one single hand (44, 45). A similar balance also exists with the sense of agency (46). Disembodiment (of limbs) and reduced agency (over actions) are clinical features of persons with passivity symptoms, so performance on such measures are of particular interest.

In order to assess the third type of body representation (body schema), the current study employed the hand laterality task (47). In this task, participants are asked to make a judgment regarding whether an image of a hand is that of a right or left hand by mentally rotating their own hand to match the hand on the screen. Both response times and accuracy are recorded. Evidence that imagined movements are dependent upon the body schema and include findings that performance on this task is influenced by the same biophysical constraints that underlie performed actions (48). A recent study shows that schizophrenia individuals ($n = 13$) were impaired on the task (49), although an analysis of passivity symptoms was not conducted.

AIMS AND HYPOTHESES

In the current study, we studied body representations in 53 individuals with schizophrenia and 48 healthy controls on the validated projected-hand illusion (50, 51) and the hand laterality task (47). Individuals with schizophrenia were clustered into subgroups based upon their lifetime history of passivity symptoms. The research questions were as follows: (1) what is the pattern of performance on measures of body schema, body image, and the sense of agency in individuals with schizophrenia compared to controls?; (2) does the evidence point to a stable trait for schizophrenia (no difference between clinical subgroups) or to quantitative differences depending on the passivity symptom profile? Our hypotheses are that body representation distortions will be present in varying degrees in the clinical population: individuals who are currently symptomatic (with passivity symptoms) will have the most severe abnormalities on all body representations, and those with a past history of symptoms, by virtue of their trait vulnerability, will have greater abnormalities than those with no history of symptoms and healthy controls but less than those who are currently symptomatic.

MATERIALS AND METHODS

PARTICIPANTS

The patient sample included individuals with schizophrenia or schizoaffective disorder (53 total, 36 males) recruited from the research database of the WA Family Study of Schizophrenia (52, 53). All patients met both ICD-10 and DSM-IV criteria for a lifetime diagnosis of schizophrenia or schizoaffective disorder, and were community outpatients not currently admitted into a psychiatric hospital and were treated with psychotropic medication. Exclusion criteria included comorbid organic brain disease or substance-use disorder that could account for the psychotic symptoms or language difficulties.

Healthy controls (48 total, 24 males) were recruited through community advertising. Potential controls were excluded if they had a history of a psychotic disorder, or if any of their first-degree relatives had been diagnosed with schizophrenia, schizophrenia-spectrum, or bipolar affective disorder.

The study protocol was explained to all participants and written informed consent was obtained. The study was approved by the North Metropolitan Mental Health Service Human Research Ethics Committee and conformed to the appropriate regulatory standards.

CLINICAL EVALUATION

Clinical evaluation was conducted with the Scales for the Assessment of Positive and Negative Symptoms [SAPS and SANS; (54, 55)]. Passivity symptoms were assessed using the Passivity Symptoms Interview (PSI) (56) with selected items from the Schedule for Clinical Assessment in Neuropsychiatry [SCAN, Version 2.1; items: 17.008, 18.005–18.010, 18.012–18.017, see Ref. (57)]. All symptoms were rated in accordance with stringent definitions and criteria assessed for lifetime history and presence in the last 4 weeks as determined by self-reports and case-note reviews. Patients were rated as having current passivity symptoms (current group) if they reported two or more such symptoms in the past 4 weeks ($n = 20$). Patients were rated as "Past" ($n = 12$) if they had a positive rating of at least two passivity symptoms in the past but not within the past 4 weeks or "Never" ($n = 21$) if they had never experienced these symptoms during any period. Independent classification of patients into groups was conducted by two of the investigators (Kyran T. Graham and Flavie Waters) and rated based on consensus.

EXPERIMENTAL TASKS

Hand illusion

Each participant sat in front of a table with a Fujitsu 17″ color monitor embedded horizontally in the top, with both hands resting on top of the table. The right hand was hidden behind a removable curtain. An image of this hand was captured by an analog camera (AVC-561, AVTECH, Taiwan) and transmitted to the monitor via an analog delay line (DL1B-5379, Ovation Systems Ltd., UK). The real hand and the image of the hand were separated by 15 cm. A photograph of the set-up used can be seen in **Figure 1**. There were two delay conditions in the illusion; *synchronous* (<10 ms video feedback) and *asynchronous* (an additional imposed 500 ms delay). Participant were exposed to each condition once (3 min each), with the order of presentation being counter-balanced across participants. A 20-item questionnaire assessing the subjective experience of the illusion was administered after each condition (46); adapted from Ref. (43). Items relating to the component Deafference were not included as the component does not pertain to body representations. Each item was rated on a 7-point Likert scale ranging from −3 (strongly disagree) to +3 (strongly agree). A recent PCA (46) identified that the following components could be extracted from the questionnaire, assessing body image ("Disembodiment of own hand" and "Embodiment of the 'Other' hand"), and the sense of agency ("Agency over the 'Other' hand," and "Loss of agency over own hand") in both *synchronous* and *asynchronous* conditions. **Table 1** shows the 20 items (Embodiment items 1–8, Disembodiment 13–17, Agency 9–10, and Loss of agency 11–12).

Hand laterality task

For each trial, a picture of a hand, palm down, was displayed on a computer screen (47). Participants were instructed to indicate if the hand was a left or right hand by pressing an appropriate key on a keyboard. Each picture was either a left or right hand and rotated by either 0°, 90° medially, 90° laterally, or 180°. There were six repeats of each hand/rotation combination for a total of 48 trials per participant. The stimuli were presented in a random order. Participants were instructed not to make major movements of their hands or heads while making the judgments. Four practice trials with feedback were given to each participant before commencing the main experiment. The experiment was produced using E-Prime 1.2 software (Psychology Software Tools, Pittsburgh, PA, USA). In order to rule out possible abnormalities in mental rotation, a similar task was conducted in which the letter F was displayed instead of a hand. The letter was either oriented normally or mirrored along the vertical axis. The same number of trials of letter and rotation combinations was used as the hand laterality task. For both tasks, accuracy and response time were recorded.

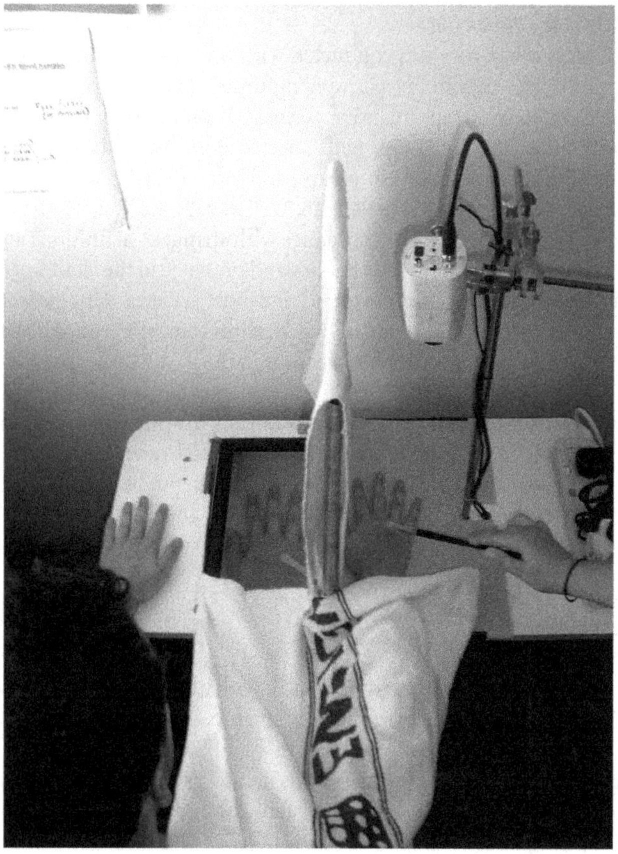

FIGURE 1 | Photograph of the projected-hand illusion is shown.

COGNITIVE TASKS

The Wechsler Test of Adult Reading (WTAR) (58) was included as a measure of pre-morbid intelligence. Trail Making Test Form A (TMTA) (59) provided a measure of speed of processing. The Digit Span (DS) provided a measure of attention span (forward span) and working memory (backward span) (59).

STATISTICAL METHODS

All statistical analyses and figures were completed using the statistical software R [version 3.0.1; Ref. (60)], and the packages "nlme" (61) and "car" (62). Analyses were performed using linear mixed-effects models with the mean score on the relevant subscale as the dependent variable, delay condition (*synchronous* or *asynchronous*) was the within-subjects variable, group (Controls, Current, Past, or Never) as the between-subjects variable and participant as the random effects term. Similarly, for the hand laterality task, separate models were created for (a) mean accuracy (% incorrect) and (b) mean response time (seconds). For these, group was the between-subjects independent variable and rotation (0°, 90° medial, 90° lateral, and 180°) was the within-subjects variable. Performance (% incorrect and response

Table 1 | Questionnaire items used during the projected-hand illusion.

It seemed like...	Component
... I was looking directly at my own hand, rather than at an image	Embodiment
... the image began to resemble my real hand	Embodiment
... the image of the hand belonged to me	Embodiment
... the image was my hand	Embodiment
... the image was part of my body	Embodiment
... my hand was in the location where the image was	Embodiment
... the image was in the location where my hand was	Embodiment
... the touch I felt was caused by the paintbrush touching the image	Embodiment
... I could have moved the image of the hand	Agency over the image
... like I was in control of the image	Agency over the image
... I was unable to move my hand	Loss of agency over own hand
... I couldn't have moved my hand if I had wanted	Loss of agency over own hand
... I couldn't really tell where my hand was	Disembodiment
... my hand had disappeared	Disembodiment
... my hand was out of my control	Disembodiment
... my hand was moving toward the image	Disembodiment
... the image was moving toward my hand	Disembodiment

time) on each rotation for the letter rotation task was included as a covariate in these analyses. Where analysis of deviance (ANODEV) on the terms of the model revealed significant differences, interaction contrasts comparing difference in scores on each of the levels of the factor were performed, i.e., [Controls(Synch) – Controls(Asynch)] – [Current(Synch) – Current (Asynch)]. Alpha was set to 0.05.

RESULTS

PROJECTED-HAND ILLUSION

Demographic information for participants can be seen in **Table 2**. Where there were differences between groups, these data were then entered into the projected-hand illusion analyses as covariates. However, there were no significant effects of any of the covariates for the PHI data ($p > 0.1$) and so these were removed from the final model.

Schizophrenia groups combined

Performance was first examined with a comparison of people with schizophrenia as a group versus healthy controls to determine overall effects of diagnosis while maximizing power to detect an effect. SAPS and SANS scores and chlorpromazine equivalents were included as further covariates in all projected-hand illusion analyses but were removed from the final model, as none were significant. People with schizophrenia reported increased feelings of disembodiment [$F(1, 99) = 29.5$, $p < 0.0001$], and a greater loss of agency over their own hand [$F(1, 99) = 21.3$, $p < 0.0001$] compared to controls, showing greater deficits identifying the experience of their own body.

There were no main effects of group [$F(1,99) = 1.83$, $p = 0.18$] or interaction [$F(1,1498) = 2.65$, $p = 0.10$] on the embodiment of the "other" hand component [$F(1,97) = 3.63$, $p = 0.06$]. Further, there was no significant difference between groups in the sense of agency over the "other" hand [$F(1,99) = 0.19$, $p = 0.66$].

Group comparisons – body image (embodiment of image)

Analysis of deviance revealed no main effects of group on Embodiment [$F(3,97) = 0.83$, $p = 0.48$], but there was a significant main effect of delay [$F(1, 1496) = 57.8$, $p < 0.0001$], with ratings being higher in the *synchronous* condition. There was a significant interaction between group (Controls, Current, Past, and Never) and delay condition [$F(3, 1496) = 4.94$, $p = 0.002$]. Interaction contrasts revealed significant differences between Current and each of the other groups: Controls ($p = 0.001$), Never ($p = 0.04$), and Past ($p = 0.0006$). Controls and patients in the Past and Never groups demonstrated embodiment of the hand in the *synchronous* condition, which was reduced in the *asynchronous* condition. By contrast, patients in the Current group showed no difference in performance between the *synchronous* and the *asynchronous* conditions, exhibiting embodiment in both conditions (see **Figure 2A**).

Group comparisons – body image (disembodiment of own hand)

For disembodiment (**Figure 2B**), there was a main effect of group [$F(3, 97) = 13.1$, $p < 0.0001$], but not delay condition [$F(1, 892) = 1.25$, $p = 0.26$] and the interaction was not significant [$F(3, 892) = 6.78$, $p = 0.08$]. Disembodiment of own hand was significantly higher in the Past ($p < 0.0001$), Current ($p < 0.0001$), and the Never groups ($p = 0.01$), relative to controls. The Current and Past groups were marginally significantly different from each other ($p = 0.05$) but both reported higher disembodiment than the Never group (Past $p = 0.009$, Current $p = 0.04$).

Group comparisons – agency (agency over the image)

Analysis of deviance revealed no main effect of group [$F(3, 97) = 0.16$, $p = 0.92$], but there was a significant main effect of delay condition [$F(1, 292) = 19.2$, $p < 0.0001$], with an overall increase in reported agency over the "other" hand in the *synchronous* compared to *asynchronous* condition. The interaction between group and delay condition neared, but did not reach, significance [$F(3, 292) = 7.59$, $p = 0.055$]. However, given the *p*-value, it was decided that it was reasonable to perform interaction contrasts. **Figure 2C** shows that Controls, Never, and Past all demonstrated increased agency over the "other" hand,

Table 2 | Demographic information of participants.

	Controls ($n = 48$)	Never ($n = 21$)	Past ($n = 12$)	Current ($n = 20$)
Sex (M/F)[a]	24/24	14/7	10/2	12/8
Age (years)[b]	46.2 ± 1.68	42.5 ± 1.57	43.6 ± 2.84	44.0 ± 2.06
Years of education[b]	13.7 ± 0.35	12.9 ± 0.37	13.0 ± 0.54	13.7 ± 0.57
WTAR[b]	104 ± 1.9	100 ± 3.3	95 ± 3.4	96 ± 3.2*
Trail Making Test A[b]	31.9 ± 2.82	53.0 ± 7.47***	51.2 ± 11.5***	45.7 ± 8.68**
SAPS composite[b]	–	12.0 ± 2.3^^^	19.2 ± 3.5	29.2 ± 3.2
SANS composite[b]	–	21.8 ± 3.6	29.8 ± 4.7	24.7 ± 2.5
Chlorpromazine equivalents (mg)[b]	–	677 ± 121	805 ± 140	754 ± 106

Mean ± SEM of selected covariates.

[a] *Fisher's Exact Test.*

[b] *One-way ANOVA with Tukey's HSD post hoc comparisons (Bonferroni corrected).*

*Different from controls: *$p < 0.05$, **$p < 0.01$, ***$p < 0.001$.*

Different from Pass. Current: ^$p < 0.05$, ^^$p < 0.01$, ^^^$p < 0.001$.

Antipsychotic doses converted into chlorpromazine equivalents using the formulae given in (69–71).

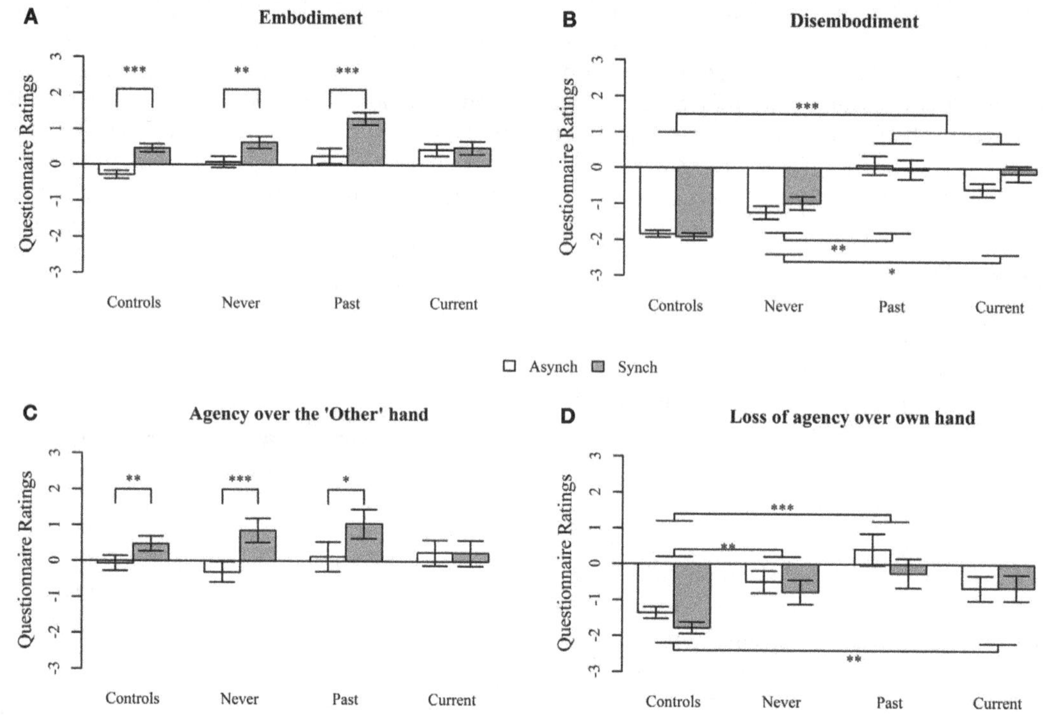

FIGURE 2 | Questionnaire responses assessing (A) Embodiment, (B) Disembodiment, (C) Agency over the "Other" hand, and (D) Loss of agency over own hand, during the projected-hand illusion after asynchronous (Asynch) and synchronous (Synch) stimulation in controls, people with schizophrenia with no history of passivity symptoms (Never), people with a past history of passivity symptoms (Past), and people with current experiences of passivity symptoms (Current). Questions were answered on a 7-point Likert scale. Data are mean ± SEM. *$p < 0.05$, **$p < 0.001$, ***$p < 0.0001$.

after *synchronous* compared to *asynchronous* stimulation (treatment contrasts; $p = 0.007$, $p = 0.002$, $p = 0.02$, respectively), while the Current group failed to demonstrate the expected decrease in the *asynchronous* condition ($p = 0.98$) and reported similar levels of agency after both *synchronous* and *asynchronous* stimulation. However, the only pairwise interaction treatment contrast that was significant was between Current and Never groups ($p = 0.009$).

Group comparisons – agency (loss of agency of own hand)

For the loss of agency of own hand component, there was a significant main effect of group [$F(3, 97) = 25.0$, $p < 0.0001$] and a significant effect of delay condition [$F(1, 293) = 3.97$, $p = 0.046$] such that loss of agency ratings were higher in the *synchronous* condition but no significant interaction [$F(3, 293) = 0.49$, $p = 0.69$]. Controls reported significantly less loss of agency over their own hand relative to the Current ($p = 0.004$), Past ($p < 0.0001$), and Never groups ($p = 0.003$), but there were no significant differences between schizophrenia groups (all $p > 0.1$; see **Figure 2D**).

HAND LATERALITY TASK

Scales for the Assessment of Positive Symptoms score, Scales for the Assessment of Negative Symptoms score, and chlorpromazine equivalents were initially included as covariates in all hand laterality analyses, but none had a significant association so they were excluded from the final model.

Schizophrenia groups combined (hand laterality task – response time)

As expected, on response time with the schizophrenia groups and healthy controls, the ANODEV displayed a significant main effect of rotation [$F(3, 700) = 460$, $p < 0.0001$] with the response time on 0° trials significantly different from 90° Medial ($p < 0.0001$), 90° Lateral ($p < 0.0001$), and 180° trials ($p < 0.0001$). There was a main effect whereby individuals with schizophrenia had longer response times across all rotations [$F(1, 99) = 17.7$, $p < 0.0001$], as well as an interaction of group and rotation [$F(3, 693) = 12.8$, $p = 0.005$], indicating a further increase in response time on the 90° lateral ($p < 0.0001$) and 180° rotations ($p < 0.0001$) compared to controls.

Schizophrenia groups combined (hand laterality task – accuracy)

There were significant positive associations between accuracy on the hand laterality task and WTAR scores [$F(1, 78) = 15.9$, $p < 0.0001$, slope = 0.26], and accuracy on the letter rotation task [$F(1, 560) = 4.91$, $p < 0.03$, slope = 0.06], so these variables were retained as covariates. There was a significant effect of rotation [$F(3, 560) = 46.2$, $p < 0.0001$]. Contrasts demonstrated that accuracy on 0° trials is not different to 90° Medial ($p = 0.53$) or 90° Lateral ($p = 0.08$) trials, but significantly different from 180° trials ($p < 0.0001$). There was no significant main effect of group (schizophrenia group versus Controls) in accuracy [$F(1, 78) = 0.14$, $p = 0.71$]. There was a significant interaction between group and rotation [$F(3, 560) = 9.13$, $p = 0.03$] due to the schizophrenia group being significantly less accurate on the 90° Lateral rotation ($p = 0.03$).

Group comparisons (hand laterality task – response times)

Response time on the letter rotation task covaried significantly with the response time on the hand rotation task [$F(1,687) = 13.9$, $p = 0.0002$, slope = 0.10]. However, all significant effects remained so with inclusion of the covariate. No other covariates, including chlorpromazine equivalents, were significant. There was a significant main effect of group on response times [$F(3, 97) = 20.6$, $p < 0.0001$]. There was also a significant interaction between group and rotation type [$F(9, 687) = 20.9$, $p = 0.01$]; response times of Current and Past were significantly longer than controls at 90° lateral ($p = 0.03$ and $p = 0.03$) and 180° rotations ($p = 0.009$ and $p = 0.005$), and Never had significantly greater response times compared to Controls at all rotations (0°, $p = 0.01$; 90° medial, $p = 0.002$; 90° lateral, $p < 0.0001$; 180°, $p < 0.0001$) (**Figure 3**).

Group comparisons (hand laterality task – accuracy)

There was a significant interaction between group and rotation [$F(9, 554) = 27.9$, $p = 0.001$], as well as a significant main effect of rotation [$F(3, 554) = 47.4$, $p < 0.0001$]. To investigate the cause of the interaction between group and rotation type, interaction treatment contrasts were performed. There were no significant group differences at 90° medial rotation (all $p > 0.3$). At 90° lateral rotations, the Current and Past (but not Never) were significantly less accurate than controls ($p = 0.006$ and 0.007, respectively). At 180° rotations, only Past were significantly less accurate than controls at 180° rotations ($p = 0.0007$). There was no main effect of group [$F(3, 76) = 0.94$, $p = 0.20$] on accuracy. In regards to the covariates, higher accuracy on the letter rotation task was associated with higher accuracy of hand laterality judgments [$F(1, 554) = 4.61$, $p = 0.01$, slope = 0.06], and a higher WTAR score was associated with higher accuracy [$F(1, 76) = 14.9$, $p = 0.002$, slope = 0.26]. All significant effects remained after inclusion of the covariates.

DISCUSSION

The main aim of the current study was to assess the integrity of body representations in individuals with schizophrenia compared to controls and the pattern of performance with regards to the presence of passivity symptoms on a body illusion and a hand laterality task.

WHAT IS THE PATTERN OF PERFORMANCE IN INDIVIDUALS WITH SCHIZOPHRENIA COMPARED TO CONTROLS?

Individuals with schizophrenia showed abnormal performance on both the hand illusion and hand laterality tasks. During the hand illusion, individuals with schizophrenia, as a group, showed increased disembodiment of their own hand, as well as a decreased sense of agency over their own hand, relative to controls.

The hand illusion, with its subjective reports, provides a particularly convenient method to examine components of body representations and self- and non-self-dimensions in one experimental set-up. The current study showed dissociation in performance by people with schizophrenia between *self*-embodiment/agency and *other*-embodiment/agency. Specifically, there was no significant difference between the schizophrenia and controls groups on embodiment and sense of agency over the "other" hand, although the clinical group was particularly impaired on trials requiring the processing of their own (self) body. This perhaps suggests that the representation of other/external people is relatively preserved in schizophrenia, but that the representation of their own body is impaired. In other words, these individuals may be particularly susceptible to disruptions in self-processes, producing a sense of disconnectedness from their own body, but that the embodiment and sense of agency over external objects/bodies are unaffected.

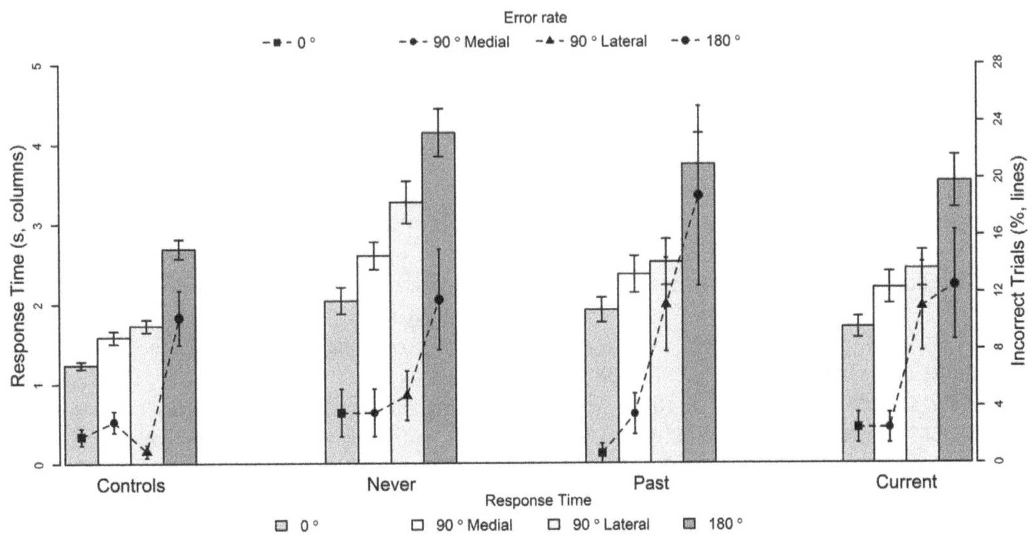

FIGURE 3 | Mean response times (seconds, columns) and inaccuracy (%, lines) of hand laterality judgments at 0°, 90° Medial, 90° Lateral, and 180° rotations for Controls, people with no history of passivity symptoms (Never), people with a past history of passivity symptoms (Past), and people with current experiences of passivity symptoms (Current). Data are mean ± SEM. See text for treatment contrasts.

In a speculative tone, the imbalance between self- and non-self-representations may give rise to distortions regarding the inference of other people's intention, perhaps triggering or increasing the vulnerability to delusions.

Disordered self-agency is a common finding in experimental tasks testing the forward model and cognitive self-monitoring models (36, 63–66). However, few studies have demonstrated disembodiment in schizophrenia. While patients frequently complain of diminished representations of the bodily self (1, 4), depersonalization and feeling of disembodiment (67, 68), and self-referential processing difficulties (66, 67), such subjective reports are rarely assessed in experimental conditions. Altogether, the current findings, using a hand illusion, provide support for anomalies in self-agency and self-ownership in this group.

Performance on the hand laterality task provided evidence of additional changes in body schema. On this task, individuals with schizophrenia took significantly longer to respond than controls. In addition, this clinical group had significantly lower accuracy on 90° lateral and 180° rotation trials. These are the most difficult trials, even in healthy groups, and performance is typically less accurate and slower than on the other trials (47). In individuals with schizophrenia, this pattern of performance on error and latency measures could not be explained simply in terms of impaired visuospatial abilities or generally slower responses, since controlling for performance on the letter rotation task with the same rotation conditions did not change the results. Given that the hand laterality task is under the same biophysical constraints as performed actions, the current results point to specific difficulties in the processes involving the synchronization of proprioceptive and tactile inputs into a representation of the body in space in schizophrenia. These findings on the hand laterality task underscore those of de Vignemont et al. ($n = 13$) (49). In contrast to the current study, however, they showed an increase in errors on all rotations in their schizophrenia group relative to controls. Their task was similar to ours, so it is likely that differences in patient characteristics or in statistical power contributed to this small difference in performance.

Together, the current findings point to deficits in sense of agency, body image, and body schema in schizophrenia. Performance on these tasks was not related to chlorpromazine equivalents, so antipsychotics dosages are an unlikely contributor to performance. Similarly, performance on the task was not correlated with other clinical or cognitive performance score. We believe that it is the first report of deficits in multiple body representations in schizophrenia.

DOES THE EVIDENCE POINT TO A STABLE TRAIT FOR SCHIZOPHRENIA (NO DIFFERENCE BETWEEN CLINICAL SUBGROUPS) OR TO QUANTITATIVE DIFFERENCES DEPENDING ON THE PASSIVITY SYMPTOM PROFILE?

If abnormal body representations represent a stable trait for schizophrenia *in toto,* then no significant differences among Current (current presence of passivity), Past (past history of passivity), and Never (no history of passivity) would be expected, although they would still perform differently from controls. Only partial evidence was found for this suggestion. Specifically, evidence for such a "stable trait" was only observed in the domain of agency, where a reduced sense of agency over one's own hand was a common feature of all three patient groups.

By contrast, performance on the other variables supported our initial hypothesis that there should be quantitative differences between people with passivity symptoms ("Current") compared to individuals with a history of these symptoms ("Past"), and individuals with no lifetime history of passivity ("Never"). Performance on tasks assessing body image suggested quantitative differences depending on the passivity symptom profile of the clinical group. Individuals with passivity symptoms (both current and past) had significantly greater changes in body image as indicated by their higher rating of items relating to disembodiment compared to the group with no history of these symptoms, who in turn reported more disembodiment compared to healthy controls.

In accordance with the above, on the hand laterality task, the Current and Past groups demonstrated reduced accuracy on judgments of the 90° lateral and 180°(Past only) rotations. This finding is in line with demonstrations of impaired performance on a task of motor imagery in people with motor passivity symptoms (37). While this points to problems in body schema, it is important to note that actions and proprioception remain largely unimpaired in this group (14, 15). This suggests that only some subcomponents of body schema are impaired, either in the access pathways to this information or in the integration with other body representations (37).

In sum, the evidence points to both general (trait) deficits in all individuals with schizophrenia (the sense of agency) and quantitative (specific) differences depending on the passivity symptom profile (body image and body schema). Questions remain, however, regarding the processes that separate individuals with current passivity symptoms from those with a history of these symptoms. Both groups show deficits in sense of agency, body image, and body schema, so these processes are not sufficient alone for passivity symptoms. What determines whether patients experience these symptoms? A clue lies in the examination of performance on the hand illusion, specifically on the asynchronous condition.

DECREASED SENSITIVITY TO TIMING DELAYS ASSOCIATED WITH PASSIVITY SYMPTOMS

On all measures of the hand illusion involving timing delays, individuals in the Current passivity group distinguished themselves from the other groups. Most remarkably, they failed to demonstrate the normal reduction in the body illusion typically seen with a 500 ms delay in visual feedback (*asynchronous* condition). This performance was specific to those in the Current group, as the other clinical groups (including the Past group) showed the expected illusory decrease on the *asynchronous* condition. In other words, individuals with passivity symptoms continued to experience illusions of embodiment and sense of agency over the "other" hand, when the other groups did not. This suggests that the temporal window that provides links between self and external stimuli is significantly, and abnormally, elongated in people with passivity symptoms. Alternatively, it is possible that the Current group uses temporal cues during multisensory integration to a lesser extent than the other groups.

The functional significance of this finding cannot be understated, given that internal timing precision is critical for a range of processes including sensory–motor awareness and self-recognition (66, 72, 73). Precise timing is needed for the synchronization of motor, cognitive, and sensory signals. It is also needed to shape sensory awareness and in the formation of causal mental associations. Specifically, voluntary actions, which are followed by a sensory event, are perceived as shifted closer together in time than they actually are, a psychological phenomenon termed intentional binding (74), which contributes toward the sense of self-agency. Abnormal internal timing mechanisms in people with passivity symptom therefore have much explanatory power for their disordered self-attribution system. Other evidence is provided by studies showing time perception impairments in individuals with schizophrenia (75, 76). Passivity symptoms studies also show dysfunctions in cognitive and motor timing. Specifically, these individuals perceive external events to be closer in time together than they are (66, 77, 78), which may impact on the integrity of self- and non-self-attribution processes.

The current hand illusion findings are particularly pertinent, because they show that individual with passivity symptoms experiences an illusory sensation of ownership and agency over an image that is spatially and temporally disjointed from the sensorimotor processes linked to their real hand. It is therefore not surprising that these individuals do not feel in control of their movements, and that they experience confusion regarding the origins of their actions and intentions. Such fragmented phenomena would lead to substantial confusion for internally generated events. If a larger window of integration was indeed closely associated with passivity symptoms, it would be expected to have impact on other behaviors and also other non-body-related illusions such as the ventriloquist illusion.

A possible mechanism might occur via dopaminergic pathways. Using an amphetamine challenge in healthy volunteers as a model of psychoses-related responses in the rubber-hand illusion, our group (44) found that amphetamine appeared to increase the temporal envelope of associability of the rubber-hand visual cues to the feel of the stroking (i.e., had a selective effect of increasing the illusion in the *asynchronous* condition) in a profile of performance, which was similar to the pattern of performance in the Current group. Together with their functional role of assigning salience to external stimuli (35), dopaminergic pathways may well contribute to confusion, and misattribution, of agency via changes in the normal temporal window for associability such that external cues become a possible source of body input.

STRENGTHS AND LIMITATIONS OF THE CURRENT STUDY

It should be noted here that the hand illusion offers significant advantage over other paradigms assessing sense of agency in schizophrenia (35, 36). Notably, subjective reports of *online and prospective* actions (e.g., "I am able to move it") in the hand illusion are superior to tasks assessing actions *retrospectively* ("I moved it"), therefore overcoming criticisms about the involvement of other cognitive processes (35), which render such retrospective predictions unreliable (36) [also see Ref. (14, 79)]. Such differentiation between prospective and retrospective assessments is thought to be significant when assessing agency reliably (35). That the items of the questionnaire of the current study assessed *prospective* agency possibly explains why there was no significant difference between the schizophrenia groups on the loss of agency over own hand questions; it would appear that the changes in agency are limited to *retrospective* agency in passivity symptoms. Confirmation of this finding could not be carried out as the current study did not assess *retrospective* agency.

A further limitation of the current study is that Current group had a significantly higher level of positive symptoms as assessed on the SAPS. It may therefore be that overall illness severity contributed to the current results, rather than the presence of passivity symptoms. However, several lines of evidence argue against this proposal: (i) there were no significant associations of SAPS scores with any of the dependent variables; (ii) SANS scores did not differ between groups; (iii) chlorpromazine equivalents did not differ between groups; and (iv) the groups did not differ from each other on cognitive performance.

CONCLUSION

To conclude, the current study demonstrated both stable traits in schizophrenia (sense of agency) and some quantitative differences depending on passivity symptom profile (body image and body schema). In addition, the presence of passivity symptoms was linked to an enduring experience of body illusion that was resistant to both spatial separation and temporal delay. Our proposal is that passivity symptoms are linked to deficits in body representations encompassing body image and body schema, changes in the sense of agency, alongside internal timing problems that contribute to excessive associability with external sensory stimuli, producing the sensation that one's actions are controlled by an external agent.

AUTHOR CONTRIBUTIONS

Kyran T. Graham conducted all participant testing, statistical analyses and wrote the first draft of the manuscript. Flavie Waters and Assen Jablenksy contributed to the conception of the project and to the design of the study. Kyran T. Graham, Mathew T. Martin-Iverson, and Nicholas P. Holmes provided input into the experimental procedures and testing. All authors contributed to manuscript drafts.

ACKNOWLEDGMENTS

This research was supported by National Health and Medical Research Grant 634328. We would like to thank Philippa Martyr and Sarah Howell for their help in the recruitment of participants and Kevin Murray and Laura Firth for their guidance and advice in regards to the statistical analysis. We would also like to thank the reviewers for their very helpful comments in the interpretation of the results.

REFERENCES

1. Schneider K. *Clinical Psychopathology.* New York: Grune & Stratton (1959).
2. Bleuler E. *Dementia Praecox or the Group of Schizophrenias [J. Zinkin trans.].* New York, NY: International Universities Press (1950).
3. Sass LA, Parnas J. Schizophrenia, consciousness, and the self. *Schizophr Bull* (2003) **29**(3):427–44. doi:10.1093/oxfordjournals.schbul.a007017
4. Parnas J. The self and intentionality in the pre-psychotic stages of schizophrenia. In: Zahavi D, editor. *Exploring the Self: Philosophical and Psychopathological Perspectives on Self-Experience.* Amsterdam: John Benjamins (2000). p. 115–47.

5. Frith CD. In: Hove E, editor. *The Cognitive Neuropsychology of Schizophrenia.* Sussex: Lawrence Erlbaum Associates (1992).
6. Frith CD. The neural basis of hallucinations and delusions. *C R Biol* (2005) **328**(2):169–75. doi:10.1016/j.crvi.2004.10.012
7. Feinberg I. Efference copy and corollary discharge: implications for thinking and its disorders. *Schizophr Bull* (1978) **4**:636–40. doi:10.1093/schbul/4.4.636
8. Wegner DM. The mind's best trick: how we experience conscious will. *Trends Cogn Sci* (2003) **7**(2):65–9. doi:10.1016/S1364-6613(03)00002-0
9. Bentall RP, Baker GA, Havers S. Reality monitoring and psychotic hallucinations. *Br J Clin Psychol* (1991) **30**(3):213–22. doi:10.1111/j.2044-8260.1991.tb00939.x
10. Synofzik M, Thier P, Lindner A. Internalizing agency of self-action: perception of one's own hand movements depends on an adaptable prediction about the sensory action outcome. *J Neurophysiol* (2006) **96**(3):1592–601. doi:10.1152/jn.00104.2006
11. Gallagher S. Neurocognitive models of schizophrenia: a neurophenomenological critique. *Psychopathology* (2004) **37**(1):8. doi:10.1159/000077014
12. Parnas J, Handest P, Sæbye D, Jansson L. Anomalies of subjective experience in schizophrenia and psychotic bipolar illness. *Acta Psychiatr Scand* (2003) **108**(2):126–33. doi:10.1034/j.1600-0447.2003.00105.x
13. Nelson B, Yung AR, Bechdolf A, McGorry PD. The phenomenological critique and self-disturbance: implications for ultra-high risk ("prodrome") research. *Schizophr Bull* (2008) **34**(2):381–92. doi:10.1093/schbul/sbm094
14. Synofzik M, Vosgerau G, Newen A. Beyond the comparator model: a multifactorial two-step account of agency. *Conscious Cogn* (2008) **17**(1):219–39.
15. Delevoye-Turrell Y, Giersch A, Danion J-M. A deficit in the adjustment of grip force responses in schizophrenia. *Neuroreport* (2002) **13**(12):1537–9. doi:10.1097/00001756-200208270-00010
16. Waters FAV, Badcock JC. First-rank symptoms in schizophrenia: reexamining mechanisms of self-recognition. *Schizophr Bull* (2010) **36**(3):510–7. doi:10.1093/schbul/sbn112
17. Coslett HB, Saffran EM, Schwoebel J. Knowledge of the human body – a distinct semantic domain. *Neurology* (2002) **59**(3):357–63. doi:10.1212/WNL.59.3.357
18. Gallagher S. *How the Body Shapes the Mind.* New York: Oxford University Press (2005).
19. Paillard J. Body schema and body image – a double dissociation in deafferented patients. In: Gantchev G, Mori S, Massion J, editors. *Motor Control, Today and Tomorrow.* Sofia: Academic Publishing House (1999). p. 197–214.
20. Schwoebel J, Coslett HB. Evidence for multiple, distinct representations of the human body. *J Cogn Neurosci* (2005) **17**(4):543–53. doi:10.1162/0898929053467587
21. Holmes NP, Spence C. Dissociating body image and body schema with rubber hands. *Behav Brain Sci* (2007) **30**(02):211–2. doi:10.1017/S0140525X07001501
22. Arzy S, Overney LS, Landis T, Blanke O. Neural mechanisms of embodiment: asomatognosia due to premotor cortex damage. *Arch Neurol* (2006) **63**(7):1022–5. doi:10.1001/archneur.63.7.1022
23. Wolpert DM, Goodbody SJ, Husain M. Maintaining internal representations the role of the human superior parietal lobe. *Nat Neurosci* (1998) **1**(6):529–33. doi:10.1038/2245
24. Biran I, Chatterjee A. Alien hand syndrome. *Arch Neurol* (2004) **61**(2):292–4. doi:10.1001/archneur.61.2.292
25. Biran I, Giovannetti T, Buxbaum L, Chatterjee A. The alien hand syndrome: what makes the alien hand alien? *Cogn Neuropsychol* (2006) **23**(4):563–82. doi:10.1080/02643290500180282
26. Coslett H. Evidence for a disturbance of the body schema in neglect. *Brain Cogn* (1998) **37**(3):527–44. doi:10.1006/brcg.1998.1011
27. Ehrsson HH, Holmes NP, Passingham RE. Touching a rubber hand: feeling of body ownership is associated with activity in multisensory brain areas. *J Neurosci* (2005) **25**(45):10564–73. doi:10.1523/JNEUROSCI.0800-05.2005
28. Ehrsson HH, Spence C, Passingham RE. That's my hand! Activity in premotor cortex reflects feeling of ownership of a limb. *Science* (2004) **305**(5685):875–7. doi:10.1126/science.1097011
29. Lau HC, Rogers RD, Haggard P, Passingham RE. Attention to intention. *Science* (2004) **303**(5661):1208–10. doi:10.1126/science.1090973
30. Farrer C, Frith CD. Experiencing oneself vs. another person as being the cause of an action: the neural correlates of the experience of agency. *Neuroimage* (2002) **15**(3):596–603. doi:10.1006/nimg.2001.1009
31. Tsakiris M, Longo MR, Haggard P. Having a body versus moving your body: neural signatures of agency and body-ownership. *Neuropsychologia* (2010) **48**(9):2740–9. doi:10.1016/j.neuropsychologia.2010.05.021
32. Blakemore S-J, Frith CD. Self-awareness and action. *Curr Opin Neurobiol* (2003) **13**(2):219–24. doi:10.1016/S0959-4388(03)00043-6
33. Haggard P. Conscious intention and motor cognition. *Trends Cogn Sci* (2005) **9**(6):290–5. doi:10.1016/j.tics.2005.04.012
34. Gallagher S. The natural philosophy of agency. *Philos Compass* (2007) **2**(2):347–57. doi:10.1111/j.1747-9991.2007.00067.x
35. Voss M, Moore J, Hauser M, Gallinat J, Heinz A, Haggard P. Altered awareness of action in schizophrenia: a specific deficit in predicting action consequences. *Brain* (2010) **133**(10):3104–12. doi:10.1093/brain/awq152
36. Synofzik M, Thier P, Leube DT, Schlotterbeck P, Lindner A. Misattributions of agency in schizophrenia are based on imprecise predictions about the sensory consequences of one's actions. *Brain* (2010) **133**(1):262–71. doi:10.1093/brain/awp291
37. Maruff P, Wilson P, Currie J. Abnormalities of motor imagery associated with somatic passivity phenomena in schizophrenia. *Schizophr Res* (2003) **60**(2–3):229–38. doi:10.1016/S0920-9964(02)00214-1
38. Priebe S, Röhricht F. Specific body image pathology in acute schizophrenia. *Psychiatry Res* (2001) **101**(3):289–301. doi:10.1016/S0165-1781(01)00214-1
39. Botvinick M, Cohen J. Rubber hands 'feel' touch that eyes see. *Nature* (1998) **391**(6669):756. doi:10.1038/3578
40. Thakkar KN, Nichols HS, McIntosh LG, Park S. Disturbances in body ownership in schizophrenia: evidence from the rubber hand illusion and case study of a spontaneous out-of-body experience. *PLoS One* (2011) **6**(10):e27089. doi:10.1371/journal.pone.0027089
41. Peled A, Ritsner M, Hirschmann S, Geva AB, Modai I. Touch feel illusion in schizophrenic patients. *Biol Psychiatry* (2000) **48**(11):1105–8. doi:10.1016/S0006-3223(00)00947-1
42. Peled A, Pressman A, Geva AB, Modai I. Somatosensory evoked potentials during a rubber-hand illusion in schizophrenia. *Schizophr Res* (2003) **64**(2–3):157–63. doi:10.1016/S0920-9964(03)00057-4
43. Longo MR, Schüür F, Kammers MP, Tsakiris M, Haggard P. What is embodiment? A psychometric approach. *Cognition* (2008) **107**(3):978–98. doi:10.1016/j.cognition.2007.12.004
44. Albrecht M, Martin-Iverson M, Price G, Lee J, Iyyalol R, Waters FAV. Dexamphetamine effects on separate constructs in the rubber hand illusion test. *Psychopharmacology* (2011) **217**(1):39–50. doi:10.1007/s00213-011-2255-y
45. Ehrsson HH. How many arms make a pair? Perceptual illusion of having an additional limb. *Perception* (2009) **38**(2):310–2. doi:10.1068/p6304
46. Graham K, Martin-Iverson MT, Holmes N, Waters FAV. The projected hand illusion: component structure in a community sample, and association with demographics, cognition and psychotic-like experiences. *Atten Percept Psychophys* (2014). doi:10.3758/s13414-014-0748-6
47. Parsons LM. Imagined spatial transformations of one's hands and feet. *Cogn Psychol* (1987) **19**(2):178–241. doi:10.1016/0010-0285(87)90011-9
48. Parsons LM. Temporal and kinetic properties of motor behavior reflected in mentally simulated action. *J Exp Psychol Hum Percept Perform* (1994) **20**(4):709–30. doi:10.1037/0096-1523.20.4.709
49. de Vignemont F, Zalla T, Posada A, Louvegnez A, Koenig O, Georgieff N, et al. Mental rotation in schizophrenia. *Conscious Cogn* (2006) **15**(2):295–309. doi:10.1016/j.concog.2005.08.001
50. Tsakiris M, Prabhu G, Haggard P. Having a body versus moving your body: how agency structures body-ownership. *Conscious Cogn* (2006) **15**(2):423–32. doi:10.1016/j.concog.2005.09.004
51. Ijsselsteijn WA, de Kort YAW, Haans A. Is this my hand I see before me? The rubber hand illusion in reality, virtual reality and mixed reality. *Presence (Camb)* (2006) **15**(4):455–64. doi:10.1162/pres.15.4.455
52. Hallmayer JF, Jablensky A, Michie P, Woodbury M, Salmon B, Combrinck J, et al. Linkage analysis of candidate regions using a composite neurocognitive phenotype correlated with schizophrenia. *Mol Psychiatry* (2003) **8**(5):511. doi:10.1038/sj.mp.4001273
53. Jablensky A. Researching psychiatry in Western Australia. *Aust N Z J Psychiatry* (2004) **38**(5):306–15. doi:10.1080/j.1440-1614.2004.01265.x
54. Andreasen NC. *The Scale for the Assessment of Positive Symptoms (SAPS).* Iowa City, IA: The University of Iowa (1984).
55. Andreasen NC. *The Scale for the Assessment of Negative Symptoms (SANS).* Iowa City, IA: The University of Iowa (1984).

56. Waters FAV, Badcock JC, Dragovic M, Jablensky A. Neuropsychological functioning in schizophrenia patients with first-rank (passivity) symptoms. *Psychopathology* (2009) **42**(1):47–58. doi:10.1159/000187634
57. Wing JK, Babor T, Brugha T, Burke J, Cooper JE, Giel R, et al. SCAN: schedules for clinical assessment in neuropsychiatry. *Arch Gen Psychiatry* (1990) **47**(6):589–93. doi:10.1001/archpsyc.1990.01810180089012
58. Wechsler D. *Wechsler Test of Adult Reading*. San Antonio, TX: Psychological Corporation (2001).
59. Lezak M, Howieson D, Loring D, Hannay H, Fischer J. *Neuropsychological Assessment*. 3rd ed. New York: Oxford University Press (1995).
60. R Core Team. *R: A Language and Environment for Statistical Computing*. 3.0. 1 ed. Vienna: R Foundation for Statistical Computing (2012).
61. Pinheiro J, Bates D, DebRoy S, Sarkar D, The R Development Core Team. *nlme: Linear and Nonlinear Mixed Effects Models. R Package Version 3.1*. (2013).
62. Fox J, Weisberg S. *An {R} Companion to Applied Regression*. 2nd ed. Thousand Oaks, CA: Sage (2011).
63. Daprati E, Franck N, Georgieff N, Proust J, Pacherie E, Dalery J, et al. Looking for the agent: an investigation into consciousness of action and self-consciousness in schizophrenic patients. *Cognition* (1997) **65**(1):71–86. doi:10.1016/S0010-0277(97)00039-5
64. Franck N, Farrer C, Georgieff N, Marie-Cardine M, Dalery J, d'Amato T, et al. Defective recognition of one's own actions in patients with schizophrenia. *Am J Psychiatry* (2001) **158**(3):454–9. doi:10.1176/appi.ajp.158.3.454
65. Cahill C, Silbersweig D, Frith C. Psychotic experiences induced in deluded patients using distorted auditory feedback. *Cognitive Neuropsychiatry* (1996) **1**(3):201–11.
66. Blakemore S-J, Smith J, Steel R, Johnstone EC, Frith CD. The perception of self-produced sensory stimuli in patients with auditory hallucinations and passivity experiences: evidence for a breakdown in self-monitoring. *Psychol Med* (2000) **30**(05):1131–9. doi:10.1017/S0033291799002676
67. Röhricht F, Priebe S. Body image in patients with acute paranoid schizophrenia. A longitudinal study. *Nervenarzt* (1996) **67**(7):602–7.
68. Röhricht F, Priebe S. Do cenesthesias and body image aberration characterize a subgroup in schizophrenia? *Acta Psychiatr Scand* (2002) **105**(4):276–82. doi:10.1034/j.1600-0447.2002.1107.x
69. Bazire S. *Psychotropic Drug Directory*. Dinton: Quay Books (2009).
70. Taylor D, Paton C, Kapur S. *The Maudsley Prescription Guidelines*. 10th ed. London: Informa Pharmaceuticals (2009).
71. Woods S. Chlorpromazine equivalent doses for the newer atypical antipsychotics. *J Clin Psychiatry* (2003) **64**(6):663–7.
72. Haggard P, Martin F, Taylor-Clarke M, Jeannerod M, Franck N. Awareness of action in schizophrenia. *Neuroreport* (2003) **14**(7):1081–5. doi:10.1097/01.wnr.0000073684.00308.c0
73. Waters FAV. Time perception and discrimination in individuals with auditory hallucinations. In: Jardri R, Cachia A, Thomas P, Pins D, editors. *The Neuroscience of Hallucinations*. New York: Springer (2013). p. 185–99.
74. Haggard P, Clark S, Kalogeras J. Voluntary action and conscious awareness. *Nat Neurosci* (2002) **5**(4):382. doi:10.1038/nn827
75. Elvevag B, McCormack T, Gilbert A, Brown GDA, Weinberger DR, Goldberg TE. Duration judgements in patients with schizophrenia. *Psychol Med* (2003) **33**(07):1249–61. doi:10.1017/S0033291703008122
76. Franck N, Posada AS, Pichon S, Haggard P. Altered subjective time of events in schizophrenia. *J Nerv Ment Dis* (2005) **193**(5):350–3. doi:10.1097/01.nmd.0000161699.76032.09
77. Spence SA. Free will in the light of neuropsychiatry. *Philos Psychiatr Psychol* (1996) **3**(2):75–90. doi:10.1353/ppp.1996.0019
78. Waters FAV, Jablensky A. Time discrimination deficits in schizophrenia patients with first-rank (passivity) symptoms. *Psychiatry Res* (2009) **167**(1–2):12–20. doi:10.1016/j.psychres.2008.04.004
79. Moore JW, Lagnado D, Deal DC, Haggard P. Feelings of control: contingency determines experience of action. *Cognition* (2009) **110**(2):279–83. doi:10.1016/j.cognition.2008.11.006

13

Prevalence of the catatonic syndrome in an acute inpatient sample

Mirella Stuivenga*[1] *and Manuel Morrens*[1,2]

[1] *Collaborative Antwerp Psychiatric Research Institute (CAPRI), University of Antwerp, Antwerp, Belgium*
[2] *Psychiatric Center Brothers Alexians, Boechout, Belgium*

Edited by:
Mihaly Hajos, Yale University School of Medicine, USA

Reviewed by:
Bernhard J. Mitterauer, Volitronics-Institute for Basic Research Psychopathology and Brain Philosophy, Austria
Pascal Sienaert, Universitair Psychiatrisch Centrum KU Leuven, Belgium

****Correspondence:***
Manuel Morrens, Collaborative Antwerp Psychiatric Institute (CAPRI), University of Antwerp, Campus Drie Eiken, Universiteitsplein 1, Antwerp B-2610, Belgium
e-mail: manuel.morrens@uantwerpen.be

Objective: In this exploratory open label study, we investigated the prevalence of catatonia in an acute psychiatric inpatient population. In addition, differences in symptom presentation of catatonia depending on the underlying psychiatric illness were investigated.

Methods: One hundred thirty patients were assessed with the Bush–Francis Catatonia Rating Scale (BFCRS), the Positive and Negative Syndrome Scale, the Young Mania Rating Scale, and the Simpson–Angus Scale. A factor analysis was conducted in order to generate six catatonic symptom clusters. Composite scores based on this principal component analysis were calculated.

Results: When focusing on the first 14 items of the BFCRS, 101 patients (77.7%) had at least 1 symptom scoring 1 or higher, whereas, 66 patients (50.8%) had at least 2 symptoms. Interestingly, when focusing on the DSM-5 criteria of catatonia, 22 patients (16.9%) could be considered for this diagnosis. Furthermore, different symptom profiles were found, depending on the underlying psychopathology. Psychotic symptomatology correlated strongly with excitement symptomatology ($r=0.528$, $p<0.001$) and to a lesser degree with the stereotypy/mannerisms symptom cluster ($r=0.289$; $p=0.001$) and the echo/perseveration symptom cluster ($r=0.185$; $p=0.035$). Similarly, manic symptomatology correlated strongly with the excitement symptom cluster ($r=0.596$; $p<0.001$) and to a lesser extent with the stereotypy/mannerisms symptom cluster ($r=0.277$; $p=0.001$).

Conclusion: There was a high prevalence of catatonic symptomatology. Depending on the criteria being used, we noticed an important difference in exact prevalence, which makes it clear that we need clear-cut criteria. Another important finding is the fact that the catatonic presentation may vary depending on the underlying pathology, although an unambiguous delineation between these catatonic presentations cannot be made. Future research is needed to determine diagnostical criteria of catatonia, which are clinically relevant.

Keywords: catatonia, psychomotor, acute psychiatric admissions, classification, schizophrenia, mood disorders

INTRODUCTION

Catatonia is a psychomotor symptom cluster characterized by a heterogeneous group of mental, motor, vegetative, and behavioral signs. The recognition of catatonia is essential since it is a syndrome that can be effectively and rapidly relieved in most cases. Whereas, the pathophysiology of catatonia is still unknown, it is clear that the psychomotor syndrome results from many etiologies (1).

Although some critics have suggested the syndrome is much more uncommon than a century ago or may even be disappearing, catatonia is still highly prevalent (2). Whereas early investigators reported catatonia in 20–50% of the schizophrenic patients (3, 4), contemporary literature demonstrates the presence of catatonia in 4–15% of schizophrenia patients (5–8). In acutely ill psychiatric inpatients higher estimates are reported, ranging between 5 and 20% (9, 10).

Most recently, the DSM-5 rightfully loosened the association between schizophrenia and catatonia that was predominant in its preceding editions and now recognizes that catatonia can be induced by different disorders (11). In the study of Pommepuy and Januel, including 607 catatonic patients, there was an average of 30.9% of all patients with a primary diagnosis of schizophrenia, whereas 43% of the patients had a mood disorder (12). The review of Caroff and colleagues shows similar results (13). Among patients with a mood disorder, catatonia can be seen in patients with a bipolar disorder with a percentage of 17–47% in mania and 0–20% in patients with a depressive episode (14, 15). In a study including patients with an unipolar depressive disorder 20% of the patients met the criteria for catatonia (16).

There are reasons to believe that the profile of catatonic symptomatology may depend on the underlying pathology (15, 17). Krüger and colleagues demonstrated that catatonia in schizophrenia was mainly characterized by abnormal movements, stereotypies, mannerisms, catalepsy, negativism, automatic obedience, and waxy flexibility, whereas, catatonic excitation was more associated with mania and catatonic inhibition more with depression (15). This notion is very intriguing since it can both have diagnostical and therapeutical implications and give clues toward future research on the underlying pathophysiology of the psychomotor syndrome.

In the present study, prevalence of catatonia in an acute psychiatric inpatient population was investigated. In addition, differences in symptom presentation of catatonia depending on the underlying psychiatric illness were investigated.

MATERIALS AND METHODS

STUDY DESIGN

In an exploratory open label study design, each patient admitted to a psychiatric intensive ward during a period of 12 months was assessed for catatonic and clinical symptomatology. The patients admitted to this department were experiencing the most acute phase of a mental illness. The department is for men and women over the age of 18 year who require a period of psychiatric intensive care. The assessments were conducted on the first day of admission in the hospital. There were no exclusion criteria for participation. All of the 130 patients who were admitted to the psychiatric intensive ward were included in the study.

PARTICIPANTS

A total group of 130 patients (female: $n = 50$; 38.5%) were tested after admission on an acute psychiatric enclosed ward. The mean age was 40.5 years (SD = 13.9; range 18–76). More than half of our patient group had a psychotic illness as a primary illness ($n = 67$; 51.5%) including 26 patients (20.0%) with schizophrenia (amongst which 3 patients with a diagnosed catatonic subtype) and 35 patients with a psychotic illness not otherwise specified (26.9%). The second most common primary diagnosis ($n = 16$; 12.3%) was a bipolar disorder, followed by substance abuse disorders ($n = 14$; 10.8%). Major depressive disorder was the main diagnosis in six patients (4.6%). Similarly, six patients received a diagnosis of personality disorder (4.6%).

Antipsychotics were taken by 56.9% of the patients ($n = 74$). Twenty-six patients (20.0%) took at least 1 first generation antipsychotic (FGA), whereas 64 patients (49.2%) took a second generation antipsychotic (SGA), 4 patients were taking lithium (3.1%), whereas 12 patients took anti-epileptics (9.2%) at the time of testing. Antidepressants were administered to 30.8% of the patients at the time of testing [SSRI ($n = 17$); SNRI ($n = 10$); TCA ($n = 2$); and others ($n = 5$)]. Finally, 40% of the patients were taking benzodiazepines (n = 52) and 6 patients took an anticholinergic agent (4.6%).

CLINICAL ASSESSMENT

All patients were assessed with the Bush–Francis Catatonia Rating Scale (BFCRS) (18), the Positive and Negative Syndrome Scale (PANSS) (19), the Young Mania Rating Scale (YMRS), and the Simpson–Angus Scale (SAS).

The BFCRS is used to recognize and score catatonic signs and symptoms. It measures the severity of 23 catatonic signs. By scoring the first 14 items of the BFCRS, the instrument can be used as a screening tool. If two or more of the BFCRS signs are present, the presence of catatonia can be considered. Items of the BFCRS are scored on a 0–3 point scale. The PANSS is a widely used medical scale for measuring symptom severity of patients with schizophrenia. Scores ranging from 1 to 7 are given on 30 different symptoms in three subscales (positive scale 7 items, negative scale 7 items, general psychopathology scale 16 items), with total score ranging from 30 to 210. In order to measure depressive symptoms we used a depression-subscale of the PANSS (PANSS-dep) including items depression, anxiety and guilt feelings. The YMRS is a rating scale to assess manic symptoms. The scale has 11 items and is based on the patient's subjective report of his or her clinical condition over the previous 48 h. Additional information is based upon clinical observations made during the course of the clinical interview. The SAS is used to measure extrapyramidal symptoms. It is composed of 10 items and signs.

RESULTS

CATATONIA SYMPTOMATOLOGY

Catatonic symptomatology was highly prevalent in our patient sample. When focusing on the first 14 items of the BFCRS, which are suggested for using the instrument as a screening tool, 101 patients (77.7%) had at least 1 symptom scoring 1 or higher, whereas 66 patients (50.8%) had at least 2 symptoms. Interestingly, when focusing on the DSM-5 criteria of catatonia (at least 3 out of 12 selected symptoms), 22 patients (16.9%) fulfill the diagnostic criteria, which still implied a high prevalence rate, but drastically lower than when using the BFCRS-criteria, and interestingly and unexpectedly, also lower than with the DSM-IV-TR criteria (see **Table 1**).

In our patient sample, the most prevalent catatonic symptoms were excitement ($n = 49$; 37.7%), perseveration ($n = 32$; 24.6%), impulsivity ($n = 31$; 23.8%), and verbigeration ($n = 31$; 23.8%), whereas, a grasp reflex or waxy flexibility could not be observed in any of the patients. Similarly, catatonic symptoms such as mitgehen ($n = 3$; 2.3%), gegenhalten ($n = 2$; 1.5%), or ambitendency ($n = 3$; 2.3%) could only seldomly be observed (see **Table 2**).

A factor analysis (Principal Component Analysis, varimax rotation) was conducted in order to generate catatonic symptom clusters. Given that items grasp reflex and waxy flexibility had a zero variance, these items were excluded from the analysis. This yielded six symptom clusters (see **Table 3**): a negative factor including immobility/stupor, mutism, staring, posturing, rigidity, negativism, withdrawal, gegenhalten, and ambitendency; a stereotypy/mannerism factor including stereotypy,

Table 1 | Prevalence of catatonia in an acute psychiatric patient sample according to different criteria.

	DSM-IV (20)	DSM-V (11)	BFCRS (18)	Fink and Taylor (21, 22)
Psychotic disorder	19 (28.4%)	14 (20.9%)	48 (71.6%)	9 (13.4%)
Mood disorder	7 (31.8%)	5 (22.7%)	17 (77.3%)	5 (22.7%)
Substance use disorder	1 (7.1%)	0 (0%)	3 (21.4%)	0 (0%)
Another diagnosis	5 (18.5%)	3 (11.1%)	14 (51.9%)	2 (7.4%)
Total patient group	32 (24.6%)	22 (16.9%)	82 (63.1%)	16 (12.3%)

Table 2 | Scores on the individual items of the BFCRS.

	Score = 0 (absent symptom)	Score = 1	Score = 2	Score = 3	Patients with symptom (*N*)
Excitement	81	35	14	0	49
Immobility/stupor	107	18	5	0	23
Mutism	117	4	6	3	13
Staring	101	22	5	2	29
Posturing/catalepsy	112	11	4	3	18
Grimacing	119	11	0	0	11
Echopraxia/echolalia	126	3	1	0	4
Stereotypy	104	19	6	1	26
Mannerisms	114	7	7	2	16
Verbigeration	99	17	12	2	31
Rigidity	115	13	2	0	15
Negativism	124	5	1	0	6
Waxy flexibility	130	0	0	0	0
Withdrawal	107	12	6	5	23
Impulsivity	99	13	18	0	31
Automatic obedience	121	4	5	0	9
Mitgehen	127	0	0	3	3
Gegenhalten	128	0	0	2	2
Ambitendency	127	0	0	3	3
Grasp reflex	130	0	0	0	0
Perseveration	98	0	0	32	32
Combativeness	112	15	2	1	18
Autonomic abnormality	116	13	1	0	14

mannerisms, and mitgehen; an echo/perseveration factor including echophenomena, verbigeration, and perseveration; an excitement factor encompassing items excitement, impulsivity, and combativeness; a grimacing factor only including that specific item, and finally, an autonomic factor including autonomic abnormalities and, strangely, automatic obedience. Composite scores based on this principal component analysis were calculated.

CLINICAL SYMPTOMATOLOGY

All patients completed the PANSS. Out of the total patient group, 88 (67.7%) had a PANSS-pos score higher than 14 reflecting a symptom state that was higher than dubious and 51 patients (39.2%) had at least mild psychotic symptomatology (i.e., a PANSS-pos score of 21 or higher). Similarly, all patients completed a YMRS: 29 patients (22.3%) had a score of 20 or higher, reflecting (hypo)manic symptomatology whereas only 34 patients (26.2%) had an absent of manic symptomatology (i.e., a maximum score of 6).

TO WHAT EXTENT IS THE CATATONIC SYMPTOMATOLOGY DETERMINED BY THE UNDERLYING DIAGNOSIS?

The total patient sample was divided in four groups: patients with a psychotic disorder ($n = 67$; 51.5%), patients with a mood disorder ($n = 22$; 16.9%; composed of 16 bipolar patients and 6 patients with a major depressive disorder), patients with a substance use disorder (SUD; $n = 14$; 10.8%), and patients with another diagnosis (patients-OD; $n = 27$; 20.8%).

Patients with a psychotic or mood disorder as a primary diagnosis had the most prominent catatonic symptom profiles (see **Figure 1**).

Compared to patients with a SUD or the patient-OD group psychotic patients tended to score higher on the stereotypy/mannerism symptom cluster (SUD: $p = 0.044$; patient-OD: $p = 0.076$), the negative symptom cluster (SUD: $p = 0.069$; patient-OD: $p = 0.121$), and on the excitement symptom cluster (SUD: $p = 0.021$; patient-OD: $p = 0.063$). No differences between the psychosis group and the combined mood disorder group could be seen. However, when only the bipolar patients entered analyses, these patients had significant more excitement symptoms ($p = 0.015$) than the patients with a psychotic illness, whereas, the latter group had significantly more excitement symptoms compared to the major depressive disorder group ($p = 0.029$). Very similar results were found after controlling for extrapyramidal symptomatology by use of the total score on the SAS. These results could mostly be explained by the fact that the SUD- and patient-OD groups hardly showed any catatonic symptomatology.

Psychotic symptomatology correlated strongly with excitement symptomatology ($r = 0.528$, $p < 0.001$) and to a lesser degree with the stereotypy/mannerisms symptom cluster ($r = 0.289$; $p = 0.001$) and the echo/perseveration symptom cluster ($r = 0.185$; $p = 0.035$). Similarly, manic symptomatology as assessed by the YMRS correlated strongly with the excitement symptom cluster ($r = 0.596$; $p < 0.001$) and to a lesser extent with the stereotypy/mannerisms symptom cluster ($r = 0.277$,

Table 3 | Factor analysis (principal component analysis), varimax rotation on the items of the BFCRS[a].

	Negative factor	**Stereotypy/mannerisms factor**	**Echo/perseveration factor**	**Excitement factor**	**Grimacing factor**	**Autonomic factor**
Excitement	−0,320	0,509	0,070	**0,442**	0,070	−0,156
Immobility/stupor	**0,836**	−0,06	0,096	−0,135	−0,019	−0,143
Mutism	**0,837**	0,013	−0,068	−0,069	0,047	−0,177
Staring	**0,790**	0,140	0,086	−0,111	0,055	0,105
Posturing/catalepsy	**0,900**	0,007	−0,038	−0,037	0,006	−0,094
Grimacing	−0,065	0,142	−0,046	0,180	**0,637**	−0,065
Echopraxia/echolalia	−0,092	−0,209	**0,756**	−0,066	0,204	−0,247
Stereotypy	−0,074	**0,830**	0,096	0,008	−0,026	−0,005
Mannerisms	0,139	**0,608**	−0,071	0,215	0,053	0,138
Verbigeration	0,109	0,188	0,727	0,070	−0,149	0,270
Rigidity	**0,777**	0,069	0,146	0,096	−0,034	0,183
Negativism	**0,663**	0,115	0,033	0,137	0,490	0,257
Withdrawal	**0,665**	−0,129	−0,199	0,004	−0,219	−0,103
Impulsivity	0,112	0,492	0,134	**0,399**	0,192	0,030
Automatic obedience	−0,047	0,068	0,010	0,154	−0,068	**0,714**
Mitgehen	0,075	**0,688**	−0,018	−0,403	0,270	−0,127
Gegenhalten	**0,678**	−0,016	0,164	0,280	−0,041	0,053
Ambitendency	**0,650**	0,223	0,004	−0,069	0,545	0,068
Perseveration	0,243	0,348	**0,560**	−0,036	−0,403	0,09
Combativeness	0,006	0,068	−0,050	**0,728**	0,147	−0,018
Autonomic Abnormality	−0,033	−0,109	0,042	−0,285	0,053	**0,660**

[a]Items waxy flexibility and grasp reflex were excluded from this analysis, because of the zero variance on these items. Composite scores based on this principal component analysis (symptoms scores in bold) were calculated.

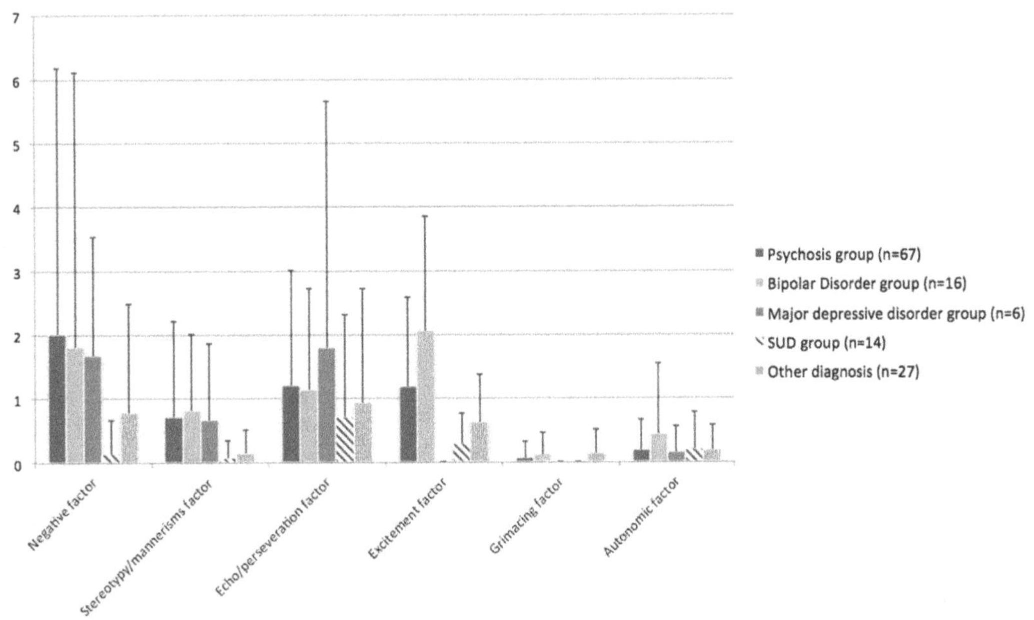

FIGURE 1 | Distribution of catatonic signs.

$p = 0.001$). It should be noted that the PANSS-pos subscale and the YMRS strongly intercorrelated ($r = 0.695$; $p < 0.011$), which undoubtedly confounded these results.

A PANSS-dep was calculated including items depression, anxiety, and guilt feelings. Kontaxakis and colleagues found this subscale to intercorrelate with the Hamilton Depression subscale (23).

PANSS-dep was inversely correlated with the grimacing factor ($r = -0.288$; $p = 0.001$) and tended toward an inversely correlation with the excitement factor ($r = -0.170$; $p = 0.054$), suggesting that depressive patients had these catatonic symptoms to a lesser degree than their non-depressed peers.

The total score on the SAS also correlated with the negative catatonia symptomatology ($r = 0.350$; $p < 0.001$) and with the echo/perseveration symptoms ($r = 0.318$; $p < 0.001$), which suggests that catatonic symptoms and extrapyramidal symptoms could not clearly be delineated from each other in our patient sample.

DISCUSSION

Out of the 130 patients that were admitted to an enclosed psychiatric ward, 101 patients (77.7%) had at least 1 symptom, whereas 66 patients (50.8%) had at least 2 symptoms when screened for catatonia symptoms, irrespective of the underlying diagnosis. In other words, catatonic symptomatology was highly prevalent in our patient population, although in most cases mildly. The most prevalent catatonic symptoms were excitement ($n = 49$; 37.7%), perseveration ($n = 32$; 24.6%), impulsivity ($n = 31$; 23.8%), and verbigeration ($n = 31$; 23.8%).

Our current findings demonstrate the presence of at least one symptom that is labeled as being catatonic by the BFCRS in most of the patients admitted to an enclosed psychiatric ward. In other studies, catatonia has been reported in 5–20% of acutely ill patients admitted to psychiatric units (9, 10, 18, 21, 24–26). In these studies, different criteria to diagnose catatonia were used, which renders a comparison between different studies on the prevalence of catatonia more difficult. For example, in the study of Lee, DSM-criteria were used to classify catatonia (24). When we used the latest DSM-criteria, only 16.9% of the patients ($n = 22$) could be considered as being catatonic. In the study of Ungvari, the diagnosis was made in the presence of four or more signs or symptoms with at least one having a score "2" or above on the BFCRS (26), which again, are more strict criteria than those used in our study. Fink and Taylor made their own diagnostic criteria with emphasis on the duration of the catatonic symptoms (22). Consequently, these divergent findings raise two interesting points. Depending on which criteria are being used, the more strict DSM-criteria versus the more liberal criteria suggested by Bush and colleagues (i.e., two items on the BFCRS), very different prevalence rates were found, which clearly emphasizes the shortcomings caused by a lack of clear-cut criteria (27). Of note, the DSM-5 criteria for catatonia appear to be even more strict than those of its predecessor, even if all 12 items, which were clustered in five categories in the DSM-IV can now be scored separately. This is mainly due to the fact that now three instead of two items have to be present. On the other hand, the high prevalence of symptoms using the BFCRS-criteria was mostly explained by the presence of mild symptomatology, whereas, more severe symptoms were present in a minority of our sample. Consequently, our results seem to point out that catatonic features, and more broadly psychomotor symptoms, may deserve a dimensional approach, much like cognitive symptoms associated with these psychiatric illnesses (27). It should also be noted that the most prevalent catatonic symptoms were not the strictly motor symptoms, which mostly seem associated with the traditional view on catatonia. Cognitive symptoms like perseveration and affective symptoms like excitement were the most prevalent and their validity and specificity as catatonic features should be questioned, especially in the more mild presentations. The unknown pathophysiology may contribute to the different views on catatonia. An unifying pathogenesis of catatonia that explains all motor, vegetative, and behavioral symptoms remains elusive. As a result, an unclear clinical concept of catatonia exists with the use of different diagnostical criteria and different rating scales to score catatonic symptomatology.

In our study, no significant differences in overall prevalence of catatonia between the psychosis group and the combined mood disorder group could be seen. Other studies also show that the syndrome is highly prevalent in both psychotic and mood disorders (17). Several studies found that the frequency of catatonia as part of schizophrenia varies with a range between 4 and 15% (5–8). Slightly higher prevalence rates have been shown in mood disorders with prevalence rates of 10–25% in bipolar disorder and up to 20% of patients with an unipolar depressive disorder (14–16, 22). However, again, different criteria for catatonia were used in these studies.

Different catatonia symptom profiles were found, depending on the underlying psychopathology. Psychotic patients tended to score higher on the stereotypy/mannerism symptom cluster, the negative symptom cluster, and the excitement symptom cluster compared to patients with a substance use disorder and patients with another diagnosis, but not compared to patients with mood disorders. In this line, psychotic symptomatology correlated strongly with excitement symptomatology and to a lesser degree with the stereotypy/mannerisms symptom cluster and the echo/perseveration symptom cluster. Similarly, manic symptomatology correlated strongly with the excitement symptom cluster and to a lesser extent with the stereotypy/mannerisms symptom cluster. Kraepelin already suggested that catatonia had a different symptomatology depending on the underlying pathology. Partly in line with our results, he described that negativism and mannerism were mainly associated to dementia praecox (4). Similarly, Schneider compared patients with catatonic (schizophrenic) and manic excitement, respectively and found that schizophrenic agitated patients displayed more blocking, waxy flexibility, stereotyped speech, mutism, and negativism (28). In a study of catatonic adolescents, automatic obedience and stereotypies were significantly more associated with schizophrenic than they were with non-schizophrenic catatonia (29). Finally, Krüger and colleagues found that catatonic chronic schizophrenia is mainly associated with catalepsy, waxy flexibility, and volitional disturbances such as automatic obedience and negativism, as well as mannerisms and abnormal involuntary movements such as grimacing, jerky movements, and stereotypies. In contrast, manic patients mainly displayed catatonic excitement, whereas, depressed patients were characterized by catatonic inhibition in terms of stupor, mutism, and rigidity (15). This was also in line with our findings, since symptoms of excitement and combativeness was significantly more present in the manic patients sample and significantly less in the depressed group, when compared to the psychotic patients sample.

Some limitations of our study should be pointed out. First, the impact of medication could be a confounding factor in our study.

A vast number of patients were taking benzodiazepines at the time of testing, which could have masked more severe presentations of the catatonic syndrome. Another limitation of the study is the lack of a depression scale. To overcome this limitation, we used the PANSS-dep but a dedicated depression scale would have been more elegant. Moreover, the sample size was rather small, especially in some subgroups. Larger scale trials are needed to replicate our findings.

In conclusion, there was a high prevalence of catatonic symptomatology. Remarkably, there is an important difference in exact prevalence depending on the criteria being used, which makes it clear that we need clear-cut criteria. Another important finding is the fact that the catatonic presentation may vary depending on the underlying pathology, although an unambiguous delineation between these catatonic presentations cannot be made. Future research is needed to determine diagnostical criteria of catatonia, which are clinically relevant.

AUTHOR CONTRIBUTION

All authors met ICMJE criteria and all those who fulfilled those criteria were listed as authors. All authors had access to the study data and made the final decision about where to present these data.

ACKNOWLEDGMENTS

The authors thank the study participants, without whom the study would never have been accomplished.

REFERENCES

1. Dhossche DM, Stoppelbein L, Rout UK. Etiopathogenesis of catatonia: generalizations and working hypotheses. *J ECT* (2010) **26**:253–8. doi:10.1097/YCT.0b013e3181fbf96d
2. Mahendra B. Where have all the catatonics gone? *Psychol Med* (1981) **11**:669–71. doi:10.1017/S0033291700041155
3. Bleuler E. *Dementia Praecox or Group of Schizophrenias* [1911]. New York, NY: International Universities Press (1950).
4. Kraepelin E. *Dementia Praecox and Paraphrenia*. Edinburgh: E&S Livingstone (1919). 331 p.
5. Deister A, Marneros A. Prognostic value of initial subtype in schizophrenic disorders. *Schizophr Res* (1994) **12**:145–57. doi:10.1016/0920-9964(94)90072-8
6. Ungvari GS, Leung SK, Ng FS, Cheung H-K, Leung T. Schizophrenia with prominent catatonic features ('catatonic schizophrenia'): I. Demographic and clinical correlates in the chronic phase. *Prog Neuropsychopharmacol Biol Psychiatry* (2005) **29**:27–38. doi:10.1016/j.pnpbp.2004.08.007
7. Beratis S, Gabriel J, Hoidas S. Age at onset in subtypes of schizophrenic disorders. *Schizophr Bull* (1994) **20**:287–96. doi:10.1093/schbul/20.2.287
8. Kleinhaus K, Harlap S, Perrin MC, Manor O, Weiser M, Harkavy-Friedman JM, et al. Catatonic schizophrenia: a cohort prospective study. *Schizophr Bull* (2012) **38**:331–7. doi:10.1093/schbul/sbq087
9. Fink M, Taylor MA. The catatonia syndrome. *Arch Gen Psychiatry* (2009) **66**:1173–7. doi:10.1001/archgenpsychiatry.2009.141
10. Van Harten PN. [Catatonia: a syndrome to be remembered]. *Tijdschr Psychiatr* (2005) **6**:371–82.
11. American Psychiatric Association. *Diagnostic and Statistical Manual of Mental Disorders, Fifth Edition*. Washington, DC: American Psychiatric Association (2013).
12. Pommepuy N, Januel D. [Catatonia: resurgence of a concept. A review of the international literature]. *Encephale* (2002) **28**:481–92.
13. Caroff SN, Mann SC, Francis A, Fricchione GL. *Catatonia. From Psychopathology to Neurobiology*. London: American Psychiatric Publishing (2004). 248 p.
14. Bräunig P, Krüger S, Shugar G. Prevalence and clinical significance of catatonic symptoms in mania. *Compr Psychiatry* (1998) **39**:35–46. doi:10.1016/S0010-440X(98)90030-X
15. Krüger S, Bagby RM, Höffler J, Bräunig P. Factor analysis of the catatonia rating scale and catatonic symptom distribution across four diagnostic groups. *Compr Psychiatry* (2003) **44**:472–82. doi:10.1016/S0010-440X(03)00108-1
16. Starkstein SE, Petracca G, Tesón A, Chemerinski E, Merello M, Migliorelli R, et al. Catatonia in depression: prevalence, clinical correlates, and validation of a scale. *J Neurol Neurosurg Psychiatry* (1996) **60**:326–32. doi:10.1136/jnnp.60.3.326
17. Usman DM, Olubunmi OA, Taiwo O, Taiwo A, Rahman L, Oladipo A. Comparison of catatonia presentation in patients with schizophrenia and mood disorders in Lagos, Nigeria. *Iran J Psychiatry* (2011) **6**:7–11.
18. Bush G, Fink M, Petrides G, Dowling F, Francis A. Catatonia. I. Rating scale and standardized examination. *Acta Psychiatr Scand* (1996) **93**:129–36. doi:10.1111/j.1600-0447.1996.tb09814.x
19. Kay SR, Fiszbein A, Opler LA. The positive and negative syndrome scale (PANSS) for schizophrenia. *Schizophr Bull* (1987) **13**:261–76. doi:10.1093/schbul/13.2.261
20. American Psychiatric Association. *Diagnostic and Statistical Manual of Mental Disorders, Fourth Edition*. Washington, DC: American Psychiatric Association (2000).
21. Fink M, Taylor MA. *Catatonia: A Clinician's Guide to Diagnosis and Treatment*. Cambridge: Cambridge University prEss (2003). 256 p.
22. Taylor MA, Fink M. Catatonia in psychiatric classification: a home of its own. *Am J Psychiatry* (2003) **160**:1233–41. doi:10.1176/appi.ajp.160.7.1233
23. Kontaxakis VP, Havaki-Kontaxaki BJ, Stamouli SS, Margariti MM, Collias CT, Christodoulou GN. Comparison of four scales measuring depression in schizophrenic inpatients. *Eur Psychiatry* (2000) **15**:274–7. doi:10.1016/S0924-9338(00)00232-7
24. Lee JW, Schwartz DL, Hallmayer J. Catatonia in a psychiatric intensive care facility: incidence and response to benzodiazepines. *Ann Clin Psychiatry* (2000) **12**:89–96. doi:10.3109/10401230009147094
25. Rosebush PI, Hildebrand AM, Furlong BG, Mazurek MF. Catatonic syndrome in a general psychiatric inpatient population: frequency, clinical presentation, and response to lorazepam. *J Clin Psychiatry* (1990) **51**:357–62.
26. Ungvari GS, Leung CM, Wong MK, Lau J. Benzodiazepines in the treatment of catatonic syndrome. *Acta Psychiatr Scand* (1994) **89**(4):285–8. doi:10.1111/j.1600-0447.1994.tb01515.x
27. Morrens M, Docx L, Walther S. Beyond boundaries: in search of an integrative view on motor symptoms in schizophrenia. *Front Psychiatry* (2014) **5**:145. doi:10.3389/fpsyt.2014.00145
28. Schneider K. Uber Wesen und Bedeutung katatonischer Symptome. *Zeitschrift fur die gesamte Neurol und Psychiatr* (1914) **22**:486–505. doi:10.1007/BF02869176
29. Cohen D, Nicolas JD, Flament MF, Périsse D, Dubos PF, Bonnot O, et al. Clinical relevance of chronic catatonic schizophrenia in children and adolescents: evidence from a prospective naturalistic study. *Schizophr Res* (2005) **76**:301–8. doi:10.1016/j.schres.2005.01.014

14

Physical activity in schizophrenia is higher in the first episode than in subsequent ones

Sebastian Walther*, Katharina Stegmayer, Helge Horn, Nadja Razavi, Thomas J. Müller and Werner Strik

University Hospital of Psychiatry, Bern, Switzerland

Edited by:
Mihaly Hajos, Yale University School of Medicine, USA

Reviewed by:
Manuel Morrens, University of Antwerp, Belgium
Fabian U. Lang, Ulm University, Germany

***Correspondence:**
Sebastian Walther, University Hospital of Psychiatry, Bolligenstrasse 111, Bern 60 3000, Switzerland
e-mail: walther@puk.unibe.ch

Schizophrenia is frequently associated with abnormal motor behavior, particularly hypokinesia. The course of the illness tends to deteriorate in the first years. We aimed to assess gross motor activity in patients with a first episode ($n = 33$) and multiple episodes ($n = 115$) of schizophrenia spectrum disorders using wrist actigraphy. First episode patients were younger, had higher motor activity and reduced negative symptom severity. Covarying for age, chlorpromazine equivalents, and negative symptoms, first episode patients still had higher motor activity. This was also true after excluding patients with schizophreniform disorder from the analyses. In first episode patients, but not in patients with multiple episodes, motor activity was correlated with antipsychotic dosage. In conclusion, after controlling for variables related to disorder chronicity, patients with first episodes were still more active than patients with multiple episodes. Thus, reduced motor activity is a marker of deterioration in the course of schizophrenia spectrum disorders.

Keywords: actigraphy, antipsychotic, negative symptoms, hypokinesia, psychosis

INTRODUCTION

The first episode is of particular interest to schizophrenia research because it allows assessing the clinical presentation in the absence of factors related to illness chronicity. Longitudinal studies have demonstrated a strong decline in function and quality of life during the first 2–5 years. Despite vast heterogeneity in illness course, the condition during initial episode has some predictive value (1).

Motor abnormalities are intrinsic to schizophrenia and have been reported throughout the whole course of the disorder irrespective of medication status (2–6). Particularly, psychomotor slowing impacts cognitive performance and outcome (7). Objective measures acquired with actigraphy have established hypokinesia in schizophrenia, which is correlated with negative symptom severity (8–10). However, objectively assessed gross motor activity has not been tested in first episode patients. Even though 67% of unmedicated first episode patients present with at least one motor sign (11), first episode patients tend to present with less or comparably severe negative symptoms as patients with multiple episodes (12, 13). Thus, the current study aimed to test whether physical activity as measured by wrist actigraphy would differ between first episode and multiple episode patients with schizophrenia spectrum disorders. Furthermore, we aimed to explore the association of physical activity with antipsychotic dosage and negative syndrome severity in both groups. We hypothesized that physical activity was higher in first episode patients compared to multiple episode patients, as functional decline often occurs within the early course of the disorder (1).

MATERIALS AND METHODS

PATIENTS

To explore differences between patients with a first vs. multiple episodes on physical activity, we pooled data from previous and ongoing studies applying actigraphy in schizophrenia spectrum disorders (9, 14–19). A total of 148 patients with schizophrenia spectrum disorders were included (first episode $n = 33$, multiple episodes $n = 115$). The patients with multiple episodes had on average 7.9 episodes (SD = 6.2). Diagnoses were given according to DSM-IV criteria after thorough clinical examination and review of all case files by board certified psychiatrists. The local mental health care system ensures that most of the patients are admitted to our clinic in every psychotic episode requiring inpatient treatment, allowing the collection of reliable diagnostic information. In a proportion of studies that contributed data to this analysis, the diagnoses were ascertained by structured clinical interviews such as SCID and MINI (27% of cases). Diagnoses given included paranoid schizophrenia (33% of first episode vs. 55% of multiple episode patients), catatonic schizophrenia (12 vs. 11%), disorganized schizophrenia (0 vs. 16%), schizoaffective disorder (6 vs. 5%), and schizophreniform disorder (49 vs. 13%) with significant differences between groups ($\chi^2 = 21.7, df = 1, p < 0.001$). Patients were excluded in case of substance abuse other than nicotine, medical conditions affecting physical activity, and epilepsy. Physical activity was recorded approximately 2 weeks after admission to the psychiatric department. At the same time, psychopathology was assessed using the positive and negative syndrome scale (PANSS) (20). Most patients were medicated (71% received atypical antipsychotics, 18% received mixed medication of typical and atypical antipsychotics, 6% received only typical antipsychotics, and 5% were medication-free at the time of our assessments). Chlorpromazine equivalents (CPZ) of the current antipsychotic pharmacotherapy were calculated according to Woods (21). In addition, diazepam equivalents (DE) were calculated according to Ashton (22). The protocols of the studies applying wrist actigraphy in schizophrenia spectrum disorders had been approved by the local ethics committee and participants provided written informed consent prior to study inclusion.

ACTIGRAPHY

Participants wore an actigraph (Actiwatch, Cambridge Neurotechnology, Inc., Cambridge, UK) for 24 consecutive hours at the wrist of the non-dominant arm. The piezoelectric sensor converts acceleration into movement counts. Data were sampled in 2 s intervals. Participants provided sleep log information and information on recording pauses (due to showering or bathing). Only the data collected during wakeful periods of the 24 h recording time were analyzed. Activity counts were averaged to provide the activity level (AL) in counts/h.

STATISTICAL ANALYSES

Demographic and clinical parameters were compared between groups by one-way ANOVAs and χ^2-tests. Since groups differed in the PANSS negative syndrome subscale score, age, and CPZ dosage, these variables were entered as covariates in an ANCOVA of AL. Furthermore, as the group of first episode patients included a large proportion of patients with schizophreniform disorder, we recalculated the ANCOVA excluding all patients with schizophreniform disorder. In order to test the additional effects of illness duration and benzodiazepine administration, we recalculated the ANCOVA first including duration of illness, negative symptoms, and CPZ as covariate and second including duration of illness, negative symptoms, CPZ, and DE as covariates. Furthermore, we compared AL in patients with different medication types (typical antipsychotics, atypical antipsychotics, and mixed medication). Next, clinical and demographic variables were correlated with AL for both groups separately. Because of the divergent results, we also calculated the interaction of CPZ and group on AL using an ANCOVA in the whole sample. Besides the classical PANSS subscores, we also tested the five PANSS factors according to van der Gaag and colleagues (23) (positive, negative, disorganization, excitement, and emotional distress), and the avolition score (sum of items N2 + N4) according to Bervoets et al. (24). All tests were performed with SPSS 21.

RESULTS

Gender distribution was not different between groups (first episode patients 61% male, multiple episode patients 57% male, $\chi^2 = 0.175$, df = 1, $p = 0.696$).

First episode patients had increased AL, were younger, received lower doses of antipsychotics and had a trend to reduced PANSS negative scores (see **Table 1**). Furthermore, first episode patients had reduced scores in the PANSS factors negative, disorganization, and excitement (23), as well as the PANSS avolition score (24).

The difference in AL between groups remained when adding the PANSS negative syndrome subscale score, age, and CPZ as covariates ($F = 6.2$, df = 4, $p < 0.001$, $\eta^2 = 0.15$). Furthermore, including duration of illness, negative symptoms, and CPZ as covariate did not substantially alter the results ($F = 4.53$; df = 4; $p = 0.002$; $\eta = 0.12$). Moreover, differences in AL between groups remained stable with the inclusion of duration of illness, negative symptoms, CPZ, and DE as covariates ($F = 4.23$; df = 5; $p = 0.001$; $\eta = 0.13$). Likewise, the difference in AL between groups remained when all subjects with schizophreniform disorder were excluded from the ANCOVA ($F = 4.2$, df = 4, $p = 0.003$, $\eta^2 = 0.13$) with the PANSS negative syndrome subscale score, age, and CPZ as covariates.

Table 1 | Clinical and demographic characteristics.

	First episode patients (*n* = 33)	Multiple episode patients (*n* = 115)	*F*-value	*p*-Value
Activity level (counts/h)	18057 (9194)	13551 (7047)	9.7	0.002
Age (years)	31.9 (12.5)	39.6 (11.2)	15.4	<0.001
Duration of illness (years)	1.7 (3.2)	12.7 (10.2)	30.9	<0.001
CPZ (mg)	360.2 (341.2)	530.5 (399.9)	3.9	0.049
DE (mg)	6.3 (10.5)	5.0 (10.1)	0.6	0.547
PANSS positive subscale	13.4 (4.6)	15.7 (5.6)	1.5	0.226
PANSS negative subscale	15.9 (6.5)	18.1 (6.2)	3.2	0.078
PANSS total score	61.1 (15.8)	68.7 (16.2)	5.5	0.020
PANSS avolition	4.0 (2.2)	5.0 (2.2)	5.3	0.022
PANSS factor positive	16.1 (7.1)	17.7 (6.6)	1.4	0.239
PANSS factor negative	15.2 (7.8)	18.3 (7.0)	4.6	0.033
PANSS factor disorganization	20.9 (5.7)	24.2 (6.6)	6.6	0.011
PANSS factor excitement	13.2 (3.9)	15.4 (5.3)	5.1	0.026
PANSS factor emotional distress	14.7 (6.1)	16.0 (5.5)	1.4	0.242

Numbers are given as mean (SD).

Finally, AL did not differ between groups with distinct antipsychotic medication (typical, atypical antipsychotics, and mixed medication) ($F = 0.96$; df = 2; $p = 0.386$; $\eta = 0.01$).

Correlations between AL and clinical parameters are given in **Table 2**. Associations with measures of the negative syndrome were more dominant in the patients with multiple episodes. Groups differed in the correlation of CPZ and AL, with significant effects in first episode patients and no effects in patients with multiple episodes (ANCOVA of AL with intercept between CPZ and group $F = 11.3$, df = 1, $p < 0.001$, $\eta^2 = 0.07$).

DISCUSSION

In the present study, we were able to demonstrate that patients in a first episode of schizophrenia spectrum disorders have higher physical activity than patients with multiple episodes. This result held true after controlling for negative symptoms, age, dosage of antipsychotics, and administration of benzodiazepines. Furthermore, it was still evident after excluding patients with schizophreniform disorder. Thus, we are confident that there is a true difference in physical activity between the groups beyond other major differences that are related to illness duration. Of course, the magnitude of the effect was small to medium in size as there are also other factors contributing to physical activity besides age, chronicity, and negative symptoms, such as lifestyle habits and physical constitution. Still, the mean AL value of the first episode

Table 2 | Correlation between activity level and clinical parameters.

	First episode patients		Multiple episode patients	
	r	*p*	*r*	*p*
Age	−0.21	0.251	−0.19	0.038
CPZ	−0.46	0.008	0.08	0.411
DE	−0.03	0.893	−0.29	0.002
PANSS positive syndrome score	0.07	0.698	0.13	0.163
PANSS negative syndrome score	−0.02	0.910	−0.29	0.001
PANSS total score	−0.07	0.708	−0.17	0.070
PANSS avolition factor	−0.38	0.031	−0.29	0.002
PANSS positive factor	−0.05	0.784	−0.01	0.897
PANSS negative factor	−0.33	0.064	−0.32	<0.001
PANSS disorganization factor	0.32	0.073	−0.08	0.399
PANSS excitement factor	−0.04	0.835	−0.08	0.418
PANSS emotional distress factor	−0.05	0.800	−0.13	0.183

patients is close to the mean of AL reported in different samples of healthy controls, e.g., 18000–21000 counts/h (8, 15, 25). Furthermore, subjects at ultra high risk for psychosis were shown to have reduced ALs at trend level compared to matched controls (26). Thus, even though the AL of first episode patients might still be slightly reduced compared to age matched controls, AL appear comparable to those of healthy control groups with wider age ranges. Our finding is in line with the observation that motor abnormalities are present from the first episode of schizophrenia spectrum disorders but tend to deteriorate with the progression of the disorder (2, 5). Likewise, neurocognitive measures of fine motor performance have indicated impairments in first episode patients and even more in chronic patients (27). However, it remains unknown, which factors drive the reduction of physical activity in patients with multiple episodes. Clearly, negative symptoms are related to reduced physical activity (8–10). In addition, the use of catatonia rating scales such as the modified Rogers scale (28) indicated that the frequency of the item "marked underactivity" was increased in a mixed sample of schizophrenia spectrum disorder patients as compared to first episode patients (28 vs. 9%) (11, 29). In general, motor abnormalities are prevalent in the early course but increase in frequency with multiple episodes. In many instances, it is hard to disentangle the multiple causes of hypokinesia, such as catatonia, parkinsonism, or reduced volition, i.e., negative symptoms (2). If reduction of physical activity was an indicator of deterioration, it would well fit in the observation of clinical deterioration within the first 2–5 years after the onset of schizophrenia spectrum disorders (1). First evidence suggests that hypokinesia due to parkinsonism in first episode patients was predictive of poor cognitive function after 6 months (30). However, schizophrenia presents with a heterogeneous longitudinal course and deterioration of symptoms is not everyone's fate (31).

Another important finding of the present study is the interaction of antipsychotic dosage and group on AL. Whereas, in multiple episode patients, we were unable to find a correlation of AL and CPZ, increased antipsychotic dosage was related to lower AL in first episode patients. Here, we may speculate that in first episode patients in the absence of marked negative symptoms, parkinsonism, or catatonia, antipsychotic agents may exert more impact on the overall motor activity. However, this view is partly challenged by the fact that antipsychotic agents ameliorate most psychomotor impairments in previously naïve first episode patients, including hypokinesia, parkinsonism, and catatonia (11). Still, the various antipsychotic agents currently used may exert differential effects on physical activity or spontaneous, i.e., preexisting motor symptoms. So far, only few reports exist investigating the effect of different antipsychotic agents on motor behavior in previously unmedicated subjects (32). However, we found no differences of AL in patients with different medication types (typical, atypical antipsychotics, and mixed medication).

In line with previous reports, reduced motor activity was associated with negative symptoms in both first episode and chronic schizophrenia spectrum disorders (8, 9). Also, reduced tongue movements were demonstrated to correlate with negative symptoms in first episode patients (33). Likewise, hypokinesia was associated with negative symptoms in first episode patients (11). In chronic schizophrenia, various measures of hypokinesia have demonstrated correlations with negative symptom severity, particularly the initiation of movements seems affected (2, 24, 29, 34, 35). As in one previous report, the avolition component of the negative syndrome displayed strongest correlations with spontaneous motor activity (8). Thus, our data support the assumption that actigraphy may particularly well suited to assess motivational aspects of the negative syndrome. Finally, exercise interventions have regained interest in schizophrenia targeting various problems of these patients, such as metabolic, cognitive, and social problems (36). First controlled studies reported positive effects of exercise interventions on negative symptoms and working memory in schizophrenia (37).

This study has some limitations requiring discussion. We have used data from a database to answer the research question. The methods of actigraphy and PANSS assessment were the common ground. If we had to conduct a new study on this topic, we would include more standardized measures of motor function focusing on parkinsonism and catatonia. Parkinsonism and catatonia may have influenced AL (2, 38). However, both symptoms are frequently present in patients with a first psychotic episode and in patients with multiple episodes (11). Still, these symptoms might be more frequent in patients with a chronic course of the disease (14). However, treatment with antipsychotics shows a heterogeneous effect on parkinsonism and catatonia in previously antipsychotic naïve patients: in some patients, these symptoms are ameliorated by treatment, in others they tend to emerge or deteriorate during pharmacotherapy, while in a third group symptoms remain unchanged with antipsychotic medication (32). In addition, there are better scales to assess negative symptoms (39). Still, the PANSS is a commonly used instrument, which aids data interpretation. Finally, we did not measure depressive symptoms, even though, depression might affect ALs. Patients with major depression move less than healthy controls (40). Still, in a previous investigation, we found only weak associations in major depressed patients between depression severity as assessed by the Hamilton depression rating scale (HAMD) and AL (41). However, taking the emotional dysregulation factor according to van der Gaag (23) as a substitute parameter for depression, we failed to identify correlations with AL in any of the two groups.

In conclusion, we demonstrated that first episode patients have higher physical activity than patients with multiple episodes. The finding underlines that functional deterioration including reduced motor activity frequently occurs beyond the first episode. Thus, future studies should evaluate whether this reduction may be targeted by pharmacotherapy or specialized programs to promote physical exercise in schizophrenia (36, 42).

AUTHOR CONTRIBUTIONS

Dr. Sebastian Walther and Dr. Helge Horn designed the study. Dr. Sebastian Walther wrote the protocol. Drs. Nadja Razavi, Katharina Stegmayer, and Sebastian Walther recruited participants and performed assessments. Dr. Sebastian Walther performed the data analyses. All authors interpreted and discussed the findings. Dr. Sebastian Walther wrote the first draft of the manuscript. All authors contributed to the final version of the manuscript.

ACKNOWLEDGMENTS

Parts of this study received funding from the Bangerter-Rhyner Foundation (to Dr. Sebastian Walther) and the Swiss National Science Foundation (SNF grant 152619/1 to Dr. Sebastian Walther).

REFERENCES

1. McGlashan TH. Duration of untreated psychosis in first-episode schizophrenia: marker or determinant of course? *Biol Psychiatry* (1999) **46**(7):899–907. doi:10.1016/S0006-3223(99)00084-0
2. Walther S, Strik W. Motor symptoms and schizophrenia. *Neuropsychobiology* (2012) **66**(2):77–92. doi:10.1159/000339456
3. Wolff AL, O'Driscoll GA. Motor deficits and schizophrenia: the evidence from neuroleptic-naive patients and populations at risk. *J Psychiatry Neurosci* (1999) **24**(4):304–14.
4. Pappa S, Dazzan P. Spontaneous movement disorders in antipsychotic-naive patients with first-episode psychoses: a systematic review. *Psychol Med* (2009) **39**(7):1065–76. doi:10.1017/S0033291708004716
5. Whitty PF, Owoeye O, Waddington JL. Neurological signs and involuntary movements in schizophrenia: intrinsic to and informative on systems pathobiology. *Schizophr Bull* (2009) **35**(2):415–24. doi:10.1093/schbul/sbn126
6. Koning JP, Tenback DE, van Os J, Aleman A, Kahn RS, van Harten PN. Dyskinesia and parkinsonism in antipsychotic-naive patients with schizophrenia, first-degree relatives and healthy controls: a meta-analysis. *Schizophr Bull* (2010) **36**(4):723–31. doi:10.1093/schbul/sbn146
7. Morrens M, Hulstijn W, Sabbe B. Psychomotor slowing in schizophrenia. *Schizophr Bull* (2007) **33**(4):1038–53. doi:10.1093/schbul/sbl051
8. Docx L, Sabbe B, Provinciael P, Merckx N, Morrens M. Quantitative psychomotor dysfunction in schizophrenia: a loss of drive, impaired movement execution or both? *Neuropsychobiology* (2013) **68**(4):221–7. doi:10.1159/000355293
9. Walther S, Koschorke P, Horn H, Strik W. Objectively measured motor activity in schizophrenia challenges the validity of expert ratings. *Psychiatry Res* (2009) **169**(3):187–90. doi:10.1016/j.psychres.2008.06.020
10. Wichniak A, Skowerska A, Chojnacka-Wojtowicz J, Taflinski T, Wierzbicka A, Jernajczyk W, et al. Actigraphic monitoring of activity and rest in schizophrenic patients treated with olanzapine or risperidone. *J Psychiatr Res* (2011) **45**(10):1381–6. doi:10.1016/j.jpsychires.2011.05.009
11. Peralta V, Campos MS, De Jalon EG, Cuesta MJ. Motor behavior abnormalities in drug-naive patients with schizophrenia spectrum disorders. *Mov Disord* (2010) **25**(8):1068–76. doi:10.1002/mds.23050
12. Zhang XY, Chen da C, Xiu MH, Yang FD, Haile CN, Kosten TA, et al. Gender differences in never-medicated first-episode schizophrenia and medicated chronic schizophrenia patients. *J Clin Psychiatry* (2012) **73**(7):1025–33. doi:10.4088/JCP.11m07422
13. Vohs JL, Lysaker PH, Francis MM, Hamm J, Buck KD, Olesek K, et al. Metacognition, social cognition, and symptoms in patients with first episode and prolonged psychoses. *Schizophr Res* (2014) **153**(1–3):54–9. doi:10.1016/j.schres.2014.01.012
14. Bracht T, Heidemeyer K, Koschorke P, Horn H, Razavi N, Wopfner A, et al. Comparison of objectively measured motor behavior with ratings of the motor behavior domain of the Bern psychopathology scale (BPS) in schizophrenia. *Psychiatry Res* (2012) **198**(2):224–9. doi:10.1016/j.psychres.2011.12.038
15. Walther S, Federspiel A, Horn H, Razavi N, Wiest R, Dierks T, et al. Alterations of white matter integrity related to motor activity in schizophrenia. *Neurobiol Dis* (2011) **42**(3):276–83. doi:10.1016/j.nbd.2011.01.017
16. Walther S, Horn H, Razavi N, Koschorke P, Muller TJ, Strik W. Quantitative motor activity differentiates schizophrenia subtypes. *Neuropsychobiology* (2009) **60**(2):80–6. doi:10.1159/000236448
17. Walther S, Horn H, Razavi N, Koschorke P, Wopfner A, Muller TJ, et al. Higher motor activity in schizophrenia patients treated with olanzapine versus risperidone. *J Clin Psychopharmacol* (2010) **30**(2):181–4. doi:10.1097/JCP.0b013e3181d2ef6f
18. Walther S, Ramseyer F, Horn H, Strik W, Tschacher W. Less structured movement patterns predict severity of positive syndrome, excitement, and disorganization. *Schizophr Bull* (2014) **40**(3):585–91. doi:10.1093/schbul/sbt038
19. Walther S, Vanbellingen T, Muri R, Strik W, Bohlhalter S. Impaired pantomime in schizophrenia: association with frontal lobe function. *Cortex* (2013) **49**(2):520–7. doi:10.1016/j.cortex.2011.12.008
20. Kay SR, Fiszbein A, Opler LA. The positive and negative syndrome scale (PANSS) for schizophrenia. *Schizophr Bull* (1987) **13**(2):261–76. doi:10.1093/schbul/13.2.261
21. Woods SW. Chlorpromazine equivalent doses for the newer atypical antipsychotics. *J Clin Psychiatry* (2003) **64**(6):663–7. doi:10.4088/JCP.v64n0607
22. Ashton H. Toxicity and adverse consequences of benzodiazepine use. *Psychiatr Ann* (1995) **25**(3):158–65. doi:10.3928/0048-5713-19950301-09
23. van der Gaag M, Hoffman T, Remijsen M, Hijman R, de Haan L, van Meijel B, et al. The five-factor model of the positive and negative syndrome scale II: a ten-fold cross-validation of a revised model. *Schizophr Res* (2006) **85**(1–3):280–7. doi:10.1016/j.schres.2006.03.021
24. Bervoets C, Docx L, Sabbe B, Vermeylen S, Van Den Bossche MJ, Morsel A, et al. The nature of the relationship of psychomotor slowing with negative symptomatology in schizophrenia. *Cogn Neuropsychiatry* (2014) **19**(1):36–46. doi:10.1080/13546805.2013.779578
25. Walther S, Hugli S, Hofle O, Federspiel A, Horn H, Bracht T, et al. Frontal white matter integrity is related to psychomotor retardation in major depression. *Neurobiol Dis* (2012) **47**(1):13–9. doi:10.1016/j.nbd.2012.03.019
26. Mittal VA, Gupta T, Orr JM, Pelletier-Baldelli A, Dean DJ, Lunsford-Avery JR, et al. Physical activity level and medial temporal health in youth at ultra high-risk for psychosis. *J Abnorm Psychol* (2013) **122**(4):1101–10. doi:10.1037/a0034085
27. Mesholam-Gately RI, Giuliano AJ, Goff KP, Faraone SV, Seidman LJ. Neurocognition in first-episode schizophrenia: a meta-analytic review. *Neuropsychology* (2009) **23**(3):315–36. doi:10.1037/a0014708
28. Lund CE, Mortimer AM, Rogers D, McKenna PJ. Motor, volitional and behavioural disorders in schizophrenia. 1: assessment using the modified Rogers scale. *Br J Psychiatry* (1991) **158**(323–7):33–6. doi:10.1192/bjp.158.3.323
29. Peralta V, Cuesta MJ. Motor features in psychotic disorders. I factor structure and clinical correlates. *Schizophr Res* (2001) **47**(2–3):107–16. doi:10.1016/S0920-9964(00)00035-9
30. Cuesta MJ, Sanchez-Torres AM, de Jalon EG, Campos MS, Ibanez B, Moreno-Izco L, et al. Spontaneous parkinsonism is associated with cognitive impairment in antipsychotic-naive patients with first-episode psychosis: a 6-month follow-up study. *Schizophr Bull* (2014) **40**(5):1164–73. doi:10.1093/schbul/sbt125
31. Lang FU, Kosters M, Lang S, Becker T, Jager M. Psychopathological long-term outcome of schizophrenia – a review. *Acta Psychiatr Scand* (2013) **127**(3):173–82. doi:10.1111/acps.12030
32. Peralta V, Cuesta MJ. The effect of antipsychotic medication on neuromotor abnormalities in neuroleptic-naive nonaffective psychotic patients: a naturalistic study with haloperidol, risperidone, or olanzapine. *Prim Care Companion J Clin Psychiatry* (2010) **12**(2):e1–11. doi:10.4088/PCC.09m00799gry
33. Covington MA, Lunden SL, Cristofaro SL, Wan CR, Bailey CT, Broussard B, et al. Phonetic measures of reduced tongue movement correlate

with negative symptom severity in hospitalized patients with first-episode schizophrenia-spectrum disorders. *Schizophr Res* (2012) **142**(1–3):93–5. doi:10.1016/j.schres.2012.10.005

34. Docx L, Morrens M, Bervoets C, Hulstijn W, Fransen E, De Hert M, et al. Parsing the components of the psychomotor syndrome in schizophrenia. *Acta Psychiatr Scand* (2012) **126**(4):256–65. doi:10.1111/j.1600-0447.2012.01846.x
35. Ungvari GS, Leung SK, Ng FS, Cheung HK, Leung T. Schizophrenia with prominent catatonic features ('catatonic schizophrenia'): I. demographic and clinical correlates in the chronic phase. *Prog Neuropsychopharmacol Biol Psychiatry* (2005) **29**(1):27–38. doi:10.1016/j.pnpbp.2004.08.007
36. Malchow B, Reich-Erkelenz D, Oertel-Knochel V, Keller K, Hasan A, Schmitt A, et al. The effects of physical exercise in schizophrenia and affective disorders. *Eur Arch Psychiatry Clin Neurosci* (2013) **263**(6):451–67. doi:10.1007/s00406-013-0423-2
37. Oertel-Knochel V, Mehler P, Thiel C, Steinbrecher K, Malchow B, Tesky V, et al. Effects of aerobic exercise on cognitive performance and individual psychopathology in depressive and schizophrenia patients. *Eur Arch Psychiatry Clin Neurosci* (2014) **264**(7):589–604. doi:10.1007/s00406-014-0485-9
38. Morrens M, Docx L, Walther S. Beyond boundaries: in search of an integrative view on motor symptoms in schizophrenia. *Front Psychiatry* (2014) **5**:145. doi:10.3389/fpsyt.2014.00145
39. Kaiser S, Heekeren K, Simon JJ. The negative symptoms of schizophrenia: category or continuum? *Psychopathology* (2011) **44**(6):345–53. doi:10.1159/000325912
40. Walther S, Hofle O, Federspiel A, Horn H, Hugli S, Wiest R, et al. Neural correlates of disbalanced motor control in major depression. *J Affect Disord* (2012) **136**(1–2):124–33. doi:10.1016/j.jad.2011.08.020
41. Razavi N, Horn H, Koschorke P, Hugli S, Hofle O, Muller T, et al. Measuring motor activity in major depression: the association between the Hamilton depression rating scale and actigraphy. *Psychiatry Res* (2011) **190**(2–3):212–6. doi:10.1016/j.psychres.2011.05.028
42. Vancampfort D, Probst M, Sweers K, Maurissen K, Knapen J, De Hert M. Relationships between obesity, functional exercise capacity, physical activity participation and physical self-perception in people with schizophrenia. *Acta Psychiatr Scand* (2011) **123**(6):423–30. doi:10.1111/j.1600-0447.2010.01666.x

15

Psychosocial vulnerabilities to depression after acute coronary syndrome: the pivotal role of rumination in predicting and maintaining depression

Ellen-ge D. Denton[1]*, Nina Rieckmann[2], Karina W. Davidson[1] and William F. Chaplin[3]

[1] Department of Medicine, Columbia University Medical Center, New York, NY, USA
[2] Berlin School of Public Health, Charité Universitätsmedizin Berlin, Berlin, Germany
[3] Department of Psychology, St. John's University, Jamaica, NY, USA

Edited by:
Gian Mauro Manzoni, Istituto Auxologico Italiano IRCCS, Italy

Reviewed by:
Brandon Abbs, Partners Healthcare, USA
Angelo Compare, University of Bergamo, Italy

***Correspondence:**
Ellen-ge D. Denton, Department of Medicine, Columbia University College of Physicians and Surgeons, Room 309, PH9 West Wing, 622W 168th Street, New York, NY 10032, USA.
e-mail: ed2426@columbia.edu

Psychosocial vulnerabilities may predispose individuals to develop depression after a significant life stressor, such as an acute coronary syndrome (ACS). The aims are (1) to examine the interrelations among vulnerabilities, and their relation with changes in depressive symptoms 3 months after ACS, (2) to prospectively assess whether rumination interacts with other vulnerabilities as a predictor of later depressive symptoms, and (3) to examine how these relations differ between post-ACS patients who meet diagnostic criteria for depression at baseline versus patients who do not. Within 1 week after hospitalization for ACS, and again after 3 months, 387 patients (41% female, 79.6% white, mean age 61) completed the Beck Depression Inventory (BDI) and measures of vulnerabilities (lack of pleasant events, dysfunctional attitudes, role transitions, poor dyadic adjustment). Exclusion criteria were a BDI score of 5–9, terminal illness, active substance abuse, cognitive impairment, and unavailability for follow-up visits. We used hierarchical regression modeling cross-sectionally and longitudinally. Controlling for baseline (in-hospital) depression and cardiovascular disease severity, vulnerabilities significantly predicted 3 month depression severity. Rumination independently predicted increased depression severity, above other vulnerabilities ($\beta = 0.75$, $p < 0.001$), and also interacted with poor dyadic adjustment ($\beta = 0.32$, $p < 0.001$) to amplify depression severity. Among initially non-depressed patients, the effects of vulnerabilities were amplified by rumination. In contrast, in patients who were already depressed at baseline, there was a direct effect of rumination above vulnerabilities on depression severity. Although all vulnerabilities predict depression 3 months after an ACS event has occurred rumination plays a key role to amplify the impact of vulnerabilities on depression among the initially non-depressed, and maintains depression among those who are already depressed.

Keywords: psychosocial vulnerabilities, post-ACS, depression, rumination, cardiovascular disease

INTRODUCTION

In patients who have experienced an acute coronary syndrome (ACS), the risk of a major adverse cardiac event (MACE) recurrence and mortality is associated with depression (Carney et al., 2003; McGee et al., 2006; Lange and Herrmann-Lingen, 2007; Parker et al., 2008; Davidson et al., 2010; Denollet et al., 2010; Compare et al., 2011). Psychosocial vulnerabilities may predispose individuals to develop depression after a significant life stressor, such as an ACS. Previous studies have identified personality types, cognitive, interpersonal, and behavioral stressors that are related to elevated depressive symptoms after a cardiac event (Rieckmann et al., 2006; Denollet and Kupper, 2007; Gulliksson et al., 2007; Stafford et al., 2008). Grounded in the diathesis stress model, psychosocial vulnerabilities are thought to be stable person characteristics and social contexts that predispose persons to be more or less vulnerable to depression. Previous studies have identified behavioral (e.g., lack of pleasant events), interpersonal (e.g., lack of social support and attachments), and cognitive (e.g., maladaptive cognitions) vulnerabilities as correlates of depression symptoms among ACS patients (Contrada et al., 2008; Stafford et al., 2008). Rieckmann et al. (2006) showed that these vulnerabilities were independently associated with depressive status immediately after an ACS. Importantly, the vulnerabilities were only mildly to moderately correlated, and a substantial number of patients with elevated depressive symptoms had *no* psychosocial vulnerability, suggesting that the vulnerabilities were not merely the "products" of current depressive symptomatology. This finding has since been replicated using a cross-sectional design (Doyle et al., 2011). However, it is not clear whether vulnerabilities exacerbate depressive symptoms over time, or whether depressive symptoms in turn negatively impact vulnerabilities over time. Previous studies have considered the cross-sectional relations between psychosocial vulnerabilities and depression among cardiac patients (Rieckmann et al., 2006; Oxlad and Wade, 2008; Pedersen et al., 2008; Larsen and Christenfeld, 2009). However, longitudinal studies are lacking. Episodes of depression are typically relapsing/recurring and the cause of depression episodes is multifactorial (Naqvi et al., 2007; van Gestel et al., 2007). Likewise, psychosocial vulnerabilities vary and covary on a continuum throughout a lifetime (Harris, 2001; Birmaher et al., 2004; O'Sullivan, 2004; Hankin et al., 2009). The associations between psychosocial vulnerabilities and depression are not well understood for patients with cardiovascular disease and can be best understood with a prospective study.

Theories seeking to explain the role of rumination for patients with cardiovascular risk suggest that a "perseverative cognition" or rumination is associated with decreased parasympathetic activity and prolonged sympathetic activation, and thus may be the key vulnerability for explaining the underlying pathophysiology of depressive disorder and CVD risk (Brosschot et al., 2006). Nolen-Hoeksema defines rumination as the tendency to think repetitively and passively about negative emotions, focusing on symptoms of distress (Berkman et al., 2003; Brosschot et al., 2006). Ruminative responses to depressed mood involve repetitively focusing on the fact that one is depressed: on one's symptoms of depression; and on the causes, meanings, and consequences of depressive symptoms. Moreover, rumination in response to first and/or lifetime major events is not uncommon (Garnefski et al., 2003; Enns and Cox, 2005; Grant and Beck, 2010; McIntosh et al., 2010). Rumination also impairs social relations and activities (Lam et al., 2003). Ciesla and Roberts (2002) found that rumination exacerbates cognitive factors to depression. We propose to test if rumination is an independent psychosocial vulnerability for depression, and/or an amplifier of other depression vulnerabilities, predicting future depression severity, in patients with cardiovascular disease.

Though studies have evaluated psychosocial predictors of depression in cardiac patients, no study has assessed rumination as a potential predictor of later depression among ACS patients. Additionally, there are no prospective studies assessing the impact of psychosocial depression vulnerabilities after an ACS on continuing depression. Therefore the aims of this research are to (1) evaluate the interplay between depression vulnerabilities, including rumination 3 months after an ACS, (2) to predict future depressive symptoms with vulnerabilities, rumination, and their interactions, when controlling for cross-sectional associations, and (3) to compare the associations of depression vulnerabilities and rumination with future depressive symptom severity in initially depressed and non-depressed Post-ACS patients.

We propose to examine the interplay between psychosocial vulnerability and depression for cardiovascular disease patients, using two different statistical approaches. We use cross-lagged correlation analysis and depressed group versus non-depressed group comparisons to investigate the complex associations that can occur between psychosocial vulnerability and depression disease onset and maintenance. Examination of cross-lagged paths, which contain both cross-sectional and longitudinal observational analyses, allows some possible causal pathways to be ruled out, and others to be further considered in future trials or interventions. For example, if elevated depressive symptoms only longitudinally predict rumination, when first controlling for their cross-sectional association, then future studies could determine if decreasing depression decreases rumination. However, if in this same analysis we discovered that rumination does not predict later increased depression (again, controlling for their cross-sectional analysis) then we need not design rumination interventions, hoping this would improve depression. We therefore use cross-lagged correlations to examine and rule out possible causal links among psychosocial vulnerabilities and depression. We contrast the possible casual pathways to depression between the initially depressed and non-depressed patient groups. In this subgroup analysis we can observe if trait-like vulnerabilities cause and/or exacerbate the depression severity for some individuals and not others. Thus, we target the individuals who are prone to specific psychosocial vulnerabilities that potentially play a causal role in their depression symptoms versus individuals whose psychosocial vulnerabilities may prevent them from recovery.

MATERIALS AND METHODS

The Coronary Psychosocial Evaluation Study (COPES) is a set of three studies, one of which is an observational cohort that included 457 patients; average age of 61 years old who had a recent ACS. The baseline analyses are based on all 457 patients. However, 55 patients died, were re-hospitalized, or could not be found at 3 month follow-up and 15 patients did not answer enough items to justify a regression-based approach to impute their total scores from the subset of answered items, thus, the sample size for the 3 month and longitudinal analyses is 387 (85% of the initial sample).

PROCEDURE

Patients were recruited on the coronary care and cardiac care step-down units of three hospitals in New York City, NY, USA, New Jersey, and New Haven, CT, USA, between May 2003 and March 2004. The institutional review boards of each hospital approved the study and informed consent was obtained from every patient. Patients were eligible if they met the criteria for ACS (either acute MI with or without ST-segment elevation or unstable angina with documented existing coronary artery disease) verified by the study cardiologists and had scores on the Beck Depression Inventory BDI-I (Beck et al., 1961) of either 0–4 (indicating minimal depressive symptoms), or ≥ 10 (indicating at least mild depressive symptoms), assessed within 1 week after the index ACS event. Exclusion criteria were terminal illness (life expectancy <1 year), cognitive impairment, substance abuse, and unavailability for follow-up.

After enrollment, a short medical exam was conducted, and patients completed questionnaires and interviews assessing psychosocial vulnerabilities within 7 days of the hospitalization. For Spanish-speaking patients, Spanish versions of the measures were used (see Rieckmann et al., 2006). Upon 3 month follow-up, patients were given a follow-up exam, the BDI-I, and again completed all measures of psychosocial vulnerabilities.

MEASURES

Depressive symptoms

The 21 item BDI-I (Beck et al., 1961) was administered to all patients, as a measure of depression severity. Patients' responses were measured using a 4 point scale (0–3). Scores were aggregated, with higher scores indicative of elevated depression symptom severity. The BDI had good internal consistency in the present sample (Cronbach alpha = 0.91).

Cognitive vulnerability

Using the 24 item Dysfunctional Attitude Scale [DAS-24] (Power et al., 1994), we assessed maladaptive cognitive schemata. The scale measures attitudes or beliefs that represent distorted cognitive styles (i.e., "if I fail partly, it is as bad as being a complete failure"). Responses ranged from 1 (totally disagree) to 7 (totally agree). Higher scores indicate higher levels of dysfunctional attitudes. The internal consistency of the DAS at baseline and 3 month follow-up was 0.83 and 0.85, respectively.

Behavioral vulnerability

The 20 item short version of the Pleasant Events Schedule for the Elderly (PES-E; Teri and Lewinsohn, 1982) was administered to assess the lack of pleasant events or behavioral vulnerability, according to patient report. Patients reported their frequency of engaging in 20 pleasant events. Scores were recoded so that higher mean scores on this scale represented increased *in*frequency of pleasant events. The internal consistency of the PES at baseline and 3 month follow-up was 0.82 and 0.84, respectively.

Interpersonal vulnerability

Interpersonal vulnerability was assessed using two different measures. The Role Transitions scale (Markowitz et al., 2000) listed six life changing events, and asked patients to indicate whether they had experienced any of these events within the past year. Items were summed to assess the total number of role transitions, with more role transitions indicative of increased interpersonal vulnerability. Role Transitions were not stable across time (as would be expected) with a test-re-test reliability across 3 months of 0.39 ($p < 0.001$).

Patients were also administered the 15 item Dyadic Adjustment Scale (Spanier, 1976), which was not comprised of multiple item responses. Patients were asked to name (1) one person closest to them and (2) to rate the extent they agree or disagree with them on 15 important issues (i.e., handling finances, household tasks, career decisions, etc.). Patient responses ranged from 1 (always disagree) to 6 (always agree). Scores were recoded so that higher scores represent higher disagreement (i.e., poorer dyadic adjustment). Test-re-test reliability was 0.55.

Rumination

The short ruminative responses scale (Treynor et al., 2003) was administered to each patient. This scale is comprised of two subscales: Reflection (five items) and Brooding (five items). Examples of Rumination Reflection include: "I analyze recent events to understand why I am depressed" or "I write down what I am thinking and analyze it" and Rumination Brooding: "I think, what am I doing to deserve this?" or " I think, why can't I handle things better?" Patients rated their ruminative behavior using a 4-point scale, (1) never to (4) always. Higher scores indicated more rumination. The internal consistency for rumination brooding at baseline was 0.84 and 0.87 at 3 months. The internal consistency for rumination reflection at baseline was 0.77 and 0.81 at 3 months.

COVARIATES

Charlson comorbidity index

Patients were assessed using a weighted index of 22 medical conditions (Charlson et al., 1987). The score ranges from 0 to 37; the higher the score, the more the number of and severities of their co-morbid diseases.

Left ventricular ejection fraction

We used left ventricular ejection fraction (LVEF) as a measure of cardiac disease severity. Patients' LVEF was obtained from cardiac diagnostic and intervention procedure reports (e.g., echocardiogram, left ventriculogram, Multiple Gated Acquisition Scan) performed during hospitalization. Values for LVEF were categorized into 4 groups: normal (=60), mild (45–59), moderate (30–44), and severe dysfunction (<30).

ANALYSES

All predictor variables were centered. Cross-lagged correlations were used to address the cross-sectional and longitudinal associations between vulnerabilities and depression. We conducted 4 hierarchical regression analyses to identify the unique relations between each psychosocial vulnerability and depression severity, controlling for the other vulnerabilities. First, we analyzed the cross-sectional relations between 3-month psychosocial vulnerabilities and 3-month depression. Previous research with this data set had established the psychosocial vulnerability and depressive symptomology association immediately following ACS (Rieckmann et al., 2006). Thus our focus is to extend this model to 3-months and, most important consider these relations longitudinally. We analyzed the data longitudinally by regressing 3 month depression symptom severity, controlling for baseline depression severity, on the baseline psychosocial vulnerabilities, including rumination, and with rumination as a moderator for all other vulnerabilities. Finally, we considered the different impacts that psychosocial vulnerabilities and rumination may play in non-depressed and depressed patients. This allows for the differentiation between the role that psychosocial factors play in the maintenance of existing depressive symptoms, and the role they play in predicting the new onset of depressive symptoms.

In the hierarchical regression analyses, we used demographic covariates (age, sex, ethnicity, presence of partner, years of schooling, and work status), depression, medical comorbidity, and cardiac disease severity in the first step of the model. In the second step we used psychosocial vulnerabilities (dysfunctional attitudes, pleasant events, poor dyadic adjustment, and role transitions). Third, we used rumination, and finally the interaction terms (i.e., rumination × each respective vulnerability) in step four.

For the depressed and non-depressed subgroup analyses we determined the presence or absence of minor ($N = 64$)/major ($N = 48$) depression with the DISH interview (The Depression Interview and Structured Hamilton, Freedland et al., 2002). In addition, we classified patients who were prescribed an antidepressant ($N = 57$), as depressed. Thus, we compared 169 depressed patients and 288 non-depressed patients.

RESULTS

Table 1 presents the descriptive statistics for the demographic characteristics, covariates, and the variables used in the analyses. In general, depression vulnerabilities and depression severity

Table 1 | Demographic and psychosocial vulnerabilities of 457 post-acute coronary syndrome patients at baseline and 387 post-acute coronary syndrome patients at 3 months.

Variable	Baseline ($N=457$)	3 Months ($N=387$)	*p*-Value
Age, mean (SD), years	61.1 (12.47)		
Female%	41.4		
White%	79.6		
Hispanic%	10.7		
Currently living with partner%	62.1		
Currently employed%	49.9		
Education, mean (SD), years	13.65 (3.25)		
Charlson score, mean (SD)	1.37 (1.57)		
LVEF: normal ≥60%	45.1		
Depression severity (BDI), mean (SD)	8.96 (9.02)	6.88 (8.29)	<0.001
Dysfunctional attitudes (DAS), mean (SD)	78.91 (21.71)	75.39 (21.53)	<0.001
Pleasant events schedule (PES), mean (SD)	0.36 (0.28)	0.37 (0.27)	0.10
Poor dyadic adjustment (DYAD), mean (SD)	2.10 (0.77)	2.06 (0.77)	0.65
Number of role transitions (RLT), mean (SD)	0.86 (0.98)	0.72 (0.88)	0.01
Rumination brooding (RB), mean (SD)	9.76 (3.19)	9.46 (3.22)	0.01

All displayed descriptive statistics are before any transformations were applied to the scales. Paired sampled t-tests were performed to test for significant mean change in scores.

decreased across the 3 months. And this decrease reached statistical significance for depression severity, dysfunctional attitudes, number of role transitions, and rumination brooding. Reflective rumination was unrelated to depression; thus, we only report results for the rumination subscale of "rumination brooding."

With increasing age, patients had lower scores on some of the vulnerabilities (Baseline: Rumination Brooding, $r = -0.21$, $p < 0.001$; Role Transitions, $r = -0.20$, $p < 0.001$; Dyadic Adjustment Disagreement, $r = -0.15$, $p = 0.002$, 3 months: Rumination Brooding, $r = -0.23$, $p < 0.001$; Role Transitions, $r = -0.10$, $p = 0.05$; Dyadic Adjustment Disagreement, $r = -0.15$, $p = 0.002$).

Men exhibited significantly higher Dysfunctional Attitudes at baseline (Male = 82.10, SD = 20.74, Female = 74.38, SD = 22.30, $p < 0.001$) and 3 months (Male = 77.89, SD = 21.59, Female = 72.09, SD = 21.06, $p = 0.01$) than women. Women had significantly higher Rumination Brooding at 3 months; Male = 9.15, SD = 3.11, Female = 9.89, SD = 3.32, $p = 0.02$) when compared to men. Otherwise, there were no sex differences in any of the vulnerabilities.

As seen in **Table 2**, the correlations among the psychosocial vulnerabilities were low to moderate cross-sectionally, both at baseline and at 3-months. Stability across the 3 months was highest for the Dysfunctional Attitudes and Rumination Brooding. In bivariate analyses, depression severity was moderately correlated with each of the vulnerabilities (**Figure 1**).

CROSS-SECTIONAL MODEL: VULNERABILITIES ASSESSED AT 3 MONTHS AS PREDICTORS OF 3 MONTHS DEPRESSION SEVERITY

After adjustment by covariates, including baseline depression severity, 3 month psychosocial vulnerabilities were concurrently related to 3 month depression severity. As shown in **Table 3**, together, all covariates predicted 48.2% of the variance in 3 month depression [$R = 0.69$, df = 9, $F(9, 388) = 39.18$, $p < 0.001$]. An additional 10.5% of 3 month depression severity was explained by the psychosocial vulnerabilities obtained at 3 months in block 2 [$R = 0.77$, $F(13, 388) = 41.07$, $\Delta F = 23.96$, $p < 0.001$], and an additional 5.1% of 3 month depression severity was explained by rumination brooding at 3 months, in block 3 [$R = 0.80$, $F(14, 388) = 47.11$, $\Delta F = 54.41$, $p < 0.001$]. Finally, an additional 4.1% of 3 month depression severity was explained by all of the, 3 month, rumination brooding and psychosocial vulnerability interactions (dysfunctional attitudes × rumination brooding; pleasant events infrequency × rumination brooding; role transitions × rumination brooding; and poor dyadic adjustment × rumination brooding), in block 4 [$R = 0.82$, $F(18, 388) = 43.45$, $\Delta F = 11.74$, $p < 0.001$]. Interaction effects show that high rumination brooding served as a significant amplifier of infrequent pleasant events, ($\beta = 0.57$, $p = 0.06$), whereas low rumination brooding served to buffer the negative effect of poor dyadic adjustment ($\beta = 0.32$, $p < 0.001$), and dysfunctional attitudes ($\beta = 0.01$, $p = 0.003 < 0.05$), on 3 month depression severity. A fourth significant interaction effect between role transitions and rumination brooding indicates that depression severity is high if a person broods and if the person is undergoing role transitions ($\beta = -0.19$, $p = 0.04$). Depression severity is only low among patients who are neither undergoing role transitions nor brooding.

LONGITUDINAL MODEL: BASELINE VULNERABILITIES AS PREDICTORS OF 3 MONTHS DEPRESSION SEVERITY

After adjustment for covariates, including baseline depression and cardiovascular disease severity, baseline psychosocial vulnerabilities were longitudinally related to depression severity at 3 months. As shown in **Table 4**, the covariates predicted 48.5% of the variance in 3 month depression [$R = 0.70$, $F(9, 375) = 38.35$, $p < 0.001$], and an additional 1.6% of this depression severity was explained by baseline psychosocial vulnerabilities, in block 2 [$R = 0.71$, $F(13, 375) = 27.96$, $\Delta F = 2.85$, $p = 0.02$], an additional 1.2% of 3 month depression severity was explained by rumination brooding, in block 3 [$R = 0.72$, $F(14, 375) = 27.21$, $\Delta F = 9.21$, $p = 0.003$]. Finally an additional 1.4% of 3 month depression severity was explained by all of the baseline rumination brooding and psychosocial vulnerability interactions (dysfunctional attitudes × rumination brooding; pleasant events infrequency × rumination brooding; role transitions × rumination brooding; poor dyadic adjustment × rumination brooding), in block 4 [$R = 0.73$, $F(18, 375) = 22.15$, $\Delta F = 2.67$, $p = 0.03$]. The interaction between baseline poor dyadic adjustment and rumination brooding independently predicted future, 3 month depression severity ($p < 0.05$; see **Figure 2**).

Table 2 | Cross-sectional and longitudinal intercorrelations among the psychosocial vulnerabilities and rumination.

	Dysfunctional attitude	Pleasant events	Role transitions	Dyadic adjustment disagreement	Rumination brooding
Dysfunctional attitude	**0.73****	0.26**	0.19**	0.17**	0.49**
Pleasant events	0.22**	**0.65****	0.10*	0.26**	0.25**
Role transitions	0.06	0.06	**0.39****	0.09	0.22**
Dyadic adjustment disagreement	0.10	0.17**	0.13**	**0.55****	0.23**
Rumination brooding	0.38**	0.23**	0.16**	0.21**	**0.74****

*Correlates in the main diagonal are test-retest coefficients (baseline and 3 month correlates). Below and above the main diagonal are the baseline and 3 month intercorrelations, respectively. **p < 0.001.*

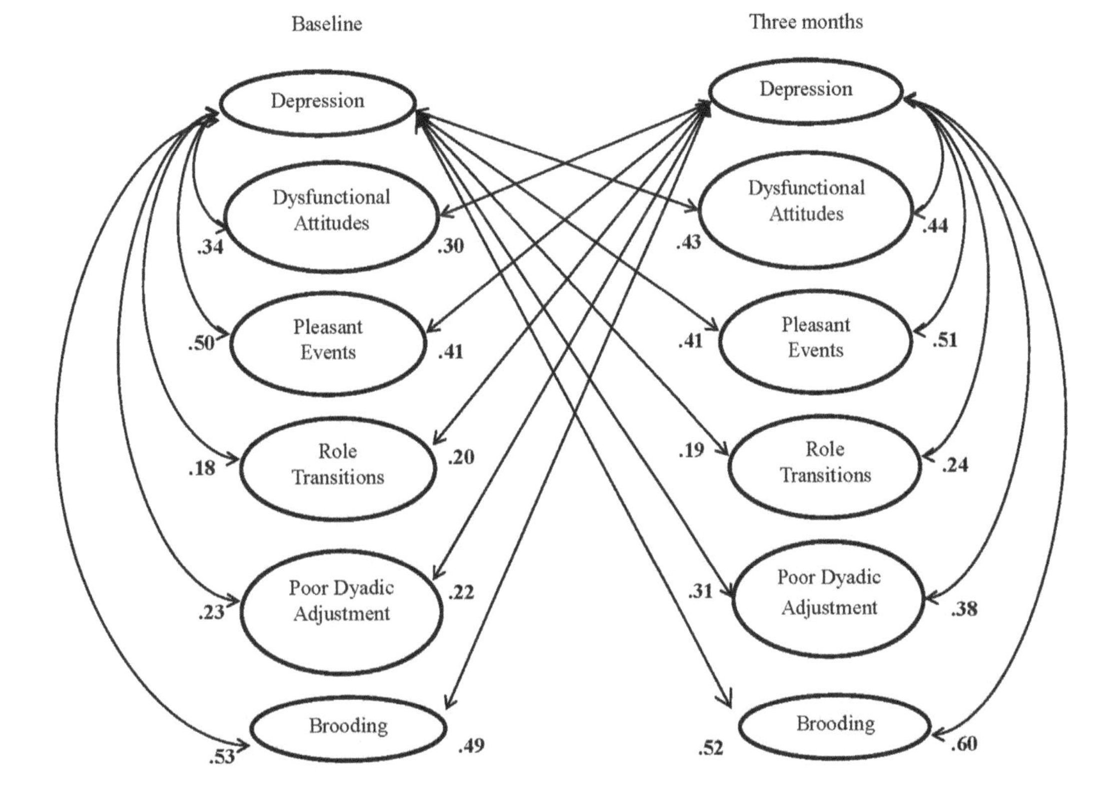

FIGURE 1 | Cross lagged correlations between depression, vulnerabilities, and rumination for baseline and 3 months. All correlations are significant at $**p < 0.001$.

SUB-GROUP DIFFERENCES BETWEEN NON-DEPRESSED AND DEPRESSED AT BASELINE

We used hierarchical regression to assess if the relation of baseline psychosocial vulnerabilities to 3 month depression severity was different for the depressed and non-depressed sub-groups. The overall moderating effect of depression status (depressed versus non-depressed subgroup) on the overall relation between baseline psychosocial vulnerabilities with 3 month depression was suggestive [$R = 0.65$, $F(17, 395) = 16.02$, $\Delta F = 2.15$, $p = 0.074$]. Moreover, the 3-way interaction, of baseline rumination × psychosocial vulnerabilities × depressed versus non-depressed subgroup status to predict 3 month depression severity was significant [$R = 0.69$, $F(15, 394) = 22.29$, $\Delta F = 11.66$, $p = 0.001$]. In exploring this effect we found that that high rumination amplified baseline vulnerabilities to depression severity for depressed patients but buffered depression severity for non-depressed patients.

We then applied the fully adjusted hierarchical model separately in the non-depressed patient sample and depressed patient sample. For depressed patients the demographic variables and covariates were significantly related to depression at 3 months [Step 1: $F(9, 125) = 12.36$, $p < 0.001$, $R^2 = 0.47$], yet, the baseline psychosocial vulnerabilities were not significant predictors of 3 month depression severity [Step 2: $\Delta F = (4, 121) = 1.06$, $p = 0.38$, $\Delta R^2 = 0.02$]. Baseline rumination brooding did directly predict 3 month depression severity for this group [Step 3: $\Delta F = (1, 120) = 6.65$, $p = 0.01$, ΔR^2 change $= 0.03$], but did not interact with baseline

Table 3 | Hierarchical regression summary of the effect of psychosocial vulnerabilities at 3 months, rumination as an independent predictor and rumination as an amplifier on 3 month depression severity, post-ACS.

	ΔR^2	B	SE(B)	p-Value
Step 1	0.48**			
Age		−0.05	0.03	0.07
Sex (1 = male; 2 = female)		−0.15	0.65	0.81
Partner (1 = yes; 2 = no)		1.16	0.67	0.8
Years of schooling		−0.28	0.10	0.01
Work status (1 = employed; 0 = unemployed)		0.29	0.73	0.69
Ethnicity (1 = Hispanic; 0 = non-Hispanic)		1.82	1.10	0.10
Baseline depression severity		0.57	0.04	<0.001
Charlson comorbidity score		0.09	0.22	0.68
LVEF		0.09	0.35	0.79
Step 2	0.11**			
Dysfunctional attitudes		0.06	0.01	<0.001
Pleasant events scale		6.58	1.16	<0.001
Role transitions		0.82	0.32	0.01
Poor dyadic adjustment		1.58	0.39	<0.001
Step 3	0.05**			
Rumination brooding		0.75	0.10	<0.001
Step 4	0.04**			
DAS × brooding		0.01	0.003	0.003
PES × brooding		0.57	0.30	0.06
RLT × brooding		−0.19	0.10	0.04
DYAD × brooding		0.32	0.08	<0.001

*DAS, dysfunctional attitudes; PES, pleasant events scale; DYAD, poor dyadic adjustment; RLT, number of role transitions. **p < 0.001.*

Table 4 | Hierarchical Regression summary of the effect of baseline psychosocial vulnerabilities, rumination as an independent predictor and rumination as an amplifier on 3 month depression severity, post-ACS.

	ΔR^2	B	SE(B)	p-Value
Step 1	0.48**			
Age		−0.04	0.03	0.26
Sex (1 = male; 2 = female)		−0.43	0.66	0.52
Partner (1 = yes; 2 = no)		1.44	0.69	0.04
Years of schooling		−0.27	0.10	0.02
Work status (1 = employed; 2 = unemployed)		0.07	0.76	0.93
Ethnicity (1 = Hispanic; 2 = non-Hispanic)		1.74	1.12	0.12
Baseline depression severity		0.58	0.04	<0.001
Charlson comorbidity score		0.28	0.23	0.23
LVEF		0.26	0.34	0.45
Step 2	0.02*			
Dysfunctional attitudes		0.03	0.02	0.07
Pleasant events scale		1.62	1.36	0.24
Role transitions		0.58	0.32	0.07
Poor dyadic adjustment		0.59	0.40	0.15
Step 3	0.01*			
Rumination brooding		0.37	0.12	0.003
Step 4	0.01*			
DAS × brooding		0.004	0.004	0.30
PES × brooding		0.24	0.39	0.54
RLT × brooding		−0.05	0.10	0.58
DYAD × brooding		0.27	0.10	0.01

*DAS, dysfunctional attitudes; PES, pleasant events scale; DYAD, poor dyadic adjustment; RLT, number of role transitions. *p < 0.05, **p < 0.001.*

psychosocial vulnerabilities when predicting 3 month depression severity [Step 4: $\Delta F = (4, 116) = 0.275, p = 0.89, \Delta R^2 = 0.01$].

A different pattern emerged for the non-depressed patients, the demographic variables and covariates were again significantly related to depression at 3 months [Step 1: $F(9, 231) = 9.42, p < 0.001, R^2 = 0.27$], however, in contrast to the depressed subgroup, the baseline psychosocial vulnerabilities emerged as significant predictors of 3 month depression severity [Step 2: $\Delta F = (4, 227) = 3.71, p = 0.01, \Delta R^2 = 0.05$]. Moreover, contrary to the results in the depressed subgroup, baseline rumination brooding did not significantly predict 3 month depression severity above baseline psychosocial vulnerabilities for the non-depressed sample [Step 3: $\Delta F = (1, 226) = 0.80, p = 0.37, \Delta R^2$ change $= 0.002$], yet did interact with the baseline psychosocial vulnerabilities for non-depressed patients [Step 4: $\Delta F = (4, 222) = 5.31, p < 0.001, \Delta R^2 = 0.06$] to exacerbate 3 month depression severity.

DISCUSSION

The purpose of this study was to extend our understanding of the relation among psychosocial depression vulnerabilities and depressive symptom severity in post-ACS patients, within a longitudinal data set. Results indicated that vulnerabilities are related to depression both cross-sectionally and longitudinally. Further, rumination brooding plays an important role as both a vulnerability and as an amplifier of other vulnerabilities for depressive symptoms after ACS. Overall, these findings replicate the results from previous cross-sectional designs that psychosocial vulnerabilities are independent correlates of depression severity among patients with cardiovascular disease (Rieckmann et al., 2006; Doyle et al., 2010). Full sample and sub-group findings are discussed in the following section. Finally, and most intriguingly vulnerabilities seem to act as precursors to depression in a non-depressed subsample at baseline and as maintaining factors for already depressed patients.

TOTAL SAMPLE: PSYCHOSOCIAL VULNERABILITIES AND DEPRESSION

Consistent with previous literature, these results show that 3 month psychosocial vulnerabilities are strong independent predictors of 3 month depression severity, controlling for the influence of cardiac disease severity, and initial depressive symptoms (Doyle et al., 2010). Psychosocial vulnerabilities explained a considerable amount of depression severity variance in the cross-sectional model illustrating the independent role of daily stressors

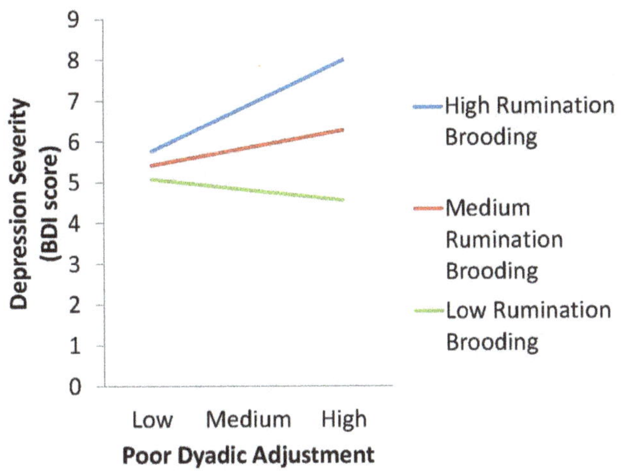

FIGURE 2 | Interaction effect of baseline poor dyadic adjustment and rumination brooding on 3 month depression severity, Post-ACS.

on depression severity. Behavioral, cognitive, and interpersonal vulnerabilities had relatively weak intercorrelations, substantiating the unique variation among psychosocial vulnerabilities in this ACS sample. Cross-lagged correlations are interpreted to suggest two important findings regarding the relation between psychosocial vulnerabilities and depression. First, the lagged correlates suggest bidirectional and stable interrelations between psychosocial vulnerabilities and depression. Second, the differential strength of correlations at each time period suggest that the psychosocial vulnerabilities and depression influence is not strong at initial cardiac presentation (baseline cross-sectional correlations in **Figure 1**); however, this influence intensifies over time (3 month cross-sectional correlations in **Figure 1**).

RUMINATION

In the total sample, we found higher rumination brooding to significantly predict future depression severity independent of the traditional psychosocial vulnerabilities. Ciesla and Roberts (2007) hypothesized rumination to be a " non-specific vulnerability" to depression, and the cardiovascular literature also identifies rumination as a risk factor to poor health outcome, explaining physiological mechanisms between depression symptoms and cardiovascular health (Brosschot et al., 2006; Larsen and Christenfeld, 2009). Also of interest is that reflective rumination was not a psychosocial vulnerability for depression. Our findings suggest that patients who reflect are at no increased risk of elevated depression symptoms.

RUMINATION AMPLIFIES DEPRESSION SEVERITY

In our total sample, rumination exacerbates depression severity when combined with cognitive, behavioral, and interpersonal stressors. The interaction effect of rumination brooding and poor dyadic adjustment (interpersonal vulnerability) independently predicted higher depression severity at 3 months. This finding demonstrates the complexity, yet importance, of close relationships and future mental health. It also supports the moderation model, coined by Ciesla and Roberts (2007). The moderation model explains that the relation between rumination and depression is conditional (Ciesla and Roberts, 2007). These authors found that level of negative cognition (cognitive vulnerability) moderated the relation between rumination and depression. Our findings extend the moderation model. In our sample, rumination brooding moderated the effect of dyadic adjustment so that high partner disagreement had no effect on depression severity at 3 months when there was no rumination brooding, with moderate rumination brooding, high levels of partner disagreement were moderately associated with depressive symptoms, and partner disagreement had the worst effect in the presence of high levels of rumination brooding.

SUBGROUP ANALYSES: PSYCHOSOCIAL VULNERABILITIES AND DEPRESSION

Perhaps the most intriguing finding of this study is that patterns of psychosocial vulnerability influence differed by initial depression group status post-ACS. Specifically, cognitive, behavioral, and interpersonal vulnerabilities appear to influence future depression symptoms in non-depressed patients, whereas rumination brooding significantly influenced future depression symptoms only among depressed patients. Rumination brooding appears to be a mechanism for *maintaining depression* for post-ACS patients who have elevated depressive symptoms at baseline. For those post-ACS patients who are not depressed, the standard psychosocial vulnerabilities – cognitive, behavioral, and interpersonal – are the ones that appear to predispose them to become depressed in the future. Thus, prevention might focus on these factors.

RUMINATION

Although we generally found (in the full sample) that rumination brooding was a unique and independent predictor of 3 month depression severity, subgroup analyses suggested a more complex process. Baseline rumination brooding independently predicted future depression severity for depressed patients, but not for non-depressed patients. Nolen-Hoeksema posits that ruminative responses prolong and intensify depressive episodes, whereas distraction from rumination response can serve as intervention, shortening, and diminishing depressive episodes (Nolen-Hoeksema, 1991; Enns and Cox, 2005). Further, the maintenance of physiological arousal for depressed cardiovascular disease patients is hypothesized to place these patients at increased risk of disease recurrence and/or mortality (Brosschot et al., 2006). We interpret our findings to indicate that rumination brooding maintains depression symptoms for patients who are already depressed. We can then speculate that clinical interventions to reduce rumination brooding symptoms can alleviate depression symptoms in those already depressed. We also found that baseline rumination brooding amplifies other psychosocial vulnerabilities in predicting future depression severity uniquely for initially non-depressed CVD patients. Thus, our study replicates the indirect and predictive effect of rumination on depression severity (Ciesla and Roberts, 2002; Ciesla and Roberts, 2007; Robinson and Alloy, 2003).

LIMITATIONS

One limitation of this study is that our participants were identified post-ACS, thus prior history of depression, depression vulnerabilities, and ruminative cognitions are not known. The interpretation of these results is in the context of an important 3 month window, or "snapshot," following an ACS event. Also, this study population may not be representative of all ACS patients, due to the exclusion of patients with BDI scores 5–9. However, this study design captures patients who are at elevated risk for ACS recurrence and mortality (those with BDI score $\geq$ 10) and demonstrates the complex interplay that depression vulnerabilities have on their recovery prognosis. Our findings are based on a vital Post-ACS recovery period and the complex role that rumination plays during this time underscores the importance of further research on this construct. Women had higher rumination brooding scores relative to men. Men had higher dysfunctional attitude scores (cognitive vulnerability) relative to women. The sex differences have theoretical and practical implications. Theoretically, gender may be a moderating determinant of depression severity. Practically, it is possible that cardiac treatment and prevention efforts can target women with increased psychosocial vulnerability and thereby reduce the risk of relatively worse recovery for women (Gulliksson et al., 2007). For men, cognitive-based interventions may be most therapeutic (Compare et al., 2011). Although we observed these gender differences in our patient sample, gender differences were not included in the overall model predicting depression severity.

CONCLUSION

The current findings suggest that cognitive, behavioral, interpersonal vulnerabilities, and rumination brooding are longitudinally associated with depression severity after an ACS. As depressive symptoms are related to the effects of rumination brooding and psychosocial vulnerabilities, CHD recovery, and treatment interventions should consider social and trait-like influences on patients' health outcome. Rumination brooding uniquely contributes as an independent and amplifying psychosocial vulnerability of depression severity. Thus it can be considered a clinical marker of 3 month depression in post-ACS patients. Based on these findings, treatment approaches for ACS patients should consider psychosocial vulnerabilities as possible contributors to CVD health outcomes.

ACKNOWLEDGMENTS

This work was supported by grants HC-25197, HL 076857, and HL 04458 from the National Heart, Lung, and Blood Institute, Bethesda, MD, USA; by an unrestricted research grant from the Hinduja Foundation, New York, NY, USA.

REFERENCES

1. Beck, A. T., Ward, C. H., Mendelson, M., Mock, J., and Erbaugh, J. (1961). An inventory for measuring depression. *Arch. Gen. Psychiatry* 4, 561–571.
2. Berkman, L. F., Blumenthal, J., Burg, M., Carney, R. M., Catellier, D., Cowan, M. J., Czajkowski, S. M., DeBusk, R., Hosking, J., Jaffe, A., Kaufmann, P. G., Mitchell, P., Norman, J., Powell, L. H., Raczynski, J. M., and Schneider- man, N. (2003). Effects of treating depression and low perceived social support on clinical events after myocardial infarction: the Enhancing Recovery in Coronary Heart Disease Patients (ENRICHD) Randomized Trial. *JAMA* 289, 3106–3116.
3. Birmaher, B., Bridge, J. A., Williamson, D. E., Brent, D. A., Dahl, R. E., Axelson, D. A., Dorn, L. D., and Ryan, N. D. (2004). Psychosocial function- ing in youths at high risk to develop major depressive disorder. *J. Am. Acad. Child Adolesc. Psychiatry* 43, 839–846.
4. Brosschot, J. F., Gerin, W., and Thayer, J. F. (2006). The perseverative cognition hypothesis: a review of worry, prolonged stress-related physiologi- cal activation, and health. *J. Psycho- som. Res.* 60, 113–124.
5. Carney, R. M., Blumenthal, J. A., Catel- lier, D., Freedland, K. E., Berkman, L. F., Watkins, L. L., Czajkowski, M., Hayano, J., and Jaffe, A. S. (2003). Depression as a risk factor for mortality after acute myocar- dial infarction. *Am. J. Cardiol.* 92, 1277–1281.
6. Charlson, M. E., Pompei, P., Ales, K. L., and MacKenzie, C. R. (1987). A new method of classifying prog- nostic co-morbidity in longitudinal studies – development and valida- tion. *J. Chronic Dis.* 40, 373–383.
7. Ciesla, J. A., and Roberts, J. E. (2002). Self-directed thought and response to treatment for depression: a pre- liminary investigation. *J. Cogn. Psy- chother.* 16, 435–453.
8. Ciesla, J. A., and Roberts, J. E. (2007). Rumination, negative cog- nition, and their interactive effects on depressed mood. *Emotion* 7, 555–565.
9. Compare, A., Germani, E., Proietti, R., and Janeway, D. (2011). Clinical psychology and cardiovascular dis- ease: an up-to-date clinical prac- tice review for assessment and treat- ment of anxiety and depression. *Clin. Pract. Epidemiol. Ment. Health* 7, 148–156.
10. Contrada, R. J., Boulifard, D. A., Hek- ler, E. B., Idler, E. L., Spruill, T. M., Labouvie, E. W., and Krause, J. (2008). Psychosocial factors in heart surgery: presurgical vul- nerability and postsurgical recovery. *Health Psychol.* 27, 309–319.
11. Davidson, K. W., Burg, M. M, Kro- nish, I. M., Shimbo, D., Detten- born, L., Mehran, R., Vorchheimer, D., Clemow, L., Schwartz, J. E., Lesperance, F., and Rieckmann, N. (2010). Association of anhedonia with recurrent major adverse car- diac events and mortality 1 year after acute coronary syndrome. *Arch. Gen. Psychiatry* 67, 480–488.
12. Denollet, J., and Kupper, N. (2007). Type-D personality, depression, and cardiac prognosis: cortisol dysregulation as a mediating mechanism. *J. Psychosom. Res.* 62, 607–609.
13. Denollet, J., Martens, E. J., Smith, O. R., and Burg, M. M. (2010). Effi- cient assessment of depressive symp- toms and their prognostic value in myocardial infarction patients. *J. Affect. Disord.* 120, 105–111.
14. Doyle, F., Conroy, R., McGee, H., and Delaney, M. (2010). Depres- sive symptoms in persons with acute coronary syndrome: specific symp- tom scales and prognosis. *J. Psycho- som. Res.* 68, 121–130.
15. Doyle, F., McGee, H. M., Conroy, R. M., and Delaney, M. (2011). What predicts depression in car- diac patients: sociodemographic fac- tors, disease severity, or theoretical vulnerabilities? *Psychol. Health* 26, 619–634.
16. Enns, M. W., and Cox, B. J. (2005). Psy- chosocial and clinical predictors of symptom persistence vs. remission in major depressive disorder. *Can. J. Psychiatry* 50, 769–777.
17. Freedland, K., Skala, J., Carney, R., Raczynski, J., Taylor, C., Mendes de Leon, C., Ironson, G., Young- blood, M., Krishnan, K. R. R., and Veith, R. (2002). The Depression Interview and Structured Hamil- ton (DISH): rationale, development, characteristics, and clinical validity. *Psychosom. Med.* 64, 897–905.
18. Garnefski, N., Boon, S., and Kraaij, V. (2003). Relationships between cognitive strategies of adolescents and depressive symptomatology across different types of life event. *J. Youth Adolesc.* 32, 401–408.
19. Grant, D. M., and Beck, J. G. (2010). What predicts the trajec- tory of rumination?: a prospective evaluation. *J. Anxiety Disord.* 24, 480–486.
20. Gulliksson, M., Burell, G., Lundin, L., Toss, H., and Svardsudd, K. (2007). Psychosocial factors during the first year after a coronary heart disease event in cases and refer- ents. Secondary Prevention in Upp- sala Primary Health Care Project (SUPRIM). *BMC Cardiovasc. Dis- ord.* 7, 36. doi:10.1186/1471-2261-7- 36
21. Hankin, B. L., Oppenheimer, C., Jen- ness, J., Barrocas, A., Shapero, B. J., and Goldband, J. (2009). Developmental origins of cog- nitive vulnerabilities to depres- sion: review of processes con- tributing to stability and change across time. *J. Clin. Psychol.* 65, 1327–1338.
22. Harris, T. (2001). Recent developments in understanding the psychosocial aspects of depression. *Br. Med. Bull.* 57, 17–32.
23. Lam, D., Schuck, N., Smith, N., Farmer, A., and Checkley, S. (2003). Response style, interpersonal diffi- culties, and social functioning in major depressive disorder. *J. Affect. Disord.* 75, 279–283.
24. Lange, H. W., and Herrmann-Lingen, C. (2007). Depressive symptoms predict recurrence of atrial fibrillation after cardioversion. *J. Psychosom. Res.* 63, 509–513.
25. Larsen, B. A., and Christenfeld, N. J. (2009). Cardiovascular disease and psychiatric comorbidity: the poten- tial role of perseverative cognition. *Cardiovasc. Psychiatry Neurol.* 2009, 791017.

26. Markowitz, J. C., Leon, A. C., Miller, N. L., Cherry, S., Clougherty, K. F., and Villalobos, L. (2000). Rater agree- ment on interpersonal psychother- apy problem areas. *J. Psychother. Pract. Res.* 9, 131–135.
27. McGee, H. M., Doyle, F., Conroy, R. M., De La Harpe, D., and Shelley, E. (2006). Impact of briefly-assessed depression on secondary prevention outcomes after acute coronary syn- drome: a one-year longitudinal sur- vey. *BMC Health Serv. Res.* 6, 9. doi:10.1186/1472-6963-6-9
28. McIntosh, E., Gillanders, D., and Rodgers, S. (2010). Rumination, goal linking, daily hassles, and life events in major depression. *Clin. Psychol. Psychother.* 17, 33–43.
29. Naqvi, T. Z., Rafique, A. M., Andreas, V., Rahban, M., Mirocha, J., and Naqvi, S. S. (2007). Predictors of depres- sive symptoms post-acute coronary syndrome. *Gend. Med.* 4, 339–351.
30. Nolen-Hoeksema, S. (1991). Responses to depression and their effects on the duration of depressive episodes. *J. Abnorm. Psychol.* 100, 569–582.
31. O'Sullivan, C. (2004). The psychosocial determinants of depression: a lifespan perspective. *J. Nerv. Ment. Dis.* 192, 585–594.
32. Oxlad, M., and Wade, T. D. (2008). Lon- gitudinal risk factors for adverse psy- chological functioning six months after coronary artery bypass graft surgery. *J. Health Psychol.* 13, 79–92.
33. Parker, G. B., Hilton, T. M., Walsh, W. F., Owen, C. A., Heruc, G. A., Olley, A., Brotchie, H., and Hadzi- Pavlovic, D. (2008). Timing is every- thing: the onset of depression and acute coronary syndrome outcome. *Biol. Psychiatry* 64, 660–666.
34. Pedersen, S. S., Denollet, J., van Ges- tel, Y. R. B. M., Serruys, P. W., and van Domburg, R. T. (2008). Clustering of psychosocial risk fac- tors enhances the risk of depres- sive symptoms 12-months post per- cutaneous coronary intervention. *Eur. J. Cardiovasc. Prev. Rehabil.* 15, 203–209.
35. Power, M., Katz, R., McGuffin, P., Dug- gan, C., Lam, D., and Beck, A. T. (1994). The Dysfunctional Attitude Scale (DAS): a comparison of forms A and B and proposals for a new subscaled version. *J. Res. Pers.* 28, 263–276.
36. Rieckmann, N., Burg, M. M., Gerin, W., Chaplin, W. F., Clemow, L., and Davidson, K. W. (2006). Depression vulnerabilities in patients with dif- ferent levels of depressive symptoms after acute coronary syndromes. *Psy- chother. Psychosom.* 75, 353–361. [IMPACT (2005) 4.966].
37. Robinson, M. S., and Alloy, L. B. (2003). Negative cognitive styles and stress-reactive rumination interact to predict depression: a prospec- tive study. *Cognit. Ther. Res.* 27, 275–292.
38. Spanier, G. B. (1976). Measuring dyadic adjustment: new scales for assessing the quality of marriage and similar dyadic adjustment disagreements. *J. Marriage Fam.* 38, 15–28.
39. Stafford, L., Jackson, H. J., and Berk, M. (2008). Cognitive-personality style as vulnerability to depression in patients with coronary artery dis- ease: roles of sociotropy and auton- omy. *Psychosom. Med.* 71, 63–69.
40. Teri, L., and Lewinsohn, P. (1982). Mod- ification of the pleasant and unpleas- ant events schedules for use with the elderly. *J. Consult. Clin. Psychol.* 50, 444–445.
41. Treynor, W., Gonzalez, R., and Nolen- Hoeksema, S. (2003). Rumination reconsidered: a psychometric analy- sis. *Cognit. Ther. Res.* 27, 247–259.
42. van Gestel, Y. R. B. M., Pedersen, S. S., van de Sande, M., de Jaegere, P. P. T., Serruys, P. W., Erdman, R. A. M., and van Domburg, R. T. (2007). Type-D personality and depressive symptoms predict anxiety 12 months post-percutaneous coro- nary intervention. *J. Affect. Disord.* 103, 197–203.

16

Cerebellar-motor dysfunction in schizophrenia and psychosis-risk: the importance of regional cerebellar analysis approaches

***Jessica A. Bernard*[1]* and Vijay A. Mittal*[1,2]**

[1] *Department of Psychology and Neuroscience, University of Colorado Boulder, Boulder, CO, USA*
[2] *Center for Neuroscience, University of Colorado Boulder, Boulder, CO, USA*

Edited by:
Manuel Morrens, University of Antwerp, Belgium

Reviewed by:
Bernhard J. Mitterauer, University of Salzburg, Austria
Sebastian Walther, University Hospital of Psychiatry, Switzerland
Manuel Morrens, University of Antwerp, Belgium

****Correspondence:***
Jessica A. Bernard, Department of Psychology and Neuroscience, University of Colorado Boulder, 345 UCB, Boulder, CO 80309-0345, USA
e-mail: jessica.bernard@colorado.edu

Motor abnormalities in individuals with schizophrenia and those at-risk for psychosis are well documented. An accumulating body of work has also highlighted motor abnormalities related to cerebellar dysfunction in schizophrenia including eye-blink conditioning, timing, postural control, and motor learning. We have also recently found evidence for motor dysfunction in individuals at ultra high-risk for psychosis (1–3). This is particularly relevant as the cerebellum is thought to be central to the cognitive dysmetria model of schizophrenia, and these overt motor signs may point to more general cerebellar dysfunction in the etiology of psychotic disorders. While studies have provided evidence indicative of motor cerebellar dysfunction in at-risk populations and in schizophrenia, findings with respect to the cerebellum have been mixed. One factor potentially contributing to these mixed results is the whole-structure approach taken when investigating the cerebellum. In non-human primates, there are distinct closed-loop circuits between the cerebellum, thalamus, and brain with motor and non-motor cortical regions. Recent human neuroimaging has supported this finding and indicates that there is a cerebellar functional topography (4), and this information is being missed with whole-structure approaches. Here, we review cerebellar-motor dysfunction in individuals with schizophrenia and those at-risk for psychosis. We also discuss cerebellar abnormalities in psychosis, and the cerebellar functional topography. Because of the segregated functional regions of the cerebellum, we propose that it is important to look at the structure regionally in order to better understand its role in motor dysfunction in these populations. This is analogous to approaches taken with the basal ganglia, where each region is considered separately. Such an approach is necessary to better understand cerebellar pathophysiology on a macro-structural level with respect to the pathogenesis of psychosis.

Keywords: cerebellum, schizophrenia, psychosis-risk, motor abnormalities, balance, timing, morphology, motor learning

INTRODUCTION

Schizophrenia is a devastating mental illness marked by a variety of symptoms, including positive symptoms (hallucinations and delusions) and negative symptoms (anhedonia and social withdrawal) (5). In addition to the classic symptoms, these patients also exhibit movement abnormalities as well as cognitive and affective dysfunction. These movement abnormalities are in a variety of domains and include dyskinesias (6), as well as psychomotor slowing, catatonia, neurological soft signs, extrapyramidal signs, and motor learning deficits (7–10). Psychosis has been studied as a spectrum disorder, with investigations of different patient groups that show some symptoms that are associated with risk. In this review, we focus on several specific groups in addition to schizophrenia, including those at psychosis-risk, a category that can refer to genetic risk, as those with a first-degree relative with the disease are at greater risk for development of schizophrenia. In this category, there are also individuals referred to as ultra high-risk (UHR), where there are recent onset or escalating range of moderate (i.e., partially formed/occurring occasionally without full conviction or related functional impairment) positive attenuated symptoms (e.g., unusual thoughts, suspiciousness, grandiosity, perceptual anomalies, and disorganized communication) associated with decreased functionality in social relationships or day-to-day life. After a diagnosis of schizophrenia, this period of attenuated symptoms is referred to as the prodromal period. However, not all those that experience these symptoms will go on to develop schizophrenia or another psychotic disorder. Finally, there are individuals diagnosed with schizotypal personality disorder, who show trait level unusual behaviors, suspiciousness, and ideas of reference. This group is also at greater than average risk for schizophrenia. Interestingly, movement abnormalities are present in these at-risk populations as well [e.g., (1, 2, 6)].

Movement abnormalities are present as early as infancy in individuals that go on to develop schizophrenia later in life [e.g., (5)], indicating that such movement abnormalities maybe associated with the disease or disease process, as opposed to being a side-effect of medication (11). Indeed, prior to the onset of schizophrenia, and certainly during infancy, individuals are less likely to be impacted by many of the confounding factors that could also further impact movement abnormalities associated with schizophrenia (e.g., anti-psychotic medications, drug, and alcohol use/abuse). These movement abnormalities are typically dyskinetic movements, and are thought to be related to the dopaminergic dysfunction in the basal ganglia (12), and have been previously reviewed elsewhere (6). Importantly, these motor abnormalities are present prior to disease onset, and continue across the disease course. Further supporting this, many movement abnormalities are seen in drug-naïve adults with schizophrenia as well (10).

In addition to the striatally mediated dyskinesias seen in schizophrenia and psychosis-risk groups (3, 6, 13–22) and the psychomotor slowing, catatonia, and parkinsonism (7–10), there is also evidence of cerebellar dysfunction in both schizophrenia, and psychosis-risk populations [e.g., Ref. (1–3, 17–21)]. The most prominent evidence of cerebellar dysfunction is with respect to its role in cognitive dysmetria (23–25). Andreasen and colleagues have demonstrated that there is abnormal functional activation in the cerebellum, thalamus, and cortex in patients with schizophrenia (23, 24), and more recently, there has been increased interest in the study of the cerebellum in these patients, particularly with respect to cerebello-thalamic connections (26). Cerebellar activation deficits exists across functional domains (27), and we refer readers to the review by Picard and colleagues for a detailed discussion of the cerebellum in schizophrenia, as it is beyond the scope of our review here (25).

The cerebellum is classically thought of as a brain structure that is important for motor control; however, there is a robust literature to indicate that the structure is also heavily involved in cognitive and affective processing (4, 28–33). As such, though the cerebellum and cerebello-thalamo-cortical circuit were first discussed in schizophrenia with respect to cognitive dysmetria, there is also a great deal of evidence to indicate that there are motor cerebellar deficits in schizophrenia in addition to the aforementioned dyskinesias, psychomotor slowing, catatonia, and parkinsonism. Indeed, there is also an emerging literature indicating that as with dyskinesias, cerebellar-motor abnormalities are also present in psychosis-risk populations [e.g., (1, 2)]. Thus, it may be that more overt cerebellar-motor dysfunction may also serve as a marker of disease and disease progression, such as has been proposed for striatal-mediated dyskinesias (6). This is particularly exciting, as the cerebellar–thalamic network represents a distinct mechanism, and may hold the potential to explain/predict heretofore poorly understood processes across the psychosis spectrum. Here, our goal is twofold. First, we provide a review of cerebellar–motor dysfunction in patients with schizophrenia as well as in psychosis-risk groups including genetic risk, UHR populations, and schizotypal individuals. Second, we provide a detailed overview of the cerebellar functional topography and weigh evidence in support of a targeted regional approach for cerebellar investigations. We suggest that more specific topographically informed approaches to investigating the cerebellum (particularly with respect to cerebellar morphology and cerebello-cortical networks) across the psychosis spectrum will yield informative results with respect to the involvement of the cerebellum in psychosis.

MOTOR CEREBELLAR DYSFUNCTION IN SCHIZOPHRENIA AND PSYCHOSIS-RISK

The cerebellum is important for motor function generally in that it is important for online monitoring of movements (34, 35). Eye-blink conditioning and postural control are both especially reliant upon the cerebellum, but it is also strongly engaged during motor learning, and it has been suggested that one of the primary functions of the cerebellum is in the precise timing of movements (36, 37). While the cerebellum is likely to be involved in many motor behaviors, several domains have been studied in greater depth in patients across the psychosis spectrum. We will discuss in turn eye-blink conditioning, postural control, timing, and motor learning. For each motor task paradigm, we will review the existing evidence indicating impairments across the psychosis spectrum, as well as any evidence that directly links these behaviors to the cerebellum [either structure or function as measured using functional magnetic resonance imaging (fMRI)] in these populations. A summary of performance for each task domain for both patients with schizophrenia and at-risk/psychosis spectrum populations is provided in **Table 1**. Finally, future directions for research in each domain will be discussed, particularly with respect to the study of psychosis.

EYE-BLINK CONDITIONING

Eye-blink conditioning is one of the simplest learning paradigms, and performance of this task is dependent upon the cerebellum (38–40). The circuits involved in eye-blink conditioning have been carefully mapped using animal models, but have also been extensively investigated in humans primarily in lesion studies, and both the deep cerebellar nuclei (particularly the interposed nuclei) and cerebellar cortex seemed to be important for task performance (38–40). In these paradigms, a puff of air is delivered to the eye, resulting in a blink response. During the conditioning phases, a tone precedes and typically co-terminates with the air-puff, resulting in conditioned responses (CRs). That is, individuals that learn the association between the tone and the air-puff that follows it blink their eyes at the sound of the tone. Because this is so heavily dependent upon the cerebellum, it is often used as an indicator of cerebellar function. In schizophrenia, there is a growing literature investigating performance on this task in patients.

Across the literature investigating patients with schizophrenia, the general finding is that patients are impaired in eye-blink conditioning, and show fewer CRs to the tone alone when compared with controls (40–47). During the paradigm, the percentage of CRs is significantly lower than that in controls. However, though this seems to be a relatively robust finding, there have been several studies that provide evidence to the contrary (48–51). Reasons for the mixed findings are unclear, but may be due to the heterogeneity of the patients included in these samples particularly with respect to medication, as well as differences in task design. Importantly, a recent investigation of neuroleptic naïve patients or patients that have been off medication for 3 weeks demonstrated eye-blink conditioning deficits suggesting that this impairment is not solely a function of medication status (46).

In addition to the lower percentage of CRs, there is also evidence in patients with schizophrenia to indicate that the timing of these responses is negatively impacted (41, 42, 45) (timing will also be discussed in further detail below). During the conditioning

Table 1 | Summary of findings across the reviewed motor domains for both patients with schizophrenia and high-risk groups.

Task domain	Schizophrenia deficits	High-risk deficits
Eye-blink conditioning	Poor conditioning: fewer conditioned responses to the presentation of a tone, which is followed by an aversive puff of air to the eye	Fewer and earlier conditioned responses in SPD
	Altered timing of responses so that eye does not close in time with the air-puff	Genetic risk populations also show fewer conditioned responses
Postural control	Greater postural sway indicative of poor postural control, associated with symptom severity	Increased postural sway in UHR individuals that is specifically associated with negative symptom severity
	Presence of the Romberg sign more common in patients	
Timing	Impairments in temporal bisection (time perception)	No evidence indicating sub-second cerebellar timing deficits
	Increased variability during temporal production (synchronization–continuation tasks)	Sub-second timing correlated with dimensions of schizotypy
Motor learning	Implicit and explicit sequence learning deficits such that patients learn, but to a lesser degree than controls	Deficits in pursuit rotor performance in UHR
	Relationships also seen with the cerebellum	No deficits on sequence learning in SPD

SPD, schizotypal personality disorder; UHR, ultra high-risk.

paradigms, the tone typically co-terminates with the onset of the air-puff to the eye. The optimal response is such that the anticipatory eye-blink that occurs as a result of the tone (CR) is timed so that the eye is closed upon the delivery of the air-puff. Brown and colleagues found that the timing of the CRs was more variable in patients with schizophrenia (42) while Bolbecker and colleagues reported less adaptive CRs as they occurred significantly earlier in patients when compared to controls (41). A similar trend level finding of earlier CRs in patients was found by Forsyth and colleagues (45).

Across the psychosis spectrum, there is also evidence to indicate impairments in eye-blink conditioning. Individuals with schizotypal personality disorder have deficits similar to patients with schizophrenia in that they show fewer CRs, and there is also a trend indicating altered (earlier) CR timing in this population (45). Most recently, Bolbecker and colleagues investigated eye-blink conditioning in a group of patients with schizophrenia, those at genetic risk, and healthy controls (52). Both the patient and genetic risk groups showed impaired associative learning as measured with CRs. The authors suggest that cerebellar abnormalities may be a marker of risk for schizophrenia (52). Furthermore, this provides additional support to indicate that these deficits are not an artifact of medication, as they are present in genetic risk groups.

Finally, it is of note that there have been several investigations of the cerebellum more directly with respect to eye-blink conditioning. First, Edwards and colleagues measured the volume of the anterior and posterior aspects of the cerebellum and investigated these volumes with respect to conditioning (43) in patients with schizophrenia and controls. Volume of the anterior cerebellum in patients was smaller than that of controls and the patients also showed impaired conditioning. However, there were no significant correlations between cerebellar volume and conditioning performance in patients with schizophrenia. In fact, the non-significant relationship in the patient group was in the opposite direction as that seen in the controls (43). The authors suggest that there are perhaps altered structure–function relationships in the cerebellum in patients with schizophrenia (43). However, further confirmation of these findings is necessary, particularly as only very large regions of the cerebellum were investigated.

Using positron emission tomography (PET), medication free patients with schizophrenia and controls were scanned during the eye-blink conditioning paradigm (46). Not only did the patient group show impaired associative learning, but they also showed decreased blood flow in the cerebellum and the thalamus. This indicates cerebellar dysfunction in the patient group along with the behavioral impairments (46). While this investigation and that of Edwards and colleagues are important first steps in linking cerebellar morphology and function to this overt motor impairment, it is also clear that more work is needed.

There are several key future directions for eye-blink-conditioning research. Most interestingly is the use of functional neuroimaging. While Parker and colleagues took advantage of PET imaging (46), recent advances in the technology used to deliver the air-puff and monitor the eye-blinks have allowed for investigations of this task using fMRI (53, 54). This approach has provided important insights into the cerebellum and eye-blink conditioning in normative development (54). Linking eye-blink conditioning to additional cognitive measures as well as symptomatology in disease populations is important. Several groups have started to investigate eye-blink conditioning with respect to cognition with mixed results (41, 45), and to our knowledge there have not yet been any investigations linking CRs with symptom severity. Such future work is important for our understanding of cerebellar contributions to disease and cognition, and will help us to better understand whether or not this motor measure is a reasonable marker of disease state. Lastly, investigations in UHR populations would also be especially informative. The work by Bolbecker and colleagues in genetic risk is an important first step (52), and the field would benefit from a replication and extension of this work in UHR individuals.

POSTURAL CONTROL

Postural control relies upon sensorimotor integration and vestibular function. The cerebellum has long been implicated in postural control (55). Patient studies in those with ataxia or cerebellar lesions show increased postural sway (poor postural control) (56), and the measurement of regional cerebral blood flow using PET imaging has also shown increases in blood flow in the cerebellum (57). Much like eye-blink conditioning, postural control can also be used as a potential indicator of cerebellar function. Indeed in healthy adults, balance has been linked to regional cerebellar volume (58), and similar associations between cerebellar volume and balance have been seen in alcoholism where cerebellar volume is negatively effected by the disease (59, 60).

Investigations of postural control in schizophrenia were initiated as far back as the 1940s. Using vestibular stimulation Angyl and Sherman (61) found deficits related to postural control in patients with schizophrenia. Though the methods to investigate postural control vary greatly in their sensitivity, the general finding is that patients with schizophrenia have impaired postural control. Earlier work in this domain relied primarily upon behavioral measures and assessments of balance such as judgment of the presence of the Romberg sign (loss of balance when the eyes are closed, arms are outstretched, and feet are in a heel-to-toe tandem position), or assessing the ability to stand heel-to-toe, or on one foot (62, 63). Presence of the Romberg sign is significantly more common in patients with schizophrenia as compared to healthy controls (62) and patients are also impaired at standing on one foot, and heel-to-toe standing, though this is further compounded in patients with schizophrenia that also have a history of alcoholism (63). Thus, in schizophrenia, these postural control deficits are present, and can increase in severity in cases of alcohol abuse.

More recent investigations have used instrumental measures of balance and quantify body sway. Such measures have a much higher degree of sensitivity in their ability to detect postural abnormalities. Postural sway is quantified, and a greater degree of sway is indicative of poorer postural control. Furthermore, these instrumental measures also allow researchers to manipulate the placement of the feet, and whether or not participants complete the task with their eyes opened or closed. Marvel and colleagues (64) were the first to use such a measure of balance to investigate postural control in patients with schizophrenia. This investigation demonstrated that patients with schizophrenia have deficits in postural control such that they sway more than controls, though they did not see any further effects of alcohol use (64). These findings were recently replicated by Kent and colleagues (65), and they demonstrated that in patients, greater postural sway was associated with worse general psychopathology symptoms. There was a similar trend with respect to negative symptoms (such as anhedonia). Importantly, in both of these investigations anti-psychotic medications do not seem to be impacting the findings (64, 65). The findings of increased sway were also replicated across a heterogeneous group of patients with psychosis, including those with schizophrenia, acute psychosis, and undefined psychotic disorder (66). It is of note, however, that an additional recent study is not consistent with these findings (67).

To our knowledge, there has been only one study investigating postural control in UHR individuals. We recently investigated whether or not adolescents and young adults at UHR for psychosis show impaired postural control as measured by increased sway area (1). We found that postural control deficits are indeed present in UHR individuals. Furthermore, greater sway area was associated with increased negative symptoms. Finally, we investigated cerebello-cortical networks using resting state connectivity MRI. Not only were cerebello-cortical networks weaker in the UHR group relative to the controls, but they were also correlated with postural sway, providing a link between cerebellar networks and behavior in this population (1).

Future directions regarding postural control across the psychosis spectrum fall into several key domains. First is the use of instrumental measures to quantify postural sway. Since Marvel and colleagues first used this method in patients with schizophrenia (64) there have been several replications. Using such methods whenever possible provides a more sensitive measure of postural control, and also allows for better comparison across investigations. Relatedly, such methods also lend themselves to more complex statistical analysis techniques, which may yield additional important information regarding postural control and schizophrenia, as demonstrated by Kent and colleagues (65). Second, additional investigations and replications of our recent findings regarding postural control deficits in UHR populations (1) are warranted. Follow-ups across disease progression in longitudinal investigations will also be especially informative. Finally, more direct links with cerebellar structure and function in patient groups are needed. While there is strong evidence in healthy individuals and in other clinical populations linking the cerebellum more directly to cerebellar structure and function (57, 58, 63), such work is lacking across the psychosis spectrum.

TIMING

The cerebellum has been implicated in timing function across multiple research domains. Assessments in cerebellar patients have indicated that these individuals are impaired in both timing production and perception (68), and more recently, these impairments have been linked more specifically to discontinuous timing tasks, such as discrete finger tapping (69). Furthermore, functional neuroimaging methods have also implicated the cerebellum in timing perception (70, 71). Overall, the cerebellum is thought to be generally very important in timing, particularly with respect to precise event timing (72). It has been suggested that the cerebellum is particularly important in timing on the sub-second scale, and that longer timing intervals (supra-second) are more cognitively mediated, and may be related to the basal ganglia (72). On the whole the cerebellum is certainly implicated in timing and this is important for a wide array of motor tasks such as finger tapping and sequence learning. With respect to schizophrenia, there is evidence to indicate that timing functions, particularly those that are purported to be cerebellar-dependent are impaired. Here, we will focus primarily on sub-second timing, as this is most closely linked to the cerebellum.

Before discussing the timing deficits seen in patients with schizophrenia, it is important to understand the more common methods to investigate timing. Broadly speaking, these paradigms fall into two categories – time perception and production. The most typical way of assessing time perception is with a temporal bisection task. During a temporal bisection task, participants are presented with anchor durations that are either long or short. Then, test durations are presented and participants are asked to determine if the test duration is closer to the long or short anchor, and timing variability and temporal precision can be quantified [e.g., (48)]. Production tasks typically involved finger tapping using a synchronization–continuation type paradigm. Participants synchronize their tapping to a tone, and the tone is then taken away while tapping continues. Tap variability, often measured as the coefficient of variation, is used to quantify timing in these paradigms [e.g., (49)]. In both cases, the intervals used can vary to include both sub- and supra-second timing.

While investigations of timing in schizophrenia are certainly nothing new, earlier work largely focused on intervals of several seconds [e.g., Ref. (50–52)], which are thought to be more cognitively demanding, and are less likely to involve the cerebellum. More recent work, however, has investigated these sub-second durations in schizophrenia. The first of these investigations was by Elvevåg and colleagues (73). This study included two tasks, a temporal bisection task, as well as a temporal generalization task where participants had to recognize a standard duration. Across both domains, patients with schizophrenia were impaired with respect to controls, and importantly, performance was not correlated with working memory abilities, nor was it strongly associated with general intelligence (73). Davalos and colleagues replicated these findings even when the time between the anchor and test durations was varied (74), and similar results are seen with stimuli in both the auditory and visual domains (75). The patient group was impaired in both domains, but the impairment was greatest for the auditory presentation of stimuli. Interestingly, deficits have also been seen in patients with schizophrenia that have first-rank symptoms (76). These individuals experience hallucinations and thoughts that they believe to be under the control of another agent. The authors suggest that these patients may have a slowed internal pacemaker such that they experience time differently. However, it is crucial to note that these differences were not present in patients without first-rank symptoms (76), though it is possible that such sub-groups may be driving the effects in other investigations.

As noted above, sub-second intervals are thought to be more reliant upon the cerebellum, while supra-second intervals rely upon other neural systems, perhaps the basal ganglia, and are postulated to be more cognitively demanding (72). While the primary focus here is on cerebellar-mediated motor behaviors, work by Carroll and colleagues comparing temporal bisection performance on sub- and supra-second durations is worth noting (77). In this investigation, the patients were impaired in both timing ranges and the authors suggest that this may be indicative of a more general timing deficit in schizophrenia (77). There were also no associations with time deficits and symptomatology. However, it is worth noting that the sub-second findings not only support the cerebellar deficits in schizophrenia, the basal ganglia, and prefrontal cortex, which are important for more cognitively mediated tasks, have long since been implicated in schizophrenia (78). Thus, the longer supra-second durations may be tapping into additional neural systems that are impacted by the disease.

The majority of timing work has been done using time perception. In the one study, we know of using a synchronization–continuation time production task, there are also deficits in patients with schizophrenia as compared to controls during both the synchronization and continuation phases (79). During this task, tapping variability was increased in patients during both task phases. Furthermore, models of timing indicated that in patients with schizophrenia the deficit was due to actual deficits in timing as opposed to task performance or implementation (79). The motor production aspects of timing production may also come into play in motor learning tasks that involve timed, sequential finger movements (please see below).

Across the psychosis spectrum and in UHR individuals there has been very little work to date on timing. In those at genetic risk, a timing deficit was found, but this study was limited to supra-second durations, and similar supra-second deficits are seen in those with high schizotypy based on the Schizotypal Personality Questionnaire (80, 81). Thus, investigations of sub-second cerebellar-mediated timing tasks are necessary in UHR populations. However, sub- and supra-second performance was correlated with schizotypy dimensions (81). Overall, it is clear that further work is needed in these populations to better understand cerebellar-mediated timing deficits.

Future directions with respect to timing deficits fall into several domains. Most importantly is the need for additional work using temporal production tasks at the sub-second level in patients with schizophrenia. Relatedly, there is a general lack of research on this domain in at-risk populations and across the psychosis spectrum. Understanding whether or not such sub-second timing deficits exist prior to the onset of formal psychosis will provide us important insight as to the range of cerebellar-motor dysfunction prior to disease. Next, translation of such tasks to the scanner environment using functional neuroimaging is warranted, as are investigations looking at associations with regional cerebellar volume. While studies in individuals with cerebellar damage (69) and those using functional neuroimaging (70, 71) have implicated the cerebellum, such measures in schizophrenia and across the psychosis spectrum will further our understanding of the nature of this timing deficit in patients. Similarly, insightful relationships with regional cerebellar volume may be gleaned, and indeed Ivry and Spencer have suggested that there may be regional contributions of the cerebellum to timing (72). Finally, more work looking at timing with respect to symptom severity is needed.

MOTOR LEARNING

Motor learning is the process by which individuals learn to use new tools or devices, and turn novel and perhaps disjointed movements into fluid performance. Examples include learning to use a new computer mouse, or putting together a sequence of movements to shoot a basketball. The process of motor learning recruits a variety of cortical and subcortical brain regions (82–87), including the cerebellum. While it is certainly not the case that the cerebellum is engaged alone in motor learning, it does seem to be a key contributor, and investigating motor learning in patients with schizophrenia and those at UHR may be especially informative for our understanding of cerebellar–motor dysfunction in psychosis.

There are several different motor learning paradigms that are most typically used, and they seem to engage slightly different regions of the cerebellum (88). Motor sequence learning typically requires participants to learn a new sequence of finger movements, and both accuracy and reaction time are compared to a random sequence of button presses. This can be done explicitly where the participant knows they are learning a sequence, or implicitly when a sequence is learned while the participant is unaware. Mirror-drawing is a form of implicit motor learning that requires participants to update their movements based on a mirror-reflection of their movements. Over multiple trials, participants are able to accurately trace complex shapes. Pursuit rotor tasks, which are also implicit, ask participants to track a target across a track pad using a mouse or joystick. The target is titrated so that the target moves with varying speed in order to ensure a standard minimum level of accuracy and time on target is calculated. Over several trials, the time on target increases, indicative of learning.

Early work investigating motor learning in schizophrenia was behavioral in nature. Deficits on a pursuit rotor task were demonstrated by Schwartz and colleagues (89). Patients with schizophrenia spent less time on the target and deficits were exacerbated by advanced age. Furthermore, these findings were not associated with medication or other movement abnormalities in the patient group, though they were weakly related to cognitive abilities. Using an implicit sequence learning task (serial reaction time task), Green and colleagues investigated motor learning in patients with schizophrenia (90). While both patients with schizophrenia and healthy controls showed overall improvement in reaction time over the course of the task, the patient group showed less learning. The authors suggested that this may be due to possible cerebellar deficits (90). Looking at both implicit and explicit sequence learning, Pederesen and colleagues found deficits in both domains relative to controls in those with first-episode schizophrenia (91). Using mirror-drawing paradigms, patients with schizophrenia have been shown to have implicit learning adaptation deficits (92–94). However, these deficits are often linked to medications in these patients.

These initial behavioral findings were soon followed up by neuroimaging investigations using functional, anatomical, structural, and connectivity methods (95–100). Though the measures of motor learning varied to some degree, with one exception (100), the behavioral findings were consistent with prior work indicating deficits in motor learning in patients with schizophrenia. In addition, these neuroimaging investigations also provide further information about what underlying brain differences may be contributing to these deficits.

Kumari and colleagues (95) showed that there are differential brain activations when comparing patients to controls, and this included both the cerebellum and regions in the basal ganglia. The patients with schizophrenia did not activate these regions, though they were activated by controls (95). The implication of the cerebellum is perhaps not surprising, and interesting given the proposed role of the cerebellum in schizophrenia. Implicit sequence learning has also been investigated in patients with schizophrenia using PET (96). The patients showed less learning over time when compared to the control participants. In the patient group, the pre-frontal cortex and cerebellum showed differential correlations with sequence learning, highlighting the importance of the cerebellum, but also the importance of investigating the interactions between the cerebellum and pre-frontal cortex. Null findings with regards to learning and the cerebellum in schizophrenia have also been reported (100). Recently, using meta-analysis, we investigated cerebellar functional activation across a variety of task domains including motor function (27). The majority of included motor studies related to finger tapping and motor sequence learning. While we cannot speak to performance in our analyses, across these studies we did find that in patients with schizophrenia cerebellar functional activation was altered relative to controls during motor tasks, indicating that perhaps patients with schizophrenia rely upon less efficient cerebellar networks and processing (27).

As noted above with respect to the findings of Marvel and colleagues (96) investigating the interactions between the cerebellum and cortex is potentially of great interest. One way to do so is with functional connectivity analyses. These analyses measure the correlations between the brain signal in different brain regions. Recently, Kasparek and colleagues (97) investigated motor sequencing abnormalities with respect to functional connectivity between the cerebellum and cortex assessed while subjects were making finger movements (finger-to-thumb opposition). Motor sequencing was indexed based on the Neurological Evaluation Scale (NES). Both patients and controls were assessed and then divided into those with sequencing abnormalities and those without, regardless of diagnosis. However, motor sequencing deficits were more common in the patient group. There were no differences between patients with schizophrenia and controls with respect to functional connectivity; but, those with motor sequencing deficits had lower functional connectivity between the cerebellum and the motor cortex (101). Though the differences were not related to diagnosis, given that motor sequencing deficits were more common in the patient group, this finding is potentially important for understanding motor learning deficits in schizophrenia, and further highlights the role of the cerebellum.

Also relying upon the NES measure of sequencing, Hüttlova and colleagues recently looked at structural connectivity of the cerebellum using diffusion tensor imaging (DTI) (98). In the patients with motor sequencing deficits, there was decreased white matter structural integrity relative to controls in the superior cerebellar peduncle, which is the primary cerebellar efferent to the thalamus, whereas in the patients without deficits, differences relative to controls were seen in the corticospinal tract. This suggests potential sub-groups within schizophrenia related to motor sequencing, but also further highlights the cerebellum in motor deficits in this patient population.

Finally, structural MRI has been used with respect to sequence learning in patients with schizophrenia (99). Volumes of the cerebellum and pre-supplementary motor area (SMA) were investigated. First, the only group differences in volume were seen in the pre-SMA, and in patients volume in this region was correlated with implicit learning. While it is notable that there were no group differences in total cerebellar volume, nor were there any cerebellar-behavior relationships, the measurement of the entire structure may be a contributing factor. In sum, across multiple studies, there seem to be relatively robust deficits in motor sequence learning and in procedural learning in patients with schizophrenia, and this is supported by meta-analysis (102). Furthermore, there is at this point at least some evidence linking these deficits to the cerebellum, along with other liable neural substrates.

Though there has been a good deal of investigation related to motor learning in patients with schizophrenia, across the psychosis spectrum this has been investigated less extensively. In schizotypal individuals relative to controls, there do not appear to be any deficits in motor sequence learning, as measured using the implicit serial reaction time task (103, 104). However, more recently, we demonstrated procedural learning deficits in UHR patients relative to controls using a pursuit rotor task (2). Furthermore, learning was associated with volume of Crus I of the cerebellum. Given the cognitive functions of this region (4), and its associations with the pre-frontal cortex (105), this is an especially interesting finding, and may perhaps be related to the differing relationships with learning seen in the pre-frontal cortex and cerebellum (96). This may be due in part to the overall difficulty of this task as more complex motor tasks recruit this region of the cerebellum (106), though we may also be tapping into cognitive deficits as well.

Future directions in motor learning research across the psychosis spectrum include the further investigation of motor learning in psychosis spectrum populations. While there have been some inroads in this domain, further research is clearly warranted. Additionally, interesting investigations using non-invasive brain stimulation to the cerebellum have been completed in healthy individuals (107, 108). This stimulation can influence motor learning in these healthy individuals, and the impact on motor learning in patients with schizophrenia or across the psychosis spectrum may be especially informative. Finally, while there has been a great deal of work looking at the functional MRI correlates of motor learning in patients with schizophrenia, inclusion of anatomical and structural connectivity measures will be especially informative, both with respect to cerebellar pathology, but also to other brain regions implicated in motor learning.

Importantly, across all of these domains medication and cognitive deficits may be impacting performance. For example, deficits in mirror-drawing seem to be largely tied to medication (92–94), and our recent findings with respect to the cerebellum and pursuit rotor implicate cognitive cerebellar regions (2). Findings of cerebellar–motor deficits in at-risk populations where anti-psychotics are less commonly used indicate that many of these deficits are not an artifact of medications. However, not all studies of at-risk groups include only anti-psychotic naïve participants, and in patient groups, medications may be exacerbating these findings. Similarly, cognitive deficits in patients with schizophrenia may also be confounding these motor findings as motor performance is certainly closely linked to cognitive function [e.g., Ref. (109, 110)].

Finally, as noted throughout, and with the exception of motor learning, across most domains evidence directly linking these motor behaviors to the cerebellum are generally lacking. As such, the implication of cerebellar dysfunction is relatively indirect. By combining these motor measures with neuroimaging techniques we can better investigate the cerebellum in psychosis. Importantly, by combining these behavioral measures with measures of cerebellar volume or function, we can more effectively establish whether or not these behaviors may serve as markers of disease, and in clinical high-risk populations, they may serve as predictive biomarkers, as recently suggested by Bolbecker and colleagues (52). However, the cerebellum is a relatively large structure that is involved in both motor and non-motor behaviors (34, 35). An understanding of the cerebellar functional topography (4, 111) is important when considering the structure and its role in disease. It is important to consider the regional and functional organization within the cerebellum when looking to link the structure to overt motor deficits seen across the psychosis spectrum.

CEREBELLAR FUNCTIONAL TOPOGRAPHY

Beginning in the mid 1980s, investigators began speculating about the non-motor role of the cerebellum (28–31, 112). Investigations in non-human primates provided additional support for this notion. Using viral tract tracing methods, distinct tracts connecting pre-frontal and primary motor regions of the cortex to the cerebellum were revealed (113–116). These closed-loop circuits provide topographically segregated connections with the cerebral cortex. Specifically, the anterior aspects of the cerebellum (largely lobule V, but also lobules IV, and VI) along with a region in the inferior posterior cerebellum (lobules VIIIa and VIIIb) were connected to the primary motor cortex. Conversely, lateral aspects of the cerebellum (Crus II) were connected to the pre-frontal cortex (113). Similar motor and pre-frontal dissociations were seen in the dorsal and ventral aspects, respectively, of the cerebellar dentate nucleus (115).

More recently, using both structural (DTI) and functional connectivity neuroimaging (fcMRI) methods, a parallel topography of connections has been demonstrated in the human brain as well. fcMRI has revealed comparable distinct motor and cognitive networks in the cerebellar hemispheres at rest, based on the correlation between the resting state brain signal in these regions (117–119), and the dorsal and ventral dentate distinction was also replicated in humans using this methodology (120). However, distinct cerebello-cortical networks go beyond just a general motor/pre-frontal (non-motor) distinction. By investigating the resting state cerebello-cortical networks of individual cerebellar lobules, Bernard and colleagues showed that on a lobular level, the cerebellum is uniquely coupled with distinct cortical regions, resulting in distinct networks (105). Further support for multiple distinct motor and non-motor cerebellar networks comes from the work of Buckner and colleagues (121) (**Figure 1A**). They created a cerebellar parcelation based on coupling with multiple cortical resting state networks of the cortex. Finally, DTI has demonstrated distinct white matter tracts connecting the cerebellum and the cortex, that nicely parallel non-human primate literature (122). Thus, the cerebellum has distinct motor and non-motor closed-loop circuits with the cerebral cortex.

While the dissociable structural and functional motor and non-motor connections between the cerebellum and the cerebral cortex provide evidence for a topographically distinct functional organization in the cerebellum, there is also additional evidence from lesion studies and functional neuroimaging. The notion of a cognitive affective syndrome due to damage in the posterior lobe of the cerebellum was initially described by Schmahmann and Sherman (31). More recently, several investigations by Stoodley and colleagues (4, 111, 124) using both meta-analysis and functional

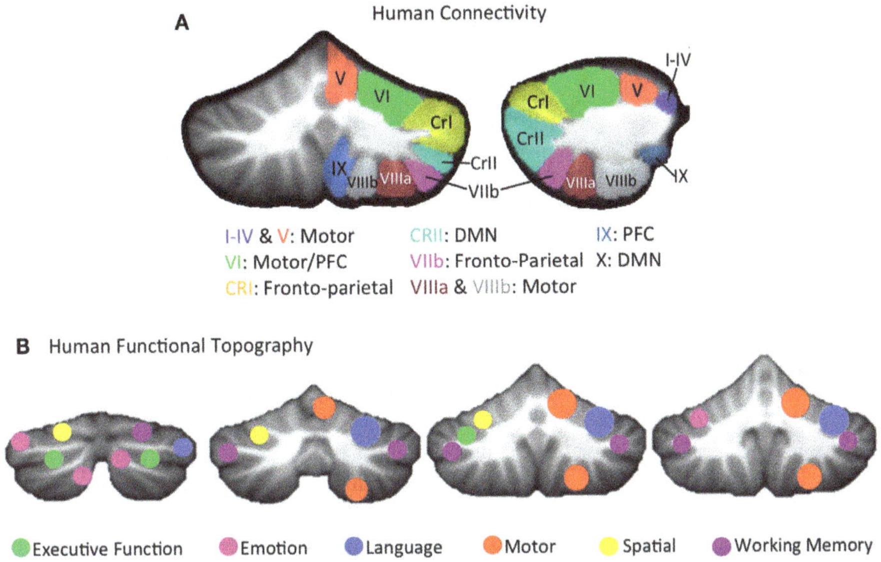

FIGURE 1 | (A) A lobular summary of resting state connectivity (left: coronal, right: sagittal) analyses conducted in humans, shown for the right cerebellar hemisphere, and concatenated across several studies (105, 121). Lobules of the right hemisphere are labeled, and general connectivity patterns are listed. The cerebellar vermis, made up of mid-line lobular aspects analogous to the hemispheres was not included, but distinct connectivity patterns, comparable to those seen in their hemispheric counterparts, have been reported (105). **(B)** A summary of the cerebellar functional topography presented on coronal slices (left to right, posterior to anterior), as demonstrated in humans using meta-analysis (4, 123) as well as functional neuroimaging (111) is provided. Verbal and spatial processing is differentially lateralized, and motor and non-motor processing patterns are relatively consistent with cerebellar sub-regions that are associated with motor and non-motor cortical regions, respectively. Motor activation was largely localized to the right hemisphere, given that only right handed individuals were included in these investigations. CRI, Crus I; CRII, Crus II; DMN, default mode network; PFC, pre-frontal cortex.

neuroimaging indicate that in addition to the closed-loop circuitry of the cerebellum, there is also a distinct topography of functional activation across different task domains (**Figure 1B**). That is, tasks such as working memory and motor tapping result in activations in distinct cerebellar regions. Likewise, language and spatial processing are lateralized as in the cortex (4, 111), and there is some evidence of a unique area active when processing emotion (4). Even within the anterior cerebellum, there appear to be sub-regions associated with distinct types of motor behavior and learning (88). Finally, in healthy individuals, regional cerebellar volume is also associated with individual differences in behavioral performance on motor and cognitive tasks in regionally specific ways (58). Importantly, there is increasing evidence to indicate that the cerebellum is processing non-motor information in many of these higher order cognitive tasks (125), and that cerebellar contributions are necessary for effective task performance, and not just an artifact of the structure's connections with the cerebral cortex (33). Given the diverse functional contributions of the cerebellum and the topographical nature of the activation associated with these task domains, the potential benefits of more targeted regional investigations are clear. Distinct cortico-cerebellar circuits and cerebellar regions may be differentially impacted in the disease state, and consideration of this putative regional variability may provide additional clarity for our understanding of the cerebellum in psychosis. Not only might this provide key insights into the motor deficits seen in schizophrenia and psychosis-risk, but it may also shed light on the various cognitive deficits that accompany the disorder.

REGIONAL CEREBELLAR INVESTIGATIONS

Converging evidence indicates that there are distinct functional sub-regions within the cerebellum making up a functional topography within the structure. Furthermore, the sub-regions of the cerebellum are part of distinct motor and non-motor cortical circuits. As such, when investigating the cerebellum it is important to consider the structure regionally. Making up approximately 10% of the total brain volume, the cerebellum is especially large to be considered as a whole. Its size, coupled with the known functional sub-regions call for a more fine-grained approach. It may be that sub-regions of the cerebellum are differentially impacted in the disease state. Not only would this approach provide important insight into the cerebellum across the psychosis spectrum, but it would also allow for comparisons across psychopathology. Cerebellar morphological differences with respect to controls have been observed in both depression and bipolar disorder (126–129). Understanding whether or not individual sub-regions or lobules are impacted differently across disease types will increase our understanding of the cerebellar contributions to psychopathology.

Post-mortem investigations provided some of the first evidence to indicate that there are cerebellar morphological differences in patients with schizophrenia with respect to controls. Differences when compared to controls have indicated reduced gyrification in the cerebellar vermis in patients (130), decreased neuronal integrity in patients, also in the cerebellar vermis (131), and there is a decrease in Purkinje cell (one of the main cerebellar cell types) density (fewer Purkinje cells) in patients with schizophrenia, as compared to controls (132). However, these results have been somewhat mixed with some groups showing no differences in patients relative to controls (133–135). These mixed findings may be because cerebellar deficits are specific to certain subtypes of schizophrenia as suggested by Lohr and colleagues (133), though regional sampling (or lack thereof) may also come into play in these investigations. Despite the mixed results, this work has provided important insights into the cerebellum in schizophrenia, particularly with respect to the underlying cytoarchitectonic pathology. That is, any possible volumetric differences seen using neuroimaging may be due to the decreased neuronal integrity and smaller number of Purkinje cells revealed in these post-mortem investigations. However, one weakness in this method is the fact that in at-risk populations (both genetic and UHR), there is a lack of post-mortem data as these individuals are typically quite young. Thus, we can only make inferences regarding cerebellar cytoarchitecture in these populations, and are reliant upon neuroimaging research.

Thanks to *in vivo* neuroimaging methods, there is increasing evidence to indicate that there are morphological differences in the cerebella of patients with schizophrenia, and there is an emerging literature indicating this in psychosis-risk as well (both UHR and genetic). However, the results thus far are relatively mixed [for a review, see Ref. (28)]. That is, in some cases, patients with schizophrenia have larger cerebellar volumes than controls, whereas in other cases, cerebellar volume in patients is decreased with respect to controls [cf. (28)]. Subsequent to the review of Shenton and colleagues, additional mixed findings with respect to cerebellar volume in schizophrenia have been revealed (136–142). The majority of these studies were methodologically similar in that they looked at the cerebellar hemispheres as a whole, and also investigated the vermis, which was often further subdivided into vermal sub-regions. The most consistent differences were found in the vermis across studies (136, 140), and the more detailed approach taken to investigating the vermis may be a contributing factor. The literature on the cerebellum in those at-risk for psychosis (UHR and genetic risk) is much smaller than that in schizophrenia, but the mixed findings persist (2, 142–144). However, they did differ methodologically, largely relying upon whole brain methods to assess gray matter. While this is not an exhaustive list of investigations of the cerebellum in schizophrenia and psychosis-risk, it is clear that the results are mixed, and while differences in study inclusion factors and subject age may contribute, we suggest that the gross measures of cerebellar volume, particularly in the hemispheres are a contributing factor.

Assessments of the cerebellum taking regional approaches are certainly the exception to the rule, and the few cases where these approaches have been used have provided interesting results. In a relatively small sample ($n = 19$), Loeher and colleagues (141) traced individual cerebellar lobules and found volumetric differences in the vermis. In childhood-onset schizophrenia, siblings, and healthy controls, Greenstein and colleagues also investigated cerebellar sub-regions (142). Though they did not look at individual lobules, they did subdivide the cerebellar hemispheres based on anatomical boundaries, providing increased detail relative to whole hemisphere analyses. In this study, the patients with schizophrenia ($n = 94$) had smaller anterior cerebellar volume, as well as smaller vermis volume when compared to controls, and they also showed differing developmental volumetric trajectories with respect to controls. Though the siblings of the patients did not differ in their regional cerebellar volumes from controls at baseline, they did show differing regional volumetric trajectories during longitudinal assessments (142). The detailed approaches taken here, along with the large sample size provide important insights with respect to cerebellar volume across the schizophrenia spectrum, and indicate that cerebellar sub-regions may be differentially impacted. As discussed above, Edwards and colleagues (43) investigated the anterior and posterior cerebellum with respect to eye-blink conditioning. They found smaller anterior cerebellar volume in patients with schizophrenia, and though there were no significant correlations with behavior in the patient group, the relationships were in the opposite direction as compared to controls. The authors as a result suggested that there may be altered structure–function relationships in schizophrenia with respect to the cerebellum and eye-blink conditioning (43). Using automatic lobular segmentation methods (58) we recently demonstrated that there are regional lobular differences in UHR adolescents and young adults (2). The anterior cerebellum and Crus I differed between the patient group and age-matched healthy controls, as did the vermis, though lobule X did not differ. Though this study was focused on specific cerebellar lobules, this provides further preliminary evidence that regional cerebellar volumetric differences may be present prior to the development of psychosis, and as we continue to longitudinally investigate these individuals, we will be able to investigate their volumetric trajectories over time. Finally, an intriguing new study looking at modularity of the cerebellum using DTI, indicates that the modular organization of the cerebellum is altered in schizophrenia (145). This finding further underscores the importance of regional approaches, as the functional architecture of the cerebellum seems to differ in schizophrenia (93), and these structural findings may underlie this (145).

It is clear that cerebellar-mediated motor behaviors are impacted in patients with schizophrenia, and across the psychosis spectrum. There are also cognitive deficits that may be linked, at least in part, to the cerebellum. From a morphological or network perspective, the contributions of the cerebellum are better understood by investigating this structure regionally. This may provide key insights into both the motor and cognitive deficits experienced by patients with schizophrenia and psychosis-risk groups. In the work summarized above, though the cerebellum is implicated in these motor deficits, direct links between morphology and performance are generally lacking. By taking a regional approach, specific hypotheses with respect to the cerebellum and motor performance can be defined and tested to better understand cerebellar-motor deficits across the psychosis spectrum. Applying this approach to procedural learning in UHR populations, we demonstrated that volume of Crus I in at-risk individuals was positively correlated with procedural learning (2). Interestingly, this motor task was associated with a more cognitive region of the cerebellum, suggesting that cognitive circuits, which are implicated in complex motor tasks (106) are perhaps also implicated in the cerebellar-motor deficits seen across the psychosis spectrum. Future investigations including regional measures of cerebellar volume with respect to motor deficits are warranted, and will likely provide important insights into the involvement of this structure in the disease state.

Most importantly, it is now much easier to investigate the cerebellum, especially morphology, on a lobular basis. While in the past such detailed analyses would require precise hand tracing of individual cerebellar lobules requiring large amounts of time and multiple raters, several recent studies have presented automatic lobular segmentation methods (58, 146, 147). These methods allow for investigators to easily compute lobular cerebellar volumes, and can be applied to large clinical samples, eliminating much of the methodological challenge associated with hand tracing. Bernard and Seidler (58) used the lobular delineations and masks originally created by Diedrichsen and colleagues as part of the SUIT atlas (148, 149). We successfully applied these methods in an investigation of adolescents and healthy controls at ultra-high risk for psychosis (2), demonstrating their utility in clinical populations, and providing important information about both regional cerebellar volume as well as motor learning in this population. Similarly, the lobular delineations available in the SUIT atlas can be used as starting seed regions for resting state connectivity analyses (1, 105, 150), and such analyses have revealed interesting differences and associations between lobular cerebellar connectivity, postural control, and symptom severity in UHR individuals (1). Finally, these regions may also serve as useful starting points for DTI analyses. Salmi and colleagues looked at cerebello-thalamo-cortical white matter networks in healthy adults (122), and similar analyses across the psychosis spectrum would be beneficial to our understanding of the role of the cerebellum in motor deficits, as well with respect to the disease state more generally.

CONCLUSION

A range of cerebellar-mediated motor tasks are impacted across the psychosis spectrum. Such motor impairments are present prior to disease onset, and may serve as a marker for pre-morbid cerebellar dysfunction. However, to date, direct links between these motor impairments and cerebellar morphology and/or cerebello-cortical networks have generally been lacking. In part, this may be due to standard approaches that treat the cerebellum as a functionally homogenous brain structure, though converging evidence indicates that there are distinct motor and non-motor functional regions within the cerebellum [e.g., Ref. (16, 23, 34, 90)]. Thus, we suggest that more specific topographically informed approaches to investigating the cerebellum (particularly with respect to cerebellar morphology and cerebello-cortical networks) across the psychosis spectrum will yield informative results with respect to the involvement of the cerebellum in psychosis. Such analyses will provide important information with respect to motor dysfunction, and they also may shed light on mixed findings with respect to cerebellar morphology. Furthermore, such an approach may provide additional insights into cognitive deficits experienced by these patient groups. That is, regional volume or functional differences may be limited to sub-regions of the cerebellum, and investigations of the structure as a whole may have masked these important findings. A better understanding of regional cerebellar morphological and functional differences will indicate whether or not there are more global or local cerebellar deficits in psychosis. Cerebellar-mediated movement abnormalities may be an overt manifestation of a more general cerebellar deficit, and regional analyses will allow this to be tested more directly. However, it is of note that these insights will be on a macro-structural level and potential underlying cellular differences and cellular contributions to pathophysiology are not assessed with these volumetric techniques. Computational models with respect of cerebellar cytoarchitectonics may be especially informative in that domain. Finally, regional approaches to investigating the cerebellum and cerebellar-motor abnormalities across disorders will allow for important comparisons resulting in a better understanding of the cerebellum across disorders.

ACKNOWLEDGMENTS

This work was supported by the National Institutes of Health (R01MH094650 to Vijay A. Mittal and F32MH102989-01 to Jessica A. Bernard). Publication of this article was funded by the University of Colorado Boulder Libraries Open Access Fund.

REFERENCES

1. Bernard JA, Dean DJ, Kent JS, Orr JM, Pelletier-Baldelli A, Lunsford-Avery J, et al. Cerebellar networks in individuals at ultra high-risk of psychosis: impact on postural sway and symptom severity. *Hum Brain Mapp* (2014) **35**:4064–78. doi:10.1002/hbm.22458
2. Dean DJ, Bernard JA, Orr JM, Pelletier-Baldelli A, Gupta T, Carol EE, et al. Cerebellar morphology and procedural learning impairment in neuroleptic-naive youth at ultrahigh risk of psychosis. *Clin Psychol Sci* (2013) **2**:152–64. doi:10.1177/2167702613500039
3. Mittal VA, Dean DJ, Bernard JA, Orr JM, Pelletier-Baldelli A, Carol EE, et al. Neurological soft signs predict abnormal cerebellar-thalamic tract development and negative symptoms in adolescents at high risk for psychosis: a longitudinal perspective. *Schizophr Bull* (2014) **40**:1204–15. doi:10.1093/schbul/sbt199
4. Stoodley CJ, Schmahmann JD. Functional topography in the human cerebellum: a meta-analysis of neuroimaging studies. *Neuroimage* (2009) **44**:489–501. doi:10.1016/j.neuroimage.2008.08.039
5. Andreasen NC, Olsen S. Negative v positive schizophrenia. *Arch Gen Psychiatry* (1982) **39**:789–94. doi:10.1001/archpsyc.1982.04290070025006
6. Mittal VA, Walker EF. Movement abnormalities: a putative biomarker of risk for psychosis. In: Ritsner MS, editor. *Neuropsychiatric Biomarkes, Endophenotypes, and Genes*. Springer Science + Business Media LLC (2009). p. 239–58.
7. Docx L, Morrens M, Bervoets C, Hulstijn W, Fransen E, De Hert M, et al. Parsing the components of the psychomotor syndrome in schizophrenia. *Acta Psychiatr Scand* (2012) **126**:256–65. doi:10.1111/j.1600-0447.2012.01846.x
8. Morrens M, Hulstijn W, Sabbe B. Psychomotor slowing in schizophrenia. *Schizophr Bull* (2007) **33**:1038–53. doi:10.1093/schbul/sbl051
9. Morrens M, Docx L, Walther S. Beyond boundaries: in search of an integrative view on motor symptoms in schizophrenia. *Front Psychiatry* (2014) **5**:145. doi:10.3389/fpsyt.2014.00145
10. Peralta V, Campos MS, De Jalón EG, Cuesta MJ. Motor behavior abnormalities in drug-naïve patients with schizophrenia spectrum disorders. *Mov Disord* (2010) **25**:1068–76. doi:10.1002/mds.23050
11. Pappa S, Dazzan P. Spontaneous movement disorders in antipsychotic-naive patients with first-episode psychoses: a systematic review. *Psychol Med* (2009) **39**:1065–76. doi:10.1017/S0033291708004716
12. Mittal VA, Daley M, Shiode MF, Bearden CE, O'Neill J, Cannon TD. Striatl volumes and dyskinetic movements in youth at high-risk for psychosis. *Schizophr Res* (2010) **123**:68–70. doi:10.1016/j.schres.2010.08.002.Striatal
13. Mittal VA, Dhruv S, Tessner KD, Walder DJ, Walker EF. The relations among putative biorisk markers in schizotypal adolescents: minor physical anomalies, movement abnormalities, and salivary cortisol. *Biol Psychiatry* (2007) **61**:1179–86. doi:10.1016/j.biopsych.2006.08.043
14. Mittal VA, Tessner KD, Trottman HD, Esterberg M, Dhrub SH, Simeonova DI, et al. Movement abnormalities and the progression of prodromal symptomatology in adolescents at risk for psychotic disorders. *J Abnorm Psychol* (2007) **116**:260–7. doi:10.1037/0021-843X.116.2.260
15. Mittal VA, Walker EF. Movement abnormalities predict conversion to axis I psychosis among prodromal adolescents. *J Abnorm Psychol* (2007) **116**:796–803. doi:10.1037/0021-843X.116.4.796
16. Mittal VA, Neumann C, Saczawa M, Walker EF. Longitudinal progression of movement abnormalities in relation to psychotic symptoms in adolescents at high risk of schizophrenia. *Arch Gen Psychiatry* (2008) **65**:165–71. doi:10.1001/archgenpsychiatry.2007.23

17. Mittal VA, Walker EF, Bearden CE, Walder D, Trottman H, Daley M, et al. Markers of basal ganglia dysfunction and conversion to psychosis: neurocognitive deficits and dyskinesias in the prodromal period. *Biol Psychiatry* (2010) **68**:93–9. doi:10.1016/j.biopsych.2010.01.021.Markers
18. Mittal VA, Walker EF. Movement abnormalities and schizophrenia in DSM-V. *Psychol Med* (2010) **40**:1581–3. doi:10.1017/S0033291710001352
19. Mittal VA, Jalbrzikowski M, Daley M, Roman C, Bearden CE, Cannon TD. Abnormal movements are associated with poor psychosocial functioning in adolescents at high risk for psychosis. *Schizophr Res* (2011) **130**:164–9. doi:10.1016/j.schres.2011.05.007
20. Mittal VA, Walker EF. Dyskinesias, tics, and psychosis: issues for the next diagnostic and statistical manual of mental disorders. *Psychiatry Res* (2013) **189**:158–9. doi:10.1016/j.psychres.2011.06.006.Dyskinesias
21. Dean DJ, Teulings H-L, Caligiuri M, Mittal VA. Handwriting analysis indicates spontaneous dyskinesias in neuroleptic naïve adolescents at high risk for psychosis. *J Vis Exp* (2014) **81**:e50852. doi:10.3791/50852.Handwriting
22. Mittal VA, Orr JM, Turner J, Pelletier AL, Dean DJ, Lunsford-Avery J, et al. Striatal abnormalities and spontaneous dyskinesias in non-clinical psychosis. *Schizophr Res* (2013) **151**:141–7. doi:10.1016/j.schres.2013.10.003
23. Andreasen NC, O'Leary DS, Cizadlo T, Arndt S, Rezai K, Ponto LL, et al. Schizophrenia and cognitive dysmetria: a positron-emission tomography study of dysfunctional prefrontal-thalamic-cerebellar circuitry. *Proc Natl Acad Sci U S A* (1996) **93**:9985–90. doi:10.1073/pnas.93.18.9985
24. Andreasen NC, Paradiso S, O'Leary DS. "Cognitive dysmetria" as an integrative theory of schizophrenia: a dysfunction in cortical-subcortical-cerebellar circuitry? *Schizophr Bull* (1998) **24**:203–18. doi:10.1093/oxfordjournals.schbul.a033321
25. Picard H, Amado I, Mouchet-Mages S, Olié J-P, Krebs M-O. The role of the cerebellum in schizophrenia: an update of clinical, cognitive, and functional evidences. *Schizophr Bull* (2008) **34**:155–72. doi:10.1093/schbul/sbm049
26. Barch DM. Cerebellar-thalamic connectivity in schizophrenia. *Schizophr Bull* (2014) **40**:1200–3. doi:10.1093/schbul/sbu076
27. Bernard JA, Mittal VA. Dysfunctional activation of the cerebellum in schizophrenia: a functional neuroimaging meta-analysis. *Clin Psychol Sci* (2014). doi:10.1177/2167702614542463
28. Leiner HC, Leiner L, Dow RS. Reappraising the cerebellum: what does the hindbrain contribute to the forebrain? *Behav Neurosci* (1989) **103**:998–1008. doi:10.1037/0735-7044.103.5.998
29. Leiner HC, Leiner L, Dow RS. Cognitive and language functions of the human cerebellum. *Trends Neurosci* (1993) **16**:444–7. doi:10.1016/0166-2236(93)90072-T
30. Leiner HC, Leiner AL, Dow RS. Does the cerebellum contribute to mental skills? *Behav Neurosci* (1986) **100**:443–54. doi:10.1037/0735-7044.100.4.443
31. Schmahmann JD, Sherman JC. The cerebellar cognitive affective syndrome. *Brain* (1998) **121**(Pt 4):561–79. doi:10.1093/brain/121.4.561
32. Chen SHA, Desmond JE. Temporal dynamics of cerebro-cerebellar network recruitment during a cognitive task. *Neuropsychologia* (2005) **43**:1227–37. doi:10.1016/j.neuropsychologia.2004.12.015
33. Desmond JE, Chen SHA, Shieh PB. Cerebellar transcranial magnetic stimulation impairs verbal working memory. *Ann Neurol* (2005) **58**:553–60. doi:10.1002/ana.20604
34. Ramnani N. The primate cortico-cerebellar system: anatomy and function. *Nat Rev Neurosci* (2006) **7**:511–22. doi:10.1038/nrn1953
35. Ito M. Control of mental activities by internal models in the cerebellum. *Nat Rev Neurosci* (2008) **9**:304–13. doi:10.1038/nrn2332
36. Spencer RMC, Ivry RB. Cerebellum and timing. In: Manto M, Schmahmann JD, Rossi F, Gruol DL, Koibuchi N, editors. *Handbook of the Cerebellum and Cerebellar Disorders*. New York: Springer (2013). p. 1201–19.
37. Keele SW, Ivry RB. Does the cerebellum provide a common computation for diverse tasks? A timing hypothesis. *Ann N Y Acad Sci* (1990) **6-8**:179–211. doi:10.1111/j.1749-6632.1990.tb48897.x
38. Kim JJ, Thompson RF. Cerebellar circuits and synaptic mechanisms involved in classical eyeblink conditioning. *Trends Neurosci* (1997) **20**:177–81. doi:10.1016/S0166-2236(96)10081-3
39. Gerwig M, Kolb FP, Timmann D. The involvement of the human cerebellum in eyeblink conditioning. *Cerebellum* (2007) **6**:38–57. doi:10.1080/14734220701225904
40. Lindquist DH, Steinmetz JE, Thompson RF. Cerebellum and eyeblink conditioning. In: Manto M, Schmahmann JD, Rossi F, Gruol DL, Koibuchi N, editors. *Handbook of the Cerebellum and Cerebellar Disorders*. Dordrecht: Springer (2013). p. 1175–90.
41. Bolbecker AR, Mehta CS, Edwards CR, Steinmetz JE, O'Donnell BF, Hetrick WP. Eye-blink conditioning deficits indicate temporal processing abnormalities in schizophrenia. *Schizophr Res* (2009) **111**:182–91. doi:10.1016/j.schres.2009.03.016
42. Brown SM, Kieffaber PD, Carroll C, Vohs JL, Tracy J, Shekhar A, et al. Eyeblink conditioning deficits indicate timing and cerebellar abnormalities in schizophrenia. *Brain Cogn* (2005) **58**:94–108. doi:10.1016/j.bandc.2004.09.011
43. Edwards CR, Newman S, Bismark A, Skosnik PD, O'Donnell BF, Shekhar A, et al. Cerebellum volume and eyeblink conditioning in schizophrenia. *Psychiatry Res* (2008) **162**:185–94. doi:10.1016/j.pscychresns.2007.06.001
44. Bolbecker AR, Steinmetz AB, Mehta CS, Forsyth JK, Klaunig MJ, Lazar EK, et al. Exploration of cerebellar-dependent associative learning in schizophrenia: effects of varying and shifting interstimulus interval on eyeblink conditioning. *Behav Neurosci* (2011) **125**:687–98. doi:10.1037/a0025150
45. Forsyth JK, Bolbecker AR, Mehta CS, Klaunig MJ, Steinmetz JE, O'Donnell BF, et al. Cerebellar-dependent eyeblink conditioning deficits in schizophrenia spectrum disorders. *Schizophr Bull* (2012) **38**:751–9. doi:10.1093/schbul/sbq148
46. Parker KL, Andreasen NC, Liu D, Freeman JH, O'Leary DS. Eyeblink conditioning in unmedicated schizophrenia patients: a positron emission tomography study. *Psychiatry Res* (2013) **214**:402–9. doi:10.1016/j.pscychresns.2013.07.006
47. Coesmans M, Röder CH, Smit AE, Koekkoek SKE, de Zeeuw CI, Frens MA, et al. Cerebellar motor learning deficits in medicated and medication-free men with recent-onset schizophrenia. *J Psychiatry Neurosci* (2014) **39**:3–11. doi:10.1503/jpn.120205
48. Sears LL, Andreasen NC, O'Leary DS. Cerebellar functional abnormalities in schizophrenia are suggested by classical eyeblink conditioning. *Biol Psychiatry* (2000) **48**:204–9. doi:10.1016/S0006-3223(00)00247-X
49. Marenco S, Weinberger DR, Schreurs BG. Single-cue delay and trace classical conditioning in schizophrenia. *Biol Psychiatry* (2003) **53**:390–402. doi:10.1016/S0002-3223(03)01506-8
50. Stevens A, Schwarz J, Schwarz B, Ruf I, Kolter T, Czekalla J. Implicit and explicit learning in schizophrenics treated with olanzapine and with classic neuroleptics. *Psychopharmacology (Berl)* (2002) **160**:299–306. doi:10.1007/s00213-001-0974-1
51. Lubow RE. Classical eyeblink conditioning and schizophrenia: a short review. *Behav Brain Res* (2009) **202**:1–4. doi:10.1016/j.bbr.2009.03.006
52. Bolbecker AR, Kent JS, Petersen IT, Klaunig MJ, Forsyth JK, Howell JM, et al. Impaired cerebellar-dependent eyeblink conditioning in first-degree relatives of individuals with schizophrenia. *Schizophr Bull* (2014) **40**:1001–10. doi:10.1093/schbul/sbt112
53. Cheng DT, Disterhoft JF, Power JM, Ellis D, Desmond JE. Neural substrates underlying human delay and trace eyeblink conditioning. *Proc Natl Acad Sci U S A* (2008) **105**:8108–13. doi:10.1073/pnas.0800374105
54. Cheng DT, Meintjes EM, Stanton ME, Desmond JE, Pienaar M, Dodge NC, et al. Functional MRI of cerebellar activity during eyeblink classical conditioning in children and adults. *Hum Brain Mapp* (2014) **35**:1390–403. doi:10.1002/hbm.22261
55. Holmes G. The cerebellum of man. *Brain* (1939) **62**:1–30. doi:10.1093/brain/62.1.1
56. Diener HC, Dichgans J, Bacher M, Gompf B. Quantification of postural sway in normals and patients with cerebellar diseases. *Electroencephalogr Clin Neurophysiol* (1984) **57**:134–42. doi:10.1016/0013-4694(84)90172-X
57. Ouchi Y, Okada H, Yoshikawa E, Nobezawa S, Futatsubashi M. Brain activation during maintenance of standing postures in humans. *Brain* (1999) **122**:329–38. doi:10.1093/brain/122.2.329
58. Bernard JA, Seidler RD. Relationships between regional cerebellar volume and sensorimotor and cognitive function in young and older adults. *Cerebellum* (2013) **12**:721–37. doi:10.1007/s12311-013-0481-z
59. Sullivan EV, Rose J, Pfefferbaum A. Physiological and focal cerebellar substrates of abnormal postural sway and tremor in alcoholic women. *Biol Psychiatry* (2010) **67**:44–51. doi:10.1016/j.biopsych.2009.08.008
60. Sullivan EV, Rohlfing T, Pfefferbaum A. Pontocerebellar volume deficits and ataxia in alcoholic men and women: no evidence for "telescoping". *Psychopharmacology (Berl)* (2010) **208**:279–90. doi:10.1007/s00213-009-1729-7
61. Angyal A, Sherman MA. Postural reactions to vestibular stimulation in schizophrenic and normal subjects. *Am J Psychiatry* (1942) **98**:857–62.

62. Ho B-C, Mola C, Andreasen NC. Cerebellar dysfunction in neuroleptic naive schizophrenia patients: clinical, cognitive, and neuroanatomic correlates of cerebellar neurologic signs. *Biol Psychiatry* (2004) **55**:1146–53. doi:10.1016/j.biopsych.2004.02.020
63. Sullivan EV, Rosenbloom MJ, Pfefferbaum A. Balance and gait deficits in schizophrenia compounded by the comorbidity of alcoholism. *Am J Psychiatry* (2004) **161**:751–5. doi:10.1176/appi.ajp.161.4.751
64. Marvel CL, Schwartz BL, Rosse RB. A quantitative measure of postural sway deficits in schizophrenia. *Schizophr Res* (2004) **68**:363–72. doi:10.1016/j.schres.2003.09.003
65. Kent JS, Hong SL, Bolbecker AR, Klaunig MJ, Forsyth JK, O'Donnell BF, et al. Motor deficits in schizophrenia quantified by nonlinear analysis of postural sway. *PLoS One* (2012) **7**:e41808. doi:10.1371/journal.pone.0041808
66. Stensdotter A-K, Wanvik AK, Lorås HW. Postural control in quiet standing with a concurrent cognitive task in psychotic conditions. *J Mot Behav* (2013) **45**:279–87. doi:10.1080/00222895.2013.791241
67. Ahlgrén-Rimpiläinen A, Lauerma H, Kähkönen S, Aalto H, Pyykkö I, Palmgren K, et al. Effect of visual information on postural control in patients with schizophrenia. *J Nerv Ment Dis* (2010) **198**:601–3. doi:10.1097/NMD.0b013e3181ea16bc
68. Ivry RB, Keele SW. Timing functions of the cerebellum. *J Cogn Neurosci* (1989) **1**:136–52. doi:10.1162/jocn.1989.1.2.136
69. Spencer RMC, Zelaznik HN, Diedrichsen J, Ivry RB. Disrupted timing of discontinuous but not continuous movements by cerebellar lesions. *Science* (2003) **300**:1437–9. doi:10.1126/science.1083661
70. Jueptner M, Rijntjes M, Weiller C, Faiss JH, Timmann D, Mueller SP, et al. Localization of a cerebellar timing process using PET. *Neurology* (1995) **45**:1540–5. doi:10.1212/WNL.45.8.1540
71. Lewis P, Miall R. Brain activation patterns during measurement of sub- and supra-second intervals. *Neuropsychologia* (2003) **41**:1583–92. doi:10.1016/S0028-3932(03)00118-0
72. Ivry RB, Spencer RMC. The neural representation of time. *Curr Opin Neurobiol* (2004) **14**:225–32. doi:10.1016/j.conb.2004.03.013
73. Elvevåg B, McCormack T, Glibert A, Brown GDA, Wienberger DR, Goldberg TE. Duration judgements in patients with schizophrenia. *Psychol Med* (2003) **33**:1249–61. doi:10.1017/S0033291703008122
74. Davalos DB, Kisley M, Ross RG. Effects of interval duration on temporal processing in schizophrenia. *Brain Cogn* (2003) **52**:295–301. doi:10.1016/S0278-2626(03)00157-X
75. Carroll CA, Boggs J, O'Donnell BF, Shekhar A, Hetrick WP. Temporal processing dysfunction in schizophrenia. *Brain Cogn* (2008) **67**:150–61. doi:10.1016/j.bandc.2007.12.005
76. Waters F, Jablensky A. Time discrimination deficits in schizophrenia patients with first-rank (passivity) symptoms. *Psychiatry Res* (2009) **167**:12–20. doi:10.1016/j.psychres.2008.04.004
77. Carroll CA, O'Donnell BF, Shekhar A, Hetrick WP. Timing dysfunctions in schizophrenia span from millisecond to several-second durations. *Brain Cogn* (2009) **70**:181–90. doi:10.1016/j.bandc.2009.02.001
78. Buchsbaum MS. The frontal lobes, basal ganglia, and temporal lobes as sites for schizophrenia. *Schizophr Bull* (1990) **16**:379–89. doi:10.1093/schbul/16.3.379
79. Carroll CA, O'Donnell BF, Shekhar A, Hetrick WP. Timing dysfunctions in schizophrenia as measured by a repetitive finger tapping task. *Brain Cogn* (2009) **71**:345–53. doi:10.1016/j.bandc.2009.06.009
80. Penney TB, Meck WH, Roberts S, Gibbon J, Erlenmeyer-Kimling L. Interval-timing deficits in individuals at high risk for schizophrenia. *Brain Cogn* (2005) **58**:109–18. doi:10.1016/j.bandc.2004.09.012
81. Lee K-H, Dixon JK, Spence S, Woodruff PWR. Time perception dysfunction in psychometric schizotypy. *Pers Individ Dif* (2006) **40**:1363–73. doi:10.1016/j.paid.2005.10.021
82. Imamizu H, Miyauchi S, Tamada T, Sasaki Y, Takino R, Pütz B, et al. Human cerebellar activity reflecting an acquired internal model of a new tool. *Nature* (2000) **403**:192–5. doi:10.1038/35003194
83. Jenkins IH, Brooks DJ, Frackowiak RSJ, Passingham FE. Motor sequence tomography learning: a study with positron. *J Neurosci* (1994) **14**(6):3775–90.
84. Doyon J, Song AW, Karni A, Lalonde F, Adams MM, Ungerleider LG. Experience-dependent changes in cerebellar contributions to motor sequence learning. *Proc Natl Acad Sci U S A* (2002) **99**:1017–22. doi:10.1073/pnas.022615199
85. Doyon J, Benali H. Reorganization and plasticity in the adult brain during learning of motor skills. *Curr Opin Neurobiol* (2005) **15**:161–7. doi:10.1016/j.conb.2005.03.004
86. Seidler RD, Noll DC, Chintalapati P. Bilateral basal ganglia activation associated with sensorimotor adaptation. *Exp Brain Res* (2006) **175**:544–55. doi:10.1007/s00221-006-0571-y
87. Schendan HE, Searl MM, Melrose RJ, Stern CE. An FMRI study of the role of the medial temporal lobe in implicit and explicit sequence learning. *Neuron* (2003) **37**:1013–25. doi:10.1016/S0896-6273(03)00123-5
88. Bernard JA, Seidler RD. Cerebellar contributions to visuomotor adaptation and motor sequence learning: an ALE meta-analysis. *Front Hum Neurosci* (2013) **7**:27. doi:10.3389/fnhum.2013.00027
89. Schwartz BL, Rosse RB, Veazey C, Deutsch SI. Impaired motor skill learning in schizophrenia: implications for corticostriatal dysfunction. *Biol Psychiatry* (1996) **39**:241–8. doi:10.1016/0006-3223(95)00130-1
90. Green MF, Kern RS, Williams O, McGurk S, Kee K. Procedural learning in schizophrenia: evidence from serial reaction time. *Cogn Neuropsychiatry* (1997) **2**:123–34. doi:10.1080/135468097396360
91. Pedersen A, Siegmund A, Ohrmann P, Rist F, Rothermundt M, Suslow T, et al. Reduced implicit and explicit sequence learning in first-episode schizophrenia. *Neuropsychologia* (2008) **46**:186–95. doi:10.1016/j.neuropsychologia.2007.07.021
92. Bédard M-A, Scherer H, Delorimier J, Stip E, Lalonde P. Differential effects of D2-and D4-blocking neuroleptics on the procedural learning of schizophrenic patients. *Can J Psychiatry* (1996) **41**:S21–4.
93. Bédard M-A, Shérer H, Stip E, Cohen H, Rodriguez J-P, Richer F. Procedural learning in schizophrenia: further consideration on the deleterious effect of neuroleptics. *Brain Cogn* (2000) **43**:31–9.
94. Scherer H, Bedard M-A, Stip E, Paquet F, Richer F, Bériault M, et al. Procedural learning in schizophrenia can reflect the pharmacologic properties of the antipsychotic treatments. *Cogn Behav Neurol* (2004) **17**:32–40. doi:10.1097/00146965-200403000-00004
95. Kumari V, Gray J, Honey GD, Soni W, Bullmore ET, Williams SCR, et al. Procedural learning in schizophrenia: a functional magnetic resonance imaging investigation. *Schizophr Res* (2002) **57**:97–107. doi:10.1016/S0920-9964(01)00270-5
96. Marvel CL, Turner BM, O'Leary DS, Johnson HJ, Pierson RK, Ponto LLB, et al. The neural correlates of implicit sequence learning in schizophrenia. *Neuropsychology* (2007) **21**:761–77. doi:10.1037/0894-4105.21.6.761
97. Kasparek T, Rehulova J, Kerkovsky M, Sprlakova A, Mechl M, Mikl M. Cortico-cerebellar functional connectivity and sequencing of movements in schizophrenia. *BMC Psychiatry* (2012) **12**:17. doi:10.1186/1471-244X-12-17
98. Hüttlova J, Kikinis Z, Kerkovsky M, Bouix S, Vu M-A, Makris N, et al. Abnormalities in myelination of the superior cerebellar peduncle in patients with schizophrenia and deficits in movement sequencing. *Cerebellum* (2014) **13**:415–24. doi:10.1007/s12311-014-0550-y
99. Exner C, Weniger G, Schmidt-Samoa C, Irle E. Reduced size of the pre-supplementary motor cortex and impaired motor sequence learning in first-episode schizophrenia. *Schizophr Res* (2006) **84**:386–96. doi:10.1016/j.schres.2006.03.013
100. Zedkova L, Woodward ND, Harding I, Tibbo PG, Purdon SE. Procedural learning in schizophrenia investigated with functional magnetic resonance imaging. *Schizophr Res* (2006) **88**:198–207. doi:10.1016/j.schres.2006.06.039
101. Kasparek T, Prikryl R, Rehulova J, Marecek R, Mikl M, Prikrylova H, et al. Brain functional connectivity of male patients in remission after the first episode of schizophrenia. *Hum Brain Mapp* (2012) **34**(3):501–752. doi:10.1002/hbm.21469
102. Siegert RJ, Weatherall M, Bell EM. Is implicit sequence learning impaired in schizophrenia? A meta-analysis. *Brain Cogn* (2008) **67**:351–9. doi:10.1016/j.bandc.2008.02.005
103. Pedersen A, Rist F. Implicit memory in schizotypal subjects and normal controls: effects of a secondary task on sequence learning. *Percept Mot Skills* (2001) **92**:349–67. doi:10.2466/pms.2001.92.2.349
104. Ferraro FR, Okerlund M. Implicit memory of nonclinicla schizotypal individuals. *Percept Mot Skills* (1995) **80**:371–6. doi:10.2466/pms.1995.80.2.371
105. Bernard JA, Seidler RD, Hassevoort KM, Benson BL, Welsh RC, Wiggins JL, et al. Resting state cortico-cerebellar functional connectivity networks: a comparison of anatomical and self-organizing map approaches. *Front Neuroanat* (2012) **6**:31. doi:10.3389/fnana.2012.00031

106. Schlerf JE, Verstynen TD, Ivry RB, Spencer RMC. Evidence of a novel somatopic map in the human neocerebellum during complex actions. *J Neurophysiol* (2010) **103**:3330–6. doi:10.1152/jn.01117.2009
107. Block H, Celnik P. Stimulating the cerebellum affects visuomotor adaptation but not intermanual transfer of learning. *Cerebellum* (2013) **12**:781–93. doi:10.1007/s12311-013-0486-7
108. Schlerf JE, Galea JM, Bastian AJ, Celnik P. Dynamic modulation of cerebellar excitability for abrupt, but not gradual, visuomotor adaptation. *J Neurosci* (2012) **32**:11610–7. doi:10.1523/JNEUROSCI.1609-12.2012
109. Anguera JA, Bernard JA, Jaeggi SM, Buschkuehl M, Benson BL, Jennett S, et al. The effects of working memory resource depletion and training on sensorimotor adaptation. *Behav Brain Res* (2013) **228**:107–15. doi:10.1016/j.bbr.2011.11.040.The
110. Anguera JA, Reuter-Lorenz PA, Willingham DT, Seidler RD. Failure to engage spatial working memory contributes to age-related declines in visuomotor learning. *J Cogn Neurosci* (2011) **23**:11–25. doi:10.1162/jocn.2010.21451
111. Stoodley CJ, Valera EM, Schmahmann JD. Functional topography of the cerebellum for motor and cognitive tasks: an fMRI study. *Neuroimage* (2012) **59**:1560–70. doi:10.1016/j.neuroimage.2011.08.065
112. Leiner HC, Leiner AL, Dow RS. The human cerebro-cerebellar system: its computing, cognitive, and language skills. *Behav Brain Res* (1991) **44**:113–28. doi:10.1016/S0166-4328(05)80016-6
113. Kelly RM, Strick PL. Cerebellar loops with motor cortex and prefrontal cortex of a nonhuman primate. *J Neurosci* (2003) **23**:8432–44.
114. Akkal D, Dum RP, Strick PL. Supplementary motor area and presupplementary motor area: targets of basal ganglia and cerebellar output. *J Neurosci* (2007) **27**:10659–73. doi:10.1523/JNEUROSCI.3134-07.2007
115. Dum RP, Strick PL. An unfolded map of the cerebellar dentate nucleus and its projections to the cerebral cortex. *J Neurophysiol* (2003) **89**:634–9. doi:10.1152/jn.00626.2002
116. Strick PL, Dum RP, Fiez JA. Cerebellum and nonmotor Function. *Annu Rev Neurosci* (2009) **32**:413–34. doi:10.1146/annurev.neuro.31.060407.125606
117. Krienen FM, Buckner RL. Segregated fronto-cerebellar circuits revealed by intrinsic functional connectivity. *Cereb Cortex* (2009) **19**:2485–97. doi:10.1093/cercor/bhp135
118. Habas C, Kamdar N, Nguyen D, Prater K, Beckmann CF, Menon V, et al. Distinct cerebellar contributions to intrinsic connectivity networks. *J Neurosci* (2009) **29**:8586–94. doi:10.1523/JNEUROSCI.1868-09.2009
119. O'Reilly JX, Beckmann CF, Tomassini V, Ramnani N, Johansen-Berg H. Distinct and overlapping functional zones in the cerebellum defined by resting state functional connectivity. *Cereb Cortex* (2010) **20**:953–65. doi:10.1093/cercor/bhp157
120. Bernard JA, Peltier SJ, Benson BL, Wiggins JL, Jaeggi SM, Buschkuehl M, et al. Dissociable functional networks of the human dentate nucleus. *Cereb Cortex* (2014) **24**:2151–9. doi:10.1093/cercor/bht065
121. Buckner RL, Krienen FM, Castellanos A, Diaz JC, Yeo BTT. The organization of the human cerebellum estimated by intrinsic functional connectivity. *J Neurophysiol* (2011) **106**(5):2322–45. doi:10.1152/jn.00339.2011
122. Salmi J, Pallesen KJ, Neuvonen T, Brattico E, Korvenoja A, Salonen O, et al. Cognitive and motor loops of the human cerebro-cerebellar system. *J Cogn Neurosci* (2010) **22**:2663–76. doi:10.1162/jocn.2009.21382
123. E KH, Chen SH, Ho MH, Desmond JE. A meta-analysis of cerebellar contributions to higher cognition from PET and fMRI studies. *Hum Brain Mapp* (2012) **35**(2):593–615. doi:10.1002/hbm.22194
124. Stoodley CJ, Schmahmann JD. Evidence for topographic organization in the cerebellum of motor control versus cognitive and affective processing. *Cortex* (2010) **46**:831–44. doi:10.1016/j.cortex.2009.11.008
125. Balsters JH, Whelan CD, Robertson IH, Ramnani N. Cerebellum and cognition: evidence for the encoding of higher order rules. *Cereb Cortex* (2013) **23**:1433–43. doi:10.1093/cercor/bhs127
126. Strakowski SM, Delbello MP, Adler CM. The functional neuroanatomy of bipolar disorder: a review of neuroimaging findings. *Mol Psychiatry* (2005) **10**:105–16. doi:10.1038/sj.mp.4001585
127. DelBello MP, Strakowski SM, Zimmerman ME, Hawkins JM, Sax KW. MRI analysis of the cerebellum in bipolar disorder: a pilot study. *Neuropsychopharmacology* (1999) **21**:63–8. doi:10.1016/S0893-133X(99)00026-3
128. Mills NP, Delbello MP, Adler CM, Strakowski SM. MRI analysis of cerebellar vermal abnormalities in bipolar disorder. *Am J Psychiatry* (2005) **162**:1530–2. doi:10.1176/appi.ajp.162.8.1530
129. Escalona PR, Early B, McDonald WM, Doraiswamy M, Shah SA, Husain MM, et al. Reduction of cerebellar volume in major depression: a controlled MRI study. *Depression* (1993) **1**:156–8. doi:10.1002/depr.3050010307
130. Schmitt A, Schulenberg W, Bernstein H-G, Steiner J, Schneider-Axmann T, Yeganeh-Doost P, et al. Reduction of gyrification index in the cerebellar vermis in schizophrenia: a post-mortem study. *World J Biol Psychiatry* (2011) **12**(Suppl 1):99–103. doi:10.3109/15622975.2011.598379
131. Deicken RF, Feiwell R, Schuff N, Soher B. Evidence for altered cerebellar vermis neuronal integrity in schizophrenia. *Psychiatry Res* (2001) **107**:125–34. doi:10.1016/S0925-4927(01)00103-2
132. Maloku E, Covelo IR, Hanbauer I, Guidotti A, Kadriu B, Hu Q, et al. Lower number of cerebellar Purkinje neurons in psychosis is associated with reduced reelin expression. *Proc Natl Acad Sci U S A* (2010) **107**:4407–11. doi:10.1073/pnas.0914483107
133. Lohr JB, Jeste DV. Cerebellar pathology in schizophrenia? A neuronometric study. *Biol Psychiatry* (1986) **21**:865–75. doi:10.1016/0006-3223(86)90259-3
134. Andersen BO, Pakkenberg B. Stereological quantitation in cerebella from people with schizophrenia stereological quantitation in cerebella from people with schizophrenia. *Br J Psychiatry* (2003) **182**:354–61. doi:10.1192/bjp.02.65
135. Andersen BB, Fabricius K, Gundersen HJG, Jelsing J, Stark K. No change in neuron numbers in the dentate nucleus of patients with schizophrenia estimated with a new stereological method – the smooth fractionator. *J Anat* (2004) **205**:313–21. doi:10.1111/j.0021-8782.2004.00337.x
136. Ichimiya T, Okubo Y, Suhara T, Sudo Y. Reduced volume of the cerebellar vermis in neuroleptic-naive schizophrenia. *Biol Psychiatry* (2001) **49**:20–7. doi:10.1016/S0006-3223(00)01081-7
137. Keller A, Castellanos FX, Vaituzis C, Jeffries NO, Giedd JN, Rapoport JL. Progressive loss of cerebellar volume in childhood-onset schizophrenia. *Am J Psychiatry* (2003) **160**:128–33. doi:10.1176/appi.ajp.160.1.128
138. Bottmer C, Bachmann S, Pantel J, Essig M, Amann M, Schad LR, et al. Reduced cerebellar volume and neurological soft signs in first-episode schizophrenia. *Psychiatry Res* (2005) **140**:239–50. doi:10.1016/j.pscychresns.2005.02.011
139. James AC, James S, Smith DM, Javaloyes A. Cerebellar, prefrontal cortex, and thalamic volumes over two time points in adolescent-onset schizophrenia. *Am J Psychiatry* (2004) **161**:1023–9. doi:10.1176/appi.ajp.161.6.1023
140. Okugawa G, Sedvall GC, Agartz I. Smaller cerebellar vermis but not hemisphere volumes in patients with chronic schizophrenia. *Am J Psychiatry* (2003) **160**:1614–7. doi:10.1176/appi.ajp.160.9.1614
141. Loeber RT, Cintron CM, Yurgelun-Todd D. Morphometry of individual cerebellar lobules in schizophrenia. *Am J Psychiatry* (2001) **158**:952–4. doi:10.1176/appi.ajp.158.987.952
142. Greenstein D, Lenroot R, Clausen L, Chavez A, Vaituzis C, Tran L, et al. Cerebellar development in childhood onset schizophrenia and non-psychotic siblings. *Psychiatry Res* (2011) **193**:131–7. doi:10.1016/j.pscychresns.2011.02.010
143. Borgwardt SJ, Riecher-Rössler A, Dazzan P, Chitnis X, Aston J, Drewe M, et al. Regional gray matter volume abnormalities in the at risk mental state. *Biol Psychiatry* (2007) **61**:1148–56. doi:10.1016/j.biopsych.2006.08.009
144. Pantelis C, Velakoulis D, McGorry PD, Wood SJ, Suckling J, Phillips LJ, et al. Neuroanatomical abnormalities before and after onset of psychosis: a cross-sectional and longitudinal MRI comparison. *Lancet* (2003) **361**:281–8. doi:10.1016/S0140-6736(03)12323-9
145. Kim D-J, Kent JS, Bolbecker AR, Sporns O, Cheng H, Newman SD, et al. Disrupted modular architecture of cerebellum in schizophrenia: a graph theoretic analysis. *Schizophr Bull* (2014) **40**:1216–26. doi:10.1093/schbul/sbu059
146. Weier K, Fonov V, Lavoie K, Doyon J, Collins DL. Rapid automatic segmentation of the human cerebellum and its lobules (RASCAL)-Implementation and application of the patch-based label-fusion technique with a template library to segment the human cerebellum. *Hum Brain Mapp* (2014) **35**:5026–39. doi:10.1002/hbm.22529
147. Park MTM, Pipitone J, Baer LH, Winterburn JL, Shah Y, Chavez S, et al. Derivation of high-resolution MRI atlases of the human cerebellum at 3T and segmentation using multiple automatically generated templates. *Neuroimage* (2014) **95C**:217–31. doi:10.1016/j.neuroimage.2014.03.037

148. Diedrichsen J, Balsters JH, Flavell J, Cussans E, Ramnani N. A probabilistic MR atlas of the human cerebellum. *Neuroimage* (2009) **46**:39–46. doi:10.1016/j.neuroimage.2009.01.045
149. Diedrichsen J. A spatially unbiased atlas template of the human cerebellum. *Neuroimage* (2006) **33**:127–38. doi:10.1016/j.neuroimage.2006.05.056
150. Bernard JA, Peltier SJ, Wiggins JL, Jaeggi SM, Buschkuehl M, Fling BW, et al. Disrupted cortico-cerebellar connectivity in older adults. *Neuroimage* (2013) **83**:103–19. doi:10.1016/j.neuroimage.2013.06.042

17

Functional and structural alterations in the cingulate motor area relate to decreased fronto-striatal coupling in major depressive disorder with psychomotor disturbances

Benny Liberg[1,2,3]*, Paul Klauser[1,4], Ian H. Harding[1,5], Mats Adler[2], Christoffer Rahm[1,6], Johan Lundberg[2], Thomas Masterman[2], Caroline Wachtler[7,8], Tomas Jonsson[3,9], Maria Kristoffersen-Wiberg[3,10], Christos Pantelis[1] and Björn Wahlund[11]

[1] Department of Psychiatry, Melbourne Neuropsychiatry Centre, The University of Melbourne, Melbourne, VIC, Australia
[2] Section of Psychiatry, Department of Clinical Neuroscience, Karolinska Institutet, Stockholm, Sweden
[3] Department of Clinical Science, Intervention and Technology (CLINTEC), Division of Medical Imaging and Technology, Karolinska Institutet, Stockholm, Sweden
[4] Monash Clinical and Imaging Neuroscience, School of Psychology and Psychiatry, Monash University, Clayton, VIC, Australia
[5] School of Psychological Sciences, Monash University, Melbourne, VIC, Australia
[6] Department of Medicine Huddinge, Karolinska Institutet, Stockholm, Sweden
[7] Primary Care Research Unit, Department of General Practice, The University of Melbourne, Melbourne, VIC, Australia
[8] Centre for Family Medicine (CeFAM), Department of Neurobiology, Care Sciences and Society, Karolinska Institutet, Stockholm, Sweden
[9] Department of Medical Physics, Karolinska University Hospital Huddinge, Stockholm, Sweden
[10] Department of Radiology, Karolinska University Hospital, Stockholm, Sweden
[11] Department of Energy and Engineering, Swedish University of Agricultural Sciences, Uppsala, Sweden

Edited by:
Sebastian Walther, University of Bern, Switzerland

Reviewed by:
Andrea Federspiel, University of Bern, Switzerland
Didier Schrijvers, University of Antwerp, Belgium

***Correspondence:**
Benny Liberg, Department of Psychiatry, Melbourne Neuropsychiatry Centre, Alan Gilbert Building, Level 3, 161 Barry Street, Carlton South, VIC 3053, Australia
e-mail: benny.liberg@gmail.com

Psychomotor disturbances are a classic feature of major depressive disorders. These can manifest as lack of facial expressions and decreased speech production, reduced body posture and mobility, and slowed voluntary movement. The neural correlates of psychomotor disturbances in depression are poorly understood but it has been suggested that outputs from the cingulate motor area (CMA) to striatal motor regions, including the putamen, could be involved. We used functional and structural magnetic resonance imaging to conduct a region-of-interest analysis to test the hypotheses that neural activation patterns related to motor production and gray matter volumes in the CMA would be different between depressed subjects displaying psychomotor disturbances ($n = 13$) and matched healthy controls ($n = 13$). In addition, we conducted a psychophysiological interaction analysis to assess the functional coupling related to self-paced finger-tapping between the caudal CMA and the posterior putamen in patients compared to controls. We found a cluster of increased neural activation, adjacent to a cluster of decreased gray matter volume in the caudal CMA in patients compared to controls. The functional coupling between the left caudal CMA and the left putamen during finger-tapping task performance was additionally decreased in patients compared to controls. In addition, the strength of the functional coupling between the left caudal CMA and the left putamen was negatively correlated with the severity of psychomotor disturbances in the patient group. In conclusion, we found converging evidence for involvement of the caudal CMA and putamen in the generation of psychomotor disturbances in depression.

Keywords: major depression, bipolar disorder, psychomotor disturbances, cingulate cortex, cingulate motor area, striatum, putamen

INTRODUCTION

Psychomotor disturbance is a cardinal feature of major depressive disorder. The severity of psychomotor disruption is clinically associated with depression severity and predicts response to certain pharmacological treatments (1–4). Psychomotor disturbances transcend illness phase and manifest as changes in interactiveness and spontaneity, alongside reductions in facial expression, body mobility, postural tone, speed of movement, and speech (5–7). Investigations of the neural correlates underpinning psychomotor disturbances remain sparse; indeed, the motor system has been relatively neglected in brain imaging studies of psychiatric disorders in general (8). However, available evidence points to metabolic deficits, neurochemical changes, and altered structural connections and functional connectivity involving large-scale brain networks that connect frontal cortical regions and subcortical (esp. basal ganglia) areas (9–24). Interactions between the striatum, frontal motor regions, and prefrontal association cortices are known to be critical to the initiation and regulation of motor output and cognitive processing (25, 26). However, the localization and relevance of brain abnormalities in these fronto-striatal systems to psychomotor disturbances observed in depression remains largely unknown.

One important target for investigation of psychomotor disturbances is the cingulate cortex. Converging evidence supporting the involvement of the cingulate cortex in the clinical expression of major depressive disorder comes through experimental studies using interventions, such as sadness induction (27), cognitive behavioral therapy (28), pharmacological probes, such as antidepressants and dopamine-modulating treatments (29, 30), or neuromodulation such as electroconvulsive therapy or transcranial magnetic stimulation (31–35). Additionally, secondary cingulate cortex lesions can also lead to a neuropsychiatric condition known as akinetic mutism that involves severe alterations of volition, psychomotor slowing, and apathy – clinical features that resemble severe major depressive disorder (36, 37).

The cingulate cortex has been suggested to integrate volition, affect, and behavior. It is located on the midline rim of the corpus callosum and is generally divided anatomically into four distinct subregions (38, 39). One of these subregions is the midcingulate region, which contains the cingulate motor area (CMA) (40, 41). The CMA is a cortical midline structure, located in the posterior frontal lobe, superior to the corpus callosum, and inferior to the supplementary motor area. The CMA has been implicated in motor behaviors with affective incentives (42) and receives neural signals from affective limbic regions, frontal executive regions, and motor regions (37, 43). A caudal subregion of the CMA has long been implicated in the execution of simple motor tasks, but only recently has its somatotopy and functional organization been determined with more spatially precise brain imaging (44–47). Functional connectivity and retrograde tracings in primates suggest inputs from caudal CMA to lateral putamen in general, and to rostral ventral putamen in particular, overlap with inputs from primary motor areas (48, 49).

There is currently no empirically validated functional anatomical model of psychomotor disturbances in major depressive disorder. However, within the anatomical framework of large-scale brain networks, Vogt proposed one such pathophysiological model in which a loss of neurons in the cortical output layer (layer V) of the cingulate cortex specifically attenuates the output from the CMA to subcortical motor regions, resulting in a paucity of internally guided movement and speech (50). Clinically, this neural disruption could be reflected in the altered response to external events and slowed movements that characterize psychomotor disturbances observed in major depressive disorder.

Using the framework of Vogt's theory of movement paucity in major depressive disorder, we hypothesized that psychomotor disturbances in major depressive disorder rely on structural and functional abnormalities in a network encompassing the CMA and striatal motor regions. We predict that participants with major depressive disorder show modifications of functional activation in left CMA and left posterior putamen during a task involving the generation of rapid right-lateralized finger movements (i.e., self-paced finger-tapping). We also anticipate that these functional alterations are accompanied by modifications of gray matter volume in both the left CMA and left putamen. Finally, the severity of both functional and structural abnormalities is predicted to correlate with the degree of observed psychomotor disturbances.

MATERIALS AND METHODS

STUDY SAMPLE

The Karolinska University Hospital and Stockholm City Council Ethics Committee approved the study protocol. Each subject gave oral and written informed consent to participate in this study. Thirteen patients with a bipolar I diagnosis ($n = 9$), bipolar II diagnosis ($n = 1$), or unipolar depression diagnosis ($n = 3$) were recruited from The Affective Disorders Unit at Psychiatry Southwest at Karolinska University Hospital in Huddinge, Sweden. All patients were experiencing a current episode of depression with a duration > 1 month and featuring psychomotor disturbances. No patient fulfilled the diagnostic criteria for concurrent mania, hypomania, or rapid cycling disorder. Thirteen healthy controls without psychiatric diagnoses were recruited. Clinical diagnoses were confirmed using a computerized version of the Structured Clinical Interview for DSM Disorders (51). All participants were right handed, had no history of neurologic illness, and had normal or corrected-to-normal visual acuity (52). All patients were on medication (**Table 1**), and all controls were drug free.

Table 1 | Sample characteristics.

Variable	Controls	Patients
Sex	6 F, 7 M; $n = 13$	9 F, 4 M; $n = 13$
Age (years)	39 (29–67)	44 (24–62)
Bipolar depression (type I, type II)		$n = 10$ ($n = 9$, $n = 1$)
Unipolar depression (recurrent, first episode)		$n = 3$ ($n = 2$, $n = 1$)
MADRS total score		28.9 (11–48)
CORE total score		17.7 (10–36)
CORE retardation items score		9.1 (3–15)
AS-18 retardation factor score		8.2 (0–12)
AS-18 depression factor score		23.2 (1–36)
AS-18 mania factor score		4.9 (0–13)
AS-18 total score		36.2 (2–58)
Lithium		$n = 4$
Typical neuroleptics (FGA)		$n = 2$
Atypical neuroleptics (SGA)		$n = 4$
Anticonvulsants		$n = 5$
Antidepressant (TCA)		$n = 1$
Antidepressant (SSRI)		$n = 1$
Antidepressant (SNRI)		$n = 5$
MAO-I		$n = 1$
Thyroxine		$n = 1$
Electroconvulsive treatment		$n = 2$

If not otherwise specified, values represent the mean and the range is given into brackets.

M/F, male/female; FGA, first-generation antipsychotics; SGA, second-generation antipsychotics; TCA, tricyclic antidepressants; SSRI, serotonin reuptake inhibitors; SNRI, serotonin-noradrenalin reuptake inhibitors; MAO-I, monoamine-oxidase inhibitors.

Depression severity was rated by Benny Liberg and Mats Adler with the Montgomery Åsberg Depression Rating Scale (53) and psychomotor disturbance was rated with the CORE scale (54). Retrospective assessment of patient files did not reveal the presence of extrapyramidal symptoms or signs in medicated patients.

Image acquisition

Participants performed finger-tapping while in the MRI-scanner, following instructions on a computer screen viewed through a head-coil mounted mirror. Before the experiment started, participants were shown how to perform finger-tapping, defined as a thumb-index finger opposition of the right hand. Participants were asked to tap as quickly as possible. The experiment had an ON/OFF design consisting of 20 s of finger-tapping followed by 20 s of rest. During the first second of each ON-period, the instruction "tap" was presented, and the screen then turned black for 19 s. Rest periods were indicated by a fixation-cross presented for 20 s. This stimulus cycle was repeated seven times. The total functional scanning time was 280 s.

A Siemens Avanto 1.5-T scanner was used to acquire blood oxygen level dependent (BOLD) sensitive T2*-weighted echo planar images. Each echo planar image comprised 22 axial slices with a resolution of 3.75 mm × 3.75 mm × 5 mm and an inter-slice interval of 1 mm. Volumes were acquired with a repetition time (TR) of 2.5 s, an echo time (TE) of 30 ms, a field-of-view of 64 mm × 64 mm, and a flip angle of 90°. The first six (dummy) volumes of each run were discarded to allow for T1 equilibration effects. A total of 112 volumes were acquired. After the functional scans had been collected, a T1-weighted anatomical image [magnetization prepared rapid acquisition gradient echo (MP-RAGE)], 128 slices; TR, 2400 ms; TE, 3.44 ms; with a voxel size of 1.3 mm × 1.3 mm × 1.3 mm] was acquired for all subjects. To rule out radiological signs of pathology, a consultant in neuroradiology (Maria Kristoffersen-Wiberg) assessed the anatomical scans of each subject.

Region-of-interest masks

We used the software GingerALE 2.3 to define the left caudal CMA mask. GingerALE allows for meta-analysis of human brain imaging studies using published co-ordinates in standard space (55). Co-ordinates were derived from a study that mapped the functional anatomy of the CMA at the single-subject level (44). Input foci data included co-ordinates in the left hemisphere that represented neural activation in the CMA during motor execution using the right hand. Significant clusters in the whole-brain analysis were determined by a (corrected using a Monte-Carlo approach) cluster significance threshold of $p \leq 0.05$. The resulting ROI mask is illustrated in **Figure 3**. The ROI mask for the putamen region connecting to the caudal motor cortex was derived from the Oxford Imanova Striatal Connectivity Atlas (seven-regions) supplied with FSL (56).

Analysis of functional activations

Imaging data were analyzed using the FSL 5.0.2 software suite [The Oxford Centre for Functional MRI of the Brain (FMRIB), Oxford University, United Kingdom]. Data processing was carried out using the fMRI Expert Analysis Tool version 5.98. Rigid-body head motion correction was first performed (57). We subsequently de-noised the data using the multivariate ICA-based classifier FIX (58, 59), based on a conservative threshold of five components. Non-brain tissue was then removed (60) and the functional data were smoothed using a Gaussian kernel set to a full-width half-maximum (FWHM) of 6 mm. To account for time differences in slice acquisition, we performed slice-timing correction using Fourier-space time series phase shifting. In addition, we normalized the grand-mean intensity of the entire four-dimensional (4D) dataset by a single multiplicative factor and filtered out physiological noise using a high-pass temporal filter set to a period of 100 s. Registration of the data to standard anatomical space was undertaken with the high-resolution structural (T1) scan using boundary-based registration with BBR, and affine linear registration with FLIRT (61). Estimated transformations were subsequently applied to the co-registered functional data. The time series of each subject was modeled using a general linear model (GLM) containing a single predictor representing the on–off time-course of the experiment, convolved with a hemodynamic response function (gamma). Parameter estimates (PEs) were calculated for all brain voxels. Correction for local autocorrelation in the time series was undertaken using FILM (62).

The subject-specific contrast (COPE) images of the finger-tapping effect were then entered into a second-level group analysis. As our patient sample had a different sex distribution than our control group, we added age and sex as covariates in the regression model to remove their potential confounding effects. We also created a 4D covariate image of gray matter using the feat_gm_prepare script. The 4D image output containing gray matter partial volume information was inserted as voxel-dependent EVs in the GLM model for each subject (63). The higher level analysis was carried out using FMRIB's local analysis of mixed effects stage 1 and stage 2 (64–66). Z (Gaussianized T/F) statistic images in the ROI analysis were thresholded using clusters determined by $Z \geq 2.3$ and a (corrected using Gaussian random field theory) cluster significance threshold of $p \leq 0.05$.

Analysis of functional connectivity

We performed a psychophysiological interaction (PPI) analysis to determine group differences in task-dependent alterations of functional coupling between the left caudal CMA and left putamen regions connected to caudal cortical motor regions. Analysis was performed in SPM8 using the preprocessed first-level data described above (preprocessed in FSL). A PPI analysis determines how the statistical dependency between the time courses of neural activation in a region-of-interest (ROI) and a targeted brain region depends on a task context (67). We extracted the BOLD time series data from each subject within a 5 mm sphere centered at the peak of the task-related group activation difference within the left CMA (see Results). At the first level of analysis, a GLM consisting of three predictors was specified: the left CMA time series data as a physiological regressor, the task-based model as psychological regressor, and the interaction term (the PPI) formed by their crossproduct. We entered first-level COPE images representing the interaction term into a second-level random effects analysis of group differences in a region of the left putamen connected to caudal cortical motor areas involved in movement. Inference was undertaken using two-sample T-tests restricted to a mask of the left putamen and corrected for multiple comparisons ($p \leq 0.05$) based on minimum cluster-extent thresholds estimated using the AlphaSim permutation procedure (REST toolbox; http://pub.restfmri.net). Simulations were run using an uncorrected voxel-level threshold of $p \leq 0.05$, across 1000 permutations, resulting in a minimum required cluster-threshold of 14 voxels ($p \leq 0.05$, corrected at the mask level).

Analysis of gray matter volume

Paul Klauser and Benny Liberg inspected every image to assess the presence of artifacts or gross anatomical abnormalities that could impact image preprocessing. We estimated gray matter volume using voxel-based morphometry (VBM) implemented in SPM8 (http://www.fil.ion.ucl.ac.uk/spm/software/spm8/). Each participant's T1-weighted anatomical scan was segmented into gray, white, and cerebrospinal fluid compartments using the VBM8 toolbox (http://dbm.neuro.uni-jena.de/vbm) set to default parameters. Native-space gray matter images were then spatially normalized to the DARTEL template in MNI standard space created from 550 healthy control subjects from the IXI-database (http://www.brain-development.org). For the generation of gray matter volumes, Jacobian determinants were used to modulate gray voxel intensities with non-linear warping only in order to preserve original gray matter volumes while discarding initial differences in brain sizes. The images were then smoothed with a 6 mm full-width-half-maximum Gaussian kernel prior to statistical analysis. A GLM was used to test for group differences in gray matter volume at each voxel within the CMA ROI mask, as implemented in Randomise (http://fsl.fmrib.ox.ac.uk/fsl/randomise). All results were corrected for multiple comparison type I error at the ROI mask level using a non-parametric cluster size-based procedure. We set the voxelwise cluster-forming threshold to $T \geq 2.5$. Then, a clusterwise p-value corrected at the ROI level was calculated from a permutation test (10,000 permutations). Age and gender were entered as covariates in the GLM.

Correlation analyses

Calculation of Spearman's Rho correlation coefficients between CORE ratings, imaging metrics, and neurobiological indices were assessed to determine associations between clinical phenomenology and brain abnormalities determined with different imaging modalities.

RESULTS

FUNCTIONAL ACTIVATION

In our group, comparison of task-related neural activation in the caudal CMA during self-paced finger-tapping, we found that patients activated the left caudal CMA more than healthy controls (cluster size: 356 voxels/2848 mm^3; $Z_{CMA} = 3.01$; $p = 0.003$, corrected at the cluster level; peak voxel: $x = -6$, $y = -10$, $z = 38$; **Figure 1**; **Table 2**).

FUNCTIONAL CONNECTIVITY

In our PPI analysis of task-related functional coupling between the caudal CMA and the posterior putamen regions connected to caudal motor regions in the frontal lobe, we found significant group differences (cluster size: 31 voxels/248 mm^3, $p = 0.02$, corrected; peak voxel: $x = -26$, $y = -6$, $z = 0$; **Figure 1**). We found that neural activation in controls showed a task-related correspondence between the left caudal CMA and left posterior putamen regions connected to caudal motor regions in the frontal lobe, whereas this relationship was absent in the patients.

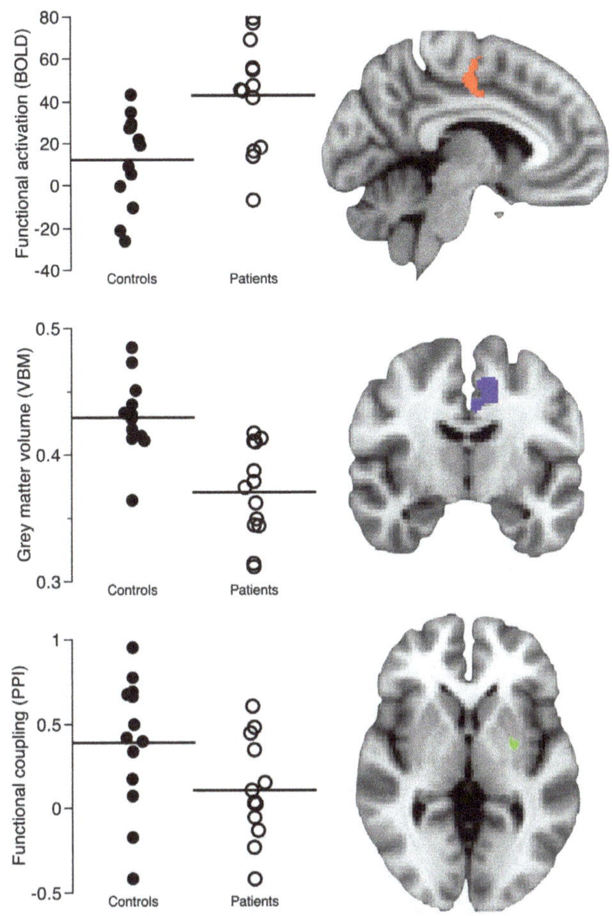

FIGURE 1 | The image shows the structural and functional imaging findings in the left caudal cingulate motor area (CMA) and putamen regions connected to caudal motor regions in the frontal lobe. The first row shows the contrast parameter estimates reflecting how patients activate the caudal cingulate motor regions more than healthy controls ($Z > 2.3$, $p = 0.05$, corrected) during self-paced finger-tapping. The second row shows decreased gray matter volume in the left CMA of patients ($T > 2.5$, $p = 0.05$, corrected). The third row shows the decreased functional coupling of the left CMA and left posterior putamen regions connected to caudal motor regions in the frontal lobe during self-paced finger-tapping ($p = 0.02$, corrected). Metrics (mean) from clusters of between-group differences in the left caudal CMA and posterior putamen were retrieved using masks comprising 356 voxels/2848 mm^3 from the functional magnetic resonance imaging analysis, 941 voxels/3176 mm^3 from the voxel-based morphometry analysis, and 31 voxels/248 mm^3 from the psychophysiological interaction analysis.

GRAY MATTER VOLUME

In our comparison of left CMA gray matter volume in patients and controls, we observed one cluster of decreased gray matter volume

Table 2 | Functional activation statistics during self-paced finger-tapping (patient > controls).

Z-max	Cluster	MNI co-ordinates			Anatomical label
		x	*y*	*z*	
3.85	1	2	−14	52	38% precentral gyrus, 36% SMA
3.66		−2	−14	50	38% SMA, 34% precentral gyrus
3.01		−6	−10	38	32% cingulate gyrus, anterior division (CMA)
2.75		4	−2	52	73% SMA
2.53		8	−2	48	49% SMA

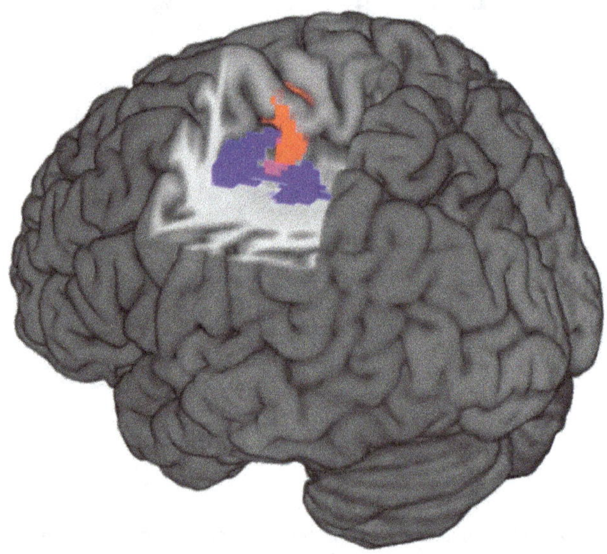

FIGURE 2 | The image shows the localization of structural and functional imaging findings in the left caudal cingulate motor. Left is left in the image. The red cluster represents increased functional activation in patients compared to controls ($Z > 2.3$, $p = 0.05$, corrected). The blue cluster represents gray matter volume decreases in patients compared to controls ($T > 2.5$, $p = 0.05$, corrected). The purple voxels represent the overlap between function and structural findings.

in the patient group that encompassed the left caudal CMA (cluster size: 941 voxels/3176 mm^3; $T_{CMA} = 6.79$; $p = 0.01$, corrected at the cluster level; peak voxel: $x = -9$, $y = 4.5$, $z = 33$; **Figures 1** and **2**).

CROSS-MODALITY RELATIONSHIPS

We found a statistically significant and negative correlation (rho: −0.57, $p = 0.002$; **Table 3**) between mean functional activation (356 voxels/2848 mm^3) and gray matter volume (941 voxels/3176 mm^3) in the left caudal CMA across both groups. There was also a statistically significant and positive correlation (rho: 0.52, $p = 0.006$, **Table 3**) between gray matter volume (941 voxels/3176 mm^3) and functional coupling of the left caudal CMA and left posterior putamen regions connected to caudal motor regions in the frontal lobe (31 voxels/248 mm^3) across both groups. The spatial overlap of between-group differences in gray matter volume and functional activation is shown in **Figure 2.**

Table 3 | Non-parametric correlations between neuroimaging modalities and clinical ratings.

Variables	Size	#Voxels (mm^3)	Rho	*p*
Functional activation – CORE (patients)	$n = 13$	356 (2848)	0.28	0.35
Functional coupling – CORE (patients)	$n = 13$	31 (248)	−0.57	0.04
Gray matter volume – CORE (patients)	$n = 13$	941 (3176)	−0.11	0.71
Gray matter volume – Functional activation	$n = 26$	941 (3176)/356 (2848)	−0.57	0.002
Gray matter volume – Functional coupling	$n = 26$	941 (3176)/31 (248)	0.52	0.006

CLINICAL CORRELATIONS

We found a statistically significant and negative correlation (rho = −0.57; $p = 0.04$, **Table 3**) between clinical ratings of psychomotor disturbances (CORE) in patients and functional coupling of the left caudal CMA and left posterior putamen regions connected to caudal motor regions in the frontal lobe (356 voxels/2848 mm^3). We did not find a significant correlation (rho = 0.39; $p = 0.18$) between CORE ratings and functional activation of the left caudal CMA (356 voxels/2848 mm^3) or between CORE ratings and gray matter volume in the left caudal CMA (rho = −0.11; $p = 0.71$; 941 voxels/3176 mm^3).

DISCUSSION

In the present study, we used structural and functional neuroimaging to investigate the contribution of the CMA to psychomotor disturbances in major depressive disorder. By combining neuroimaging modalities, we found converging evidence supporting a neural model of psychomotor disturbances that involves a fronto-striatal network contributing to motor execution. Specifically, we found that (1) patients activated the CMA more than healthy controls during right-handed self-paced finger-tapping; (2) functional coupling of the CMA and putamen was absent in patients compared to controls during task performance; (3) patients had decreased gray matter volume in the CMA; (4) clinical ratings of psychomotor disturbance in patients were negatively correlated with functional coupling of the CMA and putamen; and (5) gray matter volume of the CMA region with between-group differences was negatively correlated with functional activation, and positively correlated with functional coupling.

Our study lends experimental support to the involvement of a fronto-striatal network in the emergence of psychomotor disturbances in major depressive disorder. In our study, gray matter volume decreases were associated with decreased functional coupling of the left caudal CMA and left posterior putamen during motor execution of a right-handed self-paced finger-tapping task. The midcingulate region comprising the CMA is known to provide extensive output to skeletomotor areas, including the striatum (41). Changes in the CMA would, therefore, impact upon its

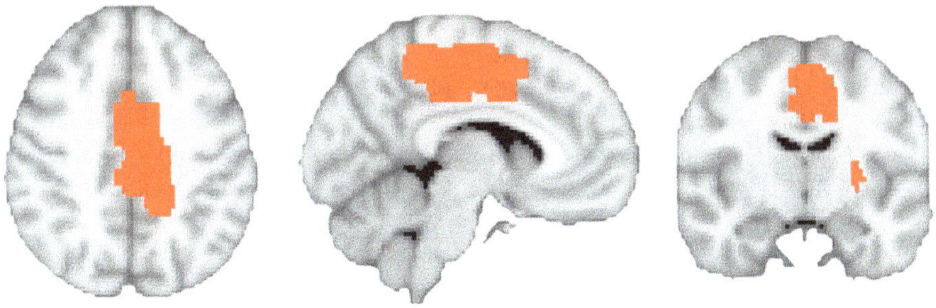

FIGURE 3 | The image shows the binarized region of interest masks defining the left caudal cingulate motor area and the left putamen regions connected to caudal motor regions in the frontal lobe.

glutamatergic inputs to subcortical motor systems and, in turn, lead to impairments in motor behavior, i.e., psychomotor disturbances. Although beyond the scope of the current study, this finding may be relevant to neuron loss in cortical layer V, from which efferent fibers are derived, in accordance with Vogt's model of motor dysfunction (50).

It is interesting to note the relative position of the clusters resulting from the functional and the structural analysis: few voxels show an overlap between the functional cluster representing increased neural activity and the structural cluster representing decreased gray matter volume in the CMA of patients (**Figure 2**). The interpretation of the spatial extent of clusters, resulting from cluster-based statistics is known to be problematic, especially when relatively low cluster-forming thresholds are used like in this study (i.e., $T > 2.5$) (68). Nevertheless, the increase of functional activation in an area that seems to be spared by gray matter volume loss may represent a less affected region or a compensatory mechanism. Compensatory cortical plasticity has been previously described after acute brain lesions but a similar mechanism could also be involved following more chronic alterations of brain networks in the context of mental illness (69).

This study conforms to previous studies that have shown paralimbic hyperactivation in major depressive disorder using both molecular metabolic imaging and functional magnetic resonance imaging with BOLD (70, 71). Hypothetically, a loss of neurons in cingulate layer V suggested by Vogt et al. (50) could arise from excess glutamate signaling with impaired plasticity and neural resilience (72). However, the BOLD signal comprises several neuronal and vascular factors that preclude a specific association of increased activation and hyperglutamatergia (73). Indirect correlational evidence for cingulate hyperglutamatergia may be inferred from the positive correlation of glutamate signaling and spontaneous neural activity of paralimbic medial frontal and posterior cingulate regions: the so-called "default-mode" network (74, 75). Several studies suggest that this network is hyperactivated in major depressive disorder (76–78). In a previous study of the bipolar disorder subgroup of this sample ($n = 9$), there was an increased activation among depressed patients in the default-mode network during motor execution (15). However, the opposite association between glutamate, functional connectivity, and depression severity has also been shown (79). Thus, we remain cautious regarding definitive interpretations of our findings in the context of the pathophysiology underlying psychomotor disturbances in major depressive disorder.

Our study has limitations. First, this is a ROI study where we had an *a priori* hypothesis involving selected brain regions in the left hemisphere known to activate during simple right-hand movements. The disadvantage of the ROI approach is that it discerns a comprehensive observation of the full large-scale neuronal networks implicated in these disturbances (80). However, our motivation for choosing the ROI approach was that our hypothesis addressed specific ideas based on previous research on the CMA in major depressive disorder. An advantage of the ROI approach is that it potentially increases the sensitivity of the neuroimaging methods we applied, and previous research suggests that ROI analyses may provide a better statistical control of both type I and type II errors than in whole-brain analyses as the ROI approach is less dependent on correction for multiple comparisons (81). This becomes even more important in smaller samples such as ours. Second, our brain imaging approach is restricted to inference from indirect monitoring of the disease underlying major depressive disorder. Functional imaging studies and anatomical mapping advocate a limbic hyperactivation in major depressive disorder and suggest that more anterior cingulate cortex regions convey limbic signals to the CMA, which in turn suggests that our observed CMA alterations may only be a tertiary marker for a disease that alters upstream nodes in the same neural network (29, 43). The BOLD contrast mechanism itself also highlights the importance of inputs to CMA (82). Third, the CMA and putamen are both rich in ascending midbrain dopamine afferents that contribute to the initiation, preparation, execution, and control of movement (56, 83). Six patients in our sample were treated with antipsychotic medication that affects dopamine transmission in both regions. This could potentially lead to misrepresentative and biased results. However, neuroimaging metrics in these six individuals were distributed across the whole patient sample, and there were no outliers in the patient group with respect to functional activation, gray matter volume, or functional coupling. Fourth, there are many types of motor behavior, and it is possible that finger-tapping does not engage identical fronto-striatal networks in the same way as more elaborate motor behavior. The strength of the finger-tapping task is that it is sensitive to pathology in fronto-striatal neurocircuitry and is considered to measure a defined entity: motor speed (84). Fifth, the BOLD signal in the

CMA may be subject to noise due to partial volume effects because of the spatial resolution of our functional scans. This contributes to a possible source of error in our PPI analysis. Finally, given the small sample size of our groups, the GLM may not provide the best fit of our second-level data. However, we analyzed our data at second level using a mixed effects analysis (FMRIB's Local Analysis of Mixed Effects stage 1 and stage 2) similar to a vast majority of comparable functional imaging studies. In order to confirm the validity of our results, we also re-analyzed data at second level with Randomise for non-parametric inference while using an identical statistical threshold. The spatial extent of those statistically significant results was close to identical regarding the CMA cluster of between-group differences. We would like to reiterate that even if the GLM does not provide the best fit for our second level analysis, the corrected p-value calculated by Randomise is valid, regardless the distribution of our data.

CONCLUSION

Our data are cross-sectional but implicates the possibility of a chain of events where primary neural hyperactivation in paralimbic regions has secondary effects on gray matter volume in fronto-striatal networks involved in movement. In our study, functional activation was negatively correlated with gray matter volume, which suggests an association between paralimbic hyperactivation and gray matter alterations. The positive correlation between gray matter volume and functional coupling supports the notion of diminished cortical output via layer V to subcortical regions that are involved in motor control. The functional coupling was also negatively correlated with clinical ratings, which suggests a role of decreased functional connectivity within fronto-striatal networks in the emergence of clinical psychomotor disturbances in major depressive disorder. Thus, our results propose an involvement of the CMA in the generation of psychomotor disturbances in a major depressive disorder. Our data also suggest the possibility of elucidating the causality of these events by using an experimental longitudinal study design and analyses of directional effective connectivity within these networks during motor performance.

AUTHOR CONTRIBUTIONS

All authors made substantial contributions to the conception and design of this work. Benny Liberg and Mats Adler collected the original data. Benny Liberg, Paul Klauser, and Ian H. Harding performed the analyses. All authors contributed to the interpretation of data for this work. Benny Liberg, Paul Klauser, and Ian H. Harding drafted the manuscript, which all authors critically revised for important intellectual content. All authors approved the final version of the manuscript. All authors agree to be accountable for all aspects of the work in ensuring that questions related to the accuracy or integrity of any part of the work are appropriately investigated and resolved.

ACKNOWLEDGMENTS

We thank Kerstin Eriksson at the MRI Unit, Radiology Clinic, Karolinska University Hospital Huddinge for clinical assistance during scanning. We thank Andrew Zalesky for valuable comments on methodology. We also thank staff members of the Section of Affective Disorders, the Southwest Psychiatric Clinic (PSSV), Stockholm County Council, for assistance with recruiting patients. Benny Liberg received funding from Svenska Läkaresällskapet (The Swedish Society of Medicine, SLS-403101), the Southwest Psychiatric Clinic (PSSV), Stockholm County Council, and the Strategic Research Committee, Karolinska Institutet/Stockholm County Council, Sweden. Paul Klauser was supported by the Swiss National Science Foundation and the Swiss Society for Medicine and Biology Scholarships (ID: 148384). Professor Christos Pantelis was supported by a NHMRC Senior Principal Research Fellowship, Australia (ID: 628386).

REFERENCES

1. Buyukdura JS, McClintock SM, Croarkin PE. Psychomotor retardation in depression: biological underpinnings, measurement, and treatment. *Prog Neuropsychopharmacol Biol Psychiatry* (2011) **35**(2):395–409. doi:10.1016/j.pnpbp.2010.10.019
2. Schrijvers D, Hulstijn W, Sabbe BG. Psychomotor symptoms in depression: a diagnostic, pathophysiological and therapeutic tool. *J Affect Disord* (2008) **109**(1–2):1–20. doi:10.1016/j.jad.2007.10.019
3. Sobin C, Mayer L, Endicott J. The motor agitation and retardation scale: a scale for the assessment of motor abnormalities in depressed patients. *J Neuropsychiatry Clin Neurosci* (1998) **10**(1):85–92.
4. Sobin C, Sackeim HA. Psychomotor symptoms of depression. *Am J Psychiatry* (1997) **154**(1):4–17.
5. Berk M, Dodd S, Kauer-Sant'anna M, Malhi GS, Bourin M, Kapczinski F, et al. Dopamine dysregulation syndrome: implications for a dopamine hypothesis of bipolar disorder. *Acta Psychiatr Scand Suppl* (2007) (434):41–9. doi:10.1111/j.1600-0447.2007.01058.x
6. Malhi GS, Berk M. Does dopamine dysfunction drive depression? *Acta Psychiatr Scand Suppl* (2007) (433):116–24. doi:10.1111/j.1600-0447.2007.00969.x
7. Parker G, Hadzi-Pavlovic D, Brodaty H, Boyce P, Mitchell P, Wilhelm K, et al. Psychomotor disturbance in depression: defining the constructs. *J Affect Disord* (1993) **27**(4):255–65. doi:10.1016/0165-0327(93)90049-P
8. Kupferschmidt DA, Zakzanis KK. Toward a functional neuroanatomical signature of bipolar disorder: quantitative evidence from the neuroimaging literature. *Psychiatry Res* (2011) **193**(2):71–9. doi:10.1016/j.pscychresns.2011.02.011
9. Bracht T, Federspiel A, Schnell S, Horn H, Hofle O, Wiest R, et al. Cortico-cortical white matter motor pathway microstructure is related to psychomotor retardation in major depressive disorder. *PLoS One* (2012) **7**(12):e52238. doi:10.1371/journal.pone.0052238
10. Caligiuri MP, Brown GG, Meloy MJ, Eberson SC, Kindermann SS, Frank LR, et al. An fMRI study of affective state and medication on cortical and subcortical brain regions during motor performance in bipolar disorder. *Psychiatry Res* (2003) **123**(3):171–82. doi:10.1016/S0925-4927(03)00075-1
11. Lohr JB, Caligiuri MP. Abnormalities in motor physiology in bipolar disorder. *J Neuropsychiatry Clin Neurosci* (2006) **18**(3):342–9. doi:10.1176/appi.neuropsych.18.3.342
12. Exner C, Lange C, Irle E. Impaired implicit learning and reduced pre-supplementary motor cortex size in early-onset major depression with melancholic features. *J Affect Disord* (2009) **119**(1–3):156–62. doi:10.1016/j.jad.2009.03.015
13. Hickie IB, Naismith SL, Ward PB, Little CL, Pearson M, Scott EM, et al. Psychomotor slowing in older patients with major depression: relationships with blood flow in the caudate nucleus and white matter lesions. *Psychiatry Res* (2007) **155**(3):211–20. doi:10.1016/j.pscychresns.2007.01.006
14. Liberg B, Adler M, Jonsson T, Landen M, Rahm C, Wahlund LO, et al. The neural correlates of self-paced finger tapping in bipolar depression with motor retardation. *Acta Neuropsychiatr* (2013) **25**(1):43–51. doi:10.1111/j.1601-5215.2012.00659.x
15. Liberg B, Adler M, Jonsson T, Landen M, Rahm C, Wahlund LO, et al. Motor imagery in bipolar depression with slowed movement. *J Nerv Ment Dis* (2013) **201**(10):885–93. doi:10.1097/NMD.0b013e3182a5c2a7
16. Marchand WR, Lee JN, Suchy Y, Johnson S, Thatcher J, Gale P. Aberrant functional connectivity of cortico-basal ganglia circuits in major depression. *Neurosci Lett* (2012) **514**(1):86–90. doi:10.1016/j.neulet.2012.02.063

17. Marchand WR, Lee JN, Thatcher GW, Jensen C, Stewart D, Dilda V, et al. A functional MRI study of a paced motor activation task to evaluate frontal-subcortical circuit function in bipolar depression. *Psychiatry Res* (2007) **155**(3):221–30. doi:10.1016/j.pscychresns.2007.03.003
18. Marchand WR, Lee JN, Thatcher J, Thatcher GW, Jensen C, Starr J. A preliminary longitudinal fMRI study of frontal-subcortical circuits in bipolar disorder using a paced motor activation paradigm. *J Affect Disord* (2007) **103**(1–3):237–41. doi:10.1016/j.jad.2007.01.008
19. Walther S, Hugli S, Hofle O, Federspiel A, Horn H, Bracht T, et al. Frontal white matter integrity is related to psychomotor retardation in major depression. *Neurobiol Dis* (2012) **47**(1):13–9. doi:10.1016/j.nbd.2012.03.019
20. Bench CJ, Friston KJ, Brown RG, Frackowiak RS, Dolan RJ. Regional cerebral blood flow in depression measured by positron emission tomography: the relationship with clinical dimensions. *Psychol Med* (1993) **23**(3):579–90. doi:10.1017/S0033291700025368
21. Dolan RJ, Bench CJ, Liddle PF, Friston KJ, Frith CD, Grasby PM, et al. Dorsolateral prefrontal cortex dysfunction in the major psychoses; symptom or disease specificity? *J Neurol Neurosurg Psychiatry* (1993) **56**(12):1290–4. doi:10.1136/jnnp.56.12.1290
22. Brody AL, Saxena S, Mandelkern MA, Fairbanks LA, Ho ML, Baxter LR. Brain metabolic changes associated with symptom factor improvement in major depressive disorder. *Biol Psychiatry* (2001) **50**(3):171–8. doi:10.1016/S0006-3223(01)01117-9
23. Mayberg HS, Lewis PJ, Regenold W, Wagner HN Jr. Paralimbic hypoperfusion in unipolar depression. *J Nucl Med* (1994) **35**(6):929–34.
24. Meyer JH, McNeely HE, Sagrati S, Boovariwala A, Martin K, Verhoeff NP, et al. Elevated putamen D(2) receptor binding potential in major depression with motor retardation: an [11C]raclopride positron emission tomography study. *Am J Psychiatry* (2006) **163**(9):1594–602. doi:10.1176/appi.ajp.163.9.1594
25. Frey SH, Fogassi L, Grafton S, Picard N, Rothwell JC, Schweighofer N, et al. Neurological principles and rehabilitation of action disorders: computation, anatomy, and physiology (CAP) model. *Neurorehabil Neural Repair* (2011) **25**(5 Suppl):6S–20S. doi:10.1177/1545968311410940
26. Rizzolatti G, Luppino G. The cortical motor system. *Neuron* (2001) **31**(6):889–901. doi:10.1016/S0896-6273(01)00423-8
27. Mayberg HS, Liotti M, Brannan SK, McGinnis S, Mahurin RK, Jerabek PA, et al. Reciprocal limbic-cortical function and negative mood: converging PET findings in depression and normal sadness. *Am J Psychiatry* (1999) **156**(5):675–82.
28. McGrath CL, Kelley ME, Holtzheimer PE, Dunlop BW, Craighead WE, Franco AR, et al. Toward a neuroimaging treatment selection biomarker for major depressive disorder. *JAMA Psychiatry* (2013) **70**(8):821–9. doi:10.1001/jamapsychiatry.2013.143
29. Seminowicz DA, Mayberg HS, McIntosh AR, Goldapple K, Kennedy S, Segal Z, et al. Limbic-frontal circuitry in major depression: a path modeling metanalysis. *Neuroimage* (2004) **22**(1):409–18. doi:10.1016/j.neuroimage.2004.01.015
30. Austin MP, Mitchell P, Hadzi-Pavlovic D, Hickie I, Parker G, Chan J, et al. Effect of apomorphine on motor and cognitive function in melancholic patients: a preliminary report. *Psychiatry Res* (2000) **97**(2–3):207–15. doi:10.1016/S0165-1781(00)00222-5
31. Liston C, Chen AC, Zebley BD, Drysdale AT, Gordon R, Leuchter B, et al. Default mode network mechanisms of transcranial magnetic stimulation in depression. *Biol Psychiatry* (2014) **76**(7):517–26. doi:10.1016/j.biopsych.2014.01.023
32. Ohnishi T, Hayashi T, Okabe S, Nonaka I, Matsuda H, Iida H, et al. Endogenous dopamine release induced by repetitive transcranial magnetic stimulation over the primary motor cortex: an [11C]raclopride positron emission tomography study in anesthetized macaque monkeys. *Biol Psychiatry* (2004) **55**(5):484–9. doi:10.1016/j.biopsych.2003.09.016
33. Ohnishi T, Matsuda H, Imabayashi E, Okabe S, Takano H, Arai N, et al. rCBF changes elicited by rTMS over DLPFC in humans. *Suppl Clin Neurophysiol* (2004) **57**:715–20. doi:10.1016/S1567-424X(09)70412-X
34. Paillere Martinot ML, Martinot JL, Ringuenet D, Galinowski A, Gallarda T, Bellivier F, et al. Baseline brain metabolism in resistant depression and response to transcranial magnetic stimulation. *Neuropsychopharmacology* (2011) **36**(13):2710–9. doi:10.1038/npp.2011.161
35. McCormick LM, Yamada T, Yeh M, Brumm MC, Thatcher RW. Antipsychotic effect of electroconvulsive therapy is related to normalization of subgenual cingulate theta activity in psychotic depression. *J Psychiatr Res* (2009) **43**(5):553–60. doi:10.1016/j.jpsychires.2008.08.004
36. Tengvar C, Johansson B, Sorensen J. Frontal lobe and cingulate cortical metabolic dysfunction in acquired akinetic mutism: a PET study of the interval form of carbon monoxide poisoning. *Brain Inj* (2004) **18**(6):615–25. doi:10.1080/02699050310001622806
37. Paus T. Primate anterior cingulate cortex: where motor control, drive and cognition interface. *Nat Rev Neurosci* (2001) **2**(6):417–24. doi:10.1038/35077500
38. Palomero-Gallagher N, Vogt BA, Schleicher A, Mayberg HS, Zilles K. Receptor architecture of human cingulate cortex: evaluation of the four-region neurobiological model. *Hum Brain Mapp* (2009) **30**(8):2336–55. doi:10.1002/hbm.20667
39. Yu C, Zhou Y, Liu Y, Jiang T, Dong H, Zhang Y, et al. Functional segregation of the human cingulate cortex is confirmed by functional connectivity based neuroanatomical parcellation. *Neuroimage* (2011) **54**(4):2571–81. doi:10.1016/j.neuroimage.2010.11.018
40. Picard N, Strick PL. Motor areas of the medial wall: a review of their location and functional activation. *Cereb Cortex* (1996) **6**(3):342–53. doi:10.1093/cercor/6.3.342
41. Vogt BA, Berger GR, Derbyshire SW. Structural and functional dichotomy of human midcingulate cortex. *Eur J Neurosci* (2003) **18**(11):3134–44. doi:10.1111/j.1460-9568.2003.03034.x
42. Shima K, Tanji J. Role for cingulate motor area cells in voluntary movement selection based on reward. *Science* (1998) **282**(5392):1335–8. doi:10.1126/science.282.5392.1335
43. Morecraft RJ, Van Hoesen GW. Convergence of limbic input to the cingulate motor cortex in the rhesus monkey. *Brain Res Bull* (1998) **45**(2):209–32. doi:10.1016/S0361-9230(97)00344-4
44. Amiez C, Petrides M. Neuroimaging evidence of the anatomo-functional organization of the human cingulate motor areas. *Cereb Cortex* (2014) **24**(3):563–78. doi:10.1093/cercor/bhs329
45. Procyk E, Wilson CR, Stoll FM, Faraut MC, Petrides M, Amiez C. Midcingulate motor map and feedback detection: converging data from humans and monkeys. *Cereb Cortex* (2014). doi:10.1093/cercor/bhu213
46. Picard N, Strick PL. Imaging the premotor areas. *Curr Opin Neurobiol* (2001) **11**(6):663–72. doi:10.1016/S0959-4388(01)00266-5
47. Paus T, Petrides M, Evans AC, Meyer E. Role of the human anterior cingulate cortex in the control of oculomotor, manual, and speech responses: a positron emission tomography study. *J Neurophysiol* (1993) **70**(2):453–69.
48. Habas C. Functional connectivity of the human rostral and caudal cingulate motor areas in the brain resting state at 3T. *Neuroradiology* (2010) **52**(1):47–59. doi:10.1007/s00234-009-0572-1
49. Takada M, Tokuno H, Hamada I, Inase M, Ito Y, Imanishi M, et al. Organization of inputs from cingulate motor areas to basal ganglia in macaque monkey. *Eur J Neurosci* (2001) **14**(10):1633–50. doi:10.1046/j.0953-816x.2001.01789.x
50. Vogt BA, Fountolakis KN, Samaras D, Kövari E, Vogt LJ, Hof PR. Cingulate neuropathological substrates of depression. In: Vogt BA, editor. *Cingulate Neurobiology and Disease.* Oxford: Oxford University Press (2009). p. xxxiv, 829.
51. First MB, Spitzer RL, Gibbon M, Williams JB. *Structured Clinical Interview for DSM-IV-TR Axis I Disorders, Research Version, Patient Edition (SCID-I/P).* 4th ed. New York: Biometrics Research Department, New York State Psychiatric Institute (2001).
52. Oldfield RC. The assessment and analysis of handedness: the Edinburgh inventory. *Neuropsychologia* (1971) **9**(1):97–113. doi:10.1016/0028-3932(71)90067-4
53. Asberg M, Montgomery SA, Perris C, Schalling D, Sedvall G. A comprehensive psychopathological rating scale. *Acta Psychiatr Scand Suppl* (1978) (271):5–27. doi:10.1111/j.1600-0447.1978.tb02357.x
54. Hickie I, Mason C, Parker G. Comparative validity of two measures of psychomotor function in patients with severe depression. *J Affect Disord* (1996) **37**(2–3):143–9. doi:10.1016/0165-0327(95)00087-9
55. Turkeltaub PE, Eden GF, Jones KM, Zeffiro TA. Meta-analysis of the functional neuroanatomy of single-word reading: method and validation. *Neuroimage* (2002) **16**(3 Pt 1):765–80. doi:10.1006/nimg.2002.1131
56. Tziortzi AC, Haber SN, Searle GE, Tsoumpas C, Long CJ, Shotbolt P, et al. Connectivity-based functional analysis of dopamine release in the striatum using diffusion-weighted MRI and positron emission tomography. *Cereb Cortex* (2014) **24**(5):1165–77. doi:10.1093/cercor/bhs397
57. Jenkinson M, Bannister P, Brady M, Smith S. Improved optimization for the robust and accurate linear registration and motion correction of brain images. *Neuroimage* (2002) **17**(2):825–41. doi:10.1006/nimg.2002.1132

58. Griffanti L, Salimi-Khorshidi G, Beckmann CF, Auerbach EJ, Douaud G, Sexton CE, et al. ICA-based artefact removal and accelerated fMRI acquisition for improved resting state network imaging. *Neuroimage* (2014) **95**:232–47. doi:10.1016/j.neuroimage.2014.03.034
59. Salimi-Khorshidi G, Douaud G, Beckmann CF, Glasser MF, Griffanti L, Smith SM. Automatic denoising of functional MRI data: combining independent component analysis and hierarchical fusion of classifiers. *Neuroimage* (2014) **90**:449–68. doi:10.1016/j.neuroimage.2013.11.046
60. Smith SM. Fast robust automated brain extraction. *Hum Brain Mapp* (2002) **17**(3):143–55. doi:10.1002/hbm.10062
61. Jenkinson M, Smith S. A global optimisation method for robust affine registration of brain images. *Med Image Anal* (2001) **5**(2):143–56. doi:10.1016/S1361-8415(01)00036-6
62. Woolrich MW, Ripley BD, Brady M, Smith SM. Temporal autocorrelation in univariate linear modeling of FMRI data. *Neuroimage* (2001) **14**(6):1370–86. doi:10.1006/nimg.2001.0931
63. Oakes TR, Fox AS, Johnstone T, Chung MK, Kalin N, Davidson RJ. Integrating VBM into the general linear model with voxelwise anatomical covariates. *Neuroimage* (2007) **34**(2):500–8. doi:10.1016/j.neuroimage.2006.10.007
64. Woolrich MW, Behrens TE, Beckmann CF, Jenkinson M, Smith SM. Multilevel linear modelling for FMRI group analysis using Bayesian inference. *Neuroimage* (2004) **21**(4):1732–47. doi:10.1016/j.neuroimage.2003.12.023
65. Woolrich MW, Jbabdi S, Patenaude B, Chappell M, Makni S, Behrens T, et al. Bayesian analysis of neuroimaging data in FSL. *Neuroimage* (2009) **45**(1 Suppl):S173–86. doi:10.1016/j.neuroimage.2008.10.055
66. Beckmann CF, Jenkinson M, Smith SM. General multilevel linear modeling for group analysis in FMRI. *Neuroimage* (2003) **20**(2):1052–63. doi:10.1016/S1053-8119(03)00435-X
67. Friston KJ, Buechel C, Fink GR, Morris J, Rolls E, Dolan RJ. Psychophysiological and modulatory interactions in neuroimaging. *Neuroimage* (1997) **6**(3):218–29. doi:10.1006/nimg.1997.0291
68. Woo CW, Krishnan A, Wager TD. Cluster-extent based thresholding in fMRI analyses: pitfalls and recommendations. *Neuroimage* (2014) **91**:412–9. doi:10.1016/j.neuroimage.2013.12.058
69. Nudo RJ. Recovery after brain injury: mechanisms and principles. *Front Hum Neurosci* (2013) **7**:887. doi:10.3389/fnhum.2013.00887
70. Wessa M, Houenou J, Paillere-Martinot ML, Berthoz S, Artiges E, Leboyer M, et al. Fronto-striatal overactivation in euthymic bipolar patients during an emotional go/nogo task. *Am J Psychiatry* (2007) **164**(4):638–46. doi:10.1176/appi.ajp.164.4.638
71. Agid Y, Buzsaki G, Diamond DM, Frackowiak R, Giedd J, Girault JA, et al. How can drug discovery for psychiatric disorders be improved? *Nat Rev Drug Discov* (2007) **6**(3):189–201. doi:10.1038/nrd2217
72. Schloesser RJ, Martinowich K, Manji HK. Mood-stabilizing drugs: mechanisms of action. *Trends Neurosci* (2012) **35**(1):36–46. doi:10.1016/j.tins.2011.11.009
73. Logothetis NK, Pfeuffer J. On the nature of the BOLD fMRI contrast mechanism. *Magn Reson Imaging* (2004) **22**(10):1517–31. doi:10.1016/j.mri.2004.10.018
74. Hu Y, Chen X, Gu H, Yang Y. Resting-state glutamate and GABA concentrations predict task-induced deactivation in the default mode network. *J Neurosci* (2013) **33**(47):18566–73. doi:10.1523/JNEUROSCI.1973-13.2013
75. Enzi B, Duncan NW, Kaufmann J, Tempelmann C, Wiebking C, Northoff G. Glutamate modulates resting state activity in the perigenual anterior cingulate cortex – a combined fMRI-MRS study. *Neuroscience* (2012) **227**:102–9. doi:10.1016/j.neuroscience.2012.09.039
76. Greicius MD, Flores BH, Menon V, Glover GH, Solvason HB, Kenna H, et al. Resting-state functional connectivity in major depression: abnormally increased contributions from subgenual cingulate cortex and thalamus. *Biol Psychiatry* (2007) **62**(5):429–37. doi:10.1016/j.biopsych.2006.09.020
77. Grimm S, Boesiger P, Beck J, Schuepbach D, Bermpohl F, Walter M, et al. Altered negative BOLD responses in the default-mode network during emotion processing in depressed subjects. *Neuropsychopharmacology* (2009) **34**(4):932–43. doi:10.1038/npp.2008.81
78. Kuhn S, Gallinat J. Resting-state brain activity in schizophrenia and major depression: a quantitative meta-analysis. *Schizophr Bull* (2013) **39**(2):358–65. doi:10.1093/schbul/sbr151
79. Horn DI, Yu C, Steiner J, Buchmann J, Kaufmann J, Osoba A, et al. Glutamatergic and resting-state functional connectivity correlates of severity in major depression – the role of pregenual anterior cingulate cortex and anterior insula. *Front Syst Neurosci* (2010) **4**:33. doi:10.3389/fnsys.2010.00033
80. Phillips ML, Swartz HA. A critical appraisal of neuroimaging studies of bipolar disorder: toward a new conceptualization of underlying neural circuitry and a road map for future research. *Am J Psychiatry* (2014) **171**(8):829–43. doi:10.1176/appi.ajp.2014.13081008
81. Poldrack RA. Region of interest analysis for fMRI. *Soc Cogn Affect Neurosci* (2007) **2**(1):67–70. doi:10.1093/scan/nsm006
82. Logothetis NK, Pauls J, Augath M, Trinath T, Oeltermann A. Neurophysiological investigation of the basis of the fMRI signal. *Nature* (2001) **412**(6843):150–7. doi:10.1038/35084005
83. Allman JM, Hakeem A, Erwin JM, Nimchinsky E, Hof P. The anterior cingulate cortex. The evolution of an interface between emotion and cognition. *Ann N Y Acad Sci* (2001) **935**:107–17. doi:10.1111/j.1749-6632.2001.tb03476.x
84. Shimoyama I, Ninchoji T, Uemura K. The finger-tapping test. A quantitative analysis. *Arch Neurol* (1990) **47**(6):681–4. doi:10.1001/archneur.1990.00530060095025

18

Alcohol and relatively pure cannabis use, but not schizotypy, are associated with cognitive attenuations

Daniela A. Herzig[1,2,3] *, David J. Nutt[4] and Christine Mohr[1,5]

[1] Department of Experimental Psychology, University of Bristol, Bristol, UK
[2] Institute for Response-Genetics, University of Zurich, Kilchberg, Switzerland
[3] Clienia AG Littenheid, Littenheid, Switzerland
[4] Neuropsychopharmacology Unit, Imperial College London, London, UK
[5] Faculté des Sciences Sociales et Politiques, Institut de Psychologie, Université de Lausanne, Lausanne, Switzerland

Edited by:
Caroline Gurvich, Monash University, Australia

Reviewed by:
John Gigg, University of Manchester, UK
Bernhard J. Mitterauer, Volitronics-Institute for Basic Research Psychopathology and Brain Philosophy, Austria

Correspondence:
Daniela A. Herzig, Clienia AG Littenheid, Littenheid, Switzerland
e-mail: daniela.herzig@clienia.ch

Elevated schizotypy relates to similar cognitive attenuations as seen in psychosis and cannabis/polydrug use. Also, in schizotypal populations cannabis and polydrug (including licit drug) use are enhanced. These cognitive attenuations may therefore either be a behavioral marker of psychotic (-like) symptoms or the consequence of enhanced drug use in schizotypal populations. To elucidate this, we investigated the link between cognitive attenuation and cannabis use in largely pure cannabis users (35) and non-using controls (48), accounting for the potential additional influence of both schizotypy and licit drug use (alcohol, nicotine). Cognitive attenuations commonly seen in psychosis were associated with cannabis and alcohol use, but not schizotypy. Future studies should therefore consider (i) non-excessive licit substance use (e.g., alcohol) in studies investigating the effect of cannabis use on cognition and (ii) both enhanced illicit and licit substance use in studies investigating cognition in schizotypal populations.

Keywords: polydrug use, licit drug use, cognition, schizotypy, psychosis-proneness

INTRODUCTION

Cannabis sativa (marijuana) is currently the most widely used illegal substance in Europe (1). Past year cannabis use was reported by about 11.2% of all 15–34 year olds (1). This elevated prevalence rate (when compared to other illicit drug use) is concerning, because cannabis use might go along with both cognitive attenuation (2, 3) and mental health problems, in particular psychosis (4–9). Yet, only a minority of cannabis users (CU) will develop psychotic illnesses (5–7, 10). Therefore, other factors likely influence adverse consequences associated with cannabis use (9, 11).

Here, we focused on the supposedly negative implications of cannabis use on cognitive functioning while accounting for individuals' schizotypy and associated licit drug use. We did so based on the following reasoning. On the one hand, relatively pure CU (i.e., no regular drug use other than marihuana, cigarettes, or alcohol) have attenuated cognitive functioning compared to non-users (3), e.g., in verbal working memory (12), verbal short-term memory (13), and mental flexibility (3, 14). On the other hand, as detailed below, schizotypal personality features are not only part of the psychosis dimension but also associate with cognitive attenuations, cannabis use, as well as licit drug use.

The schizotypy approach assumes that psychotic symptoms exist along a continuum, with severest symptoms occurring in schizophrenia and mild sub-clinical ones in schizotypal individuals from the general population (15). Schizotypy is commonly assessed using self-report questionnaires (16, 17). Scores on these questionnaires can be commonly divided into symptom dimensions known from patients, e.g., consisting of positive schizotypy (e.g., magical thinking, unusual experiences), negative schizotypy (e.g., anhedonia), and cognitive disorganization [e.g., odd speech and behavior; (16, 18)]. When it comes to laboratory measures, high as compared to low schizotypes yield relatively impaired cognitive performance, e.g., in working memory (19, 20), cognitive flexibility (21), and verbal short-term memory (22, 23). Most relevant to our reasoning, high schizotypy goes along with elevated substance use of, e.g., cannabis (24–28), nicotine, and alcohol (26, 29). Similarly, an elevated drug use has been reported in schizophrenia when compared to healthy controls (2, 6, 30–34).

Given the above described interrelationships, it is possible that the link between cannabis and cognition is influenced by individuals' schizotypal features and/or additional licit drug use. The latter reasoning is particularly likely given that CU show higher consumption of nicotine and/or alcohol when compared to non-users (35, 36). Studies that assessed all three variables (cognition, cannabis use, and schizotypy) found that CU showed both worse cognitive performance and higher schizotypy scores (24, 37), and that only in CU schizotypal symptoms correlated with worse cognitive performance (37). When it comes to licit drug use, the available information is even scarcer, as these studies did not report on a potential effect of licit (nicotine, alcohol) drug use (24, 37). We therefore investigated the link between cognitive attenuation and cannabis use in largely pure CU and non-cannabis users (nCU), accounting for the potential additional influence of both schizotypy and licit drug use (alcohol, nicotine).

We expected that both illicit and licit drug use might be more important than schizotypy to explain variance in cognitive performance (38–40). If schizotypy would additionally or instead explain variance in cognitive performance, we would expect the cognitive disorganization dimension (25–27) and/or positive schizotypy dimension (24, 41, 42) to be more relevant than the negative schizotypy dimension (27, 37, 42–44) that frequently resulted in heterogeneous findings.

MATERIALS AND METHODS

PARTICIPANTS

We recruited participants via advertisements looking for both pure CU (see also screening section) and non-nicotine consuming nCU. Advertisements were distributed at the local University and its vicinity on paper and electronically. We also used a local website ("Gumtree"). We recruited 83 healthy native English-speaking participants [35 CU (23 males) and 48 nCU (20 males)]. Participants either received monetary compensation for travel expenses or course credits. The University of Bristol ethics committee approved this study. All participants provided written informed consent prior participation.

SCREENING

In both groups (CU, nCU), people were excluded if they reported excessive alcohol use (>50 units of alcohol/week for men, >35 units of alcohol/women), alcohol use within 12 h prior to testing, a neurological, psychological, or psychiatric history, or visual problems (including dyslexia). Prior to study inclusion, participants were alerted that we would ask for a urine sample for drug screening. We then asked about illegal substance use within the past 3 months. To encourage honest responding, volunteers were kept unaware of the drug spectrum assessed with the urine test (it detected cannabis metabolites until about 2 weeks after its consumption). To ensure recruitment of largely pure CU, participants were excluded if they indicated regular illicit drug use (apart from cannabis) in the past 3 months (more than twice) and/or use within 2 weeks prior testing. Participants were also asked about their cannabis and nicotine use habits (e.g., average amount of times cannabis used/cigarettes per week) in the past 30 days prior testing. Data with a negative drug test were not excluded if CU self-reported occasional use (on average 1–2 times/week within the past 30 days), and/or indicated regular or frequent use (on average >2 times/week in the past 30 days), but not within the past 2 weeks (45). If regular or frequent CU indicated use within the past 2 weeks, participants with a negative drug test were excluded from further analysis. The healthy nCU were excluded if they reported nicotine and cannabis use in the past 30 days, and if they showed a positive drug test.

PROCEDURE

Participants were firstly screened by means of the procedure outlined above. Subsequently, participants came to the local department for a 1 h testing session. The CU were asked to abstain prior testing from (i) cannabis use at least 2 h and (ii) nicotine use 30 min. We chose this abstinence period for cannabis, because general psychotropic effects seem to taper off 2–3 h post-consumption (46). In the case of nicotine, acute effects on cognition seem observable within 15–35 min of nicotine consumption [e.g., Ref. (47, 48)]. After having provided written informed consent, participants underwent the urine test before continuing to the testing session. Participants first completed the drug and schizotypy questionnaires, before performing the cognitive tasks. Participants performed the tasks outlined below as well as a handedness questionnaire and a lateralized lexical decision task. Results from the latter will be presented elsewhere. Task order was randomized between participants. Finally, participants were debriefed and reimbursed for their time.

QUESTIONNAIRES

Schizotypy

The Oxford-Liverpool Inventory of Feelings and Experiences (17, 49) is a 159-item self-report instrument consisting of the following sub-scales: positive schizotypy (unusual experiences = UnEx, 30 items), negative schizotypy (Introvertive Anhedonia = IntAn, 27 items), and cognitive disorganization (= CogDis, 24 items). Finally, 23 items assess impulsive non-conformity (ImpNC). Normative values can be found in Mason et al. (17, 49). We did not account for IntAn and ImpNC in this study, because of the heterogeneity in findings in the former case (see Introduction) and because ImpNC does not represent a schizotypy dimension (17).

Drug questions

Participants reported on their prior drug use (lifetime, past year, and past month drug use), e.g., their alcohol, cigarette, cannabis, cocaine, amphetamine, hallucinogen, opiate, and prescribed drug use. Items were taken from the national household survey on drug abuse (50). This questionnaire taps into seven DSM-IV criteria for drug dependence (past 12 months) by asking if people (1) spent a lot of time obtaining, using, or recovering from the drug, (2) experienced a marked increase in amount and frequency of drug use, (3) experienced a marked decrease in the drug effect, and (4) gave up or reduced important social, occupational, or recreational activities due to drug use. It also asks if people experienced (5) drug-induced psychological problems (such as depressive mood), (6) drug-induced physical problems, and (7) a persistent desire for the drug or unsuccessful attempts to stop drug use. For each positive answer, participants received 1 point (maximum score 7) with higher values indicating higher substance use severity. Participants also indicated the average amount of joints/cigarettes per week they used within the past 30 days. For this reason, it is possible that current non-smokers (no tobacco use within the past month) receive a nicotine severity score $\neq 0$ if they have smoked within the past 12 months (this only concerned 2 of the 48 non-smokers).

BEHAVIORAL MEASURES: COGNITIVE FUNCTIONING

Trail making task

The trail making task (TMT) assessed executive functioning (51, 52). In the TMT A, participants connected numbered circles in chronological order (1–25) by drawing a line, as fast as possible. In the subsequent TMT B, participants saw circles containing numbers or letters. They drew a line as quickly as possible in chronological order switching between numbers and letters, i.e., from 1 to A, from A to 2, from 2 to B, etc. The RT for both versions was recorded. The TMT-index (RT version B minus version A) was used as an estimate of cognitive flexibility (53). Norm values are available from Tombaugh (54).

Verbal short-term memory (story-recall/logical memory)

We used a subtest of the revised version of the Wechsler adult intelligence scale (55). The experimenter read out a 60 words story. The participant was asked immediately afterwards to recall as many details as possible (maximum of 23 possible points). Normative data for young adults and university samples can be found in Bowden et al. (56) and Ivison (57), respectively.

Verbal working memory (two-back task)

Comparable to previous reports (58, 59), participants saw 64 sequentially presented digits (ranging from 1 to 9) in the middle of the computer screen (white on black background, font Arial, size 16). Participants had to press a given response key when the current digit (n) was identical to the digit n-2 (target trials). In all non-target trials, participants had to press another response key. Response key allocation was counterbalanced between participants. A third of the trials ($n = 20$) were target trials, and the remaining trials were non-target trials [$n = 44$; e.g., 59]. To increase task difficulty, we added intrusion trials. These were included to prevent restarting memorization after each successful target identification. Consequently, targets could occur twice in a row. Each stimulus appeared for 2000 ms, with an inter-stimulus interval of 500 ms (60) before the next digit appeared. Participants had to respond within 2500 ms, otherwise the trial was counted as an omission. All participants performed 16 practice trials. We measured the percentage of the correctly identified targets, as well as mean RTs for correct trials (59, 61).

As an additional note, we also measured a computerized Go NoGo task. Due to an overall ceiling performance, we omitted this task from further analysis.

DATA ANALYSIS

To determine if cannabis use affects cognitive functioning, we conducted separate univariate ANOVAs with group (CU, nCU) as between-subjects factor on the following measures: percentage of correct responses [(number of correctly identified target stimuli × 100)/total of targets] and RT in the two-back task, TMT-index, and the percentage of correctly identified units in the story-recall task [(number of correctly identified units × 100)/total of units)].

To determine effects of drug use and schizotypy on cognition, we firstly investigated the demographic characteristics of our population. We found sex differences between drug groups (see Results for details). We then correlated all variables with the outcome measures to preselect variables for the regression model (see Results for details). Neither age nor schizotypy significantly correlated with the cognitive measures. Due to the previous literature (see Introduction), we nevertheless kept UnEx scores and CogDis scores for the hierarchical regressions as follows: sex was entered in the first step, schizotypy (UnEx scores, CogDis scores) in the second step, and drug use severity (nicotine, alcohol, and cannabis) in the third step. Severity was preferred over frequency due to the former measure's relevance to clinical addiction. Exploratory analysis confirmed that drug use severity was more important than drug use frequency in the current regression analyses. Thus, three blocks of predictors were entered in nested blocks, meaning that each subsequent block contained all prior predictors and the additional predictors from the current block. Presentation of results only includes the new predictors entered, for economy of presentation. All tolerance values were above 0.2 (62) and all independent variables were mean-centered. Thus, multi-collinearity between the independent variables was considered negligible. The dependent variables were (i) percentage correctly identified targets and mean RT for correctly identified targets and non-targets in the two-back task; (ii) TMT-index; and (iii) percentage of correctly recalled units in the story-recall task.

Kolmogorov–Smirnov tests for the groups separately revealed normal distribution for all behavioral measures. All p-values were two-tailed and the α-level was set at 0.05.

RESULTS

PARTICIPANTS

We identified 35 CU (out of 83 healthy native English-speakers). On average (±SD), CU smoked 11.14 joints per week (±12.16), a frequency that can be classified as heavy use [>5 joints per week; (63)]. The last cannabis consumption was on average more than 24 h ago (114.37 ± 143.02 h) with 4 CU reporting cannabis use 2–6 h before testing. When only individuals are considered whose last cannabis consumption was more than 6 h ago, the results stayed largely the same. Age of cannabis use onset was at 15.46 years of age (±1.87 years). Within the CU group, 13 individuals were educated to college level (37%), 1 to secondary school (3%), and 21 to university degrees (60%). Of the 48 nCU, 12 individuals had college degrees (25%) and 36 had university degrees (75%). A chi-square test indicated that the two groups did not differ from each other in terms of highest finished education level [$\chi^2(df = 2) = 3.03$, $p = 0.22$]. A chi-square test on sex distributions showed that significantly more males ($n = 23$) were in the CU group as compared to the nCU group [$n = 20$; $\chi^2(df = 1) = 4.69$, $p = 0.03$].

We also compared schizotypy sub-scale scores to a previous normative sample (17) via calculations of Cohen's d (64) with values of ±0.2/±0.5/±0.8 being indicative of a small/medium/large effect size, respectively. As can be seen from **Table 1**, schizotypy values were largely comparable to normative data, as no large effect sizes were found. A medium effect size was indicated for UnEx, with higher values in the normative sample as compared to the current sample (see **Table 1**).

As can be seen from **Table 2**, the groups (CU, nCU) were comparable in age. However, CU as compared to nCU scored higher on UnEx (as a trend), nicotine, cannabis, and alcohol use severity

Table 1 | Means, SDs, and effect sizes (Cohen's *d*), comparing the values of the normative sample with the current sample.

Questionnaire	Norm values ($N = 508$)		Current sample ($N = 83$)		Cohen's d
	Mean	SD	Mean	SD	
O-LIFE: UnEx[a]	9.70	6.70	6.36	4.92	0.52
O-LIFE: CogDis[b]	11.60	5.80	10.61	5.28	0.17

[a] *Unusual experiences.*

[b] *Cognitive disorganization.*

(since nCU were screened for weekly cannabis and cigarette use, the comparisons between nCU and CU were not conducted for these variables).

COGNITIVE FUNCTIONING

Group comparisons

The separate univariate ANOVAs on the outcome measures revealed that CU performed significantly worse in the story-recall task, and slightly worse on the working memory task as compared to nCU (**Table 3**). The results for the remaining outcome variables were not significant (**Table 3**).

Regression analyses

The initial correlation analyses between task performances, schizotypy sub-scale scores, age, and drug measures revealed that neither age nor schizotypy related to cognitive functioning (all p-values >0.10, see **Table 4**). Accordingly, age was not further considered. UnEx and CogDis on the other hand were included as *a priori* predictions were formulated based on the published literature (see Introduction and Data Analysis).

The significant results from the subsequent regression analyses (see Data Analysis for further details) can be seen in **Table 5**. With regard to the control variables, we found that sex predicted verbal short-term memory. *Post hoc* independent t-tests revealed that women were significantly better than men in the story-recall task [women: $66.63 \pm 12.08\%$, men: $m = 58.54 \pm 15.39\%$; $t(81) = 2.65$, $p = 0.01$]. Entering schizotypy in the second step explained no additional variance on top of sex (see **Table 5**). Drug use severity in the third step predicted significant amounts of variance in the outcome measures. Here, higher alcohol use severity predicted lower working memory performance, and higher cannabis use severity predicted reduced verbal short-term memory on top of sex and schizotypy (**Table 5**).

Table 2 | Age, schizotypy, and drug use statistics comparing CU and nCU.

Variables	CU[c] ($N=35$)		nCU[d] ($N=48$)		t	p
	Mean	SD	Mean	SD		
Age	22.51	5.63	21.67	3.56	0.84	0.40
UnEx[a]	7.63	6.04	5.44	3.71	1.90	**0.06**
CogDis[b]	10.46	5.75	10.73	4.97	−0.23	0.82
Cigarettes/week	24.66	28.67	n/a	n/a	n/a	n/a
Joints/week	11.14	12.16	n/a	n/a	n/a	n/a
Nicotine use severity	1.94	1.86	0.08	0.45	5.78	**0.00**
Cannabis use severity	2.97	1.95	0.00	0.00	9.03	**0.00**
Alcohol use severity	2.29	1.84	1.31	1.42	2.72	**0.01**

[a] *Unusual experiences.*
[b] *Cognitive disorganization.*
[c] *Cannabis users.*
[d] *Cannabis non-users.*
Values were compared between groups (CU, nCU) using independent t-tests (statistical results are shown in this table; t-values, df= 81, p-values). Significant group differences are highlighted in bold, trends in gray.

DISCUSSION

We investigated whether pure cannabis use hampers cognitive performance, or whether cognitive attenuation is also, or even better explained by associated licit drug use and psychotic-like features (schizotypy). For this purpose, we tested cognitive functions commonly associated with drug use and schizotypy in CU and nCU. The main findings were that (i) CU as compared to nCU performed worse on story recall and slightly worse on the two-back task, but not on the TMT, (ii) CU scored higher than nCU on positive schizotypy (as a trend), and drug use other than cannabis, (iii) regression analyses showed that enhanced cannabis use predicted decreased verbal short-term memory, whereas enhanced alcohol use predicted reduced working memory performance, (iv) none of the schizotypy sub-scales explained any additional variance in cognitive functioning. The implications of these findings are discussed below.

ROLE OF CANNABIS USE SEVERITY

Our results showed that CU performed worse than nCU on tasks measuring verbal short-term memory (story recall), and higher cannabis use severity was associated with worse performance in this task. Our results also showed that these relatively negative cognitive implications were not associated with individuals' self-reported schizotypy. The observation that worse story recall is

Table 3 | Descriptive and statistical values for the cognitive measures, comparing perfomance of CU and nCU.

Variables	CU[b] ($N=35$)		nCU[c] ($N=48$)		F(1,81)	p	Partial η^2
	Mean	SD	Mean	SD			
Two-back % target correct	86.00	13.49	90.52	8.07	3.62	**0.06**	0.04
Two-back mean RT	822.57	164.00	821.42	205.92	0.00	0.98	<0.01
TMT[a] index	23.77	13.58	23.56	16.58	0.00	0.95	<0.01
Story-recall % correct	55.90	14.78	67.21	12.19	14.55	**<0.01**	0.15

[a] *Trail making task.*
[b] *Cannabis users.*
[c] *Cannabis non-users.*
Values were compared with univariate ANOVAs, and significant values are highlighted in bold, trends in gray.

associated with cannabis use is in line with previous studies (3, 13, 46). However, story recall (verbal memory) was the only task that was affected by cannabis use, whereas relatively impaired performance on another cognitive task (working memory as assessed with the two-back task) was related to enhanced alcohol use instead. Previous studies have indicated that cannabis use has a negative impact on working memory performance (46, 65) and mental flexibility (3, 66) as well. Our findings suggest that these previous findings on cannabis use were potentially confounded by concomitant non-excessive alcohol use (3, 67).

Despite some evidence that cannabis use is still associated with cognitive impairments after adjusting for alcohol use (68), independent studies (8, 36) report that CU tend to consume higher amounts of other drugs as well. This additional drug use, as frequently not assessed, might lead to misleading conclusions about cannabis effects on cognition. Particularly licit drug use like alcohol seems to be a relevant confounding factor. For instance, whereas in some studies alcohol use is either statistically controlled for (63) or subjects with alcohol abuse are excluded from participating (13, 14), other studies do not account for this variable (24, 69, 70, 71). Moreover, alcohol and cannabis are thought to exert comparable effects on cognition, i.e., cognitive attenuation in verbal memory (72–74), cognitive flexibility (75, 76), and working memory (77–79). Future studies should consider (non-excessive) licit drug use as a potential confounding factor when investigating the effects of cannabis use on cognition.

Table 4 | Correlations between potential predictor variables and cognitive measures.

Variables	Two-back task % target correct	Two-back task mean RT	TMT[c] index	Story-recall % correct
Age	−0.06	−0.16	−0.08	−0.03
UnEx[a]	−0.08	0.06	0.08	−0.03
CogDis[b]	0.02	−0.01	−0.04	−0.07
Nicotine use severity	**−0.24***	0.08	0.04	**−0.41*****
Cannabis use severity	**−0.27***	0.14	0.10	**−0.47*****
Alcohol use severity	**−0.29****	**0.40*****	**0.28****	−0.07

[a] *Unusual experiences.*
[b] *Cognitive disorganization.*
[c] *Trail making task.*
**Significant at $p \leq 0.05$.*
***Significant at $p \leq 0.01$.*
****Significant at $p \leq 0.001$.*
Significant values are highlighted in bold.

ROLE OF SCHIZOTYPY

Of additional significance was the observation that schizotypy did not explain variance in most cognitive tasks. We do not think that this finding can be explained by deviant features of our sample, because we replicated many previous observations, i.e., that CU as compared to nCU scored slightly higher on measures of positive schizotypy (24, 27, 28, 41, 42, 44). The observation that schizotypy was not importantly related to cognitive functioning would indicate that the impairments in, e.g., working memory (19, 20), cognitive flexibility (21), and verbal memory (22, 23) may be influenced by individuals' concomitant drug use.

Unfortunately, the above mentioned studies did not report on drug use (19, 21–23, 80), or only screened for substance use history without specifying the substances controlled for (20, 81). It is thus possible that substances (e.g., illicit as well as licit) influenced the relationship between schizotypal symptoms and the cognitive functions assessed in these experiments (38–40). In particular, our results suggest that cannabis may be more relevant than schizotypy for cognitive attenuations in verbal short-term memory, and alcohol may be more relevant than schizotypy for cognitive attenuations in working memory (82).

The specific cannabis effects on story recall, but not on the two-back or TMT may also suggest that not all cognitive functions are equally sensitive to cannabis-related attenuations. Even though many studies observe CU to show impairments compared to nCU on tasks measuring working memory (46) and mental flexibility (3, 66), this may not always be the case (71, 83). In fact, different

Table 5 | Significant results (including trends in gray) from the regression analyses assessing the effect of sex (step 1), schizotypy (UnEx[a], CogDis[b]; step 2), and drug use severity (nicotine, alcohol, and cannabis; step 3) on cognitive measures.

Outcome variables	Step	Significant predictor	β-value	Total R^2	ΔR^2	F for ΔR^2
Two-back % target correct	3	Alcohol	−0.25*	0.15**	0.14**	4.25**
Two-back mean RT	1	Sex	−0.21[†]	0.04[†]	0.04[†]	3.61[†]
	3	Alcohol	0.39***	0.18**	0.13**	4.03**
Story-recall % correct	1	Sex	0.28**	0.08**	0.08**	7.02**
	3	Cannabis	−0.41**	0.30***	0.21***	7.46***

[†] *$p \leq 0.10$.*
**Significant at $p \leq 0.05$.*
***Significant at $p \leq 0.01$.*
****Significant at $p \leq 0.001$.*
[a] *Unusual experiences.*
[b] *Cognitive disorganization.*

meta-analyses draw inconsistent conclusions about which cognitive functions qualify as cognitive markers, or endophenotypes for pathological changes. Findings are inconsistent in CU and along the schizophrenia spectrum, with some studies pointing to verbal memory impairments in both populations (65, 84–86), some pointing to cognitive flexibility impairments (86, 87), and others reporting consistent working memory impairments in both patients with psychosis and CU (65, 85, 86). Alternatively, higher THC-content of used cannabis may relate to more prominent cognitive attenuations (88). Therefore, future studies should report the type and/or strength of cannabis used to improve reliability of findings.

Admittedly, all these complex functions tap into a variety of cognitive sub-functions. For this reason, to increase reliability of findings across studies and populations, the research community might consider behavioral markers that are less complex in their cognitive demands (89–92). Additionally, the pathophysiology of psychotic disorders is currently unknown, and the disorders are quite heterogeneous in their phenotypic expression. Consequently, we may increase the reliability of findings by accounting for seemingly related as well as unrelated factors potentially influencing the relationship between cannabis, cognition, and psychosis (-risk). For instance, studies could consider different yet potentially equally relevant personality traits such as those tapping on the autism spectrum (93) or the bipolar spectrum (94, 95). Beyond personality, studies could consider genetic predisposition (96), IQ (97), and neurochemical peculiarities such as dopamine receptor availability (98, 99) that may influence the effect cannabis exerts on cognition. Such factors are also relevant for the link between psychosis and drug use, e.g., genetic predisposition (100, 101), IQ (102–104), and neurochemical peculiarities (99). At present, it is impossible to account for all putatively influential variables, and hence additional studies need to be conducted to replicate our and similar findings, be it clinical, experimental, and/or epidemiological studies.

STUDY LIMITATIONS AND FUTURE RESEARCH

In the catchment area of our study, the "binge drinking culture" reflects on the high acceptance for alcohol use (105). Consequently, we refrained from pre-selecting participants according to their alcohol use, as the recruitment of pure CU (rather than polydrug users) turned out to be challenging, and was not facilitated by the modest incentives we could offer. Likewise, controlling for the co-use of nicotine seemed even more unavoidable, because cannabis is mostly used in combination with nicotine (106). Yet, controlling for nicotine could have been relevant, because nicotine itself might counteract the effects of cannabis on cognition (33, 107–109). We therefore suggest that future studies should elucidate the role of nicotine and cannabis more directly.

The gender composition differed between groups, a difference common to studies such as the current one. This gender difference could have also affected the group differences in story recall. Typically, females perform better on verbal short-term memory tasks than males (110), a finding also observed here. Since the nCU group consisted of more females than the CU, this group difference could alternatively explain the worse story recall in CU. However, since cannabis use related to worse story-recall performance on top of sex in the regression analysis, we deem it unlikely that the group differences are solely due to effects associated with the unequal sex distribution. Nevertheless, future studies on drug use and cognition should aim to control for sex differences.

A final, frequently mentioned study limitation is the sample size, also relevant to the conducted analyses. For regression analyses, the guidelines for recommended sample sizes vary, from using $50 + 8\times N$ variables (111–113) to 10 participants per predictor variable (114). Obviously, a larger sample size would always be advisable. Yet, our sample size matches sample sizes in other studies reporting on preselected minority samples of (relatively) pure drug users (3). A potential reason could be firstly, that these individuals are either extremely difficult to motivate, or secondly, that pure users of drugs are a rarity, at least in our study region. The difficulty of finding pure CU may also be reflected in population descriptions over the last 30 years; many studies inferred on the influence of cannabis use on cognition and mental health risk without necessarily ensuring that individuals did not also consume other licit and illicit drugs. We thus face the future challenge to disentangle the impact of a specific drug use or synergetic drug uses on cognition and mental health (115–117).

Finally, cognitive attenuations related to cannabis use seem more overt in heavy as compared to moderate or light users (14, 118, 119). A higher frequency of cannabis use in our sample might have exacerbated the reported cognitive attenuations. Though definitions for heavy use may vary (118, 119), the frequency of cannabis use (joints/week) in our sample seems to indicate heavy use according to a previous report on pure CU (63). To note, our data point to a negligible influence of frequency of pure cannabis use (see Materials and Methods).

CONCLUSION

While pure cannabis and alcohol use seem associated with adverse effects on cognition, other risk factors (e.g., nicotine use) might also be relevant. Schizotypy, on the other hand, seems unrelated to cognitive attenuation. Results stress the importance to control for additional substance use (and non-excessive use in particular), whether illicit or licit, when assessing the effect of schizotypal symptoms and/or cannabis use on cognition. Moreover, heterogeneity of cannabis-related attenuations of specific cognitive functions may be avoided by controlling for additional factors potentially influencing the relationship between cannabis, cognition, and psychosis (-risk).

AUTHOR CONTRIBUTIONS

All authors significantly contributed to the conception or design of the work, the analysis, and interpretation of data for the work, as well as revising it critically for important intellectual content. Dr. Daniela A. Herzig was additionally involved in the data acquisition and drafting the first version of the manuscript. All authors approve of the final version of the manuscript, therefore, ensuring that questions related to the accuracy or integrity of any part of the work are appropriately investigated and resolved.

ACKNOWLEDGMENTS

Participant payment was provided by the University of Bristol. Part of the payment was derived from Prof. Christine Mohr's personal budget at the University of Bristol, and part from the University of Bristol Psychopharmacology Unit. The funding source had no additional role other than financial support. All authors contributed in a significant way to the manuscript and all authors have read and approved the final manuscript. There are no conflicts of interest with the present manuscript. The author would also like to thank Prof. Marcus Munafo and Dr. Stanley Zammit for their support, in particular, their aid when acquiring ethical approval for this study.

REFERENCES

1. European Monitoring Centre for Drugs and Drug Addiction. *European Drug Report 2014: Trends and Developments* (2014). Available from: http://www.emcdda.europa.eu/publications/edr/trends-developments/2014
2. Barkus E, Murray RM. Substance use in adolescence and psychosis: clarifying the relationship. *Annu Rev Clin Psychol* (2010) **6**:365–89. doi:10.1146/annurev.clinpsy.121208.131220
3. Fernández-Serrano MJ, Pérez-García M, Verdejo-García A. What are the specific vs. generalized effects of drugs of abuse on neuropsychological performance? *Neurosci Biobehav Rev* (2011) **35**:377–406. doi:10.1016/j.neubiorev.2010.04.008
4. Arseneault L, Cannon M, Poulton R, Murray R, Caspi A, Moffitt TE. Cannabis use in adolescence and risk for adult psychosis: longitudinal prospective study. *Br Med J* (2002) **325**:1212–3. doi:10.1136/bmj.325.7374.1212
5. van Os J, Bak M, Hanssen M, Bijl RV, De Graaf R, Verdoux H. Cannabis use and psychosis: a longitudinal population-based study. *Am J Epidemiol* (2002) **156**:319–27. doi:10.1093/aje/kwf043
6. Zammit S, Allebeck P, Andreasson S, Lundberg I, Lewis G. Self reported cannabis use as a risk factor for schizophrenia in Swedish conscripts of 1969: historical cohort study. *Br Med J* (2002) **325**:1199–201. doi:10.1136/bmj.325.7374.1199
7. Casadio P, Fernandes C, Murray RM, Di Forti M. Cannabis use in young people: the risk for schizophrenia. *Neurosci Biobehav Rev* (2011) **35**:1779–87. doi:10.1016/j.neubiorev.2011.04.007
8. Schimmelmann BG, Conus P, Cotton S, Kupferschmid S, Mcgorry PD, Lambert M. Prevalence and impact of cannabis use disorders in adolescents with early onset first episode psychosis. *Eur Psychiatry* (2012) **27**:463–9. doi:10.1016/j.eurpsy.2011.03.001
9. Parakh P, Basu D. Cannabis and psychosis: have we found the missing links? *Asian J Psychiatr* (2013) **6**:281–7. doi:10.1016/j.ajp.2013.03.012
10. Manrique-Garcia E, Zammit S, Dalman C, Hemmingsson T, Andreasson S, Allebeck P. Cannabis, schizophrenia and other non-affective psychoses: 35 years of follow-up of a population-based cohort. *Psychol Med* (2012) **42**:1321–8. doi:10.1017/S0033291711002078
11. Moore THM, Zammit S, Lingford-Hughes A, Barnes TRE, Jones PB, Burke M, et al. Cannabis use and risk of psychotic or affective mental health outcomes: a systematic review. *Lancet* (2007) **370**:319–28. doi:10.1016/S0140-6736(07)61162-3
12. Solowij N, Battisti R. The chronic effects of cannabis on memory in humans: a review. *Curr Drug Abuse Rev* (2008) **1**:81–98. doi:10.2174/1874473710801010081
13. Wagner D, Becker B, Gouzoulis-Mayfrank E, Daumann J. Interactions between specific parameters of cannabis use and verbal memory. *Prog Neuropsychopharmacol Biol Psychiatry* (2010) **34**:871–6. doi:10.1016/j.pnpbp.2010.04.004
14. Pope HG, Yurgelun-Todd D. The residual cognitive effects of heavy marijuana use in college students. *JAMA* (1996) **275**:521–7. doi:10.1001/jama.275.7.521
15. Meehl PE. Schizotaxia, schizotypy, schizophrenia. *Am Psychol* (1962) **17**:827–38. doi:10.1037/h0041029
16. Raine A. The SPQ: a scale for the assessment of schizotypal personality based on DSM-III-R criteria. *Schizophr Bull* (1991) **17**:555–64. doi:10.1093/schbul/17.4.555
17. Mason O, Claridge G, Jackson M. New scales for the assessment of schizotypy. *Pers Individ Dif* (1995) **18**:7–13. doi:10.1016/0191-8869(94)00132-C
18. Liddle PF. The symptoms of chronic schizophrenia. A re-examination of the positive-negative dichotomy. *Br J Psychiatry* (1987) **151**:145–51. doi:10.1192/bjp.151.2.145
19. Park S, McTigue K. Working memory and the syndromes of schizotypal personality. *Schizophr Res* (1997) **26**:213–20. doi:10.1016/S0920-9964(97)00051-0
20. Pflueger MO, Gschwandtner U, Stieglitz R-D, Riecher-Rössler A. Neuropsychological deficits in individuals with an at risk mental state for psychosis – working memory as a potential trait marker. *Schizophr Res* (2007) **97**:14–24. doi:10.1016/j.schres.2007.09.003
21. Giraldez SL, Caro MI, Rodrigo AML, Pineiro MP, Gonzalez JLB. Assessment of essential components of schizotypy by means of neurocognitive measures. *Psicothema* (1999) **11**:477–94.
22. Langdon R, Coltheart M. Recognition of metaphor and irony in young adults: the impact of schizotypal personality traits. *Psychiatry Res* (2004) **125**:9–20. doi:10.1016/j.psychres.2003.10.005
23. Simon AE, Cattapan-Ludewig K, Zmilacher S, Arbach D, Gruber K, Dvorsky DN, et al. Cognitive functioning in the schizophrenia prodrome. *Schizophr Bull* (2007) **33**:761–71. doi:10.1093/schbul/sbm018
24. Skosnik PD, Spatz-Glenn L, Park S. Cannabis use is associated with schizotypy and attentional disinhibition. *Schizophr Res* (2001) **48**:83–92. doi:10.1016/S0920-9964(00)00132-8
25. Barkus E, Lewis S. Schizotypy and psychosis-like experiences from recreational cannabis in a non-clinical sample. *Psychol Med* (2008) **38**:1267–76. doi:10.1017/S0033291707002619
26. Esterberg ML, Goulding SM, Mcclure-Tone EB, Compton MT. Schizotypy and nicotine, alcohol, and cannabis use in a non-psychiatric sample. *Addict Behav* (2009) **34**:374–9. doi:10.1016/j.addbeh.2008.11.007
27. Cohen AS, Buckner JD, Najolia GM, Stewart DW. Cannabis and psychometrically-defined schizotypy: use, problems and treatment considerations. *J Psychiatr Res* (2011) **45**:548–54. doi:10.1016/j.jpsychires.2010.08.013
28. Fridberg DJ, Vollmer JM, O'Donnell BF, Skosnik PD. Cannabis users differ from non-users on measures of personality and schizotypy. *Psychiatry Res* (2011) **186**:46–52. doi:10.1016/j.psychres.2010.07.035
29. Larrison AL, Briand KA, Sereno AB. Nicotine, caffeine, alcohol and schizotypy. *Pers Individ Dif* (1999) **27**:101–8. doi:10.1016/S0191-8869(98)00217-7
30. Cantor-Graae E, Nordström LG, Mcneil TF. Substance abuse in schizophrenia: a review of the literature and a study of correlates in Sweden. *Schizophr Res* (2001) **48**:69–82. doi:10.1016/S0920-9964(00)00114-6
31. de Leon J, Diaz FJ, Rogers T, Browne D, Dinsmore L. Initiation of daily smoking and nicotine dependence in schizophrenia and mood disorders. *Schizophr Res* (2002) **56**:47–54. doi:10.1016/S0920-9964(01)00217-1
32. Mastrigt S, Addington J, Addington D. Substance misuse at presentation to an early psychosis program. *Soc Psychiatry Psychiatr Epidemiol* (2004) **39**:69–72. doi:10.1007/s00127-004-0713-0
33. Kumari V, Postma P. Nicotine use in schizophrenia: the self medication hypotheses. *Neurosci Biobehav Rev* (2005) **29**:1021–34. doi:10.1016/j.neubiorev.2005.02.006
34. Gregg L, Barrowclough C, Haddock G. Reasons for increased substance use in psychosis. *Clin Psychol Rev* (2007) **27**:494–510. doi:10.1016/j.cpr.2006.09.004
35. Grant BF, Pickering R. The relationship between cannabis use and DSM-IV cannabis abuse and dependence: results from the national longitudinal alcohol epidemiologic survey. *J Subst Abuse* (1998) **10**:255–64. doi:10.1016/S0899-3289(99)80141-2
36. Degenhardt L, Hall W, Lynskey M. The relationship between cannabis use and other substance use in the general population. *Drug Alcohol Depend* (2001) **64**:319–27. doi:10.1016/S0376-8716(01)00130-2
37. Mass R, Bardong C, Kindl K, Dahme B. Relationship between cannabis use, schizotypal traits, and cognitive function in healthy subjects. *Psychopathology* (2001) **34**:209–14. doi:10.1159/000049309
38. Herzig DA, Tracy J, Munafò M, Mohr C. The influence of tobacco consumption on the relationship between schizotypy and hemispheric asymmetry. *J Behav Ther Exp Psychiatry* (2010) **41**:397–408. doi:10.1016/j.jbtep.2010.04.003
39. Herzig DA, Mohr C. Stressing schizotypy: the modulating role of stress-relieving behaviours and intellectual capacity on functional hemispheric asymmetry. *Laterality* (2012) **18**(2):152–78. doi:10.1080/1357650X.2011.638638
40. Herzig DA, Brooks R, Mohr C. Inferring about individual drug and schizotypy effects on cognitive functioning in polydrug using mephedrone users before and after clubbing. *Hum Psychopharmacol* (2013) **28**:168–82. doi:10.1002/hup.2307
41. Verdoux H, Sorbara F, Gindre C, Swendsen JD, Van Os J. Cannabis use and dimensions of psychosis in a nonclinical population of female subjects. *Schizophr Res* (2003) **59**:77–84. doi:10.1016/S0920-9964(01)00401-7

42. Compton MT, Chien V, Bollini A. Associations between past alcohol, cannabis, and cocaine use and current schizotypy among first-degree relatives of patients with schizophrenia and non-psychiatric controls. *Psychiatr Q* (2009) **80**:143–54. doi:10.1007/s11126-009-9102-x
43. Bailey EL, Swallow BL. The relationship between cannabis use and schizotypal symptoms. *Eur Psychiatry* (2004) **19**:113–4. doi:10.1016/j.eurpsy.2003.12.001
44. Skosnik PD, Park S, Dobbs L, Gardner WL. Affect processing and positive syndrome schizotypy in cannabis users. *Psychiatry Res* (2008) **157**:279–82. doi:10.1016/j.psychres.2007.02.010
45. Solowij N, Michie PT, Fox AM. Differential impairments of selective attention due to frequency and duration of cannabis use. *Biol Psychiatry* (1995) **37**:731–9. doi:10.1016/0006-3223(94)00178-6
46. Ranganathan M, D'Souza D. The acute effects of cannabinoids on memory in humans: a review. *Psychopharmacology* (2006) **188**:425–44. doi:10.1007/s00213-006-0508-y
47. Le Houezec J, Halliday R, Benowitz N, Callaway E, Naylor H, Herzig K. A low dose of subcutaneous nicotine improves information processing in non-smokers. *Psychopharmacology* (1994) **114**:628–34. doi:10.1007/BF02244994
48. Ernst M, Heishman SJ, Spurgeon L, London ED. Smoking history and nicotine effects on cognitive performance. *Neuropsychopharmacology* (2001) **25**:313–9. doi:10.1016/S0893-133X(01)00257-3
49. Mason O, Claridge G. The oxford-Liverpool inventory of feelings and experiences (O-LIFE): further description and extended norms. *Schizophr Res* (2006) **82**:203–11. doi:10.1016/j.schres.2005.12.845
50. United States Department of Health and Human Services. *National Household Survey on Drug Abuse.* MI: Substance Abuse and Mental Health Services Administration. Office of Applied Studies. Inter-university Consortium for Political and Social Research (1998). Available from: www.icpsr.umich.edu
51. Army Individual Test Battery. *Manual of Directions and Scoring.* Washington, DC: War Department, Adjutant General's Office (1944).
52. Reitan RM, Wolfson D. *The Halstead-Reitan Neuropsychological Test Battery: Theory and Clinical Interpretation.* Tucson, AZ: Neuropsychology Press (1985).
53. Lezak MD. *Neuropsychological Assessment.* 3rd ed. New York, NY: Oxford (1995).
54. Tombaugh TN. Trail making test A and B: normative data stratified by age and education. *Arch Clin Neuropsychol* (2004) **19**:203–14. doi:10.1016/S0887-6177(03)00039-8
55. Wechsler D. *Manual for the Wechsler Memory Scale – Revised.* San Antonio, TX: The Psychological Corporation (1987).
56. Bowden SC, Carstairs JR, Shores EA. Confirmatory factor analysis of combined Wechsler adult intelligence scale – revised and Wechsler memory scale – revised scores in a healthy community sample. *Psychol Assess* (1999) **11**:339–44. doi:10.1037/1040-3590.11.3.339
57. Ivison D. Logical memory in the Wechsler memory scales: does the order of passages affect difficulty in an university sample? *Clin Neuropsychol* (1993) **7**:215–8. doi:10.1080/13854049308401525
58. Owen AM, Mcmillan KM, Laird AR, Bullmore E. N-back working memory paradigm: a meta-analysis of normative functional neuroimaging studies. *Hum Brain Mapp* (2005) **25**:46–59. doi:10.1002/hbm.20131
59. Schoofs D, Preuß D, Wolf OT. Psychosocial stress induces working memory impairments in an N-back paradigm. *Psychoneuroendocrinology* (2008) **33**:643–53. doi:10.1016/j.psyneuen.2008.02.004
60. Barch DM, Sheline YI, Csernansky JG, Snyder AZ. Working memory and prefrontal cortex dysfunction: specificity to schizophrenia compared with major depression. *Biol Psychiatry* (2003) **53**:376–84. doi:10.1016/S0006-3223(02)01674-8
61. Jonides J, Schumacher EH, Smith EE, Lauber EJ, Awh E, Minoshima S, et al. Verbal working memory load affects regional brain activation as measured by PET. *J Cogn Neurosci* (1997) **9**:462–75. doi:10.1162/jocn.1997.9.4.462
62. Menard S. *Applied logistic regression analysis.* Thousand Oaks, CA: Sage (1995).
63. Fried PA, Watkinson B, Gray R. Neurocognitive consequences of marihuana – a comparison with pre-drug performance. *Neurotoxicol Teratol* (2005) **27**:231–9. doi:10.1016/j.ntt.2004.11.003
64. Cohen J. A power primer. *Psychol Bull* (1992) **112**:155–9. doi:10.1037/0033-2909.112.1.155
65. Crean RD, Crane NA, Mason BJ. An evidence-based review of acute and long-term effects of cannabis use on executive cognitive functions. *J Addict Med* (2011) **5**:1–8. doi:10.1097/ADM.0b013e31820c23fa
66. Lundqvist T. Cognitive consequences of cannabis use: comparison with abuse of stimulants and heroin with regard to attention, memory and executive functions. *Pharmacol Biochem Behav* (2005) **81**:319–30. doi:10.1016/j.pbb.2005.02.017
67. Zeigler DW, Wang CC, Yoast RA, Dickinson BD, Mccaffree MA, Robinowitz CB, et al. The neurocognitive effects of alcohol on adolescents and college students. *Prev Med* (2005) **40**:23–32. doi:10.1016/j.ypmed.2004.04.044
68. Medina KL, Hanson KL, Schweinsburg AD, Cohen-Zion M, Nagel BJ, Tapert SF. Neuropsychological functioning in adolescent marijuana users: subtle deficits detectable after a month of abstinence. *J Int Neuropsychol Soc* (2007) **13**:807–20. doi:10.1017/S1355617707071032
69. Barratt E, Beaver W, White R, Blakeney P, Adams P. The effects of the chronic use of marijuana on sleep and perceptual-motor performance in humans. In: Lewis MF, editor. *Current Research in Marijuana.* New York: Academic Press (1972). p. 163–93.
70. Pope HG Jr, Gruber AJ, Yurgelun-Todd D. The residual neuropsychological effects of cannabis: the current status of research. *Drug Alcohol Depend* (1995) **38**:25–34. doi:10.1016/0376-8716(95)01145-O
71. Grant JE, Chamberlain SR, Schreiber L, Odlaug BL. Neuropsychological deficits associated with cannabis use in young adults. *Drug Alcohol Depend* (2012) **121**:159–62. doi:10.1016/j.drugalcdep.2011.08.015
72. Petros TV, Kerbel N, Beckwith BE, Sacks G, Sarafolean M. The effects of alcohol on prose memory. *Physiol Behav* (1985) **35**:43–6. doi:10.1016/0031-9384(85)90169-6
73. Parada M, Corral M, Caamaño-Isorna F, Mota N, Crego A, Holguín SR, et al. Binge drinking and declarative memory in university students. *Alcohol Clin Exp Res* (2011) **35**:1475–84. doi:10.1111/j.1530-0277.2011.01484.x
74. Poltavski DV, Marino JM, Guido JM, Kulland A, Petros TV. Effects of acute alcohol intoxication on verbal memory in young men as a function of time of day. *Physiol Behav* (2011) **102**:91–5. doi:10.1016/j.physbeh.2010.10.007
75. Guillot CR, Fanning JR, Bullock JS, Mccloskey MS, Berman ME. Effects of alcohol on tests of executive functioning in men and women: a dose response examination. *Exp Clin Psychopharmacol* (2010) **18**:409–17. doi:10.1037/a0021053
76. Lyvers M, Tobias-Webb J. Effects of acute alcohol consumption on executive cognitive functioning in naturalistic settings. *Addict Behav* (2010) **35**:1021–8. doi:10.1016/j.addbeh.2010.06.022
77. Weissenborn R, Duka T. Acute alcohol effects on cognitive function in social drinkers: their relationship to drinking habits. *Psychopharmacology (Berl)* (2003) **165**:306–12. doi:10.1007/s00213-002-1281-1
78. Yücel M, Lubman DI, Solowij N, Brewer WJ. Understanding drug addiction: a neuropsychological perspective. *Aust N Z J Psychiatry* (2007) **41**:957–68. doi:10.1080/00048670701689444
79. Crego A, Rodriguez-Holguín S, Parada M, Mota N, Corral M, Cadaveira F. Reduced anterior prefrontal cortex activation in young binge drinkers during a visual working memory task. *Drug Alcohol Depend* (2010) **109**:45–56. doi:10.1016/j.drugalcdep.2009.11.020
80. Tsakanikos E, Claridge G. More words, less words: verbal fluency as a function of 'positive' and 'negative' schizotypy. *Pers Individ Dif* (2005) **39**:705–13. doi:10.1016/j.paid.2005.02.019
81. Koychev I, Mcmullen K, Lees J, Dadhiwala R, Grayson L, Perry C, et al. A validation of cognitive biomarkers for the early identification of cognitive enhancing agents in schizotypy: a three-center double-blind placebo-controlled study. *Eur Neuropsychopharmacol* (2012) **22**:469–81. doi:10.1016/j.euroneuro.2011.10.005
82. Thoma RJ, Monnig MA, Lysne PA, Ruhl DA, Pommy JA, Bogenschutz M, et al. Adolescent substance abuse: the effects of alcohol and marijuana on neuropsychological performance. *Alcohol Clin Exp Res* (2011) **35**:39–46. doi:10.1111/j.1530-0277.2010.01320.x
83. Solowij N, Stephens RS, Roffman RA, Babor T, Kadden R, Miller M, et al. Cognitive functioning of long-term heavy cannabis users seeking treatment. *JAMA* (2002) **287**:1123–31. doi:10.1001/jama.287.9.1123
84. Heinrichs RW. Meta-analysis and the science of schizophrenia: variant evidence or evidence of variants? *Neurosci Biobehav Rev* (2004) **28**:379–94. doi:10.1016/j.neubiorev.2004.06.003
85. Solowij N, Michie PT. Cannabis and cognitive dysfunction: Parallels with endophenotypes of schizophrenia? *J Psychiatry Neurosci* (2007) **32**:30–52.
86. Mesholam-Gately RI, Giuliano AJ, Goff KP, Faraone SV, Seidman LJ. Neurocognition in first-episode schizophrenia: a meta-analytic review. *Neuropsychology* (2009) **23**:315–36. doi:10.1037/a0014708

87. Sitskoorn MM, Aleman A, Ebisch SJH, Appels MCM, Kahn RS. Cognitive deficits in relatives of patients with schizophrenia: a meta-analysis. *Schizophr Res* (2004) **71**:285–95. doi:10.1016/j.schres.2004.03.007
88. Solowij N, Pesa N. Cannabis and cognition: Short- and long-term effects. In: Castle DJ, Murray RM, D'Souza CD, editors. *Marijuana and Madness.* (Vol. 2), Cambridge: Cambridge University Press (2012). p. 91–102.
89. Silverstein SM, Raulin ML, Pristach EA, Pomerantz JR. Perceptual organization and schizotypy. *J Abnorm Psychol* (1992) **101**:265–70. doi:10.1037/0021-843X.101.2.265
90. Cadenhead KS, Geyer MA, Braff DL. Impaired startle-prepulse inhibition and habituation in patients with schizotypal personality disorder. *Am J Psychiatry* (1993) **150**:1862–7.
91. Ettinger U, Kumari V, Crawford TJ, Corr PJ, Das M, Zachariah E, et al. Smooth pursuit and antisaccade eye movements in siblings discordant for schizophrenia. *J Psychiatr Res* (2004) **38**:177–84. doi:10.1016/S0022-3956(03)00105-5
92. Cappe C, Herzog MH, Herzig DA, Brand A, Mohr C. Cognitive disorganisation in schizotypy is associated with deterioration in visual backward masking. *Psychiatry Res* (2012) **200**:652–9. doi:10.1016/j.psychres.2012.07.001
93. Dinsdale NL, Hurd PL, Wakabayashi A, Elliot M, Crespi BJ. How are autism and schizotypy related? Evidence from a non-clinical population. *PLoS One* (2013) **8**:e63316. doi:10.1371/journal.pone.0063316
94. Schürhoff F, Laguerre A, Szöke A, Méary A, Leboyer M. Schizotypal dimensions: continuity between schizophrenia and bipolar disorders. *Schizophr Res* (2005) **80**:235–42. doi:10.1016/j.schres.2005.07.009
95. Claridge G, Blakey S. Schizotypy and affective temperament: relationships with divergent thinking and creativity styles. *Pers Individ Dif* (2009) **46**:820–6. doi:10.1016/j.paid.2009.01.015
96. Ho B-C, Wassink TH, Ziebell S, Andreasen NC. Cannabinoid receptor 1 gene polymorphisms and marijuana misuse interactions on white matter and cognitive deficits in schizophrenia. *Schizophr Res* (2011) **128**:66–75. doi:10.1016/j.schres.2011.02.021
97. Pope HG, Gruber AJ, Hudson JI, Cohane G, Huestis MA, Yurgelun-Todd D. Early-onset cannabis use and cognitive deficits: what is the nature of the association? *Drug Alcohol Depend* (2003) **69**:303–10. doi:10.1016/S0376-8716(02)00334-4
98. Bossong MG, Van Berckel BN, Boellaard R, Zuurman L, Schuit RC, Windhorst AD, et al. Delta 9-tetrahydrocannabinol induces dopamine release in the human striatum. *Neuropsychopharmacology* (2009) **34**:759–66. doi:10.1038/npp.2008.138
99. Kuepper R, Morrison PD, Van Os J, Murray RM, Kenis G, Henquet C. Does dopamine mediate the psychosis-inducing effects of cannabis? A review and integration of findings across disciplines. *Schizophr Res* (2010) **121**:107–17. doi:10.1016/j.schres.2010.05.031
100. Caspi A, Moffitt TE, Cannon M, Mcclay J, Murray R, Harrington H, et al. Moderation of the effect of adolescent-onset cannabis use on adult psychosis by a functional polymorphism in the catechol-O-methyltransferase gene: longitudinal evidence of a gene X environment interaction. *Biol Psychiatry* (2005) **57**:1117–27. doi:10.1016/j.biopsych.2005.01.026
101. Estrada G, Fatjo-Vilas M, Munoz MJ, Pulido G, Minano MJ, Toledo E, et al. Cannabis use and age at onset of psychosis: further evidence of interaction with COMT Val158Met polymorphism. *Acta Psychiatr Scand* (2011) **123**:485–92. doi:10.1111/j.1600-0447.2010.01665.x
102. Matheson S, Langdon R. Schizotypal traits impact upon executive working memory and aspects of IQ. *Psychiatry Res* (2008) **159**:207–14. doi:10.1016/j.psychres.2007.04.006
103. Leeson VC, Barnes TRE, Hutton SB, Ron MA, Joyce EM. IQ as a predictor of functional outcome in schizophrenia: a longitudinal, four-year study of first-episode psychosis. *Schizophr Res* (2009) **107**:55–60. doi:10.1016/j.schres.2008.08.014
104. Khandaker GM, Barnett JH, White IR, Jones PB. A quantitative meta-analysis of population-based studies of premorbid intelligence and schizophrenia. *Schizophr Res* (2011) **132**:220–7. doi:10.1016/j.schres.2011.06.017
105. Shelton N, Savell E. The geography of binge drinking: the role of alcohol-related knowledge, behaviours and attitudes. Results from the health survey for England 2007. *Health Place* (2011) **17**:784–92. doi:10.1016/j.healthplace.2011.02.004
106. Baggio S, Deline S, Studer J, Mohler-Kuo M, Daeppen J-B, Gmel G. Routes of administration of cannabis used for nonmedical purposes and associations with patterns of drug use. *J Adolesc Health* (2014) **54**:235–40. doi:10.1016/j.jadohealth.2013.08.013
107. Adler LE, Hoffer LD, Wiser A, Freedman R. Normalization of auditory physiology by cigarette smoking in schizophrenic patients. *Am J Psychiatry* (1993) **150**:1856–61.
108. Zabala A, Eguiluz JI, Segarra R, Enjuto S, Ezcurra J, Pinto AG, et al. Cognitive performance and cigarette smoking in first-episode psychosis. *Eur Arch Psychiatry Clin Neurosci* (2009) **259**:65–71. doi:10.1007/s00406-008-0835-6
109. Heishman SJ, Kleykamp B, Singleton E. Meta-analysis of the acute effects of nicotine and smoking on human performance. *Psychopharmacology* (2010) **210**:453–69. doi:10.1007/s00213-010-1848-1
110. Kaushanskaya M, Marian V, Yoo J. Gender differences in adult word learning. *Acta Psychol* (2011) **137**:24–35. doi:10.1016/j.actpsy.2011.02.002
111. Green SB. How many subjects does it take to do a regression analysis. *Multivariate Behav Res* (1991) **26**:499–510. doi:10.1207/s15327906mbr2603_7
112. Tabachnik BG, Fidell LS. *Using Multivariate Statistics.* Needham, MA: Allyn and Bacon (2001).
113. Field AP. *Discovering Statistics Using SPSS.* London: Sage (2009).
114. Harris RJ. *A Primer of Multivariate Statistics.* New York, NY: Academic Press (1985).
115. Perez-Reyes M, Hicks RE, Bumberry J, Robert Jeffcoat A, Cook CE. Interaction between marihuana and ethanol: effects on psychomotor performance. *Alcohol Clin Exp Res* (1988) **12**:268–76. doi:10.1111/j.1530-0277.1988.tb00193.x
116. Ronen A, Chassidim HS, Gershon P, Parmet Y, Rabinovich A, Bar-Hamburger R, et al. The effect of alcohol, THC and their combination on perceived effects, willingness to drive and performance of driving and non-driving tasks. *Accid Anal Prev* (2010) **42**:1855–65. doi:10.1016/j.aap.2010.05.006
117. Ramaekers J, Theunissen E, De Brouwer M, Toennes S, Moeller M, Kauert G. Tolerance and cross-tolerance to neurocognitive effects of THC and alcohol in heavy cannabis users. *Psychopharmacology* (2011) **214**:391–401. doi:10.1007/s00213-010-2042-1
118. Block RI, Ghoneim MM. Effects of chronic marijuana use on human cognition. *Psychopharmacology* (1993) **110**:219–28. doi:10.1007/BF02246977
119. Bolla KI, Brown K, Eldreth D, Tate K, Cadet JL. Dose-related neurocognitive effects of marijuana use. *Neurology* (2002) **59**:1337–43. doi:10.1212/01.WNL.0000031422.66442.49

19

Neurophysiological correlates of configural face processing in schizotypy

Rachel A. Batty[1,2]*, Andrew J. P. Francis[2], Hamish Innes-Brown[3], Nicole R. Joshua[4] and Susan L. Rossell[1,5,6]

[1] Brain and Psychological Sciences Research Centre (BPsyC), Faculty of Health, Arts and Design, Swinburne University of Technology, Melbourne, VIC, Australia
[2] School of Health Science, Psychology, RMIT University, Bundoora, VIC, Australia
[3] The Bionics Institute, Melbourne, VIC, Australia
[4] Pearson Clinical Assessment, Melbourne, VIC, Australia
[5] Cognitive Neuropsychiatry Laboratory, Monash-Alfred Psychiatry Research Centre (MAPrc), The Alfred Hospital and Central Clinical School Monash University, Melbourne, VIC, Australia
[6] Psychiatry, St. Vincents Hospital, Melbourne, VIC, Australia

Edited by:
Caroline Gurvich, Monash University, Australia

Reviewed by:
Caroline Gurvich, Monash University, Australia
Giorgio Fuggetta, University of Leicester, UK

***Correspondence:**
Rachel A. Batty, Neuroimaging Facility, Brain and Psychological Sciences Research Centre, Faculty of Health, Arts, and Design, P.O. Box 218, Hawthorn, VIC 3122, Australia
e-mail: rachel.ann.batty@gmail.com

Background: Face processing impairment in schizophrenia appears to be underpinned by poor configural (as opposed to feature-based) processing; however, few studies have sought to characterize this impairment electrophysiologically. Given the sensitivity of event-related potentials to antipsychotic medications, and the potential for neurophysiological abnormalities to serve as vulnerability markers for schizophrenia, a handful of studies have investigated early visual P100 and face-selective N170 in "at risk" populations. However, this is the first known neurophysiological investigation of configural face processing in a non-clinical schizotypal sample.

Methods: Using stimuli designed to engage configural processing in face perception (upright and inverted Mooney and photographic faces), P100 and N170 components were recorded in healthy individuals characterized by high ($N = 14$) and low ($N = 14$) schizotypal traits according to the Oxford–Liverpool Inventory of Feelings and Experiences.

Results: High schizotypes showed significantly reduced N170 amplitudes to inverted photographic faces. Typical N170 latency and amplitude inversion effects (delayed and enhanced N170 to inverted relative to upright photographic faces, and enhanced amplitude to upright versus inverted Mooney faces), were demonstrated by low, but not high, schizotypes. No group differences were shown for P100 analyses.

Conclusions: The findings suggest that neurophysiological deficits in processing facial configurations (N170) are apparent in schizotypy, while the early sensory processing (P100) of faces appears intact. This work adds to the mounting evidence for analogous neural processing anomalies at the healthy end of the psychosis continuum.

Keywords: schizotypy, configural processing, face processing, N170, P100

INTRODUCTION

Given the social cognitive anomalies characteristic of schizophrenia, emotion processing has received substantial research attention (1–6). Overwhelmingly, significant impairments in emotion perception are reported (7), and these appear present and stable from pre-onset to chronic multi-episode patients (2). A more recent line of inquiry has suggested that deficient facial emotion processing in schizophrenia may be underpinned by basic visuoperceptual deficits (8, 9), although electrophysiological evidence of this is not always demonstrated. Studies using neutral face stimuli have verified a primary deficit in the processing of configural information (described below), with a relative overreliance on facial feature processing by patients with schizophrenia (10, 11), and in ultra-high risk individuals (12). This appears to extend to non-face processing as well (11, 13), supporting a generalized bias for local relative to global perceptual processing.

In the context of face perception, configural processing refers to (i) the basic detection of the face formation (i.e., eyes above nose above mouth; first-order relations), (ii) the uniting of these as a gestalt or whole image (holistic processing), and (iii) an assessment of the spatial relationships between facial features, thought to underlie identity processing (second-order relations) [see Ref. (14, 15)]. The disruption of configural processing when a face is inverted produces the "face-inversion effect" (FIE) (16): upside-down faces are more difficult to perceive, discriminate, and recognize, demonstrated by a decrease in accuracy and increase in reaction times (RT) compared with upright faces, first reported by Yin (17). The FIE has been researched extensively [e.g., Ref. (14, 16, 18, 19)], and in schizophrenia the effect is often absent, aligned with evidence for a configural processing deficit (20–22), however, see Ref. (23) for evidence of the FIE in patients).

The different stages of face processing are reflected by the P100 and N170 event-related potentials (ERPs). The P100 component is an occipitally distributed positive deflection, with a typical peak latency between 80 and 120 ms, and is associated with early stages of visual information processing (24, 25). The N170 component is maximal over the ventral occipitotemporal cortex with a peak latency between 140 and 200 ms post stimulus onset. N170 amplitude is consistently larger for faces compared to other objects, and for this reason has been considered "face-selective" (26–28). Various attempts have been made to define N170 face-specificity further, for instance, in response to eyes only (26, 29, 30), facial emotion (31–34), and identity encoding (28). One group has even argued controversially against N170 face selectivity (35), however, most evidence points toward an index of face-specific early cortical processing (36–41).

The N170 is also modulated by configural face processing, with effects reported in response to whole faces, but not half faces (42), schematic faces that provide spatial face configuration but no distinguishable featural face information (i.e., first-order configural information) (14, 43) and two-tone Mooney faces (44) that rely on holistic processing (global gestalt) to be perceived (14, 45, 46). Reliable modulation of the N170 component is also demonstrated by the FIE: upside-down faces consistently elicit a delayed latency and enhanced amplitude over usual N170 occipitotemporal electrodes, relative to upright faces (14, 26, 43, 47). This is generally regarded as further evidence of N170 sensitivity to configural face information. Although the N170 effects in response to the inversion of schematic and Mooney faces are less consistent, a delayed and reduced N170 to upside-down schematic faces (14, 48), and reduced N170 amplitude to upside-down Mooney faces (45, 46) have been shown.

Reductions in P100 amplitude to various visual stimuli have been demonstrated in patients with schizophrenia (49–51) as well as in unaffected first-degree relatives (52), those with an "at risk" mental state (53), in schizotypy (54), and in non-pathological healthy individuals prone to visual hallucinations (55). This suggests an association between schizophrenia and impoverished visual input, and is supported by existing patient deficits in attention (56–58), as well as visual scan paths characterized by fewer visual fixations, longer duration of fixations/saccades, and smaller saccade amplitudes (21, 59, 60). However, P100 deficits have not always been reported in patient studies (13, 61–64), or in schizotypy (25). It is also noteworthy that P100 effects have typically been recorded in response to basic visual stimuli (i.e., isolated gray/white check images and line drawings) (50–52, 65, 66), with only a handful of studies demonstrating P100 deficits to (emotional) face stimuli in patients (49, 67), and in those at risk for psychosis (53). Last, antipsychotic agents have known effects on neural activation (68, 69). An increase in P100 latency during visual discrimination has previously been shown following an acute dose of bromazepam (70).

In contrast, N170 studies in schizophrenia, although few, have consistently demonstrated reduced N170 amplitude (34, 49, 63, 67, 71), and delayed N170 latency (49) relative to healthy samples. However, N170 amplitude reductions have only been shown in an at-risk population by one study (53), with no evidence for N170 effects reported in first-degree relatives (34), and in individuals prone to visual hallucinations (55). This is surprising given the hereditary nature and spectrum account of psychosis. Shared neurocognitive deficits are commonplace in healthy yet prone individuals (72–76), and the potential for neural markers to serve as endophenotypes in schizophrenia has been established [e.g., Ref. (77, 78)]. Thus, further evidence is necessary to determine whether face processing deficits illustrated neurophysiologically at N170 in patients are shared by individuals prone to psychosis.

Moreover, with rare exception [i.e., Ref. (55, 79)], the N170 literature has notably used emotional face stimuli (34, 49, 53, 63, 67, 71, 80). Thus, more evidence for the ERP correlates of configural face processing, without the potentially confounding positive and negative valence information, is also necessary. Given the established effect of pharmacological agents on neural activation (68–70), individuals prone to psychosis, and medication naïve, provide an ideal method of investigating analogous neural processing deficits (73, 74, 81–85), without concern for medication, and other potential confounds introduced by clinical samples (i.e., long-term hospitalization, social isolation) (82, 86). With this in mind, schizotypy provides a valuable model of investigation. To our knowledge, the N170 response in schizotypy has not yet been reported.

This study aimed to expand on existing literature by avoiding emotionally laden stimuli and clinical confounds while recording neural markers of face processing. Using stimuli designed to engage configural processing in face perception (upright and inverted Mooney and photographic faces), we sought to determine the ERP correlates (P100, N170 components) of configural face processing in schizotypy. We expected that, in high schizotypes, reduced P100 amplitudes would indicate impoverished visuosensory input, whereas reduced N170 amplitudes would indicate impaired face processing. Anomalous ERP responses to (i) Mooney faces, and (ii) inverted stimuli of both types, would provide evidence of configurally specific face processing deficits.

MATERIALS AND METHODS

PARTICIPANTS

Thirty participants (15 male), between ages 18 and 55 years were recruited from RMIT University, Melbourne and the Mental Health Research Institute (MHRI) participant database. Two (1 male) were excluded from the N170 analyses due to (i) inadequate accepted trials (inverted Mooney stimuli), and (ii) a corrupted data file ($M = 27.24$ years, SD = 7.48, 14 male). A third was removed from the P100 analyses due to poor quality recording on principal electrode OZ ($M = 27.20$ years, SD = 7.62, 14 male). All had normal or corrected to normal visual acuity, IQ within the average range [National Adult Reading Test IQ; NART; (87)], no concurrent alcohol or substance abuse, and no personal or family history of psychopathology (self-report).

Schizotypal personality

The Oxford–Liverpool Inventory of Feelings and Experiences [O-LIFE; (88)] was completed as a measure of psychosis-proneness for each participant. The O-LIFE is a 159 yes/no item self-report questionnaire, which measures four distinct schizotypy

Table 1 | Demographic characteristics of high and low schizotypy.

	Mean (Standard Deviation)			
	P100		**N170**	
	Low schizotypy ($n = 13$)	**High schizotypy ($n = 14$)**	**Low schizotypy ($n = 14$)**	**High schizotypy ($n = 14$)**
Age	30.16 (9.69)	24.45 (3.54)*	30.03 (9.32)	24.46 (3.54)*
Gender (M/F)	6/7	8/6	6/8	8/6
NART IQ	108.15 (8.65)	104.29 (8.11)#	108.43 (8.37)	104.29 (8.11)†
O-LIFE scales				
Unusual experiences	4.46 (5.36)	7.64 (5.89)	4.14 (5.29)	7.64 (5.89)
Cognitive disorganization	**4.46 (2.30)**	**12.57 (4.27)*** **	**4.21 (2.39)**	**12.57 (4.27)*** **
Introvertive anhedonia	2.00 (1.29)	5.43 (3.03)***	1.93 (1.27)	5.43 (3.03)***
Impulsive non-conformity	6.31 (2.94)	9.36 (3.30)*	6.14 (2.88)	9.36 (3.30)**

O-LIFE; Oxford–Liverpool Inventory of Feelings and Experiences (88). High and low schizotypy was defined by the Cognitive Disorganization dimension (M[SD] values in bold font).

The significant age difference reflects an outlier (n = 1) in the low schizotypy group (results did not change when this outlier was removed).

****$p < 0.001$; **$p < 0.01$; *$p < 0.05$.*

#$p = 0.24$ †$p = 0.20$.

dimensions with high internal consistency: unusual experiences ($\alpha = 0.89$), cognitive disorganization ($\alpha = 0.87$), introvertive anhedonia ($\alpha = 0.82$), and impulsive non-conformity ($\alpha = 0.77$) (89). A median split of the O-LIFE Cognitive Disorganization dimension defined high/low schizotypy groups. Cognitive Disorganization includes deficits in attention, concentration, decision making, and social anxiety, and the scale was deemed most appropriate because it assesses traits that reflect these cognitive deficits as well as the positive symptoms of psychosis (88, 90)[1]. Moreover, self-face recognition failures correlate with cognitive perceptual/disorganized schizotypy dimensions (90). Groups were matched on NART IQ (see **Table 1**).

FACE RECOGNITION TASKS

Two computerized tasks (20 min duration) were completed during electroencephalographic (EEG) recording. These were counterbalanced, and stimulus order was randomized for each participant. A short break was given after each 10 min block. Task One stimuli were a series of 40 original Mooney faces (44). These were digitally manipulated and repeated to create four separate conditions: *upright face, inverted face, upright disorganized face,* and *inverted disorganized face*[2]. A total of 640 stimuli were presented, with 160 per condition. Twelve[3] neutral grayscale photographic faces were used as Task Two stimuli [Ekman and Friesen series, (91)]. The same four conditions as in Task One were created, with a total of 576 stimuli presented (144 per condition).

All participants were shown a printed example of each condition type prior to the task. They fixated on central fixation cross with a random duration from between 800 and 1200 ms between stimuli, and were shown the images for 200 ms (stimuli were thus on screen for the duration of the critical time period for both P100 and N170). Using a two-button control, participants indicated when they saw either an intact (left button) or disorganized (right button) face. Accuracy and RTs were recorded. These data were submitted to repeated measures analysis of variance (ANOVA) with task (Mooney and photographic faces) and orientation (upright and inverted) as within-subjects factors, and schizotypy (high and low) as the between subjects factor.

ELECTROPHYSIOLOGICAL ACQUISITION AND DATA PROCESSING

Electroencephalographic activity was recorded continuously from 64 scalp sites (10/20 International system, *Neuroscan 4.2*, amplified using *SynAmps2* system). Recording sites included eight midline electrodes (FPZ, FZ, FCZ, CZ, CPZ, PZ, POZ, OZ), 28 electrodes over each hemisphere (FP1/FP2, AF3/AF4, AF7/AF8, F1/F2, F3/F4, F5/F6, F7/F8, FC1/FC2, FC3/FC4, FC5/FC6, FT7/FT8, C1/C2, C3/C4, C5/C6, T7/T8, CP1/CP2, CP3/CP4, CP5/CP6, TP7/TP8, P1/P2, P3/P4, P5/P6, P7/P8, PO3/PO4, PO5/PO6, PO7/PO8, O1/O2, CB1/CB2), and the left and right mastoids. A nose reference was used during acquisition and an average reference montage was calculated offline. The midline electrode between FPZ and FZ served as the ground. Electrooculogram (EOG) was measured at FP1.

Signals were amplified 20,000× and digitized at a sampling rate of 1000 Hz with a band-pass filter of 0.1–100 Hz (24 dB/octave; zero phase shift). Digital codes were sent from the stimulus-presentation computer, and response button-press, to mark the onset and type of each stimulus, and the participant response, respectively. Movement-contaminated EEG sections were discarded, and continuous data files were corrected for eye-blinks and divided into epochs from 100 ms pre-stimulus to 500 ms post-stimulus. Following baseline correction, epochs with artifacts that exceeded ±100 μV were rejected. Only trials with the correct

[1]The remaining three dimensions reflect positive and negative, but not cognitive, symptoms.

[2]The disorganized stimuli were included to provide a task and are not relevant to analyses.

[3]Tasks one and two had an imbalance of original stimuli due to the availability of images from the Ekman and Friesen series (91). The total number presented per condition was matched as closely as possible.

Table 2 | Mean (SD) accepted trials per condition.

	Mooney		Photographic	
	Upright	**Inverted**	**Upright**	**Inverted**
P100 analyses				
Low schizotypy	122.85	73.08	109.46	109.38
	(60.40)	(44.78)	(59.26)	(53.64)
High schizotypy	131.93	80.43	137.86	106.07
	(65.81)	(48.95)	(70.97)	(28.58)
N170 analyses				
Low schizotypy	123.21	75.07	110.64	106.57
	(58.04)	(43.70)	(57.11)	(52.60)
High schizotypy	131.93	80.43	137.86	106.07
	(65.81)	(48.95)	(70.97)	(28.58)

Reduced accepted trials for P100 analyses reflects the removal of a dataset (n = 1) due to poor quality recording on principal electrode OZ.

behavioral responses ($N > 20$ p/condition)[4] were included and filtered at 0.5–35 Hz (24 dB/octave; zero phase shift) (**Table 2**). ERPs were created by averaging together stimuli of the same condition subtype.

DATA ANALYSIS

Component P100 was measured as the maximal positive deflection between 80 and 120 ms (25) at electrodes O1, OZ, and O2 [established optimal occipital scalp sites; (25, 51, 53, 67, 70)]. Peak latencies and amplitudes from baseline were submitted to repeated measures ANOVA, with task (Mooney and photographic faces) and orientation (upright and inverted) as within-subjects factors. The N170 was measured as the maximal negative deflection between 140 and 200 ms (14, 28, 45) at PO7 and PO8 (41, 48). Peak N170 latencies and amplitudes from baseline were submitted to repeated measures ANOVA, with task (Mooney and photographic faces), orientation (upright and inverted), and hemisphere (left and right) as within-subjects factors. High and low schizotypy served as the between subject factor for all analyses. The Greenhouse–Geisser epsilon correction factor was applied to account for possible effects of non-sphericity where appropriate. To further investigate amplitude differences at N170, independent sample *t*-tests were run using the mean amplitude across PO7/PO8 components. Relationships between ERP data and O-LIFE scores were investigated by Spearman's correlation coefficients.

RESULTS

BEHAVIORAL DATA

An adequate number of trials remained for all but one participant. Two others had accepted trials in the 20s, and the remainder had >37 (**Table 2**). The accuracy and RT data are presented in **Table 3**. Participants correctly identified a greater number of photographic than Mooney faces; $F(1,26) = 146.77$, $p < 0.001$, $\eta_p^2 = 0.85$ and a greater number of upright than inverted faces; $F(1,26) = 147.77$, $p < 0.001$, $\eta_p^2 = 0.85$. A task × orientation interaction reflected a large decline in accuracy for the inverted Mooney faces, not shown to the inverted photographic faces; $F(1,26) = 124.47$, $p < 0.001$, $\eta_p^2 = 0.85$. These findings were mirrored by RTs: participants responded faster to photographic than Mooney faces; $F(1,26) = 62.68$, $p < 0.001$, $\eta_p^2 = 0.85$ and faster to upright than inverted faces; $F(1,26) = 197.99$, $p < 0.001$, $\eta_p^2 = 0.85$. A task × orientation interaction once again reflected much slower responses to inverted Mooney faces; $F(1,26) = 24.94$, $p < 0.001$, $\eta_p^2 = 0.85$. Neither accuracy nor RT differentiated the schizotypy groups: accuracy, task $p = 0.33$, orientation $p = 0.64$; and RTs, task $p = 0.76$, orientation $p = 0.58$ (**Table 3**).

Table 3 | Mean (SD) accuracy and reaction times per condition.

	Mooney		Photographic	
	Upright	**Inverted**	**Upright**	**Inverted**
% correct				
Low schizotypy	87.2	53.9	96.9	94.7
	(4.7)	(17.7)	(2.8)	(6.0)
High schizotypy	83.8	48.3	97.2	94.4
	(12.6)	(18.9)	(2.6)	(4.7)
RTs (ms)				
Low schizotypy	696.1	809.8	638.2	687.2
	(99.7)	(128.9)	(91.4)	(106.9)
High schizotypy	690.4	791.1	632.5	681.9
	(56.5)	(97.0)	(58.7)	(49.7)

EVENT-RELATED POTENTIALS

P100

Mean (SD) amplitudes and latencies are presented in **Table 4**, and grand-averaged waveforms are illustrated in **Figure 1**. P100 latency was increased for inverted relative to upright faces at electrode O1; $F(1,25) = 6.22$, $p = 0.02$, $\eta_p^2 = 0.85$. Larger amplitudes were shown to photographic than Mooney faces at all three occipital sites: (i) O1; $F(1,25) = 10.20$, $p = 0.004$, $\eta_p^2 = 0.85$ (ii) OZ; $F(1,25) = 10.81$, $p = 0.003$, $\eta_p^2 = 0.85$ (iii) O2; $F(1,25) = 8.68$, $p = 0.007$, $\eta_p^2 = 0.85$. Greater amplitude to inverted versus upright faces was shown at electrode O2 only; $F(1,25) = 14.74$, $p = 0.001$, $\eta_p^2 = 0.85$ (trend level at OZ, $p = 0.06$). No differences between schizotypal groups were shown for P100 latency: (i) O1; $p = 0.85$, (ii) OZ; $p = 0.54$, (iii) O2; $p = 0.61$, or P100 amplitude: (i) O1; $p = 0.19$, (ii) OZ; $p = 0.63$, (iii) O2; $p = 0.35$. No other significant P100 effects were shown.

N170

Latency. Mean (SD) amplitude and latency to upright and inverted stimuli for both tasks are shown in **Table 5**, and N170 waveforms at P07/08 are shown in **Figure 2**. Earlier N170 latencies were shown to photographic ($M = 154.72$ ms, SD = 10.06), than to Mooney ($M = 174.63$ ms, SD = 10.33) faces: $F(1,26) = 79.52$, $p < 0.001$, $\eta_p^2 = 0.85$ and to upright ($M = 163.02$ ms, SD = 8.68) than inverted ($M = 166.33$ ms, SD = 8.61) faces: $F(1,26) = 18.67$,

[4] Due to the difficulty of perceiving a Mooney face in the inverted position, 20 trials were considered a reasonable cut-off.

Table 4 | P100 Mean (SD) amplitude and latency per condition and electrode.

	Mooney						Photographic					
	Upright			Inverted			Upright			Inverted		
	O1	OZ	O2	O1	OZ	O2	O1	OZ	O2	O1	OZ	O2
Latency (ms)												
Low schizotypy	103.08	98.62	102.38	106.38	97.23	101.00	102.08	100.23	101.85	105.92	97.38	102.92
	(11.28)	(6.61)	(11.36)	(12.43)	(8.08)	(12.39)	(9.10)	(9.86)	(8.74)	(7.57)	(9.28)	(7.94)
High schizotypy	107.21	94.29	104.93	108.79	97.00	106.43	100.50	101.07	101.43	102.93	95.50	101.21
	(9.70)	(7.15)	(11.50)	(9.56)	(8.27)	(10.77)	(8.22)	(8.90)	(7.60)	(9.44)	(8.21)	(6.34)
Amplitude (μV)												
Low schizotypy	6.75	2.59	5.31	6.84	2.46	6.50	8.62	3.75	7.91	8.56	4.90	8.31
	(3.72)	(2.70)	(2.19)	(2.95)	(2.45)	(3.33)	(3.56)	(3.19)	(3.04)	(4.23)	(3.72)	(2.99)
High schizotypy	5.66	2.61	5.24	5.84	2.61	6.36	6.26	2.80	6.03	6.67	3.90	6.73
	(2.79)	(2.53)	(2.41)	(2.79)	(2.31)	(3.48)	(3.21)	(2.64)	(2.72)	(3.34)	(2.42)	(3.16)

Low schizotypy (n = 13), high schizotypy (n = 14).

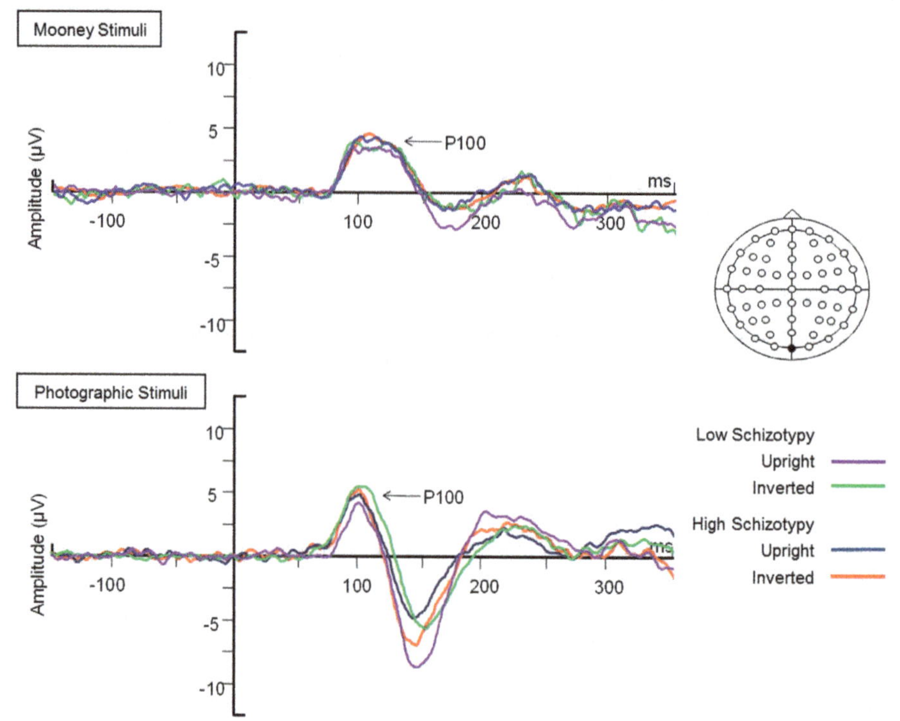

FIGURE 1 | Grand-averaged P100 waveforms at electrode OZ. Upright and inverted stimuli presentations across groups are compared for both tasks. A bird's eye view of the electrode montage is shown with the plotted electrode shaded black. Negative polarity is plotted downward.

$p < 0.001$, $\eta_p^2 = 0.85$. A task × orientation interaction demonstrated similar latencies to upright and inverted Mooney faces, whereas upright photographic faces were marked by earlier latencies relative to inverted photographic faces: $F(1,26) = 8.83$, $p = 0.006$, $\eta_p^2 = 0.85$ (see **Table 5**). The left hemisphere showed earlier latencies ($M = 162.54$ ms, SD = 9.54), than the right ($M = 163.50$ ms, SD = 9.09) to upright faces, whereas this effect was reversed for inverted faces where earlier latencies were shown in the right hemisphere ($M = 165.20$ ms, SD = 9.38) versus left ($M = 167.46$ ms, SD = 9.36): orientation × hemisphere interaction, $F(1,26) = 4.69$, $p = 0.04$, $\eta_p^2 = 0.85$. While there was no main effect for schizotypy group ($p = 0.63$), a group × orientation interaction was shown. The low schizotypy group had earlier latencies for upright relative to inverted faces; however,

Table 5 | N170 Mean (SD) amplitude and latency per condition and electrode.

	Mooney				Photographic			
	Upright		Inverted		Upright		Inverted	
	PO7	PO8	PO7	PO8	PO7	PO8	PO7	PO8
Latency (ms)								
Low schizotypy	173.57	174.64	179.86	177.14	151.79	150.79	158.64	157.29
	(12.07)	(9.83)	(11.27)	(13.33)	(7.91)	(10.37)	(9.13)	(11.50)
High schizotypy	173.79	176.29	173.29	168.43	151.00	152.29	158.07	157.93
	(11.90)	(14.13)	(13.50)	(10.79)	(15.37)	(15.33)	(11.68)	(9.96)
Amplitude (μV)								
Low schizotypy	−6.13	−6.78	−5.25	−5.25	−8.10	−8.79	−11.21	−12.89
	(3.81)	(3.61)	(4.13)	(4.46)	(4.91)	(3.77)	(3.98)	(4.12)
High schizotypy	−3.98	−4.08	−3.96	−4.07	−6.55	−7.57	−8.02	−9.55
	(3.34)	(3.69)	(2.36)	(2.85)	(4.46)	(6.19)	(4.56)	(6.01)

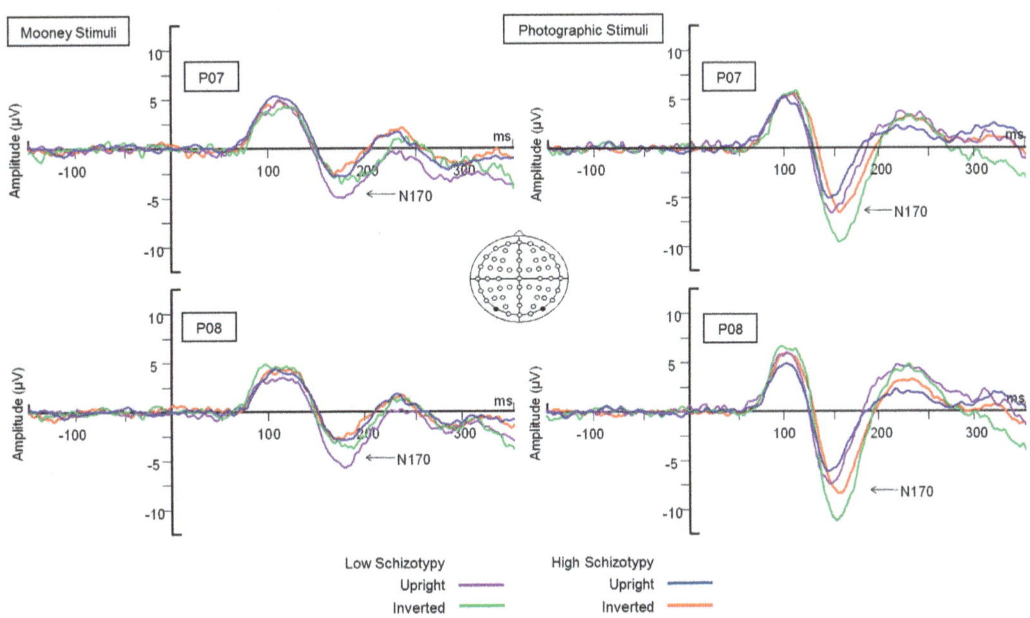

FIGURE 2 | Grand-averaged N170 waveforms at electrodes PO7 and PO8. Upright and inverted stimuli presentations across groups are compared for both tasks. A bird's eye view of the electrode montage is shown with the plotted electrodes shaded black. Negative polarity is plotted downward.

the high schizotypy group had comparable latencies across orientations: $F(1,26) = 8.41$, $p = 0.007$, $\eta_p^2 = 0.85$ (see **Table 5**; **Figure 3**). A task × orientation × group interaction was at trend level ($p = 0.067$).

Amplitude. Greater N170 amplitude was shown to photographic ($M = -9.08\,\mu V$, $SD = 4.34$) than to Mooney ($M = -4.94\,\mu V$, $SD = 3.36$) faces: $F(1,26) = 46.18$, $p < 0.001$, $\eta_p^2 = 0.85$ and to inverted ($M = -7.53\,\mu V$, $SD = 3.48$) relative to upright ($M = -6.50\,\mu V$, $SD = 3.71$) faces: $F(1,26) = 18.23$, $p < 0.001$, $\eta_p^2 = 0.85$. A task × orientation interaction also demonstrated that N170 amplitudes were greater for upright Mooney faces (relative to inverted), however, amplitudes were greater for inverted photographic faces (relative to upright): $F(1,26) = 22.15$, $p < 0.001$, $\eta_p^2 = 0.85$ (see **Table 5**). Furthermore, amplitudes were comparable across hemisphere for Mooney faces in both orientations, but greater in the right hemisphere for photographic faces, especially in the inverted orientation: task × orientation × hemisphere interaction, $F(1,26) = 4.70$, $p = 0.04$, $\eta_p^2 = 0.85$ (see **Table 5**). Again, while there was no main effect for schizotypal group ($p = 0.12$), a group × task × orientation interaction was shown: $F(1,26) = 4.87$, $p = 0.04$, $\eta_p^2 = 0.85$. The low schizotypy group demonstrated increased amplitude to upright versus inverted Mooney faces and substantially increased amplitude to inverted versus upright photographs. However, the high schizotypy group

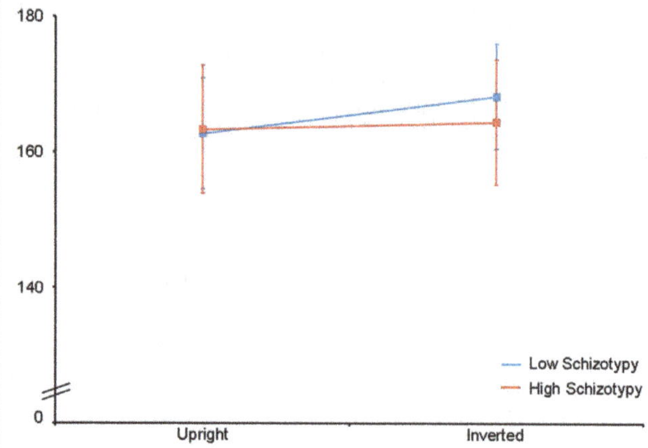

FIGURE 3 | N170 latency group x orientation interaction effect. Comparable peak latencies are shown to upright stimuli by both groups, however, high schizotypes show earlier peak latencies to inverted face stimuli (most difficult to perceive).

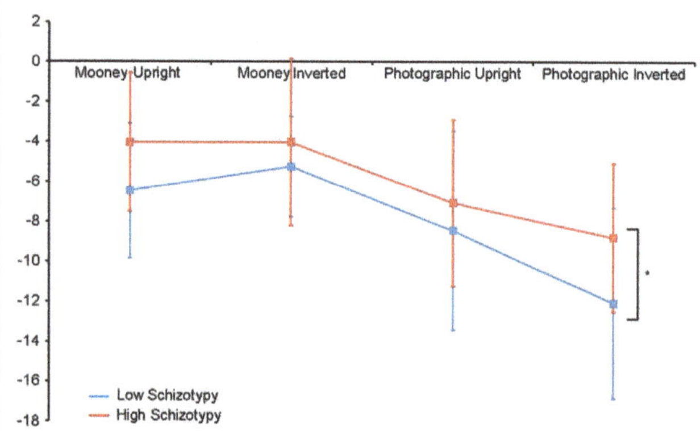

FIGURE 4 | N170 amplitude group x task x orientation interaction effect. Both high and low schizotypes showed the typical inversion effect to photographic stimuli: larger N170 amplitude to inverted versus upright photographic faces (although this difference is smaller for the high schizotypes). However, only low schizotypes showed an inversion effect to Mooney faces (reversed: smaller amplitudes to inverted compared with upright Mooney faces). High schizotypes instead showed comparable amplitude to Mooney faces irrespective of orientation. Note the overall trend for reduced amplitudes in high schizotypy. $^*p=0.05$.

demonstrated comparable amplitude to Moony faces in both orientations, and only marginally increased amplitude to inverted versus upright photographs (**Table 5**; **Figure 4**). *Post hoc* analyses using independent sample t-tests were run on the accumulated N170 mean amplitude [i.e., (PO7 + PO8)/2] for Mooney upright, Mooney inverted, photographic upright, and photographic inverted, separately. The high schizotypy group showed significantly reduced N170 amplitudes for inverted photographic faces only; $t(26) - 2.02$, $p = 0.05$, $d = 0.77$ (Mooney upright, $p = 0.07$, Mooney inverted, $p = 0.35$, and photographic upright, $p = 0.43$).

ERP CORRELATIONS WITH O-LIFE SCORES

Oxford–Liverpool Inventory of Feelings and Experiences scores from the entire sample ($n = 28$) were negatively correlated with the latency of the N170 for inverted Mooney faces, where higher scores (i.e., greater schizotypy) was associated with earlier peak latency for the inverted Mooney faces ($r = -0.38$, $p = 0.05$). No other correlations were significant.

DISCUSSION

N170 latency and amplitude main effects reflected the established literature (14, 45, 46), that is, earlier N170 latencies were demonstrated to photographic (relative to Mooney) and upright (relative to inverted) faces. This typically indicates the more efficient information processing of stimulus categories that are easier to perceive (i.e., photographic and upright faces). N170 amplitude was also larger to both photographic (relative to Mooney) and inverted (relative to upright) faces. The interaction effect clarified that peak amplitudes were greater for upright compared with upside-down Mooney faces, whereas the opposite was true for photographs: these showed the classic inversion effect of larger amplitude to upside-down compared with upright photographic faces. These amplitude effects are discussed in detail with respect to the schizotypal group differences [for more information, see (14, 45)].

Our data demonstrate that individuals high in schizotypal traits show significantly reduced N170 amplitudes to inverted photographic faces. This finding is consistent with the limited N170 literature in schizophrenia (34, 49, 63, 67, 71), and in at-risk individuals (53) where emotional face stimuli has been used. A similar, though non-significant, pattern of reduced N170 amplitude was demonstrated for the remaining three face categories (upright photographic, and upright and inverted Mooney). It is unclear why these categories did not reach significance. In a study using comparable stimuli to ours, Schwartzman et al. (55) also reported no N170 amplitude differences between individuals with high and low proneness to visual hallucinations. However, as the authors suggest, this is probably because deficits in hallucination-prone individuals are more likely to be visuo-sensory specific (as was reflected by P100 differences in their sample), and less likely to be face-specific. In schizotypy, however, neurocognitive deficits in attention, perception, social anxiety, and cognitive disorganization are shared with patients, making them more liable to face-specific deficits (88, 90). Neural processing anomalies shared by healthy individuals prone to psychosis, which are likely to be reduced in degree, may only be detected where effects are especially robust. In our study, this was demonstrated to inverted photographic faces, which are renowned for eliciting a strong amplitude response (14, 26, 43, 47).

Individuals low in schizotypal traits demonstrated the classic increase in amplitude to inverted relative to upright photographs, and an increase in amplitude to *upright* relative to inverted Mooney faces. This latter amplitude effect to Mooney faces has been shown previously, especially on trials where stimuli are recognized as a face (45, 46), which was also the case here. It has been proposed that upright photographic faces engage all three stages of configural processing; first-, holistic, and second-order (14). However, when upside-down, configural processing is disrupted and these faces are processed analytically (i.e., a part by part process using their featural information), which explains the reliably demonstrated increase in N170 amplitude in response to inversion (45). Similarly, Mooney faces containing configural (holistic/gestalt) information are only processed holistically when presented upright, accounting for a smaller N170 amplitude when compared to upright photographs. Upon inversion, however, featural information is unavailable in the Mooney face, and so analytic processing is not engaged. The subsequent difficulty of processing Mooney faces holistically when upside-down is demonstrated by the reduction in N170 amplitude (45). These typical N170 effects were expected from individuals low in schizotypal traits, and are further reflected by their earlier N170 peak latencies to upright compared with inverted faces, indicating faster face processing to upright faces.

By contrast, the high schizotypes in our study demonstrated comparable N170 amplitude to Mooney faces in both orientations, only marginally increased amplitude to inverted versus upright photographs, and comparable peak latencies across orientations to both face types. Face processing for the high schizotypes was thereby significantly less affected by orientation. Thus, this group was less affected by the disruption to configural information processing in inversion, supporting the established generalized bias for local as opposed to global perceptual processing in schizophrenia (10, 11, 13), and in psychosis prone individuals (12). This is further suggested by the relationship shown between N170 latency and O-LIFE scores for inverted Mooney faces, which indicated that the speed of information processing (latency) increased as schizotypal traits increased. Inverted Mooney faces are the most difficult stimulus category to perceive because configural information is disrupted but alternate featural processing cannot be engaged. The fact that schizotypal traits are associated with faster processing of these stimuli demonstrate further that face processing in high schizotypes is less reliant on configural processing. The generalized poor recruitment of configural information processes may further explain the overall trend for reduced N170 amplitude in this group. However, their neural response to the photographic stimuli suggests that while high schizotypes may have a bias for featural/local processing, they may not be expert in this method of processing either. If this were the case, expertise in part by part analytic processing should be shown electrophysiologically in this group in response to photographic faces. According to the existing literature, a typical, but enhanced, spike in N170 peak amplitude would be expected, and would likely exceed that of the low schizotypes in both orientations. Instead, high schizotypes showed the opposite of this: generally (though non-significantly) reduced amplitude to upright photographs and significantly reduced amplitude in response to photographic faces presented upside-down.

The P100 component is sensitive to changes in luminance and contrast (96). Thus, larger P100 amplitudes to photographic faces in our study reflects added visuosensory input compared with that of the basic black and white shaded Mooney face. Latinus and Taylor (14) have previously reported no differences in P100 latency or amplitude between photographic and Mooney face stimuli, although, they did observe an amplitude decrease to schematic faces, which supports this interpretation. In our study, the demonstrated sensitivity of P100 to orientation (i.e., reduced amplitude and increased latency for inverted versus upright stimuli) is less intuitive. Stimulus characteristics remain consistent across orientations, with more advanced stimulus discrimination not generally shown until later time windows [e.g., N170, N250; see Ref. (37)]. However, P100 may also be modulated by the allocation of attentional resources (70, 96), and it would stand to reason that attention may decline for upside-down faces over the duration of the task, which could explain this finding. Importantly, the absence of schizotypal group differences at P100, as well as the lack of relationship between P100 and O-LIFE scores, demonstrates that early visuosensory processing in high schizotypy appears intact.

Despite the aforementioned significant neurophysiological anomalies, our behavioral data reinforced the healthy status of these individuals high in schizotypal traits. Behavioral responses conformed to previous findings for both high and low schizotypes: stimuli easier to recognize (i.e., photographic and upright faces) attracted more accurate and faster responses, with the least accurate and slowest responses demonstrated for faces most difficult to perceive (i.e., inverted Mooney faces) (14, 45, 46, 55). It is not unusual that high and low schizotypes show matched behavioral performance. Semantic priming literature in schizotypy has consistently demonstrated ERP differences in high and low schizotypes that are not reflected behaviorally [e.g., Ref. (92–94)]. It has been argued that this is because behavioral measures capture later stages of processing, by which time anomalies in neural processing have been accounted for in healthy brains [see Ref. (95) for discussion].

In summary, high schizotypes demonstrated impaired face processing (N170 component), which appears to stem from a specific deficit in the configural assessment of faces, as has been shown in schizophrenia. Importantly, however, this deficit seems to be corrected by later processing, as was indicated by behavioral responses. The early visuosensory processing of faces (P100 component) looks to be intact in schizotypy, although, investigation of the P100 response to face stimuli in individuals at various stages of psychosis-proneness would be profitable. To our knowledge, this is the first study to demonstrate that neurophysiological deficits in basic face processing are present in schizotypy. This work thereby adds to the mounting evidence for analogous neural processing anomalies at the healthy end of the psychosis continuum. The N170 deficits shown by high schizotypes in our study were present without the influence of confounds commonly associated with schizophrenia samples: such as repeated hospitalization, long-term antipsychotic therapy, social isolation, chronic neuropsychological profile, and, in many cases, lowered IQ. This confirms that N170 deficits reported previously in schizophrenia samples do not stem from these confounds. The findings further suggest that face processing deficits indexed by the N170 component may constitute neural dysfunction associated with vulnerability for schizophrenia (e.g., an endophenotype). This adds to the developing profile of individuals at a high risk for the disorder and may help facilitate their early detection. Finally, the results provide further evidence of underlying neurophysiological deficits that may contribute to the poor social interaction characteristic of schizophrenia.

ACKNOWLEDGMENTS

This work was supported by RMIT University, Melbourne, VIC, Australia. The equipment used for this project was provided via a Clinical Neurobiology of Psychosis Platform grant to Susan L. Rossell; a funding platform of Neurosciences Australia. The Bionics Institute acknowledges the support it receives from the Victorian Government through its Operational Infrastructure Support Program. Thanks to all participants for their involvement.

REFERENCES

1. Bediou B, Franck N, Saoud M, Baudouin JY, Tiberghien G, Dalery J, et al. Effects of emotion and identity on facial affect processing in schizophrenia. *Psychiatry Res* (2005) **133**:149–57. doi:10.1016/j.psychres.2004.08.008
2. Comparelli A, Corigliano V, De Carolis A, Mancinelli I, Trovini G, Ottavi G, et al. Emotion recognition impairment is present early and is stable throughout the course of schizophrenia. *Schizophr Res* (2013) **143**:65–9. doi:10.1016/j.schres.2012.11.005
3. Kerr SL, Neale JM. Emotion perception in schizophrenia: specific deficit or further evidence of generalized poor performance? *J Abnorm Psychol* (1993) **105**:480–3.
4. Kring AM, Elis O. Emotion deficits in people with schizophrenia. *Annu Rev Clin Psychol* (2013) **9**:409–33. doi:10.1146/annurev-clinpsy-050212-185538
5. Tremeau F, Antonius D. Review: emotion identification deficits are associated with functional impairments in people with schizophrenia. *Evid Based Ment Health* (2012) **15**:106. doi:10.1136/ebmental-2012-100880
6. Tsui CF, Huang J, Lui SS, Au AC, Leung MM, Cheung EF, et al. Facial emotion perception abnormality in patients with early schizophrenia. *Schizophr Res* (2013) **147**:230–5. doi:10.1016/j.schres.2013.04.019
7. Kohler CG, Walker JB, Martin EA, Healey KM, Moberg PJ. Facial emotion perception in schizophrenia: a meta-analytic review. *Schizophr Bull* (2010) **36**:1009–19. doi:10.1093/schbul/sbn192
8. Norton D, McBain R, Holt DJ, Ongur D, Chen Y. Association of impaired facial affect recognition with basic facial and visual processing deficits in schizophrenia. *Biol Psychiatry* (2009) **65**:1094–8. doi:10.1016/j.biopsych.2009.01.026
9. Strauss GP, Jetha SS, Ross SA, Duke LA, Allen DN. Impaired facial affect labelling and discrimination in patients with deficit syndrome schizophrenia. *Schizophr Res* (2010) **118**:146–53. doi:10.1016/j.schres.2010.01.016
10. Joshua N, Rossell SL. Configural face processing in schizophrenia. *Schizophr Res* (2009) **112**:99–103. doi:10.1016/j.schres.2009.03.033
11. Bauser D, Thoma P, Aizenberg V, Brune M, Juckel G, Daum I. Face and body perception in schizophrenia: a configural processing deficit? *Psychiatry Res* (2012) **195**:9–17. doi:10.1016/j.psychres.2011.07.017
12. Kim HS, Shin NY, Choi J, Jung MH, Jang JH, Kang D, et al. Processing of facial configuration in individuals at ultra-high risk for schizophrenia. *Schizophr Res* (2010) **118**:81–7. doi:10.1016/j.schres.2010.01.003
13. Johnson SC, Lowery N, Kohler C, Turetsky BI. Global–local visual processing in schizophrenia: evidence for an early visual processing deficit. *Biol Psychiatry* (2005) **58**:935–46. doi:10.1016/j.biopsych.2005.04.053
14. Latinus M, Taylor MJ. Face processing stages: impact of difficulty and the separation of effects. *Brain Res* (2006) **1123**:179–87. doi:10.1016/j.brainres.2006.09.031
15. Maurer D, Grand RL, Mondloch CJ. The many faces of configural processing. *Trends Cogn Sci* (2002) **6**:255–60. doi:10.1016/S1364-6613(02)01903-4
16. Freire A, Lee K, Symons LA. The face-inversion effect as a deficit in the encoding of configural information: direct evidence. *Perception* (2000) **29**:159–70. doi:10.1068/p3012
17. Yin RK. Looking at upside-down faces. *J Exp Psychol Hum Percept Perform* (1969) **81**:141–5.
18. Eimer M. Effects of face inversion on the structural encoding and recognition of faces. Evidence from event-related brain potentials. *Brain Res Cogn Brain Res* (2000) **10**:145–58. doi:10.1016/S0926-6410(00)00038-0
19. Ingvalson EM, Wenger MJ. A strong test of the dual-mode hypothesis. *Percept Psychophys* (2005) **67**:14–35. doi:10.3758/BF03195010
20. Chambon V, Baudouin J, Franck N. The role of configural information in facial emotion recognition in schizophrenia. *Neuropsychologia* (2006) **44**:2437–44. doi:10.1016/j.neuropsychologia.2006.04.008
21. Schwartz BL, Rosse RB, Johri S, Deutsch SI. Visual scanning of facial expressions in schizophrenia. *J Neuropsychiatry Clin Neurosci* (1999) **11**:103–6.
22. Shin Y, Na MH, Ha TH, Kang D, Yoo S, Kwon JS. Dysfunction in configural face processing in patients with schizophrenia. *Schizophr Bull* (2008) **34**:538–43. doi:10.1093/schbul/sbm118
23. Schwartz BL, Marvel CL, Drapalski A, Rosse RB, Deutsch SI. Configural processing in face recognition in schizophrenia. *Cogn Neuropsychiatry* (2002) **7**:15–39. doi:10.1080/13546800143000113
24. Murray MM, Foxe JJ, Higgins BA, Javitt DC, Schroeder CE. Visuo-spatial neural response interactions in early cortical processing during a simple reaction time task: a high-density electrical mapping study. *Neuropsychologia* (2001) **39**:828–44. doi:10.1016/S0028-3932(01)00004-5
25. Vohs JL, Hetrick WP, Kieffaber PD, Bodkins M, Bismark A, Shekhar A, et al. Visual event-related potentials in schizotypal personality disorder and schizophrenia. *J Abnorm Psychol* (2008) **117**:119–31. doi:10.1037/0021-843X.117.1.119
26. Bentin S, Allison T, Puce A, Perez E, McCarthy G. Electrophysiological studies of face perception in humans. *J Cogn Neurosci* (1996) **8**:551–65. doi:10.1162/jocn.1996.8.6.551
27. George N, Jemel B, Firori N, Renault B. Face and shape repetition effects in humans: a spatio-temporal ERP study. *Neuroreport* (1997) **8**:1417–23. doi:10.1097/00001756-199704140-00019
28. Heisz JJ, Watter S, Shedden JM. Automatic face identity encoding at the N170. *Vision Res* (2006) **46**:4604–46. doi:10.1016/j.visres.2006.09.026
29. Itier RJ, Alain C, Sedore K, McIntosh AR. Early face processing specificity: it's in the eyes! *J Cogn Neurosci* (2007) **19**:1815–26. doi:10.1162/jocn.2007.19.11.1815
30. Itier RJ, Latinus M, Taylor MJ. Face, eye and object early processing: what is the face specificity? *Neuroimage* (2006) **29**:667–76. doi:10.1016/j.neuroimage.2005.07.041
31. Ashley V, Vuilleumier P, Swick D. Time course and specificity of event-related potentials to emotional expressions. *Neuroreport* (2004) **15**:211–6. doi:10.1097/00001756-200401190-00041
32. Batty M, Taylor MJ. Early processing of the six basic facial emotional expressions. *Brain Res Cogn Brain Res* (2003) **17**:613–20. doi:10.1016/S0926-6410(03)00174-5
33. Blau VC, Maurer U, Tottenham N, McCandliss BD. The face-specific N170 component is modulated by emotional facial expression. *Behav Brain Funct* (2007) **23**:3–7. doi:10.1186/1744-9081-3-7
34. Ibanez A, Riveros R, Hurtado E, Gleichgerrcht E, Urquina H, Herrera E, et al. The face and its emotion: right N170 deficits in structural processing and early emotional discrimination in schizophrenic patients and relatives. *Psychiatry Res* (2012) **195**:18–26. doi:10.1016/j.psychres.2011.07.027
35. Thierry G, Martin CD, Downing P, Pegna AJ. Controlling for interstimulus perceptual variance abolishes N170 face selectivity. *Nat Neurosci* (2007) **10**:505–11. doi:10.1038/nn1864
36. Bentin S, Taylor MJ, Rousselet GA, Itier RJ, Caldara R, Schyns PG, et al. Controlling for interstimulus perceptual variance does not abolish N170 face sensitivity. *Nat Neurosci* (2007) **10**:801–2. doi:10.1038/nn0707-801
37. Ganis G, Smith D, Schendan HE. The N170, not the P1, indexes the earliest time for categorical perception of faces, regardless of interstimulus variance. *Neuroimage* (2012) **62**:1563–74. doi:10.1016/j.neuroimage.2012.05.043
38. Itier RJ, Batty M. Neural bases of eye and gaze processing: the core of social cognition. *Neurosci Biobehav Rev* (2009) **33**:843–63. doi:10.1016/j.neubiorev.2009.02.004
39. Magnuski M, Gola M. It's not only in the eyes: nonlinear relationship between face orientation and N170 amplitude irrespective of eye presence. *Int J Psychophysiol* (2013) **89**:358–65. doi:10.1016/j.ijpsycho.2013.04.016
40. Rellecke J, Sommer W, Schacht A. Emotion effects on the N170: a question of reference? *Brain Topogr* (2013) **26**:62–71. doi:10.1007/s10548-012-0261-y
41. Schinkel S, Ivanova G, Kurths J, Sommer W. Modulation of the N170 adaptation profile by higher level factors. *Biol Psychol* (2014) **97**:27–34. doi:10.1016/j.biopsycho.2014.01.003
42. Calvo MG, Beltran D. Brain lateralization of holistic versus analytic processing of emotional facial expressions. *Neuroimage* (2014) **92**:237–47. doi:10.1016/j.neuroimage.2014.01.048
43. Eimer M, Gosling A, Nicholas S, Kiss M. The N170 component and its links to configural face processing: a rapid neural adaptation study. *Brain Res* (2011) **1376**:76–87. doi:10.1016/j.brainres.2010.12.046

44. Mooney CM. Age in the development of closure ability in children. *Can J Psychol* (1957) **11**:219–26. doi:10.1037/h0083717
45. Latinus M, Taylor MJ. Holistic processing of faces: learning effects with Mooney faces. *J Cogn Neurosci* (2005) **17**:1316–27. doi:10.1162/0898929055002490
46. George N, Jemel B, Fiori N, Chaby L, Renault B. Electrophysiological correlates of facial decision: insights from upright and upside-down Mooney-face perception. *Brain Res Cogn Brain Res* (2005) **24**:663–73. doi:10.1016/j.cogbrainres.2005.03.017
47. Itier RJ, Taylor MJ. N170 or N1? Spatiotemporal differences between object and face processing using ERPs. *Cereb Cortex* (2004) **14**:132–42. doi:10.1093/cercor/bhg111
48. Sagiv N, Bentin S. Structural encoding of human and schematic faces: holistic and part-based processes. *J Cogn Neurosci* (2001) **13**:937–51. doi:10.1162/089892901753165854
49. Caharel S, Bernard C, Thibaut F, Haouzir S, Di Maggio-Clozel C, Allio G, et al. The effects of familiarity and emotional expression on face processing examined by ERPs in patients with schizophrenia. *Schizophr Res* (2007) **95**:186–96. doi:10.1016/j.schres.2007.06.015
50. Yeap S, Kelly SP, Sehatpour P, Magno E, Garavan H, Thakore JH, et al. Visual sensory processing deficits in schizophrenia and their relationship to disease state. *Eur Arch Psychiatry Clin Neurosci* (2008) **258**:305–16. doi:10.1007/s00406-008-0802-2
51. Yeap S, Kelly SP, Thakore JH, Foxe JJ. Visual sensory processing deficits in first-episode patients with schizophrenia. *Schizophr Res* (2008) **102**:340–3. doi:10.1016/j.schres.2008.03.026
52. Yeap S, Kelly SP, Sehatpour P, Magno E, Javitt DC, Garavan H, et al. Early visual sensory deficits as endophenotypes for schizophrenia: high-density electrical mapping in clinically unaffected first-degree relatives. *Arch Gen Psychiatry* (2006) **6**:1180–8. doi:10.1001/archpsyc.63.11.1180
53. Wolwer W, Brinkmeyer J, Stroth S, Streit M, Bechdolf A, Ruhrmann S, et al. Neurophysiological correlates of impaired facial affect recognition in individuals at risk for schizophrenia. *Schizophr Bull* (2012) **38**:1021–9. doi:10.1093/schbul/sbr013
54. Bedwell JS, Chan CC, Trachik BJ, Rassovsky Y. Changes in the visual-evoked P1 potential as a function of schizotypy and background color in healthy young adults. *J Psychiatr Res* (2013) **47**:542–7. doi:10.1016/j.jpsychires.2012.12.012
55. Schwartzman D, Maravic K, Kranczioch C, Barnes J. Altered early visual processing components in hallucination-prone individuals. *Neuroreport* (2008) **19**:933–7. doi:10.1097/WNR.0b013e328301a.640
56. Baudouin JY, Martin F, Tiberghien G, Verlut I, Franck N. Selective attention to facial emotion and identity in schizophrenia. *Neuropsychologia* (2002) **40**:503–11. doi:10.1016/S0028-3932(01)00114-2
57. Breton F, Plante A, Legauffre C, Morel N, Ades J, Gorwood P, et al. The executive control of attention differentiates patients with schizophrenia, their first-degree relatives and healthy controls. *Neuropsychologia* (2011) **49**:203–8. doi:10.1016/j.neuropsychologia.2010.11.019
58. Gooding DC, Braun JG, Studer JA. Attentional network task performance in patients with schizophrenia-spectrum disorders: evidence of a specific deficit. *Schizophr Res* (2006) **88**:169–78. doi:10.1016/j.schres.2006.07.009
59. Bestelmeyer PEG, Tatler BW, Phillips LH, Fraser G, Benson PJ, St. Clair D. Global visual scanning abnormalities in schizophrenia and bipolar disorder. *Schizophr Res* (2006) **87**:212–22. doi:10.1016/j.schres.2006.06.015
60. Rosse RB, Schwartz BL, Johri S, Deutsch SI. Visual scanning of faces correlates with schizophrenia symptomatology. *Prog Neuropsychopharmacol Biol Psychiatry* (1998) **22**:971–9. doi:10.1016/S0278-5846(98)00056-6
61. Ikeda C, Kirino E, Inoue R, Arai H. Event-related potential study of illusory contour perception in schizophrenia. *Neuropsychobiology* (2011) **64**:231–8. doi:10.1159/000327706
62. Streit M, Wolwer W, Brinkmeyer J, Ihl R, Gaebel W. EEG correlates of facial affect recognition and categorisation of blurred faces in schizophrenic patients and healthy volunteers. *Schizophr Res* (2001) **49**:145–55. doi:10.1016/S0920-9964(00)00041-4
63. Turetsky BI, Kohler CG, Indersmitten T, Bhati MT, Charbonnier D, Gur RC. Facial emotion recognition in schizophrenia: when and why does it go awry? *Schizophr Res* (2007) **94**:253–63. doi:10.1016/j.schres.2007.05.001
64. Wynn JK, Lee J, Horan WP, Green MF. Using event-related potentials to explore stages of facial affect recognition deficits in schizophrenia. *Schizophr Bull* (2008) **34**:679–87. doi:10.1093/schbul/sbn047
65. Butler PD, Zemon V, Schechter I, Saperstein AM, Hoptman MJ, Lim KO, et al. Early-stage visual processing and cortical amplification deficits in schizophrenia. *Arch Gen Psychiatry* (2005) **62**:495–504. doi:10.1001/archpsyc.62.5.495
66. Foxe JJ, Doniger GM, Javitt DC. Early visual processing deficits in schizophrenia: impaired P1 generation revealed by high-density electrical mapping. *Neuroreport* (2001) **12**:3815–20. doi:10.1097/00001756-200112040-00043
67. Campanella S, Montedoro C, Streel E, Verbanck P, Rosier V. Early visual components (P100, N170) are disrupted in chronic schizophrenic patients: an event-related potentials study. *Neurophysiol Clin* (2006) **36**:71–8. doi:10.1016/j.neucli.2006.04.005
68. Anderer P, Saletu B, Semlitsch HV, Pascual-Marqui RD. Perceptual and cognitive event-related potentials in neuropsychopharmacology: methodological aspects and clinical applications (pharmaco-ERP topography and tomography). *Methods Find Exp Clin Pharmacol* (2002) **24**:121–37.
69. Pompéia S, Bueno OFA, Lucchesi LM, Manzano GM, Galduroz JCF, Tifik S. A double-dissociation of behavioral and event-related potential effects of two benzodiazepines with similar potencies. *J Psychopharmacol* (2000) **14**:288–98. doi:10.1177/026988110001400318
70. Puga F, Sampaio I, Veiga H, Ferreira C, Cagy M, Piedade R, et al. The effects of bromazepam on the early stage of visual information processing (P100). *Arq Neuropsiquiatr* (2007) **65**:955–9. doi:10.1590/S0004-282X2007000600006
71. Lynn SK, Salisbury DF. Attenuated modulation of the N170 ERP by facial expressions in schizophrenia. *Clin EEG Neurosci* (2008) **32**:108–11. doi:10.1177/155005940803900218
72. Holden C. Neuroscience. Deconstructing schizophrenia. *Science* (2003) **299**:333–5. doi:10.1126/science.299.5605.333
73. Johnstone A, Gleeson J, Rossell SL. Evidence of semantic disorganisation in schizotypy using an indirect priming task. *J Nerv Ment Dis* (2008) **196**:694–701. doi:10.1097/NMD.0b013e318183f882
74. Morgan C, Bedford N, Rossell SL. Evidence of semantic disorganisation using semantic priming in individuals with high schizotypy. *Schizophr Res* (2006) **84**:272–80. doi:10.1016/j.schres.2006.01.020
75. Myin-Germeys I, Krabbendam L, van Os J. Continuity of psychotic symptoms in the community. *Curr Opin Psychiatry* (2003) **16**:443–9. doi:10.1097/00001504-200307000-00011
76. Verdoux H, van Os J. Psychotic symptoms in non-clinical populations and the continuum of psychosis. *Schizophr Res* (2002) **54**:59–65. doi:10.1016/S0920-9964(01)00352-8
77. Goodbourn PT, Bosten JM, Bargary G, Hogg RE, Lawrance-Owen AJ, Mollon JD. Variants in the 1q21 risk region are associated with a visual endophenotype of autism and schizophrenia. *Genes Brain Behav* (2014) **13**:144–51. doi:10.1111/gbb.12096
78. Manoach DS, Agam Y. Neural markers of errors as endophenotypes in neuropsychiatric disorders. *Front Hum Neurosci* (2013) **7**:350. doi:10.3389/fnhum.2013.00.350
79. Herrmann MJ, Ellgring H, Fallgatter AJ. Early-stage face processing dysfunction in patients with schizophrenia. *Am J Psychiatry* (2004) **161**:915–7. doi:10.1176/appi.ajp.161.5.915
80. Thoma P, Soria Bauser D, Norra C, Brune M, Juckel G, Suchan B. Do you see what I feel? Electrophysiological correlates of emotional face and body perception in schizophrenia. *Clin Neurophysiol* (2014) **125**:1152–63. doi:10.1016/j.clinph.2013.10.046
81. Campo JA, Nijman H, Merckelbach H. Changes in appearance and schizotypy in normal subjects. *Acta Neuropsychiatr* (2004) **16**:138–41. doi:10.1111/j.0924-2708.2004.00065.x
82. Jahshan CS, Sergi MJ. Theory of mind, neurocognition, and functional status in schizotypy. *Schizophr Res* (2007) **89**:278–86. doi:10.1016/j.schres.2006.09.004
83. Lenzenweger MF. Schizotypy: an organising framework for schizophrenia research. *Curr Dir Psychol Sci* (2006) **15**:162–6. doi:10.1111/j.1467-8721.2006.00428.x
84. Morgan CJA, Bedford N, O'Regan A, Rossell SL. Is semantic processing impaired in individuals with high schizotypy? *J Nerv Ment Dis* (2008) **197**:232–8. doi:10.1097/NMD.0b013e31819dc.127
85. Rossler W, Riecher-Rossler A, Angst J, Murray R, Gamma A, Eich D, et al. Psychotic experiences in the general population: a twenty-year prospective community study. *Schizophr Res* (2007) **92**:1–14. doi:10.1016/j.schres.2007.01.002
86. Platek SM, Gallup GG Jr. Self-face recognition is affected by schizotypal personality traits. *Schizophr Res* (2002) **57**:81–5. doi:10.1016/S0920-9964(01)00310-3

87. Nelson HE. *The National Adult Reading Test (NART)*. Windsor: NFER (1981).
88. Mason O, Claridge GS, Jackson M. New scales for the assessment of schizotypy. *Pers Individ Dif* (1995) **18**:7–13. doi:10.1016/0191-8869(94)00132-C
89. Burch G, Steel C, Hemsley D. Oxford-Liverpool inventory of feelings and experiences: reliability in an experimental population. *Br J Clin Psychol* (1998) **37**:107–8. doi:10.1111/j.2044-8260.1998.tb01284.x
90. Laroi F, D'Argembeau A, Bredart S, van der Linden M. Face recognition failures in schizotypy. *Cogn Neuropsychiatry* (2007) **12**:554–71. doi:10.1080/13546800701707223
91. Ekman P, Friesen WV. *Pictures of Facial Affect.* Palo Alto, CA: Consulting Psychologists Press (1976).
92. Kiang J, Prugh M, Kutas M. An event-related brain potential study of schizotypal personality and associative semantic processing. *Int J Psychophysiol* (2010) **75**:119–26. doi:10.1016/j.ijpsycho.2009.10.005
93. Kostova M, Bohec AL, Blanchet A. Event-related brain potential study of expectancy and semantic matching in schizotypy. *Int J Psychophysiol* (2014) **92**:67–73. doi:10.1016/j.ijpsycho.2014.02.006
94. Wang K, Wang Y, Yan C, Wang YN, Cheung EF, Chan RC. Semantic processing impairment in individuals with schizotypal personality disorder features: a preliminary event-related potential study. *Prog Neuropsychopharmacol Biol Psychiatry* (2013) **40**:93–102. doi:10.1016/j.pnpbp.2012.08.019
95. Kutas M, Federmeier KD. Thirty years and counting: finding meaning in the N400 component of the event-related brain potential (ERP). *Annu Rev Psychol* (2011) **62**:621–47. doi:10.1146/annurev.psych.093008.131123
96. Foxe JJ, Simpson GV. Flow of activation from V1 to frontal cortex in humans. A framework for defining "early" visual processing. *Exp Brain Res* (2002) **142**:139–50. doi:10.1007/s00221-001-0906-7

20

Hyperactivity and motoric activity in ADHD: characterization, assessment, and intervention

Caterina Gawrilow [1,2,3,4] ****, Jan Kühnhausen*** [2,3]***, Johanna Schmid*** [1,4] ***and Gertraud Stadler*** [5]

[1] *Faculty of Science, Department of Psychology, Eberhard Karls Universität Tübingen, Tübingen, Germany*
[2] *German Institute for International Educational Research (DIPF), Frankfurt, Germany*
[3] *Center for Research on Individual Development and Adaptive Education of Children at Risk (IDeA), Frankfurt, Germany*
[4] *LEAD Graduate School, Eberhard Karls Universität Tübingen, Tübingen, Germany*
[5] *Psychology Department, Columbia University, New York, NY, USA*

Edited by:
Sebastian Walther, University of Bern, Switzerland

Reviewed by:
Stephan Kupferschmid, University of Bern, Switzerland
Sarah Schiebler, University of Bern, Switzerland

****Correspondence:***
Caterina Gawrilow, Faculty of Science, Psychology Department, Eberhard Karls Universität Tübingen, Schleichstraße 4, Tübingen 72076, Germany
e-mail: caterina.gawrilow@uni-tuebingen.de

The aim of the present literature review is threefold. (1) We will review theories, models, and studies on symptomatic hyperactivity and motoric activity in attention-deficit/hyperactivity disorder (ADHD). (2) Another focus will be on assessment methods that have been proven to be effective in the detection of hyperactivity and motoric activity in children, adolescents, and adults with and without ADHD and emerging areas of research in the field of ADHD. We will compare subjective methods (i.e., rating scales) and objective methods (i.e., accelerometers). (3) Finally, physical activity intervention studies aiming at a modification of activity and overactive behavior will be summarized that seem to be promising candidates for alleviating hyperactivity symptoms in children, adolescents, and adults with ADHD.

Keywords: accelerometers, bifactor models of ADHD, ADHD, hyperactivity–impulsivity, physical activity, support vector machines

INTRODUCTION

Hyperactivity and a general increase in motoric activity with respect to amount/frequency and variability of activity/movements are main symptoms of both the combined and the hyperactive–impulsive type of attention-deficit/hyperactivity disorder (ADHD). Children with ADHD fidget with hands and feet, have difficulties remaining seated, run about, or climb excessively, and have difficulties to engage in activities quietly (1). Children with ADHD show increased physical activity (PA) both during the day and the night (2). Thus, research indicates that in one-third of children with ADHD and with an even higher prevalence in adults with ADHD sleep disorders (i.e., daytime sleepiness, insomnia, delayed sleep phase syndrome, fractured sleep, restless legs syndrome, and sleep disordered breathing) are common (3). Whereas children without ADHD usually outgrow hyperactivity around the age where they enter elementary school, hyperactivity remains present in children who receive an ADHD diagnosis. This leads to severe problems during structured school activities and interactions with parents, teachers, and peers. In adolescents and adults with ADHD, hyperactivity remains as a symptom, leading to, for instance, extreme restlessness and feelings of always being on the go or driven by a motor. Hyperactivity as one of the core symptoms of ADHD is thus leading to maladaptive cognitive and social functioning and disturbed well-being.

Counterintuitively though, children and adolescents with ADHD appear to be less likely to engage in regular vigorous PA and organized sports (4). Research only begins to investigate possible barriers that might constitute underlying reasons for this physical inactivity. One of the reasons might be that due to the ADHD symptoms of inattentiveness and impulsivity, affected children are easily distracted by or respond impulsively to alternative activities [e.g., watching TV (5)]. Another reason might be that deficits in executive functions that potentially underlie the ADHD symptomatology lead to difficulties initiating and maintaining PA (4, 6). Furthermore, it seems that children are at risk for not being physically active when they receive no ADHD treatment [i.e., medication with methylphenidate, MPH (7)].

While inattentiveness as a core symptom has been investigated in numerous studies, no clear characterization of symptomatic hyperactivity and motoric activity in children, adolescents, and adults with ADHD exists. In addition, there are no guidelines for the assessment and intervention of motoric activity in ADHD (8).

Therefore, aims of the present literature review are (1) to review studies on symptomatic hyperactivity and motoric activity in ADHD on different developmental stages. This is important because hyperactivity as a symptom and its possible differentiation from other symptoms as for instance inattentiveness might alter over the lifespan. (2) Another focus will be on subjective and objective assessment methods that have been proven to be effective in the detection of hyperactivity and motoric activity in ADHD. This is important because there is a need for adequate and efficient detection methods of hyperactivity in clinical settings. As we will explain in more detail, clinical diagnoses often rely on retrospective parental and teacher reports on hyperactive behavior shown by children and adolescents. (3) Finally, PA intervention studies aiming at a change or modification of activity and overactive behavior that seem to be promising candidates for alleviating hyperactivity symptoms in ADHD will be summarized.

DIAGNOSTIC CRITERIA OF SYMPTOMATIC HYPERACTIVITY AND MOTORIC ACTIVITY IN ADHD

Hyperactivity constitutes a core symptom of ADHD that represents one of the most common disorders in childhood and adolescence, with approximately 5.3% of school-aged individuals being affected (9). The Diagnostic and Statistical Manual of Mental Disorders (DSM-5) classifies ADHD as a neurodevelopmental disorder and lists 18 symptoms on two dimensions (see **Table 1**), namely, (1) hyperactivity–impulsivity and (2) inattention that manifest in three possible main presentations: (a) predominantly hyperactive/impulsive presentation (314.01), (b) predominantly inattentive presentation (314.00), and (c) combined presentation (314.01). A diagnosis requires at least six symptoms of hyperactivity–impulsivity and/or inattention in childhood and adolescence, and at least five symptoms in adulthood to be present in two or more settings (e.g., at home, school/work, with friends) for at least six months, and to interfere with developmental level and functioning.

CURRENT PSYCHOLOGICAL THEORIES OF HYPERACTIVITY AND MOTORIC ACTIVITY IN ADHD

Several psychological theories exist that address the question of what gives rise to symptomatic hyperactivity and motoric activity in ADHD. In our review we outline three current theoretical conceptions: (1) the State Regulation Model, (2) Multiple Pathway Theories, and (3) the Dynamic Developmental Theory of ADHD.

The State Regulation Model suggests that clinical levels of ADHD symptomatology can be traced back to a deficit in keeping optimal activation states (10, 11). Building up on the cognitive-energetic theory of Sanders (12) and Sanders and van Duren (13)

Table 1 | Hyperactivity–impulsivity and inattention symptoms according to DSM-5 (1).

Hyperactivity–Impulsivity

1. Often fidgets with or taps hands or feet or squirms in seat
2. Often leaves seat in situations when remaining seated is expected (e.g., leaves his or her place in the classroom, in the office or other workplace, or in other situations that require remaining in place)
3. Often runs about or climbs in situations where it is inappropriate. (Note: In adolescents or adults, may be limited to feeling restless.)
4. Often unable to play or engage in leisure activities quietly
5. Is often "on the go," acting as if "driven by a motor" (e.g., is unable to be or uncomfortable being still for extended time, as in restaurants, meetings; may be experienced by others as being restless or difficult to keep up with)
6. Often talks excessively
7. Often blurts out an answer before a question has been completed (e.g., completes people's sentences; cannot wait for turn in conversation)
8. Often has difficulty waiting his or her turn (e.g., while waiting in line)
9. Often interrupts or intrudes on others (e.g., butts into conversations, games, or activities; may start using other people's things without asking or receiving permission; for adolescents and adults, may intrude into or take over what others are doing)

Inattention symptoms

1. Often fails to give close attention to details or makes careless mistakes in schoolwork, at work, or during other activities (e.g., overlooks or misses details, work is inaccurate)
2. Often has difficulty sustaining attention in tasks or play activities (e.g., has difficulty remaining focused during lectures, conversations, or lengthy reading)
3. Often does not seem to listen when spoken to directly (e.g., mind seems elsewhere, even in the absence of any obvious distraction)
4. Often does not follow through on instructions and fails to finish schoolwork, chores, or duties in the workplace (e.g., starts tasks but quickly loses focus and is easily sidetracked)
5. Often has difficulty organizing tasks and activities (e.g., difficulty managing sequential tasks; difficulty keeping materials and belongings in order; messy, disorganized work; has poor time management; fails to meet deadlines)
6. Often avoids, dislikes, or is reluctant to engage in tasks that require sustained mental effort [e.g., schoolwork or homework (for older adolescents and adults, preparing reports, completing forms, reviewing lengthy papers)]
7. Often loses things necessary for tasks or activities [e.g., school materials, pencils, books, tools (wallets, keys, paperwork, eyeglasses, and mobile telephones)]
8. Is often easily distracted by extraneous stimuli (for older adolescents and adults, may include unrelated thoughts).
9. Is often forgetful in daily activities (e.g., doing chores, running errands; for older adolescents and adults, returning calls, paying bills, keeping appointments)

Behavioral examples added to symptom descriptions in DSM-5 compared to DSM-IV are given in square brackets. Symptoms 1–6 from the hyperactivity–impulsivity dimension denote symptoms classed as hyperactivity. Symptoms 7–9 from the hyperactivity–impulsivity dimension denote symptoms classed as impulsivity.

the model assumes that a given person's activation level increases in situations where the presentation rate of stimuli is high, and decreases in situations where the presentation rate of stimuli is low. To reach optimal levels of performance and counteract overactivation under high stimulus presentation rates as well as underactivation under low stimulus presentation rates, the allocation of extra effort (i.e., effortful control) is necessary. Several studies at various developmental stages have shown that individuals with ADHD show greatest performance deficits compared to individuals without ADHD not under medium event rates but under fast (14, 15) and slow (15, 16) event rates when the effortful allocation of extra effort would have been necessary for optimal performance. Correspondingly, the State Regulation Model postulates ADHD symptoms, including hyperactivity, to increase or decrease relative to a given person's respective state that requires effortful control. Thus, in the context of this theoretical model, levels of hyperactivity are not seen as stable across situations but to become increasingly present under low activation states as an attempt of self-stimulation and under high activation states as a behavioral sign of overactivation.

Multiple pathway conceptions (17–19) postulate that there are several distinct developmental influences (i.e., 'pathways') that converge onto a core symptom expression of ADHD but with remaining specificities (20). Today, the most prominent multiple pathway conceptions is the Triple-Pathway Model (19) that suggests dissociable *timing*, *inhibition*, and *delay deficits* to give rise to highly heterogeneous expressions of ADHD symptoms. With regard to timing, the model suggests that individuals with ADHD display deficits in, for example, the discrimination of durations and the adequate anticipation of time intervals. Inhibition deficits refer to impaired abilities of individuals with ADHD to inhibit responses in inappropriate situations (21) such as awaiting turn in communications. Delay deficits denote the aversion and enhanced negative emotional reactions to situations characterized by (temporal) delays [e.g., Ref. (22)] such as waiting for further instructions in the classroom. Within this theoretical framework, the symptom of hyperactivity is conceptualized as a behavioral attempt to attenuate negative subjective experiences of delay where delay cannot be circumvented (23).

The Dynamic Developmental Theory of ADHD (24) suggests a hypofunctioning mesolimbic dopamine branch to underlie altered reinforcement of novel behavior and insufficient extinction of behavior that has previously been reinforced. It is assumed that the critical time frame for a reinforcer to take effect is shorter in individuals with ADHD compared to individuals without ADHD. Accordingly, socially desirable behavior is frequently not positively reinforced, and undesirable behavior not negatively reinforced in time. The theory predicts that (gradually developing) hyperactivity stems from a combination of altered positive reinforcement and deficient extinction processes, leading to an increased and accumulating number of behavioral responses that may display in excess motoric activity.

STRUCTURAL ACCOUNTS OF HYPERACTIVITY AND MOTORIC ACTIVITY IN ADHD

Despite broad consensus about what classifies as hyperactivity in the context of ADHD and several theoretical approaches to its underlying causes, the question of how the symptom relates to impulsivity and inattention has been one of the main areas of scientific debate in this research field for the last 20 years. Respective research questions are (a) is hyperactivity essentially just an expression of one underlying ADHD condition? (b) Is hyperactivity distinguishable from, yet related to impulsivity and/or inattention? (c) Or is a combination of those two perspectives possible? These questions concern our understanding of hyperactivity, how it relates to functional impairment and, by association, what kind of treatment may work and for whom. Important statistical methods to address the ongoing debate are factor analyses, which directly concern the measurement structure underlying ADHD symptoms and thus the question of coherence and distinctness between hyperactivity, impulsivity, and inattention. Factor models that have been discussed are (a) the one-factor model, which assumes one underlying unitary symptom domain, (b) the correlated factor models, which assume distinct symptom domains that are correlated, and (c) bifactor models, which incorporate both an underlying unitary symptom domain and additional specific independent symptom domains.

A one-factor model assumes that there is a single dimension underlying hyperactivity as well as impulsivity and inattention. No structural distinction is made in this model between hyperactivity and other symptom domains. However, there has been abundance of empirical evidence from factor-analytic investigations convincingly showing that this factor model does not represent an adequate conceptualization [e.g., Ref. (25–27)].

Correlated factor models emphasize the separability of hyperactivity from inattention and/or impulsivity (28). They conceptualize separate, yet related, latent constructs with either two factors (i.e., representing hyperactivity–impulsivity and inattention) or three factors (i.e., representing hyperactivity, impulsivity, and inattention) without a common core, which give rise to the phenotypic representation of ADHD.

Factor-analytic studies until the beginning of the 21st century found strong support for correlated factor models being better statistical representations of the symptom structure than the one-factor model [e.g., Ref. (29–34)]. Direct comparisons of the correlated two-factor model separating hyperactivity–impulsivity and inattention into two separate dimensions, and three-factor models separating the dimensions of hyperactivity and impulsivity besides inattention are somewhat inconclusive: Whereas many studies found support for differentiating two latent symptom dimensions (26, 29–31, 35–37), others pointed to the superior fit of models with three latent symptom dimensions that emphasize the separability of hyperactivity and impulsivity [e.g., Ref. (33, 34, 38)]. However, the more parsimonious two-factor model is usually favored because separating hyperactivity from impulsivity tends to improve the overall model fit only slightly and the latent factors of hyperactivity and impulsivity are usually highly correlated (39). Nevertheless, the question has been brought up as to whether the relative underrepresentation of symptoms of impulsivity in DSM (i.e., three) compared to the number of symptoms of hyperactivity (i.e., six; see **Table 1**) and limited psychometric properties—which limit statistical power to confirm a specific factor of impulsivity—may also explain some of the conflicting results between the studies mentioned above (30, 37, 39). Overall, it has been proposed that support for the validity of the correlated factor models comes from differential associations of the symptom domains with criterion variables of functional impairment (e.g., externalizing and internalizing behaviors). However, subscale sum scores for different symptom domains may not only represent domain specific symptom variation but also variation that can be traced to an underlying general symptom domain. Thus, such differential associations with measures of functional impairment could be compounded with influences from an underlying core symptom domain.

More recently than the one-factor model and correlated factor models, bifactor models have been proposed. They simultaneously account for both the common variance (i.e., coherence) between hyperactivity and the other core symptoms of ADHD with a latent general (g) ADHD factor, and the unique separable variance of hyperactivity, impulsivity, and inattention with specific domain factors (s) that are independent (i.e., orthogonal) from the general ADHD factor. Thus, to a greater extent than correlated factor models, bifactor models promote the common variance between symptom domains suggesting a unitary core construct underlying all ADHD symptoms, while endorsing additional covariation that manifests in orthogonal, specific symptom factors. During the last years, a number of studies have compared the more traditional correlated factor models with bifactor models and generally supported the superior model fit of the latter across a wide range of age groups (i.e., children, adolescents, adults), informants (i.e., self, parent, teacher, clinician ratings), methods of measurement (i.e., rating scales, interviews), and target populations [i.e., clinical and community samples (28, 39–48)]. Nevertheless, substantial inconsistency remains with regard to the question of whether a specific factor of hyperactivity can be distinguished from a specific factor of impulsivity (28, 40, 45, 47, 48). Just as discussed for the correlated factor models, the relative scarcity of impulsivity items may limit the power to detect a separate specific factor representing these symptoms separately from hyperactivity.

In sum, and although further studies and possibly the development of further items to assess impulsivity are needed to shed light on the question of separability between hyperactivity and impulsivity, a bifactor model framework seems to be a valid account of hyperactivity in the context of ADHD and its phenotypic representation for the following reasons: First, studies addressing the question of the development of ADHD across the lifespan reveal that it shows a substantial degree of stability and in many cases persists into adulthood (49), even though the specific symptom manifestation of this disorder may change with development [e.g., Ref. (50)]. This suggests a generic component, which lies at the core of the disorder and is stable over time, along with additional specific manifestations that may fluctuate (43). Due to the lack of a 'common core' in correlated factor models, which assume interrelated but conceptually independent symptom domains, they lack explanatory value for such a generic component. Second, quantitative genetic research (i.e., twin and adoption studies) suggest that there are sets of genes that exclusively influence hyperactivity and sets of genes that influence all domains of ADHD symptoms [(51, 52); for a review of quantitative genetic research on ADHD see (53)]. A bifactor model that represents a general ADHD symptom factor as well as independent specific symptom factors may be especially well suited to account for these findings. Third, the bifactor model has been suggested to be in line with current etiological models [e.g., Ref. (28, 43, 54)] such as multiple pathway conceptions (17–19), which postulate that there are several distinct developmental influences (i.e., 'pathways') that converge onto a core symptom expression, while specificities do remain (20).

SYMPTOMATIC HYPERACTIVITY AND MOTORIC ACTIVITY IN ADHD ON DIFFERENT DEVELOPMENTAL STAGES

Excessive motor activities are a first precursor of ADHD and often observed by parents during toddlerhood, even though they are hardly distinguishable from highly variable normative behaviors during this developmental period. Most frequently, impairing levels of hyperactivity are identified during the primary school years with a majority of children (approximately 60–85%) continuing to meet diagnostic criteria of ADHD throughout childhood and into adolescence and adulthood [e.g., Ref. (55)]. Notably, predominantly boys show symptomatic hyperactivity [e.g., Ref. (56)]. Sparse research addressing the trajectory of hyperactivity throughout development suggests a moderate stability (57). For instance, sleep problems operationalized as movements during the night (assessed by actigraphs) remain from childhood to adulthood (58). For many individuals, overt signs of hyperactivity decline from childhood into adulthood and may be confined with more subjective states such as mental restlessness, jitteriness, or impatience, indicating that the symptomatology undergoes substantial changes during the developmental course (1, 59, 60).

However, until to date, knowledge about the development of hyperactivity in the context of ADHD is limited and mainly based on retrospective self-reports of symptoms [e.g., Ref. (57)] which may well be affected by retrospective recall bias. To gain a more fine-grained understanding of the development of symptomatic hyperactivity and motoric activity across development, prospective longitudinal studies are needed that address symptom expressions as experienced by affected individuals themselves but also significant other people (e.g., parents, teachers, peers).

ASSESSMENT METHODS FOR THE DETECTION OF SYMPTOMATIC HYPERACTIVITY AND MOTORIC ACTIVITY IN ADHD

Physical activity can be assessed with a variety of measures, including subjective self-reports via survey questionnaires or more frequent daily or hourly recalls, and more objective measures such as wearable sensors (i.e., pedometers, accelerometers including those built into mobile phones, heart rate sensors), doubly labeled water, and direct observation.

So far, there is no single gold standard of measuring activity across populations (e.g., children, adolescents, adults) and across different assessment purposes [e.g., activity status in populations, relationship of activity with short-term and long-term health and well being, clinical and intervention research (61)]. With widely varying time periods assessed (from minutes to days, weeks up to several years, over the lifespan) and activity definitions regarding activity dimension and intensity, findings obtained with different activity measures can be difficult to compare. One important consideration in choosing activity measures is assessment purpose: It is important to clearly specify the research purpose as well as the exact frequency, duration, and distribution of activity of interest and then choose the appropriate study design and assessment instrument. For example, studying sedentary behavior over several years to better understand the development of obesity will likely have to recur to questionnaires; whereas a study relating micro-movements of arms and legs to concurrent ADHD symptoms over a short time period would combine several sensors on arms and legs with frequent ADHD symptom assessments.

Self-report questionnaires are still the most commonly used method for measuring activity due to their cost effective application and low participant burden. Several reviews give an overview of available measures in children and adolescents (62–65) and adults (66–68). However, several other reviews also stated concerns about the validity of self-reported activity for youth and adults without clinical diagnoses as for instance ADHD (63, 67–70). Despite mostly acceptable reliability, the validity of PA questionnaires is still low to moderate. However, the reviews identified several questionnaires that showed both good reliability and acceptable validity [e.g., FPACQ, Flemish physical activity computerized questionnaire (71); PDPAR, previous day physical activity recall (72); RPAR, recess physical activity recall (73)]. To sum up, given that the validity of self-report questionnaires is limited in youth and adults without ADHD, their validity and reliability is even more questionable in children, adolescents, and adults with ADHD. This is because problems with inattention and impulsivity interfere with accurately noticing, memorizing, and reporting activity in a questionnaire, making reliable and valid self-reports even less likely.

Sensor-based activity assessment with pedometers and accelerometers has gained popularity in research (74–76) and in everyday life over the past years. As activity sensors shrink in size and have increasingly lasting batteries, they have become widely used in activity research in children, adolescents, and adults without ADHD. Wearable sensors require some buy-in from participants, as they have to be trained how to wear them – over the hip bone, usually putting them on in the morning and taking them off at night and during water-based activities – and have to give them back at the end of the study. Pedometers often do not store wear time in addition to steps and thus miss an important confounding variable for analysis; whereas accelerometers record wear time so that it can be included in analyses. Standard cut offs for valid days are at least 10 h of daily wear time (76). Among the disadvantages of pedometers are that they miss acceleration and speed of movement that should be especially interesting for understanding hyperactivity. Among their many advantages, pedometers are affordable (i.e., participants can even keep them after the study enabling continued self-monitoring), and they allow within-person comparisons. Pedometers and accelerometers are useful for measuring habitual activity in everyday life that is hard to capture in questionnaires because it evades conscious attention. Accelerometers can record more fine-grained activity information (i.e., speed, timing of movement) that may be particularly relevant for the assessment of hyperactivity. They can also detect movement of arms and legs if worn on wrist and ankle. However, there are also disadvantages of accelerometers and pedometers: Most devices miss water-based activities (i.e., swimming) and underestimate activities that do not involve movement of the part of the body where the sensor is located, as for example rowing or cycling with an accelerometer worn at the hip (77).

Smart phones have built-in accelerometers and can be used to measure activity. However, their assessment is less precise because the phone is not consistently worn in the same position (e.g., hand, pocket, bag). In the same vein, GPS assessments can be used but again are less precise about micro-movements. Heart rate sensors provide a comprehensive method of measuring physical exertion that captures many activities, not only vertical movement. Other methods for determining activity, such as doubly labeled water, multichannel devices combining accelerometers with respiration rate, electrocardiography, or electromyography and direct observation are expensive and can be burdensome for participants and are therefore more frequently used in smaller studies within the lab.

So far, there are few studies that have used sensor-based activity assessments in children and adolescents – and even fewer in those with ADHD. Thus, particularly in individuals with ADHD the cut-off points and algorithms for counting a movement as motion and classifying activity are still being developed. However, children diagnosed with ADHD differ from those without ADHD in the amount and intensity of their movements, as has been shown with different techniques of measuring movements, such as motion tracking systems using infrared motion analysis [(78); see also Ref. (79) for the Qb test], parent and teacher rating scales (80), and accelerometers (2). This knowledge has been used to identify children with ADHD with moderate accuracy measuring their activity with accelerometers over a 2-hour period (2) and with good accuracy measuring activity for 24 h (81).

In addition to comparisons of the amount and intensity of PA over a prolonged period of time, more fine-grained analyses of movements could also be informative. Modern accelerometers provide the opportunity to obtain data measured at very high resolutions (milli-G) and at very small time intervals (100th of a second). This allows not only for a measurement of the amount of activity, but also of more detailed qualitative differences in activities. These differences can already be detected with rather short measurement times. For example, it is possible to distinguish different kinds of activities by analyzing raw accelerometer data [e.g., Ref. (82, 83)]. In these studies, accelerometer data were accurately classified into different kinds of activities using Support Vector Machines [SVMs (84, 85)]. SVMs are machine learning techniques that allow for the classification of data into different categories. The great advantage of SVMs for this purpose lies in their ability to deal with highly complex and non-linear associations between accelerometer data and the corresponding categories of activity. Therefore, SVMs are perfectly suited to classify subjects as either having or not having ADHD. In recent years, this has already been done with quite some success with the use of different kinds of data, such as EEG (86, 87), inertial measurement units [IMU (88)], and MRI data (89–91).

These considerations indicate that fine-grained data from modern accelerometers, analyzed with SVMs, could be beneficial in two respects. First, they could be used to accurately identify children with ADHD with relatively little effort, in terms of both time and money. Second, those characteristics of accelerometer data that prove to be useful for distinguishing participants with and without

ADHD could be further analyzed. By doing so, new insights about the nature of ADHD and hyperactivity could be obtained. These insights would go beyond the concept that was used in previous accelerometer studies on ADHD, namely that children with ADHD merely show higher amounts and intensities of activity. Hence, they could help to refine the concepts related to ADHD and hyperactivity (e.g., fidgeting, jitteriness), making them more objectively accessible, and less susceptible to subjective ratings.

MODIFYING ADHD AND ADHD RELATED SYMPTOMS

Vigorous PA interventions in general address several areas that are problematic for children, adolescents, and adults with ADHD. For instance, short- and long-term interventions for increasing vigorous PA have led to improved mood and improved executive functioning (i.e., neuropsychological functions as for instance inhibition, shifting/task-switching, working memory), especially to improved inhibition performance in children, adolescents, and adults (92–94). Hence, enhancing vigorous PA could be an important additional treatment option for children with ADHD, ameliorating both comorbid affective disorders and deficits in executive functioning without potential negative side effects. Children diagnosed with ADHD might particularly benefit from PA interventions treating ADHD symptoms and comorbid problems due to various reasons: (a) PA might improve children's emotional and social functioning in addition to having a positive effect on their cognitive functioning (95–97), (b) PA prevents health problems such as weight gain and obesity, which are common in children with ADHD due to impulsive behavior as for instance impulsive unhealthy snacking (98), (c) PA does not interact negatively with other therapy programs (e.g., medication with MPH, cognitive behavioral therapy), and (d) PA can easily be integrated into the everyday routine of children (e.g., in schools).

However, only few observational and single-case studies have reported improved attention and reduced hyperactivity (i.e., fidgetiness) in children with ADHD following regular PA sessions (99). Only recently, research investigated potential benefits of vigorous PA in children and adolescents with ADHD and found positive effects of various types of short- and long-term PA interventions on behavioral, (neuro-)cognitive, and comorbid symptoms associated with ADHD (99, 100). For instance, Medina et al. (101) examined the impact of running on a treadmill for 30 min in boys diagnosed with ADHD and showed improved sustained attention irrespective of medication use. More specifically, children improved on response time and vigilance in a Continuous Performance Test while decreasing in impulsivity after being physically active for 30 min. Tantillo et al. (102) tested the efficacy of treadmill walking versus quiet rest on the management of behavioral features of ADHD in 8- to 12-year-old children compared to matched comparison children. Improved motoric functions after exercise were found only in boys with ADHD. However, findings should be considered preliminary, as the sample size was rather small (i.e., 18 participants). Finally, Pontifex et al. (103) found that a single 20-min bout of exercise (i.e., again treadmill running) improved inhibitory performance and neurocognitive functions (i.e., EEG measures) in children with ADHD in particular.

Regarding long-term PA, Gapin and Etnier (99) found that higher levels of PA as measured by accelerometers were associated with better executive function performance in 18 boys with ADHD. Moderate-to-vigorous PA predicted the performance on the Tower of London planning task and was positively associated with other executive function measures. In a randomized study, Verret et al. (104) tested the effects of a moderate- to high-intensity PA program on fitness, cognitive functioning, and ADHD symptoms over 10 weeks in 21 children diagnosed with ADHD. Children in the treatment group showed better information processing and parents reported fewer attention problems as well as a lower total number of problems at follow-up than at baseline compared to children in the control group. In a pilot study, Smith et al. (105) investigated a daily 26-min continuous moderate-to-vigorous PA program before school that lasted for 8 weeks and found positive effects on inattention, hyperactive, and impulsive symptoms in children with ADHD: Response inhibition improved following the program, and ratings by parents, teachers, and program staff indicated overall improvements of motor, cognitive, and behavioral functioning in two thirds of participating children. Jensen and Kenny (106) randomly assigned 19 boys with ADHD stabilized on medication to a 20-session yoga group or a control group with cooperative activities. Both groups improved in hyperactive and impulsive behavior and the global DSM evaluation of ADHD. However, yoga decreased oppositional, restless, and impulsive behavior, and those in the yoga group who engaged in more home practice showed greater improvement for attention and affective lability.

The aforementioned studies demonstrate potential positive effects of PA interventions in children with ADHD. However, all studies are clearly underpowered and replication studies are warranted. Moreover, this claim for replication studies is underscored by a recent meta-analysis investigating the effects of acute bouts of PA in children with ADHD in laboratory and field studies, which revealed inconclusive results (107). Some laboratory studies found significant improvements on cognitive tasks (i.e., tasks measuring visual attention referring to symptomatic attention problems in ADHD and executive functions referring to underlying cognitive deficits in ADHD). One laboratory study (108) found a significant improvement in response times in a visual attention task, one study showed a maintenance of accuracy (109), and three studies showed a significant reduction of error rates but no influence on response times (103, 110, 111).

The meta-analysis also revealed that with respect to school settings, no effects of PA (i.e., as implemented in so called active lessons) on dependent variables such as measures of attention could be found. However, subgroups as elementary school children (112) seem to benefit from PA interventions. This is important because in this age group ADHD diagnoses are given frequently compared to other age groups. Furthermore, specific sports and activities as for instance coordinative exercises seem to be particularly helpful (113).

Thus, direct positive effects of acute and chronic PA interventions on ADHD symptomatic behavior including hyperactivity seem to be possible. Still, there is scarce research revealing heterogeneous results. An important research question that is still unanswered is whether there is a direct route of improving ADHD symptoms (i.e., hyperactivity) via PA or an indirect route improving for example executive function deficits leading to a subsequent improvement of ADHD symptoms. In the same vein it might also be the case that comorbid emotional deficits as for instance affective lability shown by children and adolescents with ADHD is altered via PA interventions leading to subsequent improvement of core ADHD symptoms (i.e., hyperactivity). More specifically, ADHD and affective problems are common co-morbidities in youths (114) and it might be the case that PA interventions target those affective problems and not the ADHD symptoms *per se*.

The association between vigorous PA and improved affect is well established and PA interventions have been shown to have positive effects on affect in healthy adults (115). While there is empirical evidence that children and adolescents accrue mental health benefits from PA interventions in general [e.g., Ref. (96)], until now, the specific link between physical activities and affect among children and adolescents has only been investigated in a few studies (116). A 10-year longitudinal study suggests that during adolescence, changes in leisure-time PA and negative affect are related inversely, that is, decreasing levels of PA are correlated with a rising prevalence of negative affect (117). In the same vein, a meta-analysis of studies investigating the depression-reducing effects of vigorous PA interventions on children and adolescents revealed effects in favor of the physically active group (118). Thus, vigorous PA is associated with lower levels of negative affect in children, adolescents, and adults in observational studies and randomized controlled trials.

Concretely, three studies have addressed the effects of PA on affective symptoms shown by children with ADHD so far. Jensen and Kenny (106) randomly assigned medicated boys with ADHD to a 20-session yoga condition or a control condition with cooperative leisure activities. Children in both conditions showed improvement in hyperactive and impulsive behaviors and in the global DSM evaluation of ADHD. Yoga decreased oppositional, restless, and impulsive behavior, and the children in the yoga condition who engaged in more home practicing of yoga showed greater improvement in attention and emotional stability. Kiluk et al. (119) found that participation in PA predicted less severe anxiety and depression in children with ADHD. Scores on parental reports of affect and behavior indicated that children with ADHD who participated in three or more sports displayed fewer symptoms of anxiety and depression compared to those children with ADHD who participated in fewer than three sports. Verret et al. (104) found in their exploratory but randomized study that teachers reported lower anxiety-depression scores and fewer social problems in children with ADHD after a 10-week PA program. In summary, PA interventions appear to improve not only executive functioning but also negative affect in children with and without ADHD.

SUMMARY

A bifactor model that represents a general ADHD symptom factor as well as independent specific symptom factors seems to be the best model to characterize the disorder. With regard to measuring hyperactivity as one of the ADHD symptoms only few studies have used sensor-based activity assessments in children and adolescents with ADHD. However, fine-grained accelerometer data analyzed with SVMs could potentially be useful to distinguish children with hyperactivity symptoms from those showing no hyperactivity symptoms. Moreover, further studies might also want to investigate the influence of medication (with MPH and Atomoxetine) and cognitive behavioral therapy on accelerometer data analyzed with SVMs. This is important because results could potentially inform about optimal treatments for individual children (i.e., tailored therapy). In order to gain further insight into the usefulness of PA interventions for children with motoric activity and hyperactivity as in children with diagnosed ADHD, it is important to investigate effects of PA regarding several aspects. First, the effects of everyday PA (i.e., biking to school, active lessons in school) and organized, structured sports need to be disentangled. Second, the dose–response relationship is in the need of being investigated: How often and for how long should children with ADHD take part in physical activities to receive an optimal level of their symptomatic behavior (i.e., fidgetiness in school). Third, interactions of medication with MPH or Atomoxetine and PA are understudied as well.

ACKNOWLEDGMENTS

The preparation of this paper was partly funded by the federal state government of Hesse (LOEWE initiative). We acknowledge support from Deutsche Forschungsgemeinschaft and Open Access Publishing Fund of Tuebingen University.

REFERENCES

1. American Psychiatric Association. *Diagnostic and Statistical Manual of Mental Disorders*. 5th ed. Arlington, VA: American Psychiatric Publishing (2013).
2. Wood AC, Asherson P, Rijsdijk F, Kuntsi J. Is overactivity a core feature in ADHD? Familial and receiver operating characteristic curve analysis of mechanically assessed activity level. *J Am Acad Child Adolesc Psychiatry* (2009) **48**:1023–30. doi:10.1097/CHI.0b013e3181b54612
3. Yoon SYR, Jain U, Shapiro C. Sleep in ADHD in children and adults: past present, and future. *Sleep Med Rev* (2012) **16**:371–88. doi:10.1016/j.smrv.2011.07.001
4. Cook BG, Li D, Heintrich KM. Obesity, physical activity, and sedentary behavior of youth with learning disabilities and ADHD. *J Learn Disabil* (2014). doi:10.1177/0022219413518582
5. Anderson SE, Cohen P, Naumova EN, Must A. Association of depression and anxiety disorders with weight change in a prospective community-based study of children followed up into adulthood. *Arch Pediatr Adolesc Med* (2006) **160**(3):285. doi:10.1001/archpedi.160.3.285
6. Davis C, Levitan R, Smith M, Tweed M, Curtis C. Association among overeating, overweight, and attention deficit/hyperactivity disorder: a structural equations modeling approach. *Eat Behav* (2006) **7**:266–74. doi:10.1016/j.eatbeh.2005.09.006
7. Kim J, Mutyala B, Agiovlasitis S, Fernhall B. Health behaviors and obesity among US children with attention deficit hyperactivity disorder by gender and medication use. *Prev Med* (2011) **52**(3–4):218–22. doi:10.1016/j.ypmed.2011.01.003
8. Gawrilow C, Stadler G, Langguth N, Naumann A, Boeck A. Physical activity, affect, and cognition in children with symptoms of attention deficit hyperactivity disorder. *J Atten Disord* (2013). doi:10.1177/1087054713493318
9. Polanczyk G, de Lima MS, Horta BL, Biederman J, Rohde LA. The worldwide prevalence of ADHD: a systematic review and metaregression analysis. *Am J Psychiatry* (2007) **164**(6):942–8. doi:10.1176/appi.ajp.164.6.942
10. Van der Meere J. The role of attention. In: Sandberg S, editor. *Monographs on Child and Adolescent Psychiatry* Second Edition. Cambridge: University Press (2002). p. 162–213.
11. Van der Meere J. State regulation and attention deficit hyperactivity disorder. In: Gozal D, Molfese DL, editors. *Attention Deficit Hyperactivity Disorder: from Genes to Patients*. Totawa: Humana Press Inc (2005). p. 162–213.
12. Sanders AF. Towards a model of stress and performance. *Acta Psychol* (1983) **53**:61–97. doi:10.1016/0001-6918(83)90016-1

13. Sanders AF, van Duren LL. Stimulus control of visual fixation duration in a single saccade paradigm. *Acta Psychol* (1998) **99**:163–76. doi:10.1016/S0001-6918(98)00009-2
14. Sonuga-Barke EJS. Interval length and time-use by children with AD/HD: a comparison of four models. *Journal of Abnormal Child Psychology* (2002) **30**(3):257–64.
15. Van der Meere J, Vreeling H, Sergeant J. A motor presetting study in hyperactive, learning disabled and control children. *J Child Psychol Psychiatry* (1992) **33**(8):1347–54. doi:10.1111/j.1469-7610.1992.tb00954.x
16. Scheres A, Oosterlaan J, Sergeant JA. Response execution and inhibition in children with AD/HD and other disruptive disorders: the role of behavioural activation. *J Child Psychol Psychiatry* (2001) **42**(3):347–57. doi:10.1111/1469-7610.00728
17. Nigg JT, Goldsmith HH, Sachek J. Temperament and attention deficit hyperactivity disorder: the development of a multiple pathway model. *J Clin Child Adolesc Psychol* (2004) **33**(1):42–53. doi:10.1207/S15374424JCCP3301_5
18. Sonuga-Barke EJS. The dual pathway model of AD/HD: an elaboration of neuro-developmental characteristics. *Neurosci Biobehav Rev* (2003) **27**(7):593–604. doi:10.1016/j.neubiorev.2003.08.005
19. Sonuga-Barke EJS, Bitsakou P, Thompson M. Beyond the dual pathway model: evidence for the dissociation of timing, inhibitory, and delay-related impairments in attention-deficit/hyperactivity disorder. *J Am Acad Child Adolesc Psychiatry* (2010) **49**(4):345–55. doi:10.1097/00004583-201004000-00009
20. Chen FF, West S, Sousa K. A comparison of bifactor and second-order models of quality of life. *Multivariate Behav Res* (2006) **41**(2):189–225. doi:10.1207/s15327906mbr4102_5
21. Barkley RA. *Defiant Children: A Clinician's Manual for Assessment and Parent Training*. New York: Guilford Press (1997).
22. Wilbertz G, Trueg A, Sonuga-Barke EJ, Blechert J, Philipsen A, van Elst L. Neural and psychophysiological markers of delay aversion in attention-deficit hyperactivity disorder. *J Abnorm Psychol* (2013) **122**:566–72. doi:10.1037/a0031924
23. Sonuga-Barke EJS. On dysfunction and function in psychological accounts of childhood disorder. *J Child Psychol Psychiatry* (1994) **42**:199–210.
24. Sagvolden T, Johansen EB, Aase H, Russell VA. A dynamic developmental theory of attention-deficit/hyperactivity disorder (ADHD) predominantly hyperactive/impulsive and combined subtypes. *Behav Brain Sci* (2005) **28**(3):397–419. doi:10.1017/S0140525X05000075
25. Bauermeister J, Bird H, Canino G, Rubio-Stipec M, Bravo M, Alegría M. Dimensions of attention deficit hyperactivity disorder: findings from teacher and parent reports in a community sample. *J Clin Child Psychol* (1995) **24**(3):264–71. doi:10.1207/s15374424jccp2403_3
26. DuPaul GJ, Anastopoulos AD, Power TJ, Reid R, Ikeda MJ, McGoey KE. Parent ratings of attention-deficit/hyperactivity disorder symptoms: factor structure and normative data. *J Psychopathol Behav Assess* (1998) **20**(1):83–102. doi:10.1023/A:1023087410712
27. Lahey B, Pelham W, Schaughency EA, Atkins MS, Murphy HA, Hynd G, et al. Dimensions and types of attention deficit disorder. *J Am Acad Child Adolesc Psychiatry* (1988) **27**(3):330–5. doi:10.1097/00004583-198805000-00011
28. Gibbins C, Toplak ME, Flora DB, Weiss MD, Tannock R. Evidence for a general factor model of ADHD in adults. *J Atten Disord* (2012) **16**(8):635–44. doi:10.1177/1087054711416310
29. Bauermeister J, Alegría M, Bird HR, Rubio-Stipec M, Canino G. Are attentional-hyperactivity deficits unidimensional or multidimensional syndromes? Empirical findings from a community survey. *J Am Acad Child Adolesc Psychiatry* (1992) **31**(3):423–31. doi:10.1097/00004583-199205000-00007
30. Burns GL, Boe B, Walsh JA, Sommers-Flanagan R, Teegarden LA. A confirmatory factor analysis on the DSM-IV ADHD and ODD symptoms: what is the best model for the organization of these symptoms? *J Abnorm Child Psychol* (2001) **29**(4):339–49. doi:10.1023/A:1010314030025
31. Collett BR. The factor structure of DSM-IV attention deficit-hyperactivity symptoms: a confirmatory factor analysis of the ADHD-SRS. *J Psychoeduc Assess* (2000) **18**(4):361–73. doi:10.1177/073428290001800406
32. Glutting JJ, Youngstrom EA, Watkins MW. ADHD and college students: exploratory and confirmatory factor structures with student and parent data. *Psychol Assess* (2005) **17**(1):44–55. doi:10.1037/1040-3590.17.1.44
33. Gomez R, Harvey J, Quick C, Scharer I, Harris G. DSM-IV AD/HD: confirmatory factor models, prevalence, and gender and age differences based on parent and teacher ratings of Australian primary school children. *J Child Psychol Psychiatry* (1999) **40**(2):265–74. doi:10.1111/1469-7610.00440
34. Span SA, Earleywine M, Strybel TZ. Confirming the factor structure of attention deficit hyperactivity disorder symptoms in adult, nonclinical samples. *J Psychopathol Behav Assess* (2002) **24**(2):129–36. doi:10.1023/A:1015396926356
35. Rohde LA, Barbosa G, Polanczyk G, Eizirik M, Rasmussen ER, Neuman RJ, et al. Factor and latent class analysis of DSM-IV ADHD symptoms in a school sample of Brazilian adolescents. *J Am Acad Child Adolesc Psychiatry* (2001) **40**(6):711–8. doi:10.1097/00004583-200106000-00017
36. Molina BS, Smith BH, Pelham WE. Factor structure and criterion validity of secondary school teacher ratings of ADHD and ODD. *J Abnorm Child Psychol* (2001) **29**(1):71–82. doi:10.1023/A:1005203629968
37. Wolraich M, Lambert E. Teachers' screening for attention deficit/hyperactivity disorder: comparing multinational samples on teacher ratings of ADHD. *J Abnorm Child Psychol* (2003) **31**(4):445–55. doi:10.1023/A:1023847719796
38. Pillow DR, Pelham WE, Hoza B, Molina BS, Stultz CH. Confirmatory factor analyses examining attention deficit hyperactivity disorder symptoms and other childhood disruptive behaviors. *J Abnorm Child Psychol* (1998) **26**(4):293–309. doi:10.1023/A:1022658618368
39. Ullebø AK, Breivik K, Gillberg C, Lundervold AJ, Posserud M-B. The factor structure of ADHD in a general population of primary school children. *J Child Psychol Psychiatry* (2012) **53**(9):927–36. doi:10.1111/j.1469-7610.2012.02549.x
40. Caci HM, Morin AJ, Tran A. Teacher ratings of the ADHD-RS IV in a community sample: results from the ChiP-ARD study. *J Atten Disord* (2013). doi:10.1177/1087054712473834
41. Dumenci L, McConaughy SH, Achenbach TM. A hierarchical three-factor model of inattention-hyperactivity–impulsivity derived from the attention problems syndrome of the teacher's report form. *School Psych Rev* (2004) **33**(2):287–301.
42. Gomez R, Vance A, Gomez RM. Validity of the ADHD bifactor model in general community samples of adolescents and adults, and a clinic-referred sample of children and adolescents. *J Atten Disord* (2013). doi:10.1177/1087054713480034
43. Martel MM, von Eye A, Nigg JT. Revisiting the latent structure of ADHD: is there a "g" factor? *J Child Psychol Psychiatry* (2010) **51**(8):905–14. doi:10.1111/j.1469-7610.2010.02232.x
44. Martel MM, von Eye A, Nigg J. Developmental differences in structure of attention-deficit/hyperactivity disorder (ADHD) between childhood and adulthood. *Int J Behav Dev* (2012) **36**(4):279–92. doi:10.1177/0165025412444077
45. Morin AJS, Tran A, Caci H. Factorial validity of the ADHD adult symptom rating scale in a French community sample: results from the ChiP-ARD study. *J Atten Disord* (2013). doi:10.1177/1087054713488825
46. Normand S, Flora DB, Toplak ME, Tannock R. Evidence for a general ADHD factor from a longitudinal general school population study. *J Abnorm Child Psychol* (2012) **40**(4):555–67. doi:10.1007/s10802-011-9584-5
47. Toplak ME, Pitch A, Flora DB, Iwenofu L, Ghelani K, Jain U, et al. The unity and diversity of inattention and hyperactivity/impulsivity in ADHD: evidence for a general factor with separable dimensions. *J Abnorm Child Psychol* (2009) **37**(8):1137–50. doi:10.1007/s10802-009-9336-y
48. Toplak ME, Sorge GB, Flora DB, Chen W, Banaschewski T, Buitelaar J, et al. The hierarchical factor model of ADHD: invariant across age and national groupings? *J Child Psychol Psychiatry* (2012) **53**(3):292–303. doi:10.1111/j.1469-7610.2011.02500.x
49. Faraone SV, Biederman J, Mick E. The age-dependent decline of attention deficit hyperactivity disorder: a meta-analysis of follow-up studies. *Psychol Med* (2006) **36**(2):159–65. doi:10.1017/S003329170500471X
50. Lahey B, Pelham W, Loney J, Lee SS, Willcutt E. Instability of the DSM-IV subtypes of ADHD from preschool through elementary school. *Arch Gen Psychiatry* (2005) **62**:896–902. doi:10.1001/archpsyc.62.8.896
51. Greven CU, Asherson P, Rijsdijk FV, Plomin R. A longitudinal twin study on the association between inattentive and hyperactive-impulsive ADHD symptoms. *J Abnorm Child Psychol* (2011) **39**(5):623–32. doi:10.1007/s10802-011-9513-7
52. McLoughlin G, Ronald A, Kuntsi J, Asherson P, Plomin R. Genetic support for the dual nature of attention deficit hyperactivity disorder: substantial genetic overlap between the inattentive and hyperactive-impulsive components. *J Abnorm Child Psychol* (2007) **35**(6):999–1008. doi:10.1007/s10802-007-9149-9
53. Frazier-Wood AC, Rommel AS, Kuntsi J. Attention deficit hyperactivity disorder: insight from quantitative genetic research. In: Rhee SH, Ronald A,

editors. *Behavior Genetics of Psychopathology*, Vol. 1. New York: Springer (2014). p. 1–32. doi:10.1007/978-1-4614-9509-3_1
54. Martel M, Nikolas M, Nigg JT. Executive function in adolescents with ADHD. *J Am Acad Child Adolesc Psychiatry* (2007) **46**(11):1437–44. doi:10.1097/chi.0b013e31814cf953
55. Riddle MA, Yershova K, Lazzaretto D, Paykina N, Yenokyan G, Greenhill L, et al. the preschool attention-deficit/hyperactivity disorder treatment study (PATS) 6-year follow-up. *J Am Acad Child Adolesc Psychiatry* (2013) **52**(3):264.e–78.e. doi:10.1016/j.jaac.2012.12.007
56. Larsson H, Dilshad R, Lichtenstein P, Barker ED. Developmental trajectories of DSM-IV symptoms of attention-deficit/hyperactivity disorder: genetic effects, family risk and associated psychopathology. *J Child Psychol Psychiatry* (2011) **52**(9):954–63. doi:10.1111/j.1469-7610.2011.02379.x
57. Kessler R, Green J. Structure and diagnosis of adult attention-deficit/ hyperactivity disorder: analysis of expanded symptom criteria from the adult ADHD clinical diagnostic scale. *Arch Gen Psychiatry* (2010) **67**(11):1168–78. doi:10.1001/archgenpsychiatry.2010.146
58. Gamble KL, May RS, Besing RC, Tankersly AP, Fargasaon RE. Delayed sleep timing and symptoms in adults with ADHD: a controlled actigraphy study. *Chronobiol Int* (2013) **30**:598–606. doi:10.3109/07420528.2012.754454
59. Biederman J, Mick E, Faraone SV. Age-dependent decline of symptoms of attention deficit hyperactivity disorder: impact of remission definition and symptom type. *Am J Psychiatry* (2000) **157**(5):816–8. doi:10.1176/appi.ajp.157.5.816
60. Millstein RB, Wilens TE, Biederman J, Spencer TJ. Presenting ADHD symptoms and subtypes in clinically referred adults with ADHD. *J Atten Disord* (1997) **2**(3):159–66. doi:10.4088/JCP.08m04785pur
61. Troiano RP. Large-scale applications of accelerometers: new frontiers and new questions. *Med Sci Sports Exerc* (2007) **39**(9):1501. doi:10.1097/mss.0b013e318150d42e
62. Adamo KB, Prince SA, Tricco AC, Connor-Gorber S, Tremblay M. A comparison of indirect versus direct measures for assessing physical activity in the pediatric population: a systematic review. *Int J Pediatr Obes* (2009) **4**:2–27. doi:10.1080/17477160802315010
63. Chinapaw MJ, Mokkink LB, van Poppel MN, van Mechelen W, Terwee CB. Physical activity questionnaires for youth: a systematic review of measurement properties. *Sports Med* (2010) **40**:539–63. doi:10.2165/11530770-000000000-00000
64. Kohl HW, Fulton JE, Caspersen CJ. Assessment of physical activity among children and adolescents: a review and synthesis. *Prev Med* (2000) **31**:54–76. doi:10.1006/pmed.1999.0542
65. Oliver M, Schofield GM, Kolt GS. Physical activity in preschoolers: understanding prevalence and measurement issues. *Sports Med* (2007) **37**:1045–70. doi:10.2165/00007256-200737120-00004
66. Pereira MA, Fitzergerald SJ, Gregg EW, Joswiak ML, Ryan WJ, Suminski RR, et al. A collection of physical activity questionnaires for health-related research. *Med Sci Sports Exerc* (1997) **29**:S1–205.
67. Helmerhorst HJ, Brage S, Warren J, Besson H, Ekelund U. A systematic review of reliability and objective criterion-related validity of physical activity questionnaires. *Int J Behav Nutr Phys Act* (2012) **9**(1):1–55. doi:10.1186/1479-5868-9-103
68. Van Poppel MN, Chinapaw MJ, Mokkink LB, van Mechelen W, Terwee CB. Physical activity questionnaires for adults: a systematic review of measurement properties. *Sports Med* (2010) **40**:565–600. doi:10.2165/11531930-000000000-00000
69. Prince SA, Adamo KB, Hamel ME, Hardt J, Gorber SC, Tremblay M. A comparison of direct versus self-report measures for assessing physical activity in adults: a systematic review. *Int J Behav Nutr Phys Act* (2008) **5**:56–80. doi:10.1186/1479-5868-5-56
70. Sallis JF, Saelens BE. Assessment of physical activity by self report: status, limitations, and future directions. *Res Q Exerc Sport* (2000) **71**:1–14.
71. Matton L, Wijndaele K, Duvigneaud N, Duquet W, Philippaerts R, Thomis M, et al. Reliability and validity of the Flemish physical activity computerized questionnaire in adults. *Res Q Exerc Sport* (2007) **78**:293–306. doi:10.1080/02701367.2007.10599427
72. Allor KM, Pivarnik JM. Stability and convergent validity of three physical activity assessments. *Med Sci Sports Exerc* (2001) **33**:671–6. doi:10.1097/00005768-200104000-00025
73. Martinez-Gomez D, Calabro MA, Welk GJ, Marcos A, Veiga OL. Reliability and validity of a school recess physical activity recall in Spanish youth. *Pediatr Exerc Sci* (2010) **22**:218–30.
74. Baptista F, Santos DA, Silva AM, Mota J, Santos R, Vale S, et al. Prevalence of the portuguese population attaining sufficient physical activity. *Med Sci Sports Exerc* (2012) **44**:466–73. doi:10.1249/MSS.0b013e318230e441
75. Hansen BH, Kolle E, Dyrstad SM, Holme I, Anderssen SA. Accelerometer-determined physical activity in adults and older people. *Med Sci Sports Exerc* (2012) **44**:266–72. doi:10.1249/MSS.0b013e31822cb354
76. Troiano RP, Berrigan D, Dodd KW, Masse LC, Tilert T, McDowell M. Physical activity in the United States measured by accelerometer. *Med Sci Sports Exerc* (2008) **40**:181–8. doi:10.1249/mss.0b013e31815a51b3
77. Trost SG, McIver KL, Pate RR. Conducting accelerometer-based activity assessments in field-based research. *Med Sci Sports Exerc* (2005) **37**(11):531–43. doi:10.1249/01.mss.0000185657.86065.98
78. Teicher MH, Ito Y, Glod CA, Barber NI. Objective measurement of hyperactivity and attentional problems in ADHD. *J Am Acad Child Adolesc Psychiatry* (1996) **35**:334–42. doi:10.1097/00004583-199603000-00015
79. Ramtvedt BE, Roinas E, Aabech HS, Sundet KS. Clinical gains from including both dextroamphetamine and methylphenidate in stimulant trials. *J Child Adolesc Psychopharmacol* (2013) **23**:597–604. doi:10.1089/cap.2012.0085
80. Tseng W-L, Kawabata Y, Gau SS-F, Crick NR. Symptoms of ADHD and peer functioning: a transactional model of development. *J Abnorm Child Psychol* (2014) **42**:1353–65. doi:10.1007/s10802-014-9883-8
81. Martín-Martínez D, Casaseca-de-la-Higuera P, Alberola-López S, Andrés-de-Llano J, López-Villalobos JA, Ardura-Fernández J, et al. Nonlinear analysis of actigraphic signals for the assessment of the attention-deficit/hyperactivity disorder (ADHD). *Med Eng Phys* (2012) **34**(9):1317–29. doi:10.1016/j.medengphy.2011.12.023
82. He Z, Jin L. *Activity Recognition from Acceleration Data Based on Discrete Cosine Transform and SVM*. San Antonio, TX: Proceedings of the IEEE International Conference on systems, man, and Cybernetics – SMC 2009 (2009).
83. Kühnhausen J, Leonhardt A, Dirk J, Schmiedek F. Physical activity and affect in elementary school children's daily lives. *Front Psychol* (2013) **4**:456. doi:10.3389/fpsyg.2013.00456
84. Boser BE, Guyon IM, Vapnik VN. A training algorithm for optimal margin classifiers. In: Haussler D, editor. *Proceedings of the 5th Annual ACM Workshop on Computational Learning Theory COLT'92*. Pittsburgh, PA: ACM Press (1992). p. 144–52.
85. Cortes C, Vapnik VN. Support-vector networks. *Mach Learn* (1995) **20**:273–97. doi:10.1023/A:1022627411411
86. Abibullaev B, An J. Decision support algorithm for diagnosis of ADHD using electroencephalograms. *J Med Syst* (2012) **36**:2675–88. doi:10.1007/s10916-011-9742-x
87. Mueller A, Candrian G, Kropotov JD, Ponomarev VA, Baschera GM. Classification of ADHD patients on the basis of independent ERP components using a machine learning system. *Nonlinear Biomed Phys* (2010) **4**(Suppl 1):S1. doi:10.1186/1753-4631-4-S1-S1
88. O'Mahony N, Florentino-Liano B, Carballo JJ, Baca-García E, Rodríguez AA. Objective diagnosis of ADHD using IMUs. *Med Eng Phys* (2014) **36**:922–6. doi:10.1016/j.medengphy.2014.02.023
89. Chang CW, Ho CC, Chen JH. ADHD classification by a texture analysis of anatomical brain MRI data. *Front Syst Neurosci* (2012) **6**:66. doi:10.3389/fnsys.2012.00066
90. Colby JB, Rudie JD, Brown JA, Douglas PK, Cohen MS, Shehzad Z. Insights into multimodal imaging classification of ADHD. *Front Syst Neurosci* (2012) **6**:59. doi:10.3389/fnsys.2012.00059
91. Johnston BA, Mwangi B, Matthews K, Coghill D, Konrad K, Steele JD. Brainstem abnormalities in attention deficit hyperactivity disorder support high accuracy individual diagnostic classification. *Hum Brain Mapp* (2014) **35**:5179–89. doi:10.1002/hbm.22542
92. Barenberg J, Berse T, Dutke S. Executive functions in learning processes: do they benefit from physical activity? *Educ Res Rev* (2011) **6**:208–22. doi:10.1016/j.edurev.2011.04.002
93. Best JR. Effects of physical activity on children's executive function: contributions of experimental research on aerobic exercise. *Dev Rev* (2010) **30**:331–51. doi:10.1016/j.dr.2010.08.001

94. Colcombe S, Kramer AF. Fitness effects on the cognitive function of older adults: a meta-analytic study. *Psychol Sci* (2003) **14**:125–30. doi:10.1111/1467-9280.t01-1-01430
95. Ahn S, Feweda AL. A meta-analysis of the relationship between children's physical activity and mental health. *J Pediatr Psychol* (2011) **36**:385–97. doi:10.1093/jpepsy/jsq107
96. Biddle SJH, Asare M. Physical activity and mental health in children and adolescents: a review of reviews. *Br J Sports Med* (2011) **45**:886–95. doi:10.1136/bjsports-2011-090185
97. Dunn AL, Weintraub P. Exercise in the prevention and treatment of adolescent depression: a promising but little researched intervention. *Am J Lifestyle Med* (2008) **2**(6):1–12. doi:10.1177/1559827608323225
98. Cortese S, Angriman M, Maffeis C, Isnard P, Konofal E, Lecendreux M, et al. Attention – deficit/hyperactivity disorder (ADHD) and obesity: a systematic review of the literature. *Crit Rev Food Sci Nutr* (2008) **48**:524–37. doi:10.1080/10408390701540124
99. Gapin JI, Etnier JL. The relationship between physical activity and executive function performance in children with attention-deficit hyperactivity disorder. *J Sport Exerc Psychol* (2010) **32**:753–63.
100. Gapin JI, Labban JD, Etnier JL. The effects of physical activity on attention deficit hyperactivity disorder symptoms: the evidence. *Prev Med* (2011) **52**:S70–4. doi:10.1016/j.ypmed.2011.01.022
101. Medina JA, Netto TL, Muszkat M, Medina AC, Botter D, Orbetelli R, et al. Exercise impact on sustained attention of ADHD children, methylphenidate effects. *Atten Defic Hyperact Disord* (2010) **2**(1):49–58. doi:10.1007/s12402-009-0018-y
102. Tantillo M, Kesick CM, Hynd GW, Dishman RK. The effects of exercise on children with attention-deficit hyperactivity disorder. *Med Sci Sports Exerc* (2002) **34**(2):203–12. doi:10.1097/00005768-200202000-00004
103. Pontifex MB, Saliba BJ, Raine LB, Picchietti DL, Hillman CH. Exercise improves behavioral, neurocognitive, and scholastic performance in children with attention-deficit/hyperactivity disorder. *J Pediatr* (2013) **162**:543–51. doi:10.1016/j.jpeds.2012.08.036
104. Verret C, Guay M-C, Berthiaume C, Gardiner P, Béliveau L. A physical activity program improves behavior and cognitive functions in children with ADHD: an exploratory study. *J Atten Disord* (2012) **16**:71–80. doi:10.1177/1087054710379735
105. Smith AL, Hoza B, Linnea K, McQuade JD, Tomb M, Vaughn AJ, et al. Pilot physical activity intervention reduces severity of ADHD symptoms in young children. *J Atten Disord* (2013) **17**:70. doi:10.1177/1087054711417395
106. Jensen PS, Kenny DT. The effects of yoga on the attention and behavior of boys with attention-deficit/hyperactivity disorder (ADHD). *J Atten Disord* (2004) **7**:205–16. doi:10.1177/108705470400700403
107. Janssen M, Toussaint HM, van Mechelen W, Verhagen EA. Effects of acute bouts of physical activity on children's attention: a systematic review of the literature. *Springerplus* (2014) **3**:410. doi:10.1186/2193-1801-3-410
108. Cereatti L, Casella R, Manganelli M, Pesce C. Visual attention in adolescents: facilitating effects of sport expertise and acute physical exercise. *Psychol Sport Exerc* (2009) **10**:136–45. doi:10.1016/j.psychsport.2008.05.002
109. Drollette ES, Shishido T, Pontifex MB, Hillman CH. Maintenance of cognitive control during and after walking in preadolescent children. *Med Sci Sports Exerc* (2012) **44**(10):2017–24. doi:10.1249/MSS.0b013e318258bcd5
110. Hillman CH, Pontifex MB, Raine LB, Castelli DM, Hall EE, Kramer AF. The effect of acute treadmill walking on cognitive control and academic achievement in preadolescent children. *Neuroscience* (2009) **159**(3):1044–54. doi:10.1016/j.neuroscience.2009.01.057
111. Drollette ES, Scudder MR, Raine LB, Moore RD, Saliba BJ, Pontifex MB, et al. Acute exercise facilitates brain function and cognition in children who need it most: an ERP study of individual differences in inhibitory control capacity. *Dev Cogn Neurosci* (2014) **7**:53–64. doi:10.1016/j.dcn.2013.11.001
112. Caterino MC, Polak ED. Effects of two types of activity on the performance of second-, third-, and fourth-grade students on a test of concentration. *Percept Mot Skills* (1999) **89**(1):245–8. doi:10.2466/pms.1999.89.1.245
113. Budde H, Voelcker-Rehage C, Pietrabyk-Kendziorra S, Ribeiro P, Tidow G. Acute coordinative exercise improves attentional performance in adolescents. *Neurosci Lett* (2008) **441**(2):219–23. doi:10.1016/j.neulet.2008.06.024
114. Biederman J, Ball SW, Monuteaux MC, Mick E, Spencer TJ, McCreary M, et al. (2008). New insights into the comorbidity between ADHD and major depression in adolescent and young adult females. *J Am Acad Child Adolesc Psychiatry* **47**:426–34. doi:10.1097/CHI.0b013e31816429d3
115. Conn VS. Depressive symptom outcomes of physical activity interventions: meta-analysis findings. *Ann Behav Med* **39**:128–38. doi:10.1007/s12160-010-9172-x
116. Dunton GF, Whalen CK, Jamner LD, Henker B, Floro JN. Using ecologic momentary assessment to measure physical activity during adolescence. *Am J Prev Med* (2005) **29**:281–7. doi:10.1016/j.amepre.2005.07.020
117. Nader PR, Bradley RH, Houts RM, McRitchie SL, O'Brien M. Moderate-to-vigorous physical activity from ages 9 to 15 years. *J Am Med Assoc* (2008) **300**:295–305. doi:10.1001/jama.300.3.295
118. Larun L, Nordheim LV, Ekeland E, Hagen KB, Heian F. Exercise in prevention and treatment of anxiety and depression among children and young people. *Cochrane Database Syst Rev* (2006) **3**:CD004691. doi:10.1002/14651858.CD004691.pub2
119. Kiluk BD, Weden S, Culotta VP. Sport participation and anxiety in children with ADHD. *J Atten Disord* (2009) **12**:499–506. doi:10.1177/1087054708320400

21

Motion and emotion: depression reduces psychomotor performance and alters affective movements in caregiving interactions

Katherine S. Young[1,2,3†], *Christine E. Parsons*[1,2†], *Alan Stein*[1] *and Morten L. Kringelbach*[1,2]*

[1] Department of Psychiatry, Warneford Hospital, Oxford, UK
[2] MindLab/Center of Functionally Integrative Neuroscience (CFIN), Aarhus University, Aarhus, Denmark
[3] Department of Psychology, University of California, Los Angeles (UCLA), Los Angeles, USA

Edited by:
Raymond C. K. Chan, Institute of Psychology, Chinese Academy of Sciences, China

Reviewed by:
Marian Bakermans-Kranenburg, Leiden University, Netherlands
Sebastian Herbert Scharf, F. Hoffmann-La Roche Ltd, Switzerland

***Correspondence:**
Morten L. Kringelbach, Department of Psychiatry, Warneford Hospital, Oxford OX3 7JX, UK
e-mail: morten.kringelbach@psych.ox.ac.uk

† These authors have contributed equally to this work.

Background: Impaired social functioning is a well-established feature of depression. Evidence to date suggests that disrupted processing of emotional cues may constitute part of this impairment. Beyond processing of emotional cues, fluent social interactions require that people physically move in synchronized, contingent ways. Disruptions to physical movements are a diagnostic feature of depression (psychomotor disturbance) but have not previously been assessed in the context of social functioning. Here we investigated the impact of psychomotor disturbance in depression on physical responsive behavior in both an experimental and observational setting.

Methods: In Experiment 1, we examined motor disturbance in depression in response to salient emotional sounds, using a laboratory-based effortful motor task. In Experiment 2, we explored whether psychomotor disturbance was apparent in real-life social interactions. Using mother-infant interactions as a model affective social situation, we compared physical behaviors of mothers with and without postnatal depression (PND).

Results: We found impairments in precise, controlled psychomotor performance in adults with depression relative to healthy adults (Experiment 1). Despite this disruption, all adults showed enhanced performance following exposure to highly salient emotional cues (infant cries). Examining real-life interactions, we found differences in physical movements, namely reduced affective touching, in mothers with PND responding to their infants, compared to healthy mothers (Experiment 2).

Conclusions: Together, these findings suggest that psychomotor disturbance may be an important feature of depression that can impair social functioning. Future work investigating whether improvements in physical movement in depression could have a positive impact on social interactions would be of much interest.

Keywords: depression, psychomotor performance, infant crying, social interaction, emotion

INTRODUCTION

Emotions are expressed in, and are also affected by, bodily actions and movements (Niedenthal, 2007). The notion of a reciprocal link between emotion and movement has intuitive appeal, but also considerable theoretical and empirical support. Indeed, the assertion that emotion must be understood in terms of bodily interactions with the world is a central tenet of embodied cognition approaches (Wilson, 2002). Empirical evidence shows that when an individual's movement is disrupted, so too is their emotional experience (Niedenthal et al., 2005). Disrupted movement, or psychomotor disturbance, is a core diagnostic feature of many disorders of emotion (e.g., Bauer et al., 1991; Schrijvers et al., 2008), perhaps the most apparent of which is major depressive disorder.

While the key diagnostic criteria for depression are lowered mood and anhedonia, the disorder also entails significant abnormalities in psychomotor function (Whybrow and Mendels, 1969; for review, see Sobin and Sackeim, 1997; Canbeyli, 2010). Adults with depression demonstrate decreased overall motor activity (Wehr et al., 1980; Wolff et al., 1985), slower motor response times (Schwartz et al., 1989) and disrupted gross and fine motor movements relative to comparison groups (for review, see Schrijvers et al., 2008). However, despite evidence for its pervasiveness, psychomotor disturbance is one of the least understood of the core symptoms of depression.

Emotion processing in depression, by contrast, has been the subject of extensive investigation. Adults with depression show negative biases in information processing in a variety of domains (for reviews, see Clark et al., 2009; Harmer et al., 2009) including in response to lexical and social stimuli (e.g., Joormann and Gotlib, 2006; Bistricky et al., 2011). Within the social domain, there is evidence of disrupted processing of emotions in faces

(Surguladze et al., 2005; Joormann and Gotlib, 2006; Stein et al., 2010; Arteche et al., 2011) and voices (e.g., Donovan et al., 1998; Schuetze and Zeskind, 2001; Péron et al., 2011; Young et al., 2012). Such disruptions have implications for an individual's ability to navigate the social world and there is evidence to suggest that deficits in social functioning are an important factor in the maintenance of depression (Hammen, 1997; Joiner, 2002).

Psychomotor disturbance may also have consequences for social functioning in depression. Social interactions require the ability to detect emotional content and respond contingently (Kringelbach and Rolls, 2003). A critical feature of fluent interactions is synchronized physical movements, such as imitation (Heyes, 2011). Adults spontaneously mimic a variety of behaviors, including emotional facial expressions, manual gestures, body postures, mannerisms, and speech patterns (Chartrand and Bargh, 1999). Disorders involving disrupted psychomotor abilities, such as Parkinson's disease, have been associated with disruptions to social functioning, including the ability to imitate facial expressions (Simons et al., 2003). How disruptions to emotional processing and psychomotor functioning in depression interact and potentially impact on social interactions is not currently understood.

PARENT-INFANT INTERACTIONS AS A MODEL OF AFFECTIVE SOCIAL FUNCTIONING

Parental caregiving inherently involves both reactions to emotional nonverbal cues and intricate, coordinated patterns of psychomotor activity. Parental care is frequently elicited by the sound of an infant cry, which typically evokes a strong emotional reaction in the listener (e.g., Frodi et al., 1978). Parent-infant interactions also tend to be highly synchronized, with both partners acting to maintain proximity to one another (Bowlby, 1969; Papousek and Papousek, 1989).

Previous work has shown that hearing a distressed infant's cry can specifically improve adults' ability to move in an effortful and coordinated manner (Parsons et al., 2012a). In addition, physiological reactivity to infant crying, indexed by increased heart rate, has been linked to sensitivity of maternal caregiving behavior (Del Vecchio et al., 2009; Joosen et al., 2013). Hearing infant vocalisations is also associated with early activity in the brainstem, a region that regulates autonomic function and responses to biologically salient information (Parsons et al., 2013b). Neuroimaging studies have also demonstrated increased activity in regions involved in arousal and emotion regulation (such as the amygdala and orbitofrontal cortex) when listening to infant cries (Lorberbaum et al., 1999; Swain et al., 2007; Bos et al., 2010; Kim et al., 2011). It has therefore been suggested that hearing an infant cry may induce a 'high-alert' state of autonomic arousal, where adults are physiologically primed to react to an infant's distress (Parsons et al., 2012a, 2014b).

There is much interest in the role of gender in responsiveness to infant cues given the near universal evolutionary differences in the provision of caregiving between mothers and fathers. Studies in the visual domain (responding to images of infant faces) have demonstrated that women are more sensitive than men to infant "cuteness", based on measures of explicit appraisal ("liking" ratings) and physiological reactivity (Sprengelmeyer et al., 2009; Parsons et al., 2011a; Esposito et al., 2014). However, measures of motivational salience ("wanting") have found no differences between men and women in their 'willingness to work' to view images of infants (Parsons et al., 2011a; however, see also Hahn et al., 2013). In the auditory domain, women and men are similar in their explicit appraisal of infant vocalisations, reporting similar levels of perceived distress and desire to respond (Donate-Bartfield and Passman, 1985; Leger et al., 1996; Parsons et al., 2014b,c). There is mixed evidence on whether there are gender differences in physiological reactions to infant cries, with findings demonstrating greater reactivity in women than men (Wiesenfeld et al., 1981; Furedy et al., 1989) or greater reactivity in men than women (Brewster et al., 1998; Out et al., 2010). One study to date assessing motivational salience of infant cries demonstrated no gender differences (Parsons et al., 2012a).

EVIDENCE FOR DISRUPTED SOCIAL FUNCTIONING IN POSTNATAL DEPRESSION

Postnatal depression (PND) is defined as an episode of depression experienced by parents in the early months following childbirth. It has been identified as a global health issue (Parsons et al., 2012b; Howard et al., 2014; Stein et al., 2014) because it can compromise the quality of early care the child receives (Bigelow et al., 2010). Specifically, impairments in parental sensitivity to infant cues have been observed (e.g., Lester et al., 1995). PND has also been associated with a raised risk for childhood cognitive and socio-emotional problems (van Ijzendoorn et al., 1999; Murray et al., 2010). Mothers with PND have been shown to rate cries as less perceptually salient and less likely to elicit active caregiving responses than healthy mothers (Schuetze and Zeskind, 2001). Several studies have reported that mothers with depression are less likely to initiate appropriate caregiving responses to their infant's cries than healthy mothers (Bettes, 1988; Murray et al., 1993; Schuetze and Zeskind, 2001). Disrupted sensitivity to distress in infant cries, as indexed by pitch, has also been demonstrated in both mothers with PND (Donovan et al., 1998) and adults with depression (Young et al., 2012). In addition, one recent study demonstrated that depressive symptoms were associated with lower than predicted physiological reactivity to infant crying (Riem et al., 2011). How depression impacts on motor aspects of parental sensitivity, such as the ability to move in reaction to the infant, has not been directly investigated.

STUDY AIMS

In the current study, we employed two means of exploring the relationship between depression and psychomotor functioning. First, we assessed psychomotor performance in adults with and without depression using a standardized laboratory task of effortful, precise movement (Experiment 1). Second, we assessed physical movement in real-life emotive, social interactions between mothers with their infants (Experiment 2).

EXPERIMENT 1

Experiment 1 aimed to investigate the impact of depression on two aspects of behavior important for social functioning:

emotional processing and psychomotor performance. Responding to infant distress vocalisations requires rapid, co-ordinated movement, but also recognition of the emotional salience of the sound. We hypothesized that depression might impact on performance in either of two ways. One possibility is that differential responses to emotional cues are disrupted in depression. In this case, salient emotional stimuli would no longer hold a "privileged status" and would not promote faster coordinated effortful movements. A second possibility is that psychomotor disturbance in depression disrupts the ability to move quickly in response to all cues. This would result in overall slower responses in adults with depression, compared to healthy adults. Importantly, it would be expected that enhanced psychomotor performance after exposure to infant cries would still be present.

METHODS

PARTICIPANTS

Table 1 presents participant demographic information. Twenty adults with current major depression (assessed using the Structured Clinical Interview for DSM-IV; SCID) and twenty adults without depression participated. This study was approved by the Oxfordshire Research Ethics Committee (12/07/2010). Participation was voluntary and all participants gave written informed consent.

Participants were recruited from the student and general population through poster and online advertisements. Inclusion criteria were: no medication affecting the brain (including medications for the treatment of depression or anxiety) and no self-reported hearing impairments. Six participants (three healthy and three with depression) had children, all of whom were aged over 18 months at the time of testing. Participants were identified as experiencing moderate or severe depressive symptoms if they scored greater than or equal to 13 on the Edinburgh Postnatal Depression Scale (EPDS; a cut off with high sensitivity and specificity). The EPDS has been validated for use with women outside the postnatal period (Cox et al., 1996) and fathers (Matthey et al., 2001). It has also been used in a number of studies of men outside the postnatal period (e.g., Ramchandani et al., 2008).

Participants scoring above the threshold on the EPDS were then assessed using the SCID (using the following modules: mood episodes; anxiety disorders; obsessive-compulsive and related disorders; trauma and stressor-related disorders). Assessments were carried out by a trained psychologist and a second psychologist provided additional ratings of each interview. Given the high co-morbidity of depression and anxiety symptoms (approximately 35% in this sample), only participants who received a primary diagnosis of major depressive disorder were included in the study. Participants in this study reported high levels of depressive symptoms (EPDS scores; M = 18.85, SD = 2.56), well within the range for major depression (>13, Cox et al., 1996).

Table 1 | Demographic characteristics of participants with and without depression.

	Adults with depression	Adults without depression
n (*n* male)	20 (7)	20 (8)
Age in years *M (SD)*	27.55 (7.42)	28.50 (9.83)
EPDS score *M (SD)*	18.85 (2.56)*	3.25 (3.17)
GAD-Q score *M (SD)*	9.51 (1.21)*	1.94 (2.26)

**Denotes significant group differences (two-sample t-test, $p < 0.001$).*

EXPERIMENTAL TASK

Motor performance was assessed using the "Whack-a-mole" game, which requires participants to press randomly illuminating buttons, within a predetermined time and with a specific amount of force, in order to score points. Over the course of the game, the time limit for responses gets shorter as the lights are illuminated in quicker succession. The game therefore tests the accuracy of participants' rapid, effortful responses. Participants were first familiarized with the game by playing three practice rounds of 30 s each.

Participants then played a full round of the "Whack-a-mole" game (lasting 1 min) after listening to 4.5 min of one of three types of sounds: infant cries, adult cries and bird sounds (for further details of the sound stimuli, see Parsons et al., 2012a; Young et al., 2012; Parsons et al., 2014b). This procedure was then repeated for each of the other two sound types, with the order counterbalanced across participants.

Performance was video recorded and subsequently coded. Total scores on the game were taken as a measure of accuracy. The force applied during the game was measured using a set of digital electronic scales (Salter 1036 BKDR, calibrated by the manufacturer) and coded to obtain a value for each individual button press. From this, mean, minimum and maximum pressure scores were extracted. Mean pressure was calculated as the average pressure applied during a single game and maximum and minimum pressure scores were extracted by taking the greatest and least amount of force applied, respectively. A factor analysis was performed to investigate the relationship between these dimensions (mean, maximum and minimum pressure) and whether variance might better be explained by an underlying latent variable, relating to "force" of motor responses. A 2 × 3 mixed ANOVA was used to analyze the accuracy and pressure data separately, with group as the between-subjects factor (depression, no depression) and stimulus category as the within-subjects factor (infant cry, adult cry, bird sound).

EXPERIMENT 2

In Experiment 2, we assessed whether psychomotor impairments would be apparent during naturalistic social interactions. Using observations of real-life interactions of mothers and infants, we assessed the impact of PND on aspects of a mother's physical movements towards her infant. We hypothesized that mothers with PND would show disruption to affective physical behaviors compared to mothers without PND.

METHODS

Data consisted of experimenter-coded observations of 54 mothers interacting with their infants, collected as part of a larger study of parent-infant interactions (the Oxford Parent Project, OPP).

Data in the current study was taken from an experimental session conducted with mothers and infants at 10 months postpartum. This session included assessment of maternal mental health and observation of mother-infant interactions. Approval for the OPP study was obtained from the Oxfordshire Research Ethics Committee.

PARTICIPANTS

Mothers were recruited to participate in a longitudinal observational cohort study (the Oxford Parent Project) from postnatal wards of the John Radcliffe Hospital, Oxford, UK. All mothers were aged 18 or over, spoke English, had no medical complications, were over 35 weeks gestation, and were the infants' principal caregiver. All infants had a birth weight above 2000 g. Maternal mental health was assessed using the Structured Clinical Interview for DSM Axis I disorders (SCID, research version; First et al., 2002). The SCID was conducted by a trained researcher who also provided clinician's severity ratings (CSR; Brown et al., 2001). The CSR is a scale ranging from 0–8, which indicates the level of distress or impairment associated with a specific symptom cluster (ratings of >4 indicate clinical severity).

Of the 253 participants who completed the 10-month assessment as part of the OPP, 30 were identified as fulfilling the criteria for current major depressive disorder. Of these 30 women, 27 had full ratings on all the observational dimensions being assessed in this experiment. Three were excluded because it was not possible to distinguish some of the psychomotor touch ratings assessed in this experiment. The group of 27 mothers included in this experiment had an average CSR of 5.15 ($SD = 0.95$). Participants were also assessed for other psychiatric disorders, demonstrating a substantial comorbidity of generalized anxiety disorder (GAD, 14 participants received CSR ratings >4 for GAD). The 27 participants with MDD were those who received a primary diagnosis of depression (CSR for GAD: $M = 2.81$, $SD = 2.62$). Of these participants, 13 reported that they were currently taking anti-depressant medication or receiving psychological treatment/counseling. A group of 27 mothers reporting no current psychiatric disorder (screened using the SCID) were selected to provide a control group against which to assess maternal behavior in PND. These participants were selected from the larger sample of OPP participants such that there were two groups of mothers matched as closely as possible: first for age (in years), then by socio-economic status and finally by parity (see **Table 2**).

Table 2 | Basic demographic details of participants.

	Mothers with depression	Mothers without depression
Age in years *M (SD)*	33.19 (5.61)	33.19 (5.61)
Maternal SES *M (SD)*	3.80 (4.62)	5.19 (3.92)
% primiparous mothers	41%	67%
MDD CSR *M (SD)*	5.15, 0.95	–
GAD CSR *M (SD)*	2.81, 2.62	–

Note. No significant differences in age, SES or parity were observed between groups (all p > 0.05).

INTERACTION CODING

Mother-infant interactions were recorded during 3.5 min free play sessions in which mothers were given a toy and instructed to play with their infant in any way they chose. Video tapes were subsequently coded on a number of dimensions relating to the quality of maternal responsiveness to the infant and the extent of maternal interactions. Ratings were completed by a trained researcher who was blind to the mother's mental state (see Stein et al., 2012). For the current study, a subset of coded dimensions were selected to assess features of maternal psychomotor behavior and responses to emotional stimuli. Across the larger OPP study, a subsample of tapes was coded by a second trained researcher to assess inter-rater reliability of perceived maternal behaviors. Across 25 samples, inter-rater reliability on the dimensions included in this study was high (average weighted $K = 0.72$).

Coded dimensions relating to maternal psychomotor behavior consisted of "emotional touch", "instrumental touch" and "strong control". Emotional touch was coded as the "frequency of mother-infant contact for emotional reasons (warmth, caring, affection)", on a 5-point Likert scale, ranging from 1, no touching, to 5, touching throughout most of the session. Instrumental touch was coded as "mother-infant contact for non-emotive, mechanical reasons", using the same 5-point Likert scale as for emotional touch. Strong control was coded as "the extent to which mother uses greater power or strength to override the child", on a 3-point Likert scale, ranging from 1, no strong control, to 3, consistently uses strong control.

Coded dimensions relating to maternal responses to infant cues consisted of general "maternal withdrawal" and specific "responses to vocal cues". Maternal withdrawal was coded as "mother's lack of engagement/interaction with her infant" on a 5-point Likert scale ranging from 1, very withdrawn, to 5 not at all withdrawn. Responses to vocal cues were coded as "the extent to which the mother picks up on the child's vocal cues, recognizing his/her vocalisations in an appropriate way", on a 5-point Likert scale, ranging from 1, very poor (little response to vocalisations), to 5, very good (reacting to almost all vocalisations, repeating and expanding). Ordinal data from Likert scales of coded maternal behavior were compared between mothers with and without PND using non-parametric statistical tests (independent-samples Mann-Whitney *U* tests).

EXPERIMENT 1: RESULTS

Factor analysis demonstrated that the three force measure variables were significantly positively correlated. Mean pressure scores were highly correlated with maximum pressure scores ($r = 0.91$) and minimum pressure scores ($r = 0.46$). Maximum and minimum pressure scores were also strongly correlated ($r = 0.39$). A principal components factor analysis on standardized, log-transformed scores demonstrated that all three pressure measures loaded onto one underlying "pressure factor", explaining 73.69% of the variance in the data, with an eigenvalue of 2.21. This factor reflected overall effort during the game, while also reflecting peak performance (as indexed by maximum scores) and sustained effort (minimum scores).

For the accuracy data, there was a significant main effect of group ($F_{(1,38)} = 7.37, p = 0.01, r = 0.40$) and sound type ($F_{(2,76)} =$

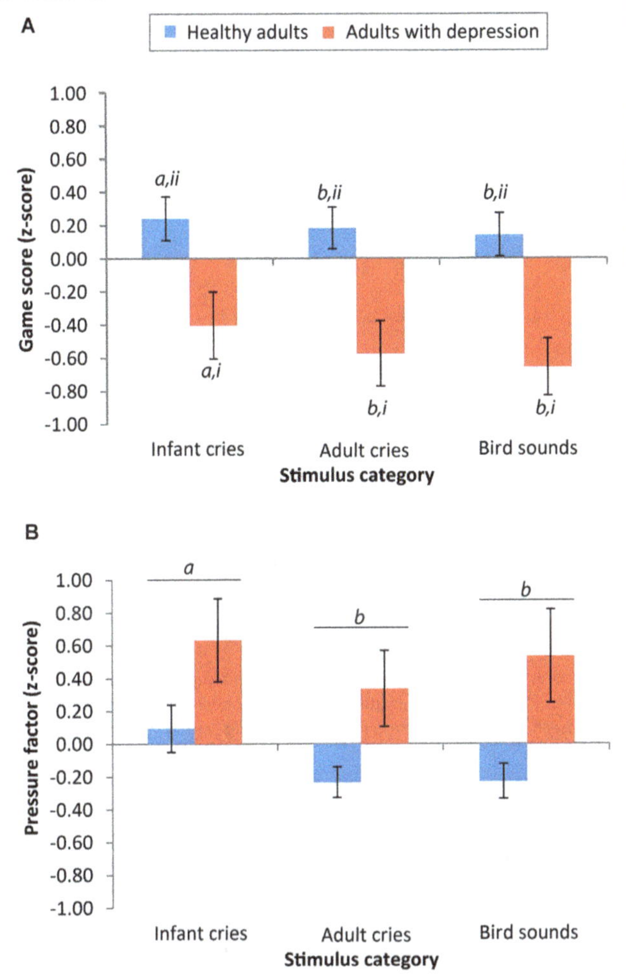

FIGURE 1 | Performance of adults with depression is significantly lower on the effortful motor task than healthy adults, but differential reactivity to salient emotional cues remains evident in both groups. **(A)** Scores from both groups were significantly higher after listening to infant cries compared to listening to adult cries or bird sounds (means with different letters are significantly different, *a* > *b*, *p* < 0.05). The mean scores of healthy adults on the "Whack-a-mole" game were significantly higher than the scores of adults with depression (means with different numerals are significantly different, *ii* > *i*, *p* < 0.05). **(B)** In both groups, pressure applied was greater after listening to infant cries compared with adult cries or bird sounds (means with different letters are significantly different, *a* > *b*, *p* < 0.05). Error bars reflect mean +/– standard error.

6.66, $p = 0.002$, $r = 0.28$), but no significant interaction between the two ($F_{(2,76)} = 1.23$, $p = 0.30$, $r = 0.13$). Across all sound categories, scores from adults with depression ($M = 35.60$, $SD = 22.05$) were significantly lower than scores from the healthy adults ($M = 55.62$, $SD = 24.52$). *Post hoc* least squares difference (LSD) comparisons showed that across both participant groups, scores on the game were significantly higher after listening to infant cries ($M = 48.63$, $SD = 26.68$) compared to adult cries ($M = 44.25$, $SD = 25.94$; $p = 0.005$) and compared to bird sounds ($M = 43.95$, $SD = 24.40$; $p = 0.002$). There was no significant difference in game scores after listening to adult cries compared to bird sounds ($p = 0.84$; see **Figure 1**).

For the pressure data, taking the "force" variable, there was no significant main effect of group ($F_{(1,34)} = 0.71$, $p = 0.41$, $r = 0.14$) but there was a significant main effect of stimulus category on pressure factor scores ($F_{(2,68)} = 3.98$, $p = 0.02$, $r = 0.24$). There was no significant interaction between group and stimulus category ($F_{(2,68)} = 0.65$, $p = 0.53$, $r = 0.10$). Participants with depression did not differ in the amount of applied pressure (pressure factor scores: $M = 0.25$, $SD = 0.95$) compared with healthy participants ($M = -0.01$, $SD = 1.04$). *Post hoc* LSD comparisons demonstrated that across both participant groups, pressure factor scores were significantly higher after listening to infant cries ($M = 0.31$, $SD = 1.03$) compared to adult cries ($M = 0.09$, $SD = 1.00$; $p < 0.001$) and compared to bird sounds ($M = 0.07$, $SD = 1.00$; $p = 0.04$). There was no significant difference in pressure applied after listening to adult cries compared to bird sounds ($p = 0.67$; see **Figure 1**).

There were no significant effects of gender on task performance as demonstrated by 2 × 2 × 3 mixed ANOVAs, with gender and participant group as between-subject factors and stimulus category as a within-subject factor. For the game score data, there was no significant main effect of gender ($F_{(1,36)} = 0.13$, $p = 0.72$), no significant interaction of gender with participant group ($F_{(1,36)} = 0.35$, $p = 0.56$) and no significant interaction of gender with stimulus category ($F_{(2,72)} = 0.1.98$, $p = 0.15$). Similarly, for the pressure factor data, there was no significant main effect of gender ($F_{(1,32)} = 1.76$, $p = 0.19$), no significant interaction of gender with participant group ($F_{(1,32)} = 0.58$, $p = 0.45$) and no significant interaction of gender with stimulus category ($F_{(2,64)} = 1.22$, $p = 0.30$).

RESULTS: EXPERIMENT 2

Significant differences in the extent of both emotional touching ($U = 247.00$, $p = 0.03$, $r = -0.32$) and the use of strong control ($U = 418.50$, $p = 0.04$, $r = 0.28$) were observed (see **Figure 2**). While the size of the effects were small to medium, mothers with PND demonstrated less emotional touching and more "strong control" compared with mothers without PND. There was no significant difference in the extent of instrumental touching ($U = 330.05$, $p = 0.69$, $r = -0.06$) between mothers with and without PND. No significant differences were observed between mothers with and without PND in coded measures of maternal withdrawal ($U = 332.50$, $p = 0.52$, $r = -0.09$) or maternal responses to infant vocal cues ($U = 122.00$, $p = 0.16$, $r = -0.23$).

DISCUSSION

These findings suggest that depression is associated with disruptions to psychomotor abilities, which could play a role in social functioning. This is supported by two converging lines of evidence. First, we found that adults with depression demonstrated reduced effortful motor performance compared with healthy adults. Despite this disruption, the performance of both groups of adults was enhanced after listening to sounds of greatest emotional salience. This highlights the persistent nature of psychomotor disruption in depression, which impacts on behavior even when reactivity to highly emotive social cues is retained. Second, we found that

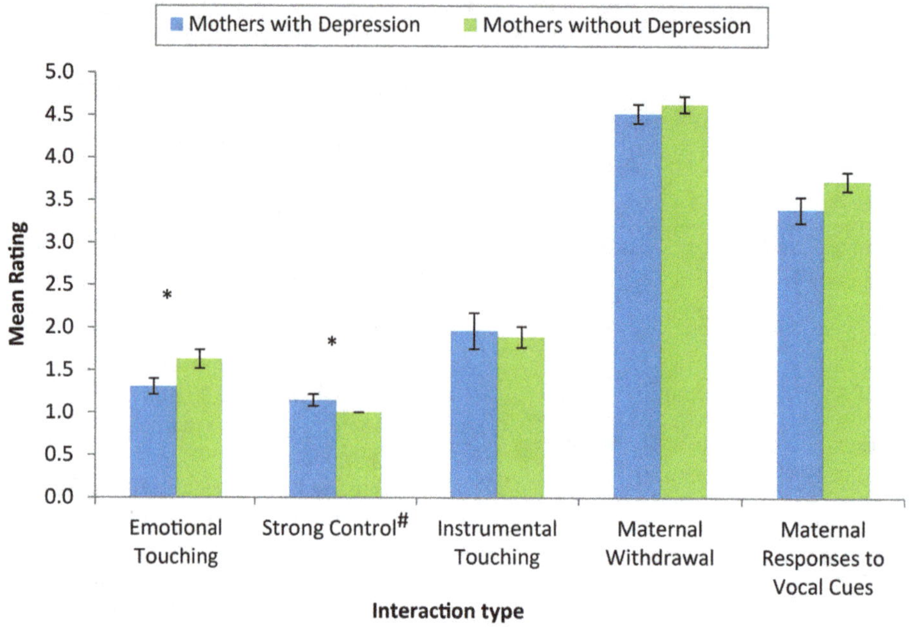

FIGURE 2 | Mean ratings of dimensions of coded interactions across mothers with and without depression. Mothers with depression showed less emotional touching and more strong control than mothers without depression. There were no significant differences between groups on instrumental touching, maternal withdrawal or maternal responses to infant vocal cues. (* Denotes significantly different values, $p < 0.05$, error bars reflect mean +/− standard error, # note that strong control was coded on a 3 point scale).

mothers with PND demonstrated altered physical movements during interactions with their infants compared with healthy mothers.

In Experiment 1, after listening to infant cries, participants' motor performance was more accurate and more forceful than after listening to adult cries or bird sounds. This suggests that hearing the highly salient sound of a distressed infant has a similarly rousing effect in adults with and without depression. Despite this reactivity to infant cries, the performance of adults with depression was impaired relative to that of healthy adults. These findings are consistent with the view that depression may have a general impact on psychomotor abilities (for review, see Schrijvers et al., 2008). In addition, there were no observed gender differences in the motivational salience of infant cries, in line with previous research (Parsons et al., 2012a).

The overall difference between the accuracy scores of the adults with and without depression was substantial. On average, healthy adults had scores that were 66% higher than adults with depression. This indicates a pervasive disruption to motor performance in adults with depression on this task. Of note, adults with depression did not differ from healthy adults in the amount of pressure applied while playing the game. This suggests that the lower overall scores of the adults with depression were a consequence of slower and less accurate movements, rather than reduced force of individual movements. While general psychomotor disturbance in depression has been widely reported (Moffoot et al., 1994; Buyukdura et al., 2011), our findings suggest two dissociable components: speed and accuracy of a movement, and the amount of force applied. Our results indicate that while the former is disrupted in depression, both components are enhanced after hearing infant cries.

The lack of enhanced motor performance after listening to adult cries suggests that while both adult and infant cries are important classes of emotional stimuli, there is something unique about the processing of infant cries. We suggest that the difference is in the communication of immediate need in infant crying, but not in adult crying. Adult crying can convey joy or sadness, depending on the context of the expression. Interpretation of genuine distress may also require other information, such as the visual cue of "tearing" (Provine et al., 2009). Our results suggest that infant cries, a class of urgent, emotional sounds, can elicit a sustained state of increased reactivity in adults with and without depression.

A physiological state that allows individuals to move with greater speed and accuracy upon hearing a distressed infant may be an adaptive mechanism that facilitates caregiving behavior. Neuroimaging studies of pain and aversion suggest that these types of mechanisms recruit affective brain areas (Lindquist and Barrett, 2012), disrupted activity in which has long been a core feature of brain models of depression (e.g., Mayberg, 1997). Studies of neural responses to infant communicative cues suggest similar networks are recruited as part of the "parental brain" (Swain et al., 2008; Bos et al., 2010; Parsons et al., 2010; Kim et al., 2011; Laurent and Ablow, 2012). One region in particular, the orbitofrontal cortex, is thought to be critically involved in the rapid processing of infant cues (Kringelbach et al., 2008; Parsons et al., 2013c). A breadth of behavioral evidence now supports the notion of privileged processing of infant cues (Sprengelmeyer et al., 2009; Parsons et al., 2011a,b, 2013a). In addition, recent evidence suggests that physical aspects of parent-infant interactions might be specifically linked to functioning of the oxytocinergic system (Weisman et al., 2013). Future studies investigating cortical and neuroendocrine processes involved in adults' behavioral responses to infant cues would further inform this emerging field.

We hypothesized that maternal PND would be associated with altered physical movements during mother-infant interactions. Previous work has demonstrated that parent-infant interactions are often disrupted in PND (e.g., Stein et al., 1991; Murray et al., 1996). In the current study, mothers with PND showed differences in key aspects of affective, physical movements during interactions with their infants compared with mothers without PND (Experiment 2). These small, but significant, differences were apparent in mothers' use of "emotional touch" and "strong control", but not in non-affective "instrumental touch", or other aspects of maternal responsiveness. Our findings, while preliminary, suggest important differences in psychomotor capacities related specifically to affective physical interactions between mother and infant.

The majority of previous work examining maternal responses to infant cries in PND has been experimental in nature (e.g., Lester et al., 1995; Donovan et al., 1998). This previous work has primarily focused on assessing specific responses to subtle differences in infant cry acoustics in experimental settings. In contrast, Experiment 2 used a naturalistic observational setting with spontaneous, idiosyncratic infant vocalisations. We found no significant disruption in maternal responses to infant cues as a category of stimuli in depression. This suggests that there may not be an obvious overall impairment in responding to infant vocalizations, at least as measured by a 5 point Likert scale. Instead, depression may impact the ability to detect and interpret subtle differences in vocal characteristics.

The specificity of differences in maternal behavior to affective aspects of physical touch is of particular interest. There is mounting neuroscientific evidence for a dissociation between "discriminative" and "affective" aspects of touch (for review, see McGlone et al., 2014). It has been demonstrated that infants are sensitive to this distinction, showing more signs of reward (i.e., smiling) to affective stroking, than to passive touch (Stack and Muir, 1990, 1992; Jean et al., 2009). Our findings suggest that depression may disrupt affective physical interactions between mother and infant. However, it is unclear at this stage whether this linked to changes in psychomotor behavior, affective processing, or some combination of the two.

Interventions targeting affective physical behavior have previously shown positive effects for infant development. Close physical skin-to-skin contact between mother and infant has been shown to confer benefits for child development in cognitive and motor outcomes (for review, see Tessier et al., 1998). Increasing skin-to-skin contact has also been shown to reduce depressive symptoms in mothers (e.g., Tessier et al., 1998; Feldman et al., 2002). The present finding of observable changes in mothers' physical movements during interactions with their infants in PND provides further impetus for exploring affective physical behavior as a target for intervention.

STRENGTHS AND LIMITATIONS

A key strength of this study is that we present evidence for functionally salient motor impairments in depression using independent experimental and observational methods, testing different samples of participants. The results from these two methods are also convergent. We demonstrate that psychomotor disturbance, apparent in current and previous laboratory based tests of motor function (e.g., Schwartz et al., 1989; Sobin and Sackeim, 1997; Schrijvers et al., 2008), can also be measured in social interaction behaviors. However, our findings are exploratory in nature, especially given that the recorded social interaction consisted of brief (3.5 min), laboratory-based mother-infant interactions. Furthermore, effect sizes were small, which is perhaps related to the three to five point scales on which touch behaviors were coded, limiting the sensitivity of this measure to subtle differences in behavior. In addition, while we assessed participants for disorders related to emotional processing, we did not specifically assess changes in other capacities (such as attention) that may have an impact on performance in the measures used. Future studies might examine individual differences in other factors related to caregiving such as empathy, parity and infant temperament (Decety and Cowell, 2014; Parsons et al., 2014a). Finally, it remains to be seen whether psychomotor disruption in depression has a similar impact on physical movements during interactions between adults.

CONCLUSION

Psychomotor disturbances and their impact on social interaction should be considered alongside other well-established deficits in social cue processing (e.g., Joormann and Gotlib, 2006; Stein et al., 2010; Arteche et al., 2011; Naranjo et al., 2011). However, our findings suggest that the role of psychomotor disturbances may have been underestimated, or at least underspecified, in prior conceptualizations of social functioning in depression. Current models of embodied emotion, which specify an intricate link between emotion and movement, lend theoretical credence to this notion. Altered movement patterns were apparent in adults with depression both in an experimental task requiring precise, co-ordinated movements, and in more naturalistic social interactions. Disrupted emotional experience, which characterizes depression, may be associated with changes in the ability to move in functionally important ways.

FINANCIAL SUPPORT

This research was supported by a Medical Research Council Studentship to Katherine S. Young, funding from the Welcome Trust, United Kingdom (Grant071571), and the TrygFonden Charitable Foundation and ERC Consolidator Grant CAREGIVING (n.615539).

ACKNOWLEDGMENTS

The authors would like to gratefully acknowledge the work of the OPP team in the collection of data presented as Experiment 2.

REFERENCES

1. Arteche, A., Joormann, J., Harvey, A., Craske, M., Gotlib, I. H., Lehtonen, A., et al. (2011). The effects of postnatal maternal depression and anxiety on the processing of infant faces. *J. Affect. Disord.* 133, 197–203. doi: 10.1016/j.jad.2011. 04.015

2. Bauer, M. S., Crits-Christoph, P., Ball, W. A., Dewees, E., McAllister, T., Alahi, P., et al. (1991). Independent assessment of manic and depressive symptoms by self-rating: scale characteristics and implications for the study of mania. *Arch. Gen. Psychiatry* 48, 807–812. doi: 10.1001/archpsyc.1991.01810330031005
3. Bettes, B. A. (1988). Maternal depression and motherese: temporal and intonational features. *Child Dev.* 59, 1089–1096. doi: 10.2307/1130275
4. Bigelow, A. E., MacLean, K., Proctor, J., Myatt, T., Gillis, R., and Power, M. (2010). Maternal sensitivity throughout infancy: continuity and relation to attachment security. *Infant Behav. Dev.* 33, 50–60. doi: 10.1016/j.infbeh.2009. 10.009
5. Bistricky, S. L., Ingram, R. E., and Atchley, R. A. (2011). Facial affect processing and depression susceptibility: cognitive biases and cognitive neuroscience. *Psychol. Bull.* 137, 998–1028. doi: 10.1037/a0025348
6. Bos, P. A., Hermans, E. J., Montoya, E. R., Ramsey, N. F., and van Honk, J. (2010). Testosterone administration modulates neural responses to crying infants in young females. *Psychoneuroendocrinology* 35, 114–121. doi: 10.1016/j.psyneuen. 2009.09.013
7. Bowlby, J. (1969). *Attachment and Loss, Vol 1: Attachment.* London: Hogarth Press. Brewster, A. L., Nelson, J. P., McCanne, T. R., Lucas, D. R., and Milner, J. S. (1998). Gender differences in physiological reactivity to infant cries and smiles in military families. *Child Abuse Negl.* 22, 775–788. doi: 10.1016/s0145- 2134(98)00055-6
8. Brown, T. A., Di Nardo, P. A., Lehman, C. L., and Campbell, L. A. (2001). Reliability of DSM-IV anxiety and mood disorders: implications for the classification of emotional disorders. *J. Abnorm. Psychol.* 110, 49–58. doi: 10.1037//0021-843x. 110.1.49
9. Buyukdura, J. S., McClintock, S. M., and Croarkin, P. E. (2011). Psychomotor retardation in depression: biological underpinnings, measurement and treatment. *Prog. Neuropsychopharmacol. Biol. Psychiatry* 35, 395–409. doi: 10. 1016/j.pnpbp.2010.10.019
10. Canbeyli, R. (2010). Sensorimotor modulation of mood and depression: an integrative review. *Behav. Brain Res.* 207, 249–264. doi: 10.1016/j.bbr.2009. 11.002
11. Chartrand, T. L., and Bargh, J. A. (1999). The chameleon effect: the perception- behavior link and social interaction. *J. Pers. Soc. Psychol.* 76, 893–910. doi: 10. 1037//0022-3514.76.6.893
12. Clark, L., Chamberlain, S. R., and Sahakian, B. J. (2009). Neurocognitive mechanisms in depression: implications for treatment. *Annu. Rev. Neurosci.* 32, 57–74. doi: 10.1146/annurev.neuro.31.060407.125618
13. Cox, J. L., Chapman, G., Murray, D., and Jones, P. (1996). Validation of the Edinburgh postnatal depression scale (EPDS) in non-postnatal women. *J. Affect. Disord.* 39, 185–189. doi: 10.1016/0165-0327(96)00008-0
14. Decety, J., and Cowell, J. M. (2014). The complex relation between morality and empathy. *Trends Cogn. Sci.* 18, 337–339. doi: 10.1016/j.tics.2014.04.008
15. Del Vecchio, T., Walter, A., and O'Leary, S. G. (2009). Affective and physiological factors predicting maternal response to infant crying. *Infant Behav. Dev.* 32, 117– 122. doi: 10.1016/j.infbeh.2008.10.005
16. Donate-Bartfield, E., and Passman, R. H. (1985). Attentiveness of mothers and fathers to their baby's cries. *Infant Behav. Dev.* 8, 385–393. doi: 10.1016/0163- 6383(85)90003-7
17. Donovan, W. L., Leavitt, L. A., and Walsh, R. O. (1998). Conflict and depression predict maternal sensitivity to infant cries. *Infant Behav. Dev.* 21, 505–517. doi: 10.1016/S0163-6383(98)90023-6
18. Esposito, G., Nakazawa, J., Ogawa, S., Stival, R., Kawashima, A., Putnick, D. L., et al. (2014). Baby, you light-up my face: culture-general physiological responses to infants and culture-specific cognitive judgements of adults. *PLoS One* 9:e106705. doi: 10.1371/journal.pone.0106705
19. Feldman, R., Eidelman, A. I., Sirota, L., and Weller, A. (2002). Comparison of skin- to-skin (kangaroo) and traditional care: parenting outcomes and preterm infant development. *Pediatrics* 110, 16–26. doi: 10.1542/peds.110.1.16
20. First, M. B., Spitzer, R. L., Gibbon, M., and Williams, J. B. W. (2002). *Structured Clinical Interview for DSM-IV-TR Axis I Disorders, Research Version, Non- Patient Edition. (SCID-I/NP).* New York: Biometrics Research, New York State Psychiatric Institute.
21. Frodi, A. M., Lamb, M. E., Leavitt, L. A., and Donovan, W. L. (1978). Fathers' and mothers' responses to infant smiles and cries. *Infant Behav. Dev.* 1, 187–198. doi: 10.1016/s0163-6383(78)80029-0
22. Furedy, J. J., Fleming, A. S., Ruble, D., Scher, H., Daly, J., Day, D., et al. (1989). Sex differences in small-magnitude heart-rate responses to sexual and infant-related stimuli: a psychophysiological approach. *Physiol. Behav.* 46, 903–905. doi: 10. 1016/0031-9384(89)90056-5
23. Hahn, A. C., Xiao, D., Sprengelmeyer, R., and Perrett, D. I. (2013). Gender differences in the incentive salience of adult and infant faces. *Q. J. Exp. Psychol. (Hove)* 66, 200–208. doi: 10.1080/17470218.2012.705860
24. Hammen, C. (1997). *Depression.* Hove, England: Psychology Press.
25. Harmer, C. J., Goodwin, G. M., and Cowen, P. J. (2009). Why do antidepressants take so long to work? A cognitive neuropsychological model of antidepressant drug action. *Br. J. Psychiatry* 195, 102–108. doi: 10.1192/bjp.bp.108.051193
26. Heyes, C. (2011). Automatic imitation. *Psychol. Bull.* 137, 463–483. doi: 10. 1037/a0022288
27. Howard, L. M., Piot, P., and Stein, A. (2014). No health without perinatal mental health. *Lancet* 384, 1723–1724. doi: 10.1016/s0140-6736(14)62040-7
28. Jean, A. D., Stack, D. M., and Fogel, A. (2009). A longitudinal investigation of maternal touching across the first 6 months of life: age and context effects. *Infant Behav. Dev.* 32, 344–349. doi: 10.1016/j.infbeh.2009.04.005
29. Joiner, T. E. J. (2002). "Depression in its interpersonal context," in *Handbook of Depression*, eds I. H. Gotlib and C. L. Hammen (New York: Guilford Press), 295– 313.
30. Joormann, J., and Gotlib, I. H. (2006). Is this happiness i see? Biases in the identification of emotional facial expressions in depression and social phobia. *J. Abnorm. Psychol.* 115, 705–714. doi: 10.1037/0021-843x.115.4.705
31. Joosen, K. J., Mesman, J., Bakermans-Kranenburg, M. J., Pieper, S., Zeskind, P. S., and van Ijzendoorn, M. H. (2013). Physiological reactivity to infant crying and observed maternal sensitivity. *Infancy* 18, 414–431. doi: 10.1111/j.1532-7078. 2012.00122.x
32. Kim, P., Feldman, R., Mayes, L. C., Eicher, V., Thompson, N., Leckman, J. F., et al. (2011). Breastfeeding, brain activation to own infant cry and maternal sensitivity. *J. Child Psychol. Psychiatry* 52, 907–915. doi: 10.1111/j.1469-7610. 2011.02406.x
33. Kringelbach, M. L., Lehtonen, A., Squire, S., Harvey, A. G., Craske, M. G., Holliday, I. E., et al. (2008). A specific and rapid neural signature for parental instinct. *PLoS One* 3:e1664. doi: 10.1371/journal.pone.0001664
34. Kringelbach, M. L., and Rolls, E. T. (2003). Neural correlates of rapid reversal learning in a simple model of human social interaction. *Neuroimage* 20, 1371– 1383. doi: 10.1016/s1053-8119(03)00393-8
35. Laurent, H. K., and Ablow, J. C. (2012). A cry in the dark: depressed mothers show reduced neural activation to their own infant's cry. *Soc. Cogn. Affect. Neurosci.* 7, 125–134. doi: 10.1093/scan/nsq091
36. Leger, D. W., Thompson, R. A., Merritt, J. A., and Benz, J. J. (1996). Adult perception of emotion intensity in human infant cries: effects of infant age and cry acoustics. *Child Dev.* 67, 3238–3249. doi: 10.2307/1131776
37. Lester, B. M., Boukydis, C. F. Z., Garcia-Coll, C. T., Peucker, M., McGrath, M. M., Vohr, B. R., et al. (1995). Developmental outcome as a function of the goodness of fit between the infant's cry characteristics and the mother's perception of her infant's cry. *Pediatrics* 95, 516–521.
38. Lindquist, K. A., and Barrett, L. F. (2012). A functional architecture of the human brain: emerging insight from the science of emotion. *Trends Cogn. Sci.* 16, 533– 540. doi: 10.1016/j.tics.2012.09.005
39. Lorberbaum, J. P., Newman, J. D., Dubno, J. R., Horwitz, A. R., Nahas, Z., Teneback, C. C., et al. (1999). Feasibility of using fMRI to study mothers responding to infant cries. *Depress. Anxiety* 10, 99–104. doi: 10.1002/(sici)1520- 6394(1999)10:3<99::aid-da2>3.0.co;2-#
40. Matthey, S., Barnett, B., Kavanagh, D. J., and Howie, P. (2001). Validation of the Edinburgh postnatal depression scale for men and comparison of item endorsement with their partners. *J. Affect. Disord.* 64, 175–184. doi: 10. 1016/s0165-0327(00)00236-6
41. Mayberg, H. S. (1997). Limbic-cortical dysregulation: a proposed model of depression. *J. Neuropsychiatry Clin. Neurosci.* 9, 471–481. doi: 10.1176/jnp. 9.3.471
42. McGlone, F., Wessberg, J., and Olausson, H. (2014). Discriminative and affective touch: sensing and feeling. *Neuron* 82, 737–755. doi: 10.1016/j.neuron.2014. 05.001
43. Moffoot, A. P. R., O'Carroll, R. E., Bennie, J., Carroll, S., Dick, H., Ebmeier, K. P., et al. (1994). Diurnal variation of mood and neuropsychological function in major depression with melancholia. *J. Affect. Disord.* 32, 257–269. doi: 10. 1016/0165-0327(94)90090-6
44. Murray, L., Fiori-Cowley, A., Hooper, R., and Cooper, P. (1996). The impact of postnatal depression and associated adversity on early mother-infant interactions and later infant outcome. *Child Dev.* 67, 2512–2526. doi: 10. 2307/1131637
45. Murray, L., Halligan, S. L., and Cooper, P. J. (2010). "Effects of postnatal depression on mother-infant interactions and child development," in *Handbook of Infant Development*, eds T. Wachs and G. Bremner (Oxford: Wiley-Blackwell), 192–220.
46. Murray, L., Kempton, C., Woolgar, M., and Hooper, R. (1993). Depressed mothers' speech to their infants and its relation to infant gender and cognitive development. *J. Child Psychol. Psychiatry* 34, 1083–1101. doi: 10.1111/j.1469- 7610.1993.tb01775.x

47. Naranjo, C., Kornreich, C., Campanella, S., Noël, X., Vandriette, Y., Gillain, B., et al. (2011). Major depression is associated with impaired processing of emotion in music as well as in facial and vocal stimuli. *J. Affect. Disord.* 128, 243–251. doi: 10. 1016/j.jad.2010.06.039
48. Niedenthal, P. M. (2007). Embodying emotion. *Science* 316, 1002–1005. doi: 10. 1126/science.1136930
49. Niedenthal, P. M., Barsalou, L. W., Winkielman, P., Krauth-Gruber, S., and Ric, F. (2005). Embodiment in attitudes, social perception and emotion. *Pers. Soc. Psychol. Rev.* 9, 184–211. doi: 10.1207/s15327957pspr0903_1
50. Out, D., Pieper, S., Bakermans-Kranenburg, M. J., and van Ijzendoorn, M. H. (2010). Physiological reactivity to infant crying: a behavioral genetic study. *Genes Brain Behav.* 9, 868–876. doi: 10.1111/j.1601-183x.2010. 00624.x
51. Papousek, M., and Papousek, H. (1989). Forms and functions of vocal matching in interactions between mothers and their precanonical infants. *First Lang.* 9, 137–157. doi: 10.1177/014272378900900603
52. Parsons, C. E., Stark, E. A., Young, K. S., Stein, A., and Kringelbach, M. L. (2013a). Understanding the human parental brain: a critical role of the orbitofrontal cortex. *Soc. Neurosci.* 8, 525–543. doi: 10.1080/17470919.2013. 842610
53. Parsons, C. E., Young, K. S., Bhandari, R., van Ijzendoorn, M. H., Bakermans- Kranenburg, M. J., Stein, A., et al. (2014a). The bonnie baby: experimentally manipulated temperament affects perceived cuteness and motivation to view infant faces. *Dev. Sci.* 17, 257–269. doi: 10.1111/desc.12112
54. Parsons, C. E., Young, K. S., Craske, M. G., Stein, A. L., and Kringelbach, M. L. (2014b). Introducing the Oxford Vocal (OxVoc) sounds database: a validated set of non-acted affective sounds from human infants, adults and domestic animals. *Front. Psychol.* 5:562. doi: 10.3389/fpsyg.2014.00562
55. Parsons, C. E., Young, K. S., Jegindø, E.-M., Vuust, P., Stein, A., and Kringelbach, M. L. (2014c). Music training and empathy positively impact adults' sensitivity to infant distress. *Front. Psychol.* 5:1440. doi: 10.3389/fpsyg.2014. 01440
56. Parsons, C. E., Young, K. S., Joensson, M., Brattico, E., Hyam, J. A., Stein, A., et al. (2013b). Ready for action: a role for the brainstem in responding to infant vocalizations. *Soc. Cogn. Affect. Neurosci.* 9, 977–984. doi: 10.1093/scan/ nst076
57. Parsons, C. E., Young, K. S., Kumari, N., Stein, A., and Kringelbach, M. L. (2011a). The motivational salience of infant faces is similar for men and women. *PLoS One* 6:e20632. doi: 10.1371/journal.pone.0020632
58. Parsons, C. E., Young, K. S., Mohseni, H., Woolrich, M. W., Thomsen, K. R., Joensson, M., et al. (2013c). Minor structural abnormalities in the infant face disrupt neural processing: a unique window into early caregiving responses. *Soc. Neurosci.* 8, 268–274. doi: 10.1080/17470919.2013.795189
59. Parsons, C. E., Young, K. S., Murray, L., Stein, A., and Kringelbach, M. L. (2010). The functional neuroanatomy of the evolving parent-infant relationship. *Prog. Neurobiol.* 91, 220–241. doi: 10.1016/j.pneurobio.2010.03.001
60. Parsons, C. E., Young, K. S., Parsons, E., Dean, A., Murray, L., Goodacre, T., et al. (2011b). The effect of cleft lip on adults' responses to faces: cross-species findings. *PLoS One* 6:e25897. doi: 10.1371/journal.pone.0025897
61. Parsons, C. E., Young, K. S., Parsons, E., Stein, A., and Kringelbach, M. L. (2012a). Listening to infant distress vocalizations enhances effortful motor performance. *Acta Paediatr.* 101, e189–e191. doi: 10.1111/j.1651-2227.2011. 02554.x
62. Parsons, C. E., Young, K. S., Rochat, T. J., Kringelbach, M. L., and Stein, A. (2012b). Postnatal depression and its effects on child development: a review of evidence from low-and middle-income countries. *Br. Med. Bull.* 101, 57–79. doi: 10. 1093/bmb/ldr047
63. Péron, J., El Tamer, S., Grandjean, D., Leray, E., Travers, D., Drapier, D., et al. (2011). Major depressive disorder skews the recognition of emotional prosody. *Prog. Neuropsychopharmacol. Biol. Psychiatry* 35, 987–996. doi: 10.1016/j.pnpbp. 2011.01.019
64. Provine, R. R., Krosnowski, K. A., and Brocato, N. W. (2009). Tearing: breakthrough in human emotional signaling. *Evol. Psychol.* 7, 52–56.
65. Ramchandani, P. G., Stein, A., O'Connor, T. G., Heron, J., Murray, L., and Evans, J. (2008). Depression in men in the postnatal period and later child psychopathology: a population cohort study. *J. Am. Acad. Child Adolesc. Psychiatry* 47, 390–398. doi: 10.1097/CHI.0b013e31816429c2
66. Riem, M. M. E., Pieper, S., Out, D., Bakermans-Kranenburg, M. J., and van Ijzendoorn, M. H. (2011). Oxytocin receptor gene and depressive symptoms associated with physiological reactivity to infant crying. *Soc. Cogn. Affect. Neurosci.* 6, 294–300. doi: 10.1093/scan/nsq035
67. Schrijvers, D., Hulstijn, W., and Sabbe, B. G. C. (2008). Psychomotor symptoms in depression: a diagnostic, pathophysiological and therapeutic tool. *J. Affect. Disord.* 109, 1–20. doi: 10.1016/j.jad.2007.10.019
68. Schuetze, P., and Zeskind, P. S. (2001). Relations between women's depressive symptoms and perceptions of infant distress signals varying in pitch. *Infancy* 2, 483–499. doi: 10.1207/s15327078in0204_06
69. Schwartz, F., Carr, A. C., Munich, R. L., Glauber, S., Lesser, B., and Murray, J. (1989). Reaction time impairment in schizophrenia and affective illness: the role of attention. *Biol. Psychiatry* 25, 540–548. doi: 10.1016/0006-3223(89)90214-x
70. Simons, G., Ellgring, H., and Smith Pasqualini, M. (2003). Disturbance of spontaneous and posed facial expressions in Parkinson's disease. *Cogn. Emot.* 17, 759–778. doi: 10.1080/02699930302280
71. Sobin, C., and Sackeim, H. A. (1997). Psychomotor symptoms of depression. *Am. J. Psychiatry* 154, 4–17. doi: 10.1176/ajp.154.1.4
72. Sprengelmeyer, R., Perrett, D. I., Fagan, E. C., Cornwell, R. E., Lobmaier, J. S., Sprengelmeyer, A., et al. (2009). The cutest little baby face: a hormonal link to sensitivity to cuteness in infant faces. *Psychol. Sci.* 20, 149–154. doi: 10.1111/j. 1467-9280.2009.02272.x
73. Stack, D. M., and Muir, D. W. (1990). Tactile stimulation as a component of social interchange: new interpretations for the still-face effect. *Br. J. Dev. Psychol.* 8, 131–145. doi: 10.1111/j.2044-835x.1990.tb00828.x
74. Stack, D. M., and Muir, D. W. (1992). Adult tactile stimulation during face-to- face interactions modulates five-month-olds' affect and attention. *Child Dev.* 63, 1509–1525. doi: 10.1111/j.1467-8624.1992.tb01711.x
75. Stein, A., Arteche, A., Lehtonen, A., Craske, M., Harvey, A., Counsell, N., et al. (2010). Interpretation of infant facial expression in the context of maternal postnatal depression. *Infant Behav. Dev.* 33, 273–278. doi: 10.1016/j. infbeh.2010. 03.002
76. Stein, A., Craske, M. G., Lehtonen, A., Harvey, A., Savage-McGlynn, E., Davies, B., et al. (2012). Maternal cognitions and mother-infant interaction in postnatal depression and generalized anxiety disorder. *J. Abnorm. Psychol.* 121, 795–809. doi: 10.1037/a0026847
77. Stein, A., Gath, D. H., Bucher, J., Bond, A., Day, A., and Cooper, P. J. (1991). The relationship between post-natal depression and mother-child interaction. *Br. J. Psychiatry* 158, 46–52. doi: 10.1192/bjp.158.1.46
78. Stein, A., Pearson, R. M., Goodman, S. H., Rapa, E., Rahman, A., McCallum, M., et al. (2014). Effects of perinatal mental disorders on the fetus and child. *Lancet* 384, 1800–1819. doi: 10.1016/S0140-6736(14)61277-0
79. Surguladze, S., Brammer, M. J., Keedwell, P., Giampietro, V., Young, A. W., Travis, M. J., et al. (2005). A differential pattern of neural response toward sad versus happy facial expressions in major depressive disorder. *Biol. Psychiatry* 57, 201– 209. doi: 10.1016/j.biopsych.2004.10.028
80. Swain, J. E., Lorberbaum, J. P., Kose, S., and Strathearn, L. (2007). Brain basis of early parent–infant interactions: psychology, physiology and in vivo functional neuroimaging studies. *J. Child Psychol. Psychiatry* 48, 262–287. doi: 10.1111/j. 1469-7610.2007.01731.x
81. Swain, J. E., Tasgin, E., Mayes, L. C., Feldman, R., Todd Constable, R., and Leckman, J. F. (2008). Maternal brain response to own baby-cry is affected by cesarean section delivery. *J. Child Psychol. Psychiatry* 49, 1042–1052. doi: 10.1111/j.1469- 7610.2008.01963.x
82. Tessier, R., Cristo, M., Velez, S., Giron, M., de Calume, Z. F., Ruiz-Palaez, J. G., et al. (1998). Kangaroo mother care and the bonding hypothesis. *Pediatrics* 102:e17. doi: 10.1542/peds.102.2.e17
83. van Ijzendoorn, M. H., Schuengel, C., and Bakermans-Kranenburg, M. J. (1999). Disorganized attachment in early childhood: meta-analysis of precursors, concomitants and sequelae. *Dev. Psychopathol.* 11, 225–249. doi: 10. 1017/s0954579499002035
84. Wehr, T. A., Muscettola, G., and Goodwin, F. K. (1980). Urinary 3-methoxy-4-hydroxyphenylglycol circadian rhythm: early timing (phase-advance) in manic-depressives compared with normal subjects. *Arch. Gen. Psychiatry* 37, 257–263. doi: 10.1001/archpsyc.1980.01780160027002
85. Weisman, O., Delaherche, E., Rondeau, M., Chetouani, M., Cohen, D., and Feldman, R. (2013). Oxytocin shapes parental motion during father–infant interaction. *Biol. Lett.* 9:20130828. doi: 10.1098/rsbl.2013. 0828
86. Whybrow, P. C., and Mendels, J. (1969). Towards a biology of depression. *Am. J. Psychiatry* 125, 1491–1500. doi: 10.1176/ajp.125.11.1491
87. Wiesenfeld, A. R., Malatesta, C. Z., and Deloach, L. L. (1981). Differential parental response to familial and unfamiliar infant distress signals. *Infant Behav. Dev.* 4, 281–295. doi: 10.1016/s0163-6383(81)80030-6
88. Wilson, M. (2002). Six views of embodied cognition. *Psychon. Bull. Rev.* 9, 625–636. doi: 10.3758/bf03196322
89. Wolff, E. A. III, Putnam, F. W., and Post, R. M. (1985). Motor activity and affective illness. The relationship of amplitude and temporal distribution to changes in affective state. *Arch. Gen. Psychiatry* 42, 288–294. doi: 10.1001/ archpsyc.1985. 01790260086010
90. Young, K. S., Parsons, C. E., Stein, A., and Kringelbach, M. L. (2012). Interpreting infant vocal distress: the ameliorative effect of musical training in depression. *Emotion* 12, 1200–1205. doi: 10.1037/a0028705

22

Neurological soft signs in the clinical course of schizophrenia: results of a meta-analysis

Silke Bachmann[1,2†], *Christina Degen*[3*†], *Franz Josef Geider*[3] *and Johannes Schröder*[3]

[1] Clienia Littenheid AG, Littenheid, Switzerland
[2] Department of Psychiatry, Psychotherapy, and Psychosomatics, University of Halle, Halle, Germany
[3] Section of Geriatric Psychiatry, Institute of Gerontology, University of Heidelberg, Heidelberg, Germany

Edited by:
Sebastian Walther, University Hospital of Psychiatry, Switzerland

Reviewed by:
Raymond C. Chan, Chinese Academy of Sciences, China
Lise Docx, University of Antwerp, Belgium

***Correspondence:**
Christina Degen, University Hospital Heidelberg, Section of Geriatric Psychiatry, Voßstraße 4, Heidelberg 69115, Germany
e-mail: christina.degen@med.uni-heidelberg.de

† Silke Bachmann and Christina Degen have contributed equally to this work.

Neurological soft signs (NSS) comprise subtle deficits in sensory integration, motor coordination, and sequencing of complex motor acts, which are typically observed in the majority of schizophrenia patients, including chronic cases and neuroleptic-naïve first-episode patients. However, recent studies clearly demonstrate that NSS are not a static feature of schizophrenia but vary in the clinical course of the disorder. This effect was investigated in a meta-analysis based on 17 longitudinal studies published between 1992 and 2012. Studies included between 10 and 93 patients with schizophrenia spectrum disorders (total number 787) with follow-up periods between 2 and 208 weeks. Beside the Neurological Examination Scale, the Cambridge Neurological Inventory and the Heidelberg NSS Scale were used to assess NSS. All but three studies found NSS to decrease in parallel with remission of psychopathological symptoms. This effect was more pronounced in patients with a remitting compared to a non-remitting, chronic course (Cohen's *d* 0.81 vs. 0.15) and was significantly correlated with length of the follow-up period ($r = -0.64$) but not with age ($r = 0.28$). NSS scores did not decrease to the level typically observed in healthy controls. From a clinical perspective, NSS may therefore be used to identify subjects at risk to develop schizophrenia and to monitor disease progression.

Keywords: NSS, schizophrenia, chronicity, course, outcome

INTRODUCTION

Neurological soft signs (NSS) refer to subtle neurological abnormalities comprising deficits in sensory integration, motor coordination, and sequencing of complex motor acts (1–3). It is generally accepted that NSS are more prevalent in schizophrenia patients compared to healthy subjects. They have consistently been demonstrated in neuroleptic-naïve first-episode patients, i.e., prior to medication exposure, supporting the assumption that NSS constitute an intrinsic feature of schizophrenia. This notion is underlined by increased NSS scores in high-risk subjects, such as relatives of schizophrenic patients, or in the unaffected co-twins of monozygotic twin-pairs discordant for schizophrenia (4–6).

Already in 1980, Torrey found NSS to be associated with more chronic and severe forms of the illness (7). Along these lines, Manschreck and Ames (1) reported significant correlations between NSS and psychopathological symptoms in a cross-sectional study. These findings led to the hypothesis that NSS are not a static feature of schizophrenia but vary in the clinical course of the disorder, which was investigated in the late 1980s and early 1990s by the Heidelberg group (3, 8). Patients with an acute exacerbation of schizophrenia were investigated on admission, the seventh day of treatment, and following remission of acute symptoms, prior to discharge. Results clearly demonstrated a decrease of NSS scores with remission of psychopathological symptoms. Similarly, the parallel decrease of NSS and psychopathological symptoms during neuroleptic treatment was confirmed in drug-naïve first-episode (FE) patients (9) and during the long-term course up to 4 years (10–12). When contrasted with healthy controls, NSS scores obtained in schizophrenia patients remained significantly higher during follow-up indicating that NSS comprise both state- and trait-features.

These findings are pivotal to our concept of NSS and indicate that cerebral sites important for motor and sensory functions are directly involved in schizophrenia. From a clinical standpoint, NSS may be used to monitor the disease process or to identify subjects with an increased liability toward schizophrenia. However, these conclusions are based on the above observation of the remission of NSS with psychopathological symptoms during the clinical course. In the present study, we therefore analyzed the development of NSS in the course of schizophrenia as it was described in longitudinal studies. We hypothesized NSS scores to decrease with remission of psychopathological symptoms and expected this effect to be more pronounced in patients with a more favorable compared to a chronic, non-remitting course of disorder.

METHODS

Studies on the longitudinal course of NSS in schizophrenia were identified by conventional bibliographic search in particular of the reference list of previous papers (13) and by a *pubmed* search performed in August 2014 using the keywords: "schizophrenia," "NSS," "course," "follow-up," "chronicity." These procedures yielded 16 relevant publications, which reported the data necessary to calculate effect sizes (Cohen's *d*). An additional data set was contributed on request (14). Studies were published between 1992 and 2012; they differed with respect to the clinical settings and the rating instruments used (**Table 1**). Eleven studies assessed NSS with the

Table 1 | Overview of studies.

Study	Follow-up (weeks)	Scale	N	Diagnostic groups	Mean age (SD)	Medication	NSS t1	NSS t2	Effect size	Psy. path t1	Psy. path t2	Effect size 2
Bachmann et al. (10)	56	HD, PANSS	39	FE (DSM-IV)	27 (7.7)	Clin. Needs	15.7 (7.1)	10.1 (7.9)	0.75	52.4 (25.6)	52 (12.4)	0.02
			22	HC	28 (3.8)		4.8 (3.3)	4.6 (3.9)	0.06	*	*	
			18	NR (DSM-IV)	*		13.8 (7.2)	13.5 (8.7)	0.04	52.6 (14.9)	63.9 (32.6)	−0.48
			21	R (DSM-IV)	*		17.3 (6.8)	7.2 (5.8)	1.60	51.4 (10)	42.6 (10.8)	0.85
Boks et al. (18)	104	NES, PANSS	29	FE (DSM-IV)	26.9 (6.3)		7.5 (7.1)	8.9 (5.5)	−0.22	*	*	*
Buchanan et al. (19)	10	NES, BPRS	16	CH (DSM-III)	34.1 (6.8)	Clozapine	16.2 (5.9)	16.8 (8.2)	−0.09	11.4 (5.8)	9.4 (5.2)	0.34
	10		15	CH (DSM-III)	34.6 (9.1)	Haloperidol	14.5 (6.3)	15.1 (7.5)	−0.09	12.6 (5.3)	12.0 (5.1)	0.12
Chen et al. (20)	156	motor CNI	93	FE (DSM-IV)	31.2 (9.6)	Haloperidol imitially	1.87 (2)	1.45 (2.2)	0.2	*	*	*
			68	HC	32 (8.4)		*	*		*	*	*
Cuesta et al. (21)	26	NES	77	FE (DSM-IV)	30.1 (10)	Risperidone or olanzapine	17.1 (9.4)	9.9 (6.8)	0.89	10.1 (3.5)[a]	1.6 (2.1)	3.04
		SAPS, SANS			30.6 (6.2)		*	*		8 (5.9)[b]	4.7 (4.9)	0.61
Emsley et al. (14)	52	NES	15	FE (DSM-IV)	28.1 (8.5)		6.2 (3.57)	5.1 (4.0)	0.3	*	*	*
Mangot and Sawant (22)	52	NES	40	FE (ICD-10)	35.5 (11.9)		8.5 (7.1)	3.3 (4.1)	0.93	*	*	*
Mayoral et al. (16)	104	NES	29	FE (DSM-IV)	15.7 (1.6)		23.2 (9.1)	19.2 (9.9)	0.42	*	*	*
			22	HC	15.2 (1.6)		12.2 (6.7)	9.7 (5.2)	0.42	*	*	*
Mayoral et al. (17)	104	NES, PANSS	69	FE (DSM-IV)	15.5 (1.8)		25.2 (9.6)	19.9 (8.1)	0.6	66.2 (17.9)	58 (23.3)	0.40
			80	HC	15.2 (1.9)		11.1 (7.2)	9.2 (5.5)	0.3	*	*	*
Mittal et al. (23)	6	Quitkin, BPRS	19	SCHIZ (DSM-III-R)	36.3 (5.4)	Haloperidol	6.3 (0.9)	5.3 (0.8)	1.18	34.3 (2.1)	22.4 (2.2)	5.53
Prikryl et al. (11)	52	NES, PANSS	92	FE (ICD-10)	25.3 (5.5)		*	*		*	*	
			20	NR	*		6.5 (4.1)	4.2 (4.1)	0.56	88.4 (19.9)	84.7 (21.6)	0.18
			72	R	*		5.3 (5.9)	2.7 (3.4)	0.56	97.6 (22.5)	43.8 (11.1)	3.20
Prikryl et al. (12)	208	NES	68	FE (ICD-10)	22.5 (5)		6.3 (5.1)	6.8 (6.6)	−0.09	97 (23.2)	51.5 (19)	2.16
			29	NR	*		6.6 (4.8)	10.1 (7.6)	−0.56	*	*	*
			39	R	*		6 (5.4)	4.4 (4.5)	0.32	*	*	*
Schröder et al. (3)	variable	HD, BPRS	27	CH (DSM-III)	36 (12.1)	Clin. needs	27.8 (9.2)	22.1 (7.1)	0.7	*	*	*
			23	R	28.9 (8.9)		23.5 (8.3)	13 (4.7)	1.61	*	*	*
Schröder et al. (8)	variable	HD, BPRS	32	CH and R (DSM-III)	32 (9)	Clin. needs	21.3 (8.3)	11.5 (5.7)	1.4	46.1 (7.3)	32.1 (5.7)	2.15
Schröder et al. (9)	4	HD, BPRS	15	FE (DSM-III-R)	29.2 (9.4)	Benperidol	16.2 (7.5)	10 (4.7)	1.02	48.1 (6.6)	35.7 (7.7)	1.75
			8	R			15.5 (7.2)	9.3 (4.6)	1.05	49.4 (7.8)	32.5 (7.2)	2.25
			7	NR			17.0 (8.5)	10.9 (5.0)	0.9	46.7 (5.2)	39.3 (7.4)	1.18
Sevincok and Topaloglu (24)	2	NES, PANSS	10	CH (DSM-IV)	24.5 (*)	Olanzapine	19.1 (13.2)	14.7 (12.5)	0.34	78.8 (19.9)	58.0 (13.1)	1.26
Whitty et al. (25)	26	NES, PANSS	79	FE (DSM-IV)	23.4 (*)		15.6 (9.7)	12.5 (7.3)	0.36	83.3 (20.1)	58.4 (15.1)	1.41

*HD, Heidelberg NSS Scale; PANSS, Positive and Negative Syndrome Scale; NES, Neurological Evaluation Scale; BPRS, Brief Psychiatric Rating Scale; CNI, Cambridge Neurological Inventory; SAPS, Scale for the assessment of positive symptoms; SANS, Scale for the assessment of negative symptoms; FE, first-episode psychosis; HC, healthy controls; NR, non-remitters; R, remitters; CH, chronic schizophrenics; SCHIZ, schizophrenia patients; [a], SAPS, [b], SANS, *, missing values.*

Neurological Examination Scale (NES) and four with the Heidelberg scale (HD). One study used the Cambridge Neurological Inventory [CNI (15)]. Two studies examined adolescents (16, 17). The latter results will be discussed separately, since the motor system has not entirely maturated at this age. Separate effect sizes were calculated for NSS and psychopathology before estimating mean effect sizes for patients with remitting and chronic courses.

RESULTS

Included studies are summarized in **Table 1**. The number of patients per study ranged between 10 and 93 (total number 787); 12 studies solely included FE patients, 2 studies focused on adolescents. Patients' clinical course was characterized as either remitting or non-remitting/chronic in eight studies; in one study only the diagnosis "schizophrenia" was conveyed. Follow-up periods ranged between 2 weeks and 4 years. In nine studies, the examination commenced during the acute psychotic episodes; in four of those a reexamining after remission of acute symptoms, prior to discharge, took place. Standardized neuroleptic treatment was prescribed in five studies, namely high potency butyrophenones (haloperidol or benperidol), risperidone, or olanzapine.

All but three studies described a decrease of NSS in the clinical course. Eleven studies included an assessment of the clinical course. Patients with remitting symptoms showed a steeper decrease of NSS scores (mean effect size: Cohen's *d* 0.81) than patients with an unfavorable or chronic course (mean effect size: Cohen's *d* 0.15), who even exhibited an increase in scores. Overall, effect sizes (Cohen's *d*) ranged between −0.56 (patients with an unfavorable course) and 1.61 (patients with a remitting course treated for an acute episode) with an overall mean effect size of Cohen's *d* 0.53. Ratings of psychopathological symptoms paralleled the development of NSS scores but were only reported in 11 of the 17 studies. Moreover, data on the distinction between negative and positive symptom scores were provided by five studies only (12, 17, 21, 23, 24). In FE patients, as a group, a moderate effect size was present (Cohen's *d* 0.42). Similar effect sizes (Cohen's *d*: 0.42–0.60) were reported in adolescent patients with FE psychosis. Effect sizes were significantly ($p < 0.05$) correlated with length of the follow-up period ($r = -0.64, p = 0.001$) but not with age ($r = 0.28$).

DISCUSSION

The present meta-analysis revealed two main findings: (i) a confirmation that NSS scores decrease in the clinical course of schizophrenia with remission of psychopathological symptoms; and (ii) an indication that this effect is more pronounced in patients with a remitting course than in those with non-remitting schizophrenia.

Despite numerous methodological differences, all but three studies found decreasing NSS scores during the clinical course with remission of acute schizophrenia symptoms. Boks et al. (18) reported NSS to increase in a group of 29 FE patients, who were investigated 2 years apart (Cohen's *d* −0.22). They assigned this effect to a subgroup of patients with a more severe form of the disorder or a regression to the mean and stressed the importance of the relatively small sample size when interpreting their findings. A marginal increase of NSS scores (Cohen's *d* −0.09) in patients with chronic schizophrenia was also reported by Buchanan and colleagues (19) in 31 patients who received haloperidol or clozapine for 10 weeks. Jahn et al. (26) identified increasing NSS scores only in a small subgroup of patients in whom symptoms deteriorated. Their study could not be included in our meta-analysis, because only median values had been documented. Prikryl et al. (12) systematically followed FE patients for 4 years and found NSS to marginally increase (Cohen's *d* −0.09) when the whole group of 68 patients was considered. This effect, however, was caused by a subgroup of patients developing chronic schizophrenia (Cohen's *d* −0.56) while NSS in those with a remitting course decreased (Cohen's *d* 0.32). A similar build-up of NSS scores has been described by Chen et al. (27) in 43 patients with chronic schizophrenia over the course of 3 years. Their study was not included here, because total NSS scores had not been provided. Taken together, effect sizes for the decrease of NSS scores ranged from Cohen's *d* 0.04 to Cohen's *d* 1.61 with an average of Cohen's *d* 0.64. The smallest effects were seen in patients with non-remitting schizophrenia (mean effect size for non-remitting patients: Cohen's *d* 0.15) while more pronounced effect sizes were observed in patients with a remitting course (mean effect size for remitting patients: Cohen's *d* 0.81). However, only eight studies assessed the clinical course while nine just characterized patients as FE or solely documented DSM diagnoses.

A most interesting question arises from the finding that the decrease of NSS and the decrease of symptoms parallel each other. Unfortunately, this relationship could not be analyzed any further by meta-analytic tools. Both NSS and psychopathology had been assessed with several different instruments, and symptom scores were not provided in several publications.

The effect sizes reported in FE studies appeared to be lower than those found in patients with a remitting and even those with a chronic course. However, only four of the available FE studies drew a distinction between remitting and non-remitting patients. In addition, the exact timing of the first examination after study intake has to be taken into account. While Prikryl and colleagues (11, 12) and Schröder et al. (9) examined NSS at or shortly after admission, i.e., in an acute psychotic state – Bachmann et al. (10) conducted the first NSS examination after clinical stabilization, before discharge. This may well have had an impact on the findings since NSS scores typically show a significant decrease with remission of the acute symptoms (3, 8). The important meta-analysis of cross-sectional NSS studies by Chan et al. (28) found effect sizes of patients vs. controls comparisons to be moderated by duration of illness. One may hypothesize that NSS continue to improve or worsen during the course following the first manifestation of the disease; a hypothesis, which conforms to the above cited studies, namely the differences, which emerged between patients with a remitting vs. a non-remitting, chronic course.

The decrease of NSS with clinical stabilization during the course was more pronounced in patients with a favorable than with a non-remitting course (3, 9, 10, 11, and 12); therefore, NSS scores could be identified as course predictors. However, even after remission of the acute illness, NSS scores remained significantly higher than in healthy controls. These findings demonstrate that NSS in schizophrenia are both trait- and state-related. NSS persistence and deterioration in patients with a chronic course of the disorder clearly point to a progression of corresponding cerebral changes as demonstrated in a recent study from the Heidelberg group (29). From a clinical perspective, NSS may therefore be used to identify subjects at risk to develop chronic schizophrenia. It is well known, that total NSS scores in schizophrenia are mainly due to motor and sensory subscores. Unfortunately, only 7 of 17 studies (10–12, 16, 17, 21, 25) reported subscores; therefore, a more detailed meta-analysis could not be performed.

A decrease of NSS scores with clinical stabilization was also reported in adolescent patients with FE psychosis (16, 17), i.e., during an age in which the motor and sensory systems are still not entirely maturated. Both studies of the Mayoral group also found a decrease of NSS in the control group over the 2-year-study period and a higher score level in patients on comparison. Authors attributed their findings to an overall developmental delay caused by rather than a direct consequence of the disease.

Potentially confounding variables include different NSS rating scales and study designs. Although different, the various NSS scales are comparable with regard to the majority of subscales and sensitivity (27); moreover, the potential impact of the respective psychometric differences is at least partially addressed by the longitudinal designs of the studies. Neuroleptic treatment was standardized in 6 of the included 17 studies only. However, the vast majority of studies discussed here report decreasing NSS in patients treated with any neuroleptic compound. Furthermore, it is known that NSS are not caused by neuroleptic medication (30, 31). In our study, a negative correlation between effect sizes and length of follow-up period was identified. It is plausible that clinical stabilization occurs in the beginning of the follow-up interval leaving mostly non-remitting patients. As a result, effect sizes of NSS decrease with length of inspected interval.

Along with this, Buchanan et al. (19) did not find meaningful or even significant differences in chronic patients receiving either clozapine or haloperidol while Schröder et al. (9) demonstrated a decrease of NSS in FE patients who received a conventional neuroleptic. As discussed above, the timing of the first examination may even have great importance, in particular as the exact starting points were not defined in a number of studies. The decrease of NSS was correlated with age, although this did not reach statistical significance. The meta-analysis of cross-sectional studies (28) did not find NSS difference scores between patients and healthy controls to be moderated by age when only studies with the NES were entered into the meta-analysis. Although both findings correspond with respect to the direction of change, the impact of age and other potential moderators as sex and education, or cognitive reserve (Urbanowitsch et al., submitted) on NSS needs to be further analyzed. Against the background of a relatively small number of studies included here, the respective methodological questions call for a large multicenter longitudinal study in FE patients. Such an endeavor would not only be suitable to dissect the decrease of NSS in the clinical course confirmed in this meta-analysis but could also serve to define the state and trait characteristics of NSS more precisely. The potential impact of motor development could be addressed in adolescent patients; moreover, neuroimaging studies could be designed to better understand the role of motor and sensory cortical sites in schizophrenia.

From a clinical standpoint, the decrease of NSS with clinical stabilization may be used to monitor disease progression or to identify subjects with an increased liability toward schizophrenia in general and more chronic, unfavorable courses in particular. As a phenomenon, NSS point at the involvement of motor and sensory cerebral sites in the disorder. Since NSS correspond to impaired motor and sensory functions like motor coordination, they can be used to further develop and optimize physical training programs, which are already part of the routine therapeutic repertoire.

ACKNOWLEDGMENTS

This study was supported by the Dietmar-Hopp Foundation, Walldorf, Germany. We are grateful to Robin Emsley/Stellenbosch, South Africa for providing his valuable data.

REFERENCES

1. Manschreck TC, Ames D. Neurologic features and psychopathology in schizophrenic disorders. *Biol Psychiatry* (1984) **19**:703–19.
2. Heinrichs DW, Buchanan RW. Significance and meaning of neurological signs in schizophrenia. *Am J Psychiatry* (1988) **145**:11–8.
3. Schröder J, Niethammer R, Geider F-J, Reitz C, Binkert M, Jauss M, et al. Neurological soft signs in schizophrenia. *Schizophr Res* (1992) **6**:25–30. doi:10.1016/0920-9964(91)90017-L
4. Niethammer R, Weisbrod M, Schiesser S, Grothe J, Maier S, Peter U, et al. Genetic Influence on laterality in schizophrenia? A twin study of neurological soft signs. *Am J Psychiatry* (2000) **157**:272–4. doi:10.1176/appi.ajp.157.2.272
5. Torrey EF, Taylor EH, Bracha HS, Bowler AE, McNeil TF, Rawlings RR, et al. Prenatal origin of schizophrenia in a subgroup of discordant monozygotic twins. *Schizophr Bull* (1994) **20**:423–32. doi:10.1093/schbul/20.3.423
6. Rossi A, De Cataldo S, Di Michele V, Manna V, Ceccoli S, Stratta P, et al. Neurological soft signs in schizophrenia. *Br J Psychiatry* (1990) **157**:735–9. doi:10.1192/bjp.157.5.735
7. Torrey EF. Neurological abnormalities in schizophrenic patients. *Biol Psychiatry* (1980) **15**:381–9.
8. Schröder J, Tittel A, Stockert A, Karr M. Memory deficits in subsyndromes of chronic schizophrenia. *Schizophr Res* (1996) **21**:19–26. doi:10.1016/0920-9964(96)00027-8
9. Schröder J, Silvestri S, Bubeck B, Karr M, Demisch S, Scherrer S, et al. D2 Dopamine receptor up-regulation, treatment response, neurological soft signs, and extrapyramidal side effects in schizophrenia: a follow-up study with ^{123}I-iodobenzamide single photon emission computed tomography in the drug-naïve state and after neuroleptic treatment. *Biol Psychiatry* (1998) **43**: 660–5.
10. Bachmann S, Bottmer C, Schröder S. Neurological soft signs in first-episode schizophrenia: a follow-up study. *Am J Psychiatry* (2005) **162**:2337–43. doi:10.1176/appi.ajp.162.12.2337
11. Prikryl R, Ceskova E, Kasparek T, Kucerova H. Neurological soft signs and their relationship to 1-year outcome in first-episode schizophrenia. *Eur Psychiatry* (2007) **22**:449–504. doi:10.1016/j.eurpsy.2007.03.012
12. Prikryl R, Ceskova E, Tronerova S, Kasparek T, Prikrylova Kucerova H, Ustohal L, et al. Dynamics of neurological soft signs and its relationship to clinical course in patients with first-episode schizophrenia. *Psychiatry Res* (2012) **200**:67–72. doi:10.1016/j.psychres.2012.03.008
13. Bachmann S, Schröder J. Neurological soft signs in schizophrenia: a review on the state- versus trait-perspective.
14. Emsley R, Turner HJ, Oosthuizen PP, Carr J. Neurological abnormalities in first-episode schizophrenia: temporal stability and clinical and outcome correlates. *Schizophr Res* (2005) **75**:35–44. doi:10.1016/j.schres.2004.06.014
15. Chen EYH, Shapleske J, Luque R, McKenna PJ, Hodges JR, Calloway SP, et al. The Cambridge Neurological Inventory: a clinical instrument for assessment of soft neurological signs in psychiatric patients. *Psychiatry Res* (1995) **56**:183–204. doi:10.1016/0165-1781(95)02535-2
16. Mayoral M, Bombin I, Zabala A, Robes O, Moreno D, Parellada M, et al. Neurological soft signs in adolescents with first-episode psychosis: two-year followup. *Psychiatry Res* (2008) **161**:344–8. doi:10.1016/j.psychres.2007.07.013
17. Mayoral M, Bombin I, Castro-Fornieles J, Gonzales-Pinto A, Otero S, Parellada M, et al. Longitudinal study of neurological soft signs in first-episode early-onset psychosis. *J Child Psychol Psychiatry* (2012) **53**:323–31. doi:10.1111/j.1469-7610.2011.02475.x

18. Boks MPM, Selten JP, Leask S, Van den Bosch RJ. The 2-year stability of neurological soft signs after a first episode of non-affective psychosis. *Eur Psychiatry* (2006) **21**:288–90. doi:10.1016/j.eurpsy.2005.09.004
19. Buchanan RW, Koeppl P, Breier A. Stability of neurological signs with clozapine treatment. *Biol Psychiatry* (1994) **36**:198–200. doi:10.1016/0006-3223(94)91225-4
20. Chen EYH, Hui CLM, Chan RCK, Dunn ELW, Miao MYK, Yeung WS, et al. A 3-year prospective study of neurological soft signs in first episode schizophrenia. *Schizophr Res* (2005) **75**:45–54. doi:10.1016/j.schres.2004.09.002
21. Cuesta MJ, Jalon EG, Campos MS, Peralta V. Cognitive effectiveness of olanzapine and risperidone in first episode psychosis. *Br J Psychiatry* (2009) **194**:439–45. doi:10.1192/bjp.bp.108.055137
22. Mangot AG, Sawant NS. First episode schizophrenia: neurological abnormalities and prognosis. *German J Psychiatry*. Reprinted from the German Journal of Psychiatry. Available from: http://www.gjpsy.uni-goettingen.de
23. Mittal VA, Hasenkamp W, Sanfilipo M, Wieland S, Angrist B, Rotrosen J, et al. Relation of neurological soft signs to psychiatric symptoms in schizophrenia. *Schizophr Res* (2007) **94**:37–44. doi:10.1016/j.schres.2007.04.017
24. Sevincok L, Topaloglu B. Neurological soft signs and positive treatment response to olanzapine in chronic schizophrenia. *Prog Neuropsychoph* (2006) **30**:141–3. doi:10.1016/j.pnpbp.2005.06.012
25. Whitty P, Clarke M, Browne S, McTique O, Kamali M, Feeney L, et al. Prospective evaluation of neurological soft signs in first-episode schizophrenia in relation to psychopathology: state versus trait phenomena. *Psychol Med* (2003) **33**:1479–84. doi:10.1017/S0033291703008225
26. Jahn T, Hubmann W, Karr M, Mohr F, Schlenker R, Heidenreich T, et al. Motoric neurological soft signs and psychopathological symptoms in schizophrenic psychoses. *Psychiatr Res* (2006) **142**:191–9. doi:10.1016/j.psychres.2002.12.003
27. Chen EYH, Kwok CL, Au JWY, Chen RYL, Lau BST. Progressive deterioration of soft neurological signs in chronic schizophrenic patients. *Acta Psychiatr Scand* (2000) **102**:342–9. doi:10.1034/j.1600-0447.2000.102005342.x
28. Chan RCK, Xu T, Heinrichs RW, Yu Y, Wang Y. Neurological soft signs in schizophrenia: a meta-analysis. *Schizophr Bull* (2009) **36**:1089–104. doi:10.1093/schbul/sbp011
29. Kong L, Bachmann S, Thomann PA, Essig M, Schröder J. Neurological soft signs and gray matter changes: a longitudinal analysis in first-episode schizophrenia. *Schizophr Res* (2012) **134**:27–32. doi:10.1016/j.schres.2011.09.015
30. Browne S, Clarke M, Gervin M, Lane A, Waddington JL, Larkin C, et al. Determinants of neurological dysfunction in first episode schizophrenia. *Psychol Med* (2000) **30**:1433–41. doi:10.1017/S003329179900286X
31. Keshavan MS, Sanders RD, Sweeney JA, Diwadkar VA, Goldstein G, Pettegrew JW, et al. Diagnostic specificity and neuroanatomical validity of neurological abnormalities in first-episode psychosis. *Am J Psychiatry* (2003) **160**:1298–304. doi:10.1176/appi.ajp.160.7.1298

23

Psychomotor retardation in elderly untreated depressed patients

Lieve Lia Beheydt[1], Didier Schrijvers[1], Lise Docx[1], Filip Bouckaert[2], Wouter Hulstijn[1] and Bernard Sabbe[1]*

[1] Collaborative Antwerp Psychiatric Research Institute (CAPRI), Antwerp University, Antwerp, Belgium
[2] University Psychiatric Center KU Leuven, Kortenberg, Belgium

Edited by:
Sebastian Walther, University Hospital of Psychiatry, Switzerland

Reviewed by:
Tobias Bracht, Cardiff University, UK
Valentin Johannes Benzing, University Hospital of Psychiatry, Switzerland

****Correspondence:***
Lieve Lia Beheydt, Medical and Health Science Department, Collaborative Antwerp Psychiatric Research Institute (CAPRI), Antwerp University, Campus Drie Eiken – gebouw R D.R.328, Universiteitsplein 1, Antwerp 2610, Belgium
e-mail: lieve.beheydt@uantwerpen.be

Background: Psychomotor retardation (PR) is one of the core features in depression according to DSM V (1), but also aging in itself causes cognitive and psychomotor slowing. This is the first study investigating PR in relation to cognitive functioning and to the concomitant effect of depression and aging in a geriatric population ruling out contending effects of psychotropic medication.

Methods: A group of 28 non-demented depressed elderly is compared to a matched control group of 20 healthy elderly. All participants underwent a test battery containing clinical depression measures, cognitive measures of processing speed, executive function and memory, clinical ratings of PR, and objective computerized fine motor skill-tests. Statistical analysis consisted of a General Linear Method multivariate analysis of variance to compare the clinical, cognitive, and psychomotor outcomes of the two groups.

Results: Patients performed worse on all clinical, cognitive, and PR measures. Both groups showed an effect of cognitive load on fine motor function but the influence was significantly larger for patients than for healthy elderly except for the initiation time.

Limitations: Due to the restrictive inclusion criteria, only a relatively limited sample size could be obtained.

Conclusion: With a medication free sample, an additive effect of depression and aging on cognition and PR in geriatric patients was found. As this effect was independent of demand of effort (by varying the cognitive load), it was apparently not a motivational slowing effect of depression.

Keywords: major depression, elderly, psychomotor retardation, cognition, copying tasks, neuropsychological assessment, medication free

INTRODUCTION

Apart from a depressed mood and lack of interest, psychomotor symptoms are core features of a major depressive episode (2). Recently, a three factor model of depression was found, representing negative effect, anhedonia, and psychomotor change (3). This psychomotor change symptom cluster has an important clinical, diagnostic, pathophysiological, and therapeutic significance in the clinical and scientific approach of Major Depressive Disorder (MDD) (4–8). Psychomotor retardation (PR) has repeatedly been denoted as an important marker of the melancholia subtype of depression (5, 9–11), and as a predictor for treatment response to several types of antidepressant treatment (5). Since psychomotor functioning is the only factor of depression that does not correlate with severity of depression and since it is not predictive for clinical outcome, it is thought to be a dimension defining a separate type (3), though not exclusively the melancholic subtype of depression. PR has been found to be present in other subtypes of depression too (11–19). However, it is not only the presence of PR that is important, the type of slowing and the cognitive share in the PR are thought to be differentiating between subtypes of depression too (20). Hence the importance of investigating psychomotor functioning in depression in relation to cognitive functioning.

Psychomotor retardation appears to be a particularly predominant symptom of late life depression, an organic subtype of geriatric depression with vascular damage of frontal–subcortical circuits and a depressive–executive dysfunction syndrome (21, 22), but also of other atypical depression presentations such as subsyndromal depression (23). As aging itself already causes a substantial psychomotor slowing in healthy elderly (24–26), elderly depressed patients could be expected to show an even more pronounced form of PR. Pier and colleagues (25) hypothesized an additive effect of aging and depression on the psychomotor performance, be it on the basis of a sample of 11 medicated patients. Bonin-Guillaume et al. (27) too found an additive PR effect in 16 patients. The retardation showed to be an addition of two different types of slowing. There was a general slowing in aging, affecting all stages of information processing, and a more specific slowing in depression, affecting the decisional stage and the neuromotor stage, but not the sensory-motor stage. It should be noted, however, that they did only investigate the reaction time and not the motor time as a measure of psychomotor speed (27). The included patients in both studies were all using psychotropic medication, i.e., antidepressants (selective serotonin re-uptake inhibitors and tricyclic antidepressants) as well as anxiolytics and confounding medication effects were observed (25, 27). Admittedly, polypharmacy is very common in elder age patients, and since these patients are also more sensitive to all kinds of adverse medication induced side-effects, differentiating between the specific effects of depression, age, and medication is particularly difficult, especially as the medication profiles of the subjects in previous studies may have been extremely divergent. Studies on PR in elderly depression are still scarce and show only partial results, because most of these have only measured PR on the basis of cognitive reaction times, without distinguishing and separating out motor slowing (27–30). The two studies that do investigate motor time include only medicated patients (25, 31). All in all, differentiated research of psychomotor symptoms in geriatric depression is still very limited and only exists in medicated clinical cohorts, so that evidence is still missing for the value of these types of symptoms as a diagnostic tool for this subgroup of depressed patients.

Psychomotor retardation not only involves motor processes, but also cognitive processes. Indeed, the term PR "not only encompasses the output of muscle contractions, but also the wider involvement of perceptual processes and cognitive-control mechanisms" (5) (p. 14). Indeed, several cognitive sub-processes contribute to the psychomotor processing. Studies on neuropsychological functioning in late life depression generally mention processing speed and executive function as the main cognitive impairments in MDD in the elderly (32, 33). Yet, PR and executive functioning are not correlated, indicating that cognitive retardation is not the sole explanation of PR (34). It has been suggested that retardation in executive function is merely the consequence of reduced processing speed (35–37). However, Sexton et al. (38) found that executive deficits could not be fully explained by general impairments in processing speed. Controlling for processing speed, Dybedal et al. (32) still found impaired executive function in elderly depressed compared to healthy controls. Considering that both processing speed and executive functioning are the cognitive hallmarks of depression, they will be treated separately here in relation to psychomotor measures. Since executive function and PR are not correlated, it would be interesting to figure out whether depression severity without interfering medication effects, has a specific impact on cognitive and psychomotor functioning, respectively.

The current study aims to measure cognitive and psychomotor functioning in a sample of unmedicated depressed elderly, applying objective psychomotor, and cognitive assessment methods. In accordance with previous studies (25, 28), it is hypothesized that unmedicated elderly depressed patients will perform worse both on the cognitive and psychomotor tasks. Different cognitive and psychomotor measures will be applied to shed a light on different cognitive factors that may influence PR, most importantly processing speed, but also inhibition and interference resistance, cognitive flexibility, and memory. With the objective measures of PR, the cognitive reaction time, i.e., the initiation time of a movement and the reinspection time, the time needed to verify the stimuli, will be separated from the motor time, i.e., the real movement time. Finally, the effect of cognitive load in PR will be tested by experimentally varying the complexity of the stimuli of the copying task to investigate the interaction of cognition and motor functioning in PR.

MATERIALS AND METHODS

STUDY POPULATION

Twenty-eight non-demented (Mini Mental State Examination Score > 24) elderly (age >60) in- and out-patients with unipolar single episode or recurrent MDD, meeting DSM-IVTR criteria (2), were compared to 20 healthy controls, matched for age, gender, education, and vascular risks (diabetes, hypertension, smoking, obesity, and hyperlipidemia). Patients with a MMSE score under 24, the consensus cut-off score for probable dementia (39–41), were excluded. Depression was identified using the DSM-IVTR criteria and the severity of depression was assessed by means of the Geriatric Depression Scale (GDS). A minimum score of 11 on the GDS was required for inclusion of patients. Patients taking medication with important psychotropic impact such as psychopharmacological treatments, but also antihistaminics and anticholinergics for instance, were excluded. For every type of disallowed or concomitant medication, the drug free period before testing was specified. For most antidepressants, a wash-out period of 1 week prior to baseline was applied, with the exception of fluoxetine (5 weeks), fluvoxamine (2 weeks), and monoamine oxidase inhibitors (2 weeks). Any anxiolytics (including benzodiazepines) and hypnotics (except Zolpidem, Zopiclone, or Zaleplon) were disallowed within the last week prior to testing. Patients and controls suffering from any medical condition [e.g., Parkinson's disease, dementia, psychotic disorders, mental retardation, substance- or alcohol abuse, organic mental disorders due to a general medical condition as defined in the DSM-IV-TR (2)] that might affect fine motor or cognitive processes were excluded, as were patients with personality disorders that might compromise the study. All participants were native Dutch speakers and had given their informed consent after the study was fully explained to them. The study was carried out consistent with the latest version of the Helsinki Declaration (42) and was approved by the medical ethics committee of the participating hospitals.

ASSESSMENTS AND TASKS

All participants performed an extensive cognitive and psychomotor test battery (see below). All testing, for patients and for healthy controls, took place in the afternoon.

Clinical assessment

Clinical depression severity was assessed using the GDS (30 items) (43) whereas the State and Trait Anxiety Inventory (STAI 1 and STAI2) (44) informed about the degree of subjective anxiety symptoms. Both tests were also applied to the controls. The 15-item Salpêtrière Retardation Rating Scale (SRRS) (45) was administered to assess the subjective, rated level of PR.

Psychomotor tasks

For the objective psychomotor assessment (46, 47), participants carried out drawing tasks. Subjects were asked to copy figures from a computer screen with the use of a special pressure-sensitive pen and a digitizer (48). A full description of the set up as shown in **Figures 1A,B** can be found in Pier et al. (25).

Line and figure copying task. In the Line Copying Task (LCT; **Figure 1A**), patients had to draw a line in one of four directions (horizontal, vertical, or one of the two diagonals) as quickly as possible. In the Figure Copying Task (FCT; **Figure 1B**), they had to copy figures consisting of four line segments with varying complexity, some were well-known letters, other were familiar figures and the third kind were less familiar patterns. The stimulus (line or figure) appeared on the screen when the participant placed the pen tip in the start circle at the bottom left of the box in which the stimulus had to be copied. As soon as participants started drawing, the figure disappeared from the screen. However, there was the possibility (which was not encouraged) to reinspect the figure by retouching the start circle. To end a trial, participants had to place the pen in the stop circle at the upper right corner of the box. Initiation time, the time between the presentation of the stimulus and the start of the first drawing movement, was measured. Also the motor time, the time from the start of the first drawing movement to the end of the last drawing movement, was calculated. In the second task, the reinspection time, the time from retouching the spot to resuming starting the drawing was also determined. Time to reinspect was not included in the motor time.

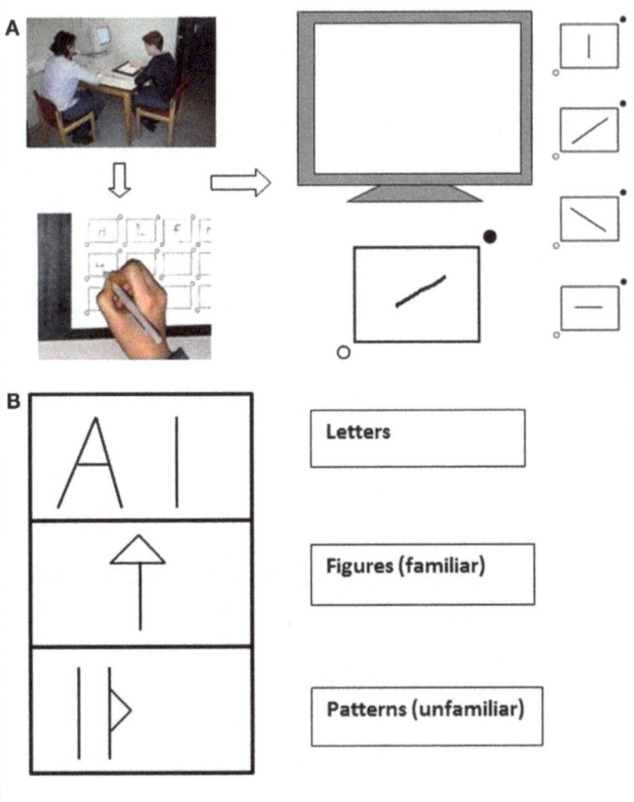

FIGURE 1 | (A,B) Set up **(A)** of the line and complex figure copying task **(B)** with pressure-sensitive digitizer.

Symbol-digit substitution test. The same recording techniques were used as with the copying tasks (49–51). This made it possible to differentiate between a cognitive and a psychomotor component apart from the general measure of information processing speed. The subjects had to substitute symbols by digits during a period of 90 s, using a key consisting of nine symbol–digit pairs. The following variables were analyzed: raw scores, i.e., the number of correct answers, matching time, representing mean pen-up time, and pause time between two successive digits (comparable to the initiation time in the copying tasks), and writing time, representing the time needed to write a digit (comparable to motor time).

Cognitive tasks

Wisconsin card sorting task. In the Wisconsin card sorting task (WCST) (52), which is primarily intended to measure cognitive flexibility, an executive function, four key cards were presented with geometric figures that vary according to three perceptual dimensions (color, form, and number). The subjects had to discover the correct sorting principle by trial and error. After each choice they got a feedback (right or wrong). Once the participant made a correct choice, this sorting principle had to be maintained across changing stimulus conditions while ignoring the other – now irrelevant – stimulus dimensions. After 10 consecutive correct matches, the classification principle changed without warning. As the WCST is not timed, sorting continued until all cards were sorted or a maximum of six correct sorting criteria had been reached. Index of the participant's performance was the number of categories completed (53–56). However, since some patients did not even complete one category, executive functions such as switching could not be measured.

Stroop color-word test. The Stroop color-word test (57, 58) is a cognitive test that requires participants to firstly read the names of colors printed in black ink (trial 1), then name printed colors (trial 2) as quickly as possible without making errors and then naming the color of a word in which it is printed (trial 3). The test measures the individual's ability to suppress task-irrelevant responses (i.e., the tendency to read the color name rather than name the color) and ability to maintain attention and concentration (59). The Stroop interference score was calculated as the time taken to name colors in trial 3 minus the time taken to name color names in trial 2. A higher Stroop interference score thus refers to the degree of interference caused by suppressing the habit of reading words in order to name colors; a higher score reflects poorer performance (59).

15-Words tests. In the 15-words task, a verbal memory task (60), subjects were presented 5 times a list of 15 words, which they had to reproduce. After an interval of 20 min, the experimenter asked to reproduce the memorized words once more. Afterward they had to recognize in a list of 30 words, which were the words they had studied. Only the sum of correct recalls has been recorded (Verbal Memory Total). The delayed recall was scored as Verbal Memory Recall. For the Verbal Memory Recognition too, only correct recognitions were scored.

STATISTICAL ANALYSIS

Statistical analysis of the data was performed using SPSS 17.00 and consisted of a General Linear Method (GLM) multivariate analysis of variance to compare the psychomotor and cognitive outcomes of the two groups. To measure the effect of cognitive load in the figure copying tasks, a GLM Repeated Measures Analysis of Variance with Group (MDD, Controls) as between-subjects factor and Complexity (letters, figures, and patterns) as within-subjects factor was performed. In addition, bivariate Pearson correlations were computed between severity of depression and the other clinical, cognitive, and psychomotor measures. Significance level was set at $p < 0.05$.

RESULTS

DEMOGRAPHIC AND CLINICAL VARIABLES

As can be seen in **Table 1**, there were no significant differences between groups on demographical variables. Patients were significantly more depressed, more anxious (as well state as trait anxiety), and showed more psychomotor retardation (SSRS) and cognitive impairment (MMSE). Severity of depression correlated with none of the cognitive and psychomotor measures, only with clinical measures of state anxiety (r GDS-STAI I = 0.524, $p = 0.006$) and slightly with the clinical rating of retardation (r GDS-SRRS = 0.418, $p = 0.047$).

COGNITIVE AND PSYCHOMOTOR PERFORMANCE

Patients performed significantly worse than controls on all cognitive measures. For an overview, see **Table 2**. The largest effects are found for the number of correct filled in items on the symbol-digit substitution test (SDST) (Cohen's $d = 1.37$) (61), the matching time of SDST (Cohen's $d = 0.94$), the Wisconsin number of categories completed (Cohen's $d = 1.40$), and the total recall of the verbal memory test (Cohen's $d = 0.96$). The measures of the perseverative errors and non-perseverative errors in the Wisconsin task had to be left out because they proved meaningless, as patients could not even complete one category. The impaired learning capacity is confirmed by the verbal memory scores. As can be seen in the table, the Stroop tasks too almost reached significance on the 0.01 level. In general, however, the significance was lowered by the difference in variance between patients and healthy controls, with a larger variance in the patient scores, except for the WCST. The latter exception can presumably be explained by a floor effect, as patients did not even manage to learn one category. The difference in SDST total correct, the measure of processing speed, reveals that a general retardation of processing speed is a central feature of elderly depression. Still on the SDST, both the matching and

Table 1 | Demographic and clinical variables of patients and controls.

	Patients ($N = 28$)	Controls ($N = 20$)	F	p	Cohen's d
Age	74.71 (7.56)	71.95 (5.14)	2.01	0.163	
Male/female	4/24	5/15	$X^2 = 0.879$	0.348	
MMSE	25.52 (3.80)	28.30 (1.38)	9.73	0.003	0.97
GDS	17.58 (4.46)	4.15 (2.50)	145.83	<0.001	3.71
STAI 1	51.93 (11.38)	34.50 (7.83)	34.98	<0.001	1.82
STAI 2	51.00 (10.25)	34.45 (7.65)	36.81	<0.001	1.83
SRRS	16.44 (8.74)	2.30 (1.92)	50.16	<0.001	2.23

Standard deviations are shown in parentheses.

Table 2 | Mean performance levels of patients and controls on cognitive and psychomotor measures.

	Patient	Control	F	P	Cohen's d
Neuropsychological tests					
SDST number correct	43.63 (9.38)	27.52 (13.46)	19.41	<0.001	1.37
SDST_matching time	3.42 (2.90)	1.47 (0.45)	8.44	0.006	0.94
SDST_writing time	1.17 (1.08)	0.66 (0.13)	4.23	0.047	0.67
Stroop card 1	63.43 (24.10)	47.32 (11.21)	7.19	0.011	0.83
Stroop interference	111.43 (110.54)	46.11 (21.42)	37.23	0.016	0.80
WCST *N* categories completed	0.65 (0.83)	2.00 (1.12)	19.16	<0.001	1.40
Verbal memory total	26.71 (11.91)	36.32 (7.77)	9.55	0.003	0.96
Verbal memory recall	4.59 (3.24)	6.63 (3.06)	4.63	0.037	0.53
Verbal memory recognition	22.72 (4.21)	25.72 (2.61)	7.15	0.011	0.86
Psychomotor tasks					
LCT_initiation time (s)	1.46 (1.00)	0.97 (0.17)	4.49	0.040	0.65
LCT_movement time (s)	0.73 (0.38)	0.47 (0.17)	7.78	0.008	0.86
FCT_initiation time (s)	2.98 (1.03)	2.60 (0.85)	1.67	0.203	0.39
FCT_reinspection time (s)	0.41 (0.66)	0.10 (0.19)	3.99	0.053	0.60
FCT_movement time (s)	3.94 (2.36)	2.38 (1.15)	7.03	0.011	0.79

Standard deviations are shown in parentheses.

the writing time were significantly higher in patients, indicating cognitive as well as psychomotor slowing on this task.

As for performance on the copying tasks, patients' initiation time was found to be impaired on the LCT, but not on the FCT, whereas movement time was significantly higher in patients than in controls on both the LCT and the FCT. Analysis reveals a more significant difference between the healthy and the depressive elderly on the movement time compared to the initiation time. Finally, patients reinspected significantly longer than controls on the FCT.

As shown in **Figure 2**, increasing figure complexity in the FCT for increased cognitive load, resulted in a significantly increased initiation time ($F = 10.38$, $p = 0.0002$) and execution time ($F = 10.721$, $p = 0.0002$) for both patients and controls and in a significantly longer reinspection time ($F = 3.89$, $p = 0.029$) in the patient group. However, the increased cognitive load affected patients' psychomotor performance more than that of controls, except for the initiation time (IT, **Figure 2A**: $F = 1.27$, $p = 0.267$, ns; MT, **Figure 2B**: $F = 10.721$, $p = 0.002$; and Reinspection, **Figure 2C**: $F = 4.98$, $p = 0.031$). Both patients and healthy controls initiated the drawing movements immediately, but the patients faltered while drawing and recurred more often to the stimuli.

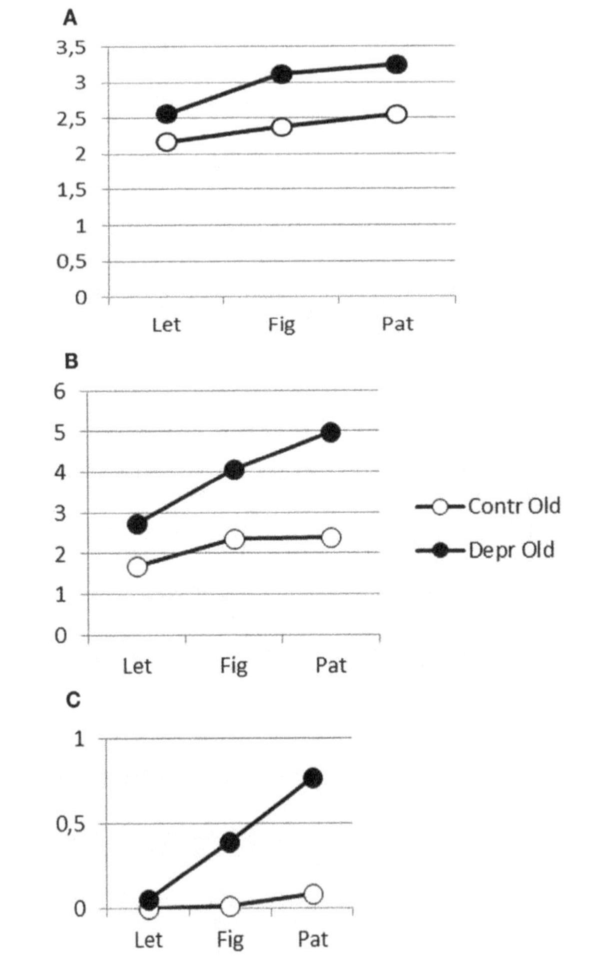

FIGURE 2 | (A–C) Differences in initiation time **(A)**, movement time **(B)**, and reinspection time **(C)** as a function of complexity between depressive patients and healthy controls.

DISCUSSION

In this study, we investigated psychomotor and cognitive performance as an effect of depression in an elderly medication free depressed sample, with both objective motor and cognitive measures. To find out the impact of a cognitive factor in PR, we experimentally varied the amount of cognitive load in psychomotor functioning. Because Tarbuck and Paykel (28), on the basis of an unmedicated sample, assumed that retardation due to age is associated with timed tasks only and that PR due to depression is associated with the complexity of the task, we chose to use a non-timed psychomotor task to see whether the difference still showed. The geriatric depressed patients (as a group) were found to be significantly slower on almost all psychomotor measures, as reflected in high SRRS scores as well as in inferior outcomes on most of the copying tasks, compared to the outcomes recorded for the matched healthy controls. In general, this is in line with previous studies in depressed samples that applied the same assessment methods, in elderly (25) and in younger patients (14, 62–64). However, the sample in this medication free population shows peculiarities of slowing that, moreover, provide valuable insights into the very specific interaction of cognitive and psychomotor slowing in the convergence of depression and aging.

When varying the complexity of figures to copy and thus varying the cognitive load, it is strikingly the motor time that shows the most significant interaction effects of group (depressive elderly versus healthy elderly) and complexity; the reinspection time is less significant, the initiation time not at all. Patients start copying immediately, irrespective of the complexity of the task. Nevertheless, in cognitive more difficult motor tasks, the movements of the depressed elderly become slower or more hesitating, with some more reinspection. Apparently, various cognitive and motor processes are involved in figure copying. Initiation times are assumed to mainly reflect the cognitive processes and encompass the attention for and the perception of the stimulus figure, as well as the storage of the representation in working memory, but also the programing and planning of the first drawing movement and the activation of motor programs that initiate the muscle to start drawing (14).

Scrutinizing the differential effect of increased task difficulty on movement time and initiation time leads to an adaptation of the notion of initiation time. Traditionally, "initiation time" has been defined as a "cognitive" time, different from "motor" time, the time of execution of the movement (14, 25, 64). The fact that more complex tasks lead to longer motor times but not to longer initiation times reveals a cognitive aspect in the motor time. The initiation time, in turn, should be perceived as a simple reaction time, a measure of general processing speed and cognitive reserve. This measure of processing speed in the performed tasks was merely measuring the time of "decision to start," which is not different for simple and complex tasks. "Decisions are made by accumulating noisy stimulus information until sufficient information for a response [for a response criterion] is obtained" (65). Admittedly, the initiation time of patients was longer compared to controls in copying simple lines. This could, however, be linked to changes in white matter integrity of the motor system (66). In a study of Walther et al. (66), patients with MDD differed from healthy controls in a loss of frontal integrity, which was linearly related to a lower activity level. An alternative explanation could be that there was already a ceiling effect of slowing of initiation time in simple tasks in patients. Slower subjects have already more influence of prefrontal executive control in simple tasks for successful performance (67). Evidence has been found indeed for different associations between structures and behavior in depressive patients and healthy controls (66). Bracht et al. found altered cortico-cortical white matter motor pathways, and concluded that these may contribute to movement initiation in MDD (68). A more refined gradation of cognitive reserve impairment can still be made by involving the motor time assessed in the copying task. The execution of a movement while planning and preparing the next is a dual task recruiting more brain regions in parallel (69). The impaired efficiency of interaction between the dorsolateral prefrontal cortex and the pre-supplementary motor area by altered white matter organization of the pathway (68) needs more prefrontal executive higher order compensation (69). We presume that this hierarchical plasticity of the brain principle with higher order integration for output with lower order deficits is also responsible for disbalanced motor control with more activation of (higher order) right orbitofrontal cortex and less activation of the (lower order) left supplemental motor area in higher activity level (70).

The predominantly dopaminergic dysregulation of cognition and motor functioning by striatal dopamine transporters (71, 72) has motivational correlates too (73), manifested in decisional anhedonia (74). Lowered mesolimbic dopamine projections in the nucleus accumbens (74) and overstimulation of nucleus accumbens adenosine receptors (75) change the GABAergic signals that relay through the ventral tegmentum, associated with motor control, and the substantia nigra, associated with reward cognition, resulting in changed effort-based decision making with decreased perceived net-value under increasing response costs (74). These response costs can be increased by task complexity or higher activity level. Limitations of these findings are the important age and sex influences in dopaminergic neuromodulating influences (72), which urge for further investigation.

Clearly, figure copying is different from the separate cognitive measures in standard cognitive testing. Even the SDST tends to reflect higher order cognitive, memory related functions more than it does psychomotor speed (14, 76). The bigger higher order executive cognitive load of searching for a number in the legend code, memorizing the found digit and subsequently performing the initiation and planning of writing the digit in the SDST and the relative easiness of writing a well-known automatized digit compared to an unknown pattern, may also explain the difference in effect size of the matching time of SDST (Cohen's $d = 0.94$) and the initiation time of the figure copying (Cohen's d LCT initiation = 0.65; Cohen's d FCT initiation = 0.39). Furthermore, patients performed worse than controls on all cognitive measures in the standard cognitive tasks. It must be remembered, however, that above all, the more cognitive executive aspects show cumulative effects of aging and depression, except in the WCST. The lack of interaction effect in the WCST is clearly a result of the missing measure of executive function due to the patients' inability to learn even one category. Measuring adaptation and perseveration thus became impossible.

All in all, the difference in slowing as a result of increasing cognitive load may be explained as an effect of cognitive aspects in psychomotor functioning. Presumably, the cognitive component of PR is different in nature and involves more motor circuitry involvement than that measured by the standard cognitive tasks.

The present results suggest that PR observed in the patient group was caused by both a cognitive and a motor factor, as, respectively, most matching times and writing times were higher in patients. In order to further scrutinize the possible cognitive effect, we compared the current results *post hoc* to the ones obtained in a similar study in an adult population of depressed medicated patients and in healthy controls (18–60 years). This way, we could also gain some insight into possible interaction effects of age and depression and we could determine whether there was a link with cognitive functioning. In **Figure 3**, we have presented the results of this *post hoc* comparison. Since adult medicated patients appear to be even less retarded than elderly depressive unmedicated patients, these results only corroborate the hypothesis of an aging effect in depression. The overall comparison in **Figure 3** reveals a clear effect of depression in all ages, both, for the cognitive measures (**Figure 3A**: F SDST matching time = 36.40, $p < 0.001$; F SDST writing time = 22.36, $p < 0.001$; F Stroop card 1 = 25.58, $p < 0.001$; F Stroop interference = 31.24, $p < 0.001$; and F WCST N categories completed = 10.54, $p = 0.001$) and for the psychomotor measures (**Figure 3A**: F LCT initiation time = 24.29, $p < 0.001$; F LCT movement time = 13.83, $p < 0.001$; F FCT initiation time = 8.54, $p = 0.004$; F FCT reinspection time = 14.71, $p < 0.001$; and F FCT movement time = 25.35, $p < 0.001$). An aging effect is equally obvious, also in both, in cognitive measures (**Figure 3A**: F SDST matching time = 29.96, $p < 0.001$; F writing time = 45.32 $p < 0.001$; F Stroop card 1 = 16.21, $p < 0.001$; F Stroop interference = 39.19, $p < 0.001$; and F WCST N categories completed = 31.21, $p < 0.001$) and in psychomotor measures (**Figure 3B**: F LCT initiation time = 8.55, $p = 0.004$; F LCT movement time = 3.22, $p = 0.074$; F FCT initiation time = 144.70, $p < 0.001$; FCT reinspection time = 19.37, $p < 0.001$; and FCT movement time = 22.02, $p < 0.001$). A calculation of possible interaction effects of aging and depression in the GLM test indicates that only the matching time and the writing time of the SDST and the Stroop interference show interaction effects (F SDST matching time = 11.80 $p = 0.001$; F SDST writing time = 9.50, $p = 0.002$; F Stroop card 1 = 1.57, $p = 0.211$; F Stroop interference = 12.65, $p < 0{,}001$; F WCST = 0.63, $p = 0.429$). In the psychomotor measures, only the reinspection time shows a slightly significant interaction effect (F LCT initiation time = 2.10, $p = 0.149$; F LCT movement time = 0.001, $p = 0.979$; F FCT initiation time = 0.04, $p = 0.837$; F FCT reinspection time = 6.35, $p = 0.12$; and F FCT movement time = 3.09, $p = 0.80$). However, this effect was not reflected in the results. The significance was diminished by the much larger variance on the reinspection times of the complex figure copying task in the elder population. Indeed, there is an overall increase of variance in the elderly, especially in psychomotor tasks where motor and cognitive aspects coincide

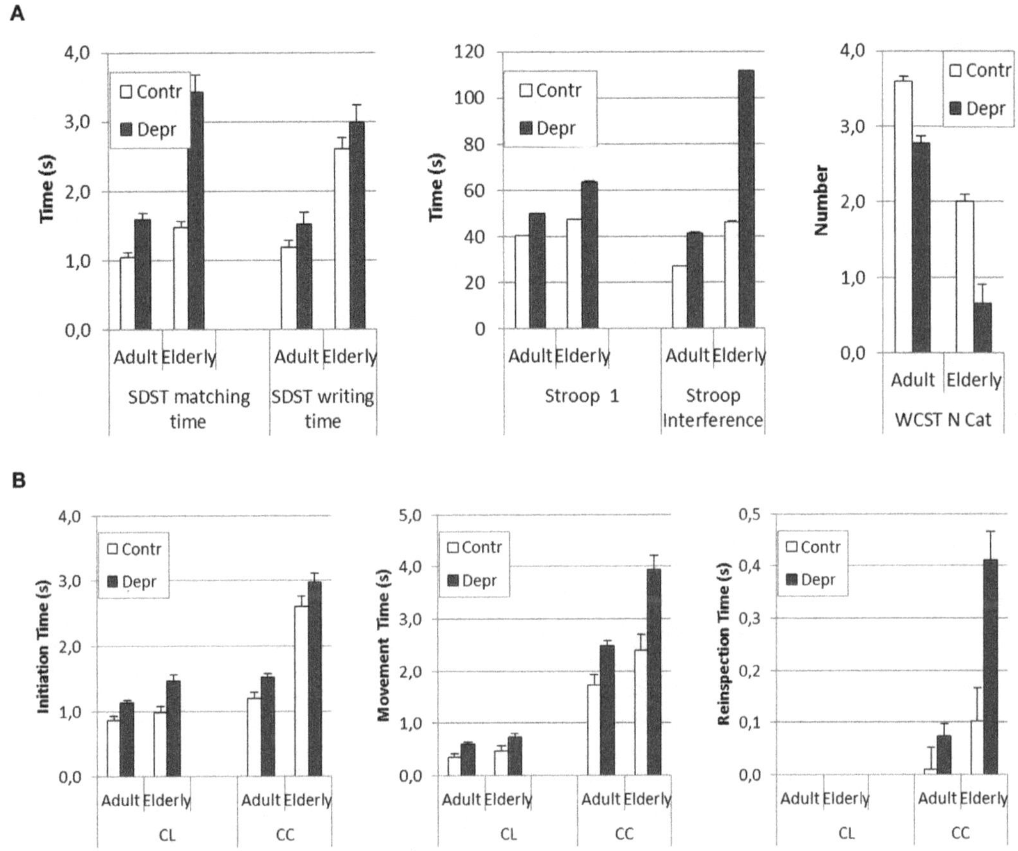

FIGURE 3 | (A,B) Comparison of psychomotor and cognitive measures between healthy and depressed elderly against the background of previous research with the same tasks in adults. Because of limited competence of the population, with the elderly the copying task consisted of just four lines, whereas with the adults a task with eight lines was used. To make the results comparable, recalculations were made for the adult scores based on the mean time for four lines. Separate times for each line were available.

(SDST matching, writing time, and complex figure reinspection). Overlooking the overall results leads to the assumption that the interaction of depression and aging reveals itself in executive functioning and in the interaction of cognitive and psychomotor functioning. The main comparison of the Cohen's *d* effect sizes in the elderly and adult group shows that the effect of depression is always bigger in elderly. The relatively small difference between the effect sizes of the adults and the elderly however, is explained by the large variance in older groups, which limits the found inter-group effects. Surprisingly, the effect sizes of initiation time of the copying tasks show the reverse direction; it is bigger in adults. Evidently, these results need to be confirmed by direct comparative research.

The present study not only confirms the results of a similar study by Pier et al. (25), it also provides a valuable contribution in its own right, as it overcomes some of the restrictions of the earlier study. Whereas, the study by Pier et al. (25) was a small sample study ($n = 11$) in which patients were taking medication that could have impacted the results, the present study is unique in that it involves only patients that are free of psychotropics. The importance of the latter condition is apparent from the fact that in the Pier et al. study (25) correlations were found between the use of antidepressants and anxiolytics on the one hand, and several psychomotor outcomes on the other. With our larger medication free sample, we succeeded in replicating the results of Pier et al. (25), corroborating their preliminary results concerning the presence of PR in elderly depressed patients, independent of medication status. Apart from that, the present study revealed an interesting difference between medicated and unmedicated patients. In comparison to the control groups (healthy aged, younger depressed), the pattern of interaction between the degree of slowing and the cognitive complexity of the task in the unmedicated elderly sample seemed to be the reverse. In the unmedicated elderly sample, PR was proportionately more visible in more complex tasks (copying more complex figures, less familiar figures) than in copying simple lines. In the medicated sample, on the contrary, the PR was more obvious in comparison with the other groups in the simple copying task than in the more complex tasks (63) (p. 24). This result is in line with the suggestion by Caligiuri et al. (20) that retardation caused by medication is predominantly neuromotor retardation, i.c. abnormal velocity, as opposed to the psychomotor slowing in depression, in which the cognitive factor is more important. Benzodiazepines, opioids, anticholinergics, but also tricyclic antidepressants (77) often elicit modest or more pronounced psychomotor or cognitive impairments (78). These findings support the diagnostic relevance of the quality of slowing in major depression, in aging and in a broad range of psychopathological disorders.

Notwithstanding the relatively small sample size, the reported effects were robust. The very restrictive inclusion criteria determining the sample size were introduced because of the high comorbidity of depression and the considerable use of medication in the elderly and because of the numerous possible cognitive – and psychomotor – side-effects of somatic and degenerative diseases. To avoid such confounding cognitive effects a selection of elderly depressive patients imposed itself. Despite the fact that such a strict selection can hardly be seen as representative for the "natural" population, it afforded a unique opportunity to rule out possible medication and comorbidity effects and to obtain an unbiased view on the differential PR effects of depression in the elderly. A limitation of this study could be that cardiovascular disease, a recognized cause of psychomotor slowing in elderly due to white matter lesions (WML) (79), was only excluded after introducing a questionnaire for the patient and the treating physician. The sample of patients was, however, too small to introduce cardiovascular disease as a covariate. MRI volume measures of WML could have provided a more objective measure of vascular risks causing neuromotor slowing (80), but the primary focus of the present investigation was to reveal the different types of slowing factors. Admittedly, Hickie et al. (79), who combined clinical, neuropsychological, magnetic resonance imaging, and single photon emission computerized tomography, found that the percentage caudate nucleus regional cerebral blood flow was associated with psychomotor slowing and presence of WML. Even if their neuropsychological measures included only reaction times and did not offer an integrated view of cognitive and motor psychomotor slowing (cf. the movement time of complex figures in the present study), they still found 25% of the variance explained by "depression." Consequently, they concluded that "while psychomotor slowing is determined in part by subcortical changes, other cortical and illness-dependent factors are likely to be relevant" (79). This result confirms the necessity of a detailed neuropsychological analysis of psychomotor functioning in the explorative stage. Such analysis is essential to unravel the complexity of the symptom of slowing and to better understand its physiopathology. Further research with more direct neurobiological measures will have to objectify relative shares of biological and functional aspects in different types of slowing. Since it has become clear that biological aspects like WML account for age-related declines, irrespective of depression (81), an interdisciplinary approach of PR in elderly depressed seems to be in order.

REFERENCES

1. American Psychiatric Association. *Diagnostic and Statistical Manual of Mental Disorders 5th ed.* Washington, DC: American Psychiatric Association (2013).
2. American Psychiatric Association. *APA Diagnostic and Statistical Manual of Mental Disorders, Fourth Edition (DSM-IV)*. Washington, DC: American Psychiatric Association (1994).
3. Vrieze E, Demyttenaere K, Bruffaerts R, Hermans D, Pizzagalli D, Sienaert P, et al. Dimensions in major depressive disorder and their relevance for treatment outcome. *J Affect Disord* (2014) **155**:35–41. doi:10.1016/j.jad.2013.10.020
4. Sobin C, Sackeim HA. Psychomotor symptoms of depression. *Am J Psychiatry* (1997) **154**:4–17. doi:10.1176/ajp.154.1.4
5. Schrijvers D, Hulstijn W, Sabbe BCG. Psychomotor symptoms in depression: a diagnostic, pathophysiological and therapeutic tool. *J Affect Disord* (2008) **109**:1–20. doi:10.1016/j.jad.2007.10.019
6. Bennabi D, Vandel P, Papaxanthis C, Pozzo T, Haffen E. Psychomotor retardation in depression: a systematic review of diagnostic, pathophysiologic, and therapeutic implications. *Biomed Res Int* (2013) **2013**:158746. doi:10.1155/2013/158746
7. Widlöcher D, Ghozlan A. The measurement of retardation in depression. In: Hindmarch I, Stonier PD, editors. *Human Psychopharmacology: Measures and Methods.* New York: Wiley (1989). 2 p.
8. Widlöcher DJ. Psychomotor retardation: clinical, theoretical, and psychometric aspects. *Psychiatr Clin North Am* (1983) **6**(1):27–40.
9. Parker G. Classifying depression: should paradigms lost be regained? *Am J Psychiatry* (2000) **157**:1195–203. doi:10.1176/appi.ajp.157.8.1195
10. Pier MPBI, Hulstijn W, Sabbe BGC. Differential patterns of psychomotor functioning in unmedicated melancholic and nonmelancholic depressed patients. *J Psychiatric Res* (2004) **38**:425–35. doi:10.1016/j.jpsychires.2003.11.008
11. Benazzi F. Psychomotor changes in melancholic and atypical depression: unipolar and bipolar-II subtypes. *Psychiatry Res* (2002) **112**(3):211–20. doi:10.1016/S0165-1781(02)00241-X
12. Gupta RK. Major depression: an illness with objective physical signs. *World J Biol Psychiatry* (2009):196–201. doi:10.1080/15622970902812072
13. Niculescu IIIAB, Akiskal HS. Proposed endophenotypes of dysthymia: evolutionary, clinical and pharmacogenomics considerations. *Mol Psychiatry* (2001) **6**(4):363–6. doi:10.1038/sj.mp.4000906
14. Schrijvers D. *Monitoring Slow Motion: Action Disturbances in Major Depressive Disorder.* Antwerpen: University of Antwerp UA Faculteit Geneeskunde (2009).
15. Smith MJ, Brebion G, Banquet JP, Cohen L. Retardation of mentation in depressives: Posner covert orientation of visual attention test. *J Affect Disord* (1995) **35**(3):107–15. doi:10.1016/0165-0327(95)00044-5
16. Widlöcher D. Retardation: a basic emotional response? In: Davis JH, Maas JW, editors. *The Affective Disorders.* Washington, DC: American Psychiatric Press (1983). p. 165–81.
17. Buyukdura J, McClintock S, Croarkin P. Psychomotor retardation in depression: biological underpinnings, measurement, and treatment. *Prog Neuropsychopharmacol Biol Psychiatry* (2011) **35**:395–409. doi:10.1016/j.pnpbp.2010.10.019
18. Akiskal HS. Dysthymia and cyclothymia a century after Kraepelin. *J Affect Disord* (2001) **62**(1–2):17–31. doi:10.1016/S0165-0327(00)00347-5
19. Blackburn IM. Mental and psychomotor speed in depression and mania. *Br J Psychiatry* (1975) **126**:329–35. doi:10.1192/bjp.126.4.329
20. Caligiuri M, Elswanger J. Motor and cognitive aspects of motor retardation in depression. *J Affect Disord* (2000) **57**:83–93. doi:10.1016/S0165-0327(99)00068-3
21. Bella R, Pennisi G, Cantone M, Palermo F, Pennisi M, Lanza G, et al. Clinical presentation and outcome of geriatric depression in subcortical ischemic vascular disease. *Gerontology* (2010) **56**(3):298–302. doi:10.1159/000272003
22. Alexopoulos GS, Meyers BS, Young RC, Kakuma T, Feder M, Einhorn A, et al. Recovery in geriatric depression. *Arch Gen Psychiatry* (1996) **53**(4):305–12. doi:10.1001/archpsyc.1996.01830040039008
23. Judd LL, Rapaport MH, Paulus MP, Brown JL. Subsyndromal symptomatic depression: a new mood disorder? *J Clin Psychiatry* (1994) **55**(4):18–28.
24. Cerella J, Rybash J, Hoyer W, Commons ML. *Adult Information Processing: Limits on Loss.* California: Academic Press (1993).
25. Pier MPBI, Hulstijn W, Sabbe BGC. Psychomotor retardation in elderly depressed patients. *J Affect Disord* (2004) **81**:73–7. doi:10.1016/j.jad.2003.08.002
26. Seidler RD, Bernard JA, Burutolu TB, Fling BW, Gordon MT, Gwin JT, et al. Motor Control and Aging: links to age-related brain structural, functional and biochemical effects. *Neurosci Biobehav Rev* (2010) **34**(5):721–33. doi:10.1016/j.neubiorev.2009.10.005
27. Bonin-Guillaume S, Hasbroucq T, Blin O. Mise en evidence d'un ralentissement psychomoteur spécifique à la depression chez le sujet agé. *Psychol Neuropsychiatr Vieil* (2008) **6**(2):137–44. doi:10.1684/pnv.2008.0121
28. Tarbuck AF, Paykel ES. Effects of major depression on the cognitive function of younger and older subjects. *Psychol Med* (1995) **25**:285–95. doi:10.1017/S0033291700036187
29. Hart RP, Kwentus JA. Psychomotor slowing and subcortical-type dysfunction in depression. *J Neurol Neurosurg Psychiatry* (1987) **50**(10):1263–6. doi:10.1136/jnnp.50.10.1263

30. Nebes RD, Halligan EM, Rosen J. Reynolds, CF3rd. Cognitive and motor slowing in Alzheimer's disease and geriatric depression. *J Int Neuropsychol Soc* (1987) **4**(5):426–34.
31. Beats BC, Sahakian BJ, Levy R. Cognitive performance in tests sensitive to frontal lobe dysfunction in the elderly depressed. *Psychol Med* (1996) **26**:591–603. doi:10.1017/S0033291700035662
32. Dybedal GS, Tanum L, Sundet K, Gaarden TL, Bjølseth TM. Neuropsychological functioning in late-life depression. *Front Psychol* (2013) **4**:381. doi:10.3389/fpsyg.2013.00381
33. Naismith SL, Norrie LM, Mowszowski L, Hickie IB. The neurobiology of depression in later-life: clinical, neuropsychological, neuroimaging and pathophysiological features. *Prog Neurobiol* (2012) **98**(1):99–143. doi:10.1016/j.pneurobio.2012.05.009
34. Baudic S, Benisty S, Dalla Barba G, Traykov L. L'atteinte des fonctions exécutives chez la personne âgèe présentant un épisode dépressif majeur unipolaire sévère: influence du ralentissement dépressif [Impairment of executive function in elderly patients with major unipolar depression: influence of psychomotor retardation]. *Psychol Neuropsychiatr Vieil* (2007) **5**(1):65–71 [Original article in French]. doi:10.1684/pnv.2007.0036
35. Butters M, Whyte E, Nebes R, Begley A, Dew M, Mulsant B, et al. The nature and determinants of neuropsychological functioning in late-life depression. *Arch Gen Psychiatry* (2004) **61**:587–95. doi:10.1001/archpsyc.61.6.587
36. Sheline YI, Barch DM, Garcia K, Gersing K, Pieper C, Welsh-Bohmer K, et al. Cognitive function in late life depression: relationships to depression severity, cerebrovascular risk factors and processing speed. *J Biol Psychiatry* (2006) **60**:58–65. doi:10.1016/j.biopsych.2005.09.019
37. Nebes RD, Butters MA, Mulsant BH, Pollock BG, Zmuda MD, Houck PR, et al. Decreased working memory and processing speed mediate cognitive impairment in geriatric depression. *Psychol Med* (2000) **30**(3):679–91. doi:10.1017/S0033291799001968
38. Sexton CE, Allan CL, Le Mausurier M, Mc Dermott LM, Kalu UG, Hermann LL, et al. Magnetic resonance imaging in late-life depression: multimodal examination of network disruption. *Arch Gen Psychiatry* (2012) **69**(7):680–9. doi:10.1001/archgenpsychiatry.2011.1862
39. Kok R, Verhey F. *Dutch Translation of the Mini Mental State Examination (Folstein et al., 1975)*. Altrecht: GGZ (2002).
40. Tombaugh TN. McIntyre. The mini-mental state examination: a comprehensive review. *J Am Geriatr Soc* (1992) **40**(9):922–35.
41. Anstey KJ, Burns RA, Birrell CL, Steel D, Kiely KM, Luszcz MA. Estimates of probable dementia prevalence from population-based surveys compared with dementia estimates based on meta-analyses. *BMC Neurol* (2010) **10**:62. doi:10.1186/1471-2377-10-62
42. World Medical Association. World Medical Association Declaration of Helsinki ethical principles for medical research involving human subjects. *JAMA* (2013) **310**(20):2191–4. doi:10.1001/jama.2013.281053
43. Yesavage JA, Brink T. Development and validation of a geriatric depression screening scale. A preliminary report. *J Psychiatr Res* (1982) **17**:37–49. doi:10.1016/0022-3956(82)90033-4
44. Spielberger CD, Gorsuch RL, Lushene PR, Vagg PR, Jacobs GA. *Test Manual for the State-Trait Anxiety Inventory*. Palo Alto, California: Consulting Psychologists Press, Inc (1983).
45. Weme de RJC, Hoeksema T, Goekoop JG. De Widlöcher remmingsschaal, een Nederlandse schaal voor het meten van psychomotore remming. *Acta Neuropsychiatr* (1996) **8**:56–63.
46. Van Hoof J, Hulstijn W, Van Mier H, Pagen M. Figure drawing and psychomotor retardation: preliminary report. *J Affect Disord* (1993) **29**:263–6. doi:10.1016/0165-0327(93)90016-D
47. Sabbe B, Hulstijn W, Van Hoof J, Tuynman Qua HG, Zitman F. Retardation in depression: assessment by means of simple motor tasks. *J Affect Disord* (1999) **55**:39–44. doi:10.1016/S0165-0327(98)00087-1
48. Maarse FJ, Janssen HJ, Dexel F. A special pen for an XY-tablet. In: Maarse FJ, Mulder LJM, Sjouw WPB, Akkerman AE, editors. *Computers in Psychology: Methods, Instrumentation and Psychodiagnostics*. Amsterdam: Swets Zeitlinger (1988). p. 133–9.
49. McLeod DR, Griffiths RR, Bigelow GE, Yingling J. An automated version of the digit symbol substitution test (DSST). *Behav Res Methods Instrum* (1982) **14**:463–6. doi:10.3758/BF03203313
50. Wechsler D. *Wechsler Adult Intelligence Scale–Revised*. San Antonio, TX: The Psychological Corporation (1981).
51. Wechsler D. *WAIS-III Administration and Scoring Manual*. San Antonio, TX: The Psychological Corporation (1997).
52. Psychological Assessment Resources. *Computerised Wisconsin Card Sort Task Version 4 (WCST)*. Lutz, Florida: Psychological Assessment Resources Inc. (2003).
53. Barceló F, Knight RT. Both random and perseverative errors underlie WCST deficits in prefrontal patients. *Neuropsychologia* (2002) **40**(3):349–56. doi:10.1016/S0028-3932(01)00110-5
54. Bardenhagen FJ, Bowden SC. Cognitive components in perseverative and nonperseverative errors on the object alternation task. *Brain Cogn* (1998) **37**(2):224–36. doi:10.1006/brcg.1997.0971
55. Greve KW, Bianchini KJ, Hartley SM, Adams D. The Wisconsin card sorting test in stroke rehabilitation: factor structure and relationship to outcome. *Arch Clin Neuropsychol* (1999) **14**(6):497–509. doi:10.1093/arclin/14.6.497
56. Greve KW, Bianchini KJ, Mathias CW, Houston RJ, Crouch JA. Detecting malingered performance with the Wisconsin card sorting test: a preliminary investigation in traumatic brain injury. *Clin Neuropsychol* (2002) **16**(2):179–91. doi:10.1076/clin.16.2.179.13241
57. Stroop J. Studies of interference in serial verbal reaction. *J Exp Psychol* (1935) **18**:643–62. doi:10.1037/h0054651
58. McLeod CM. Half a century of research on the Stroop effect: an integrative review. *Psychol Bull* (1991) **109**:163–202. doi:10.1037/0033-2909.109.2.163
59. Dodrill CB. A neuropsychological battery for epilepsy. *Epilepsia* (1978) **19**(6):611–23. doi:10.1111/j.1528-1157.1978.tb05041.x
60. Saan RJ, Deelman BG. *De 15-woordentest A en B (een voorlopige handleiding)*. Groningen: Afdeling Neuropsychologie AZG (1986).
61. Cohen J. A power primer. *Psychol Bull* (1992) **112**(1):155–9. doi:10.1037/0033-2909.112.1.155
62. Sabbe B, Hulstijn W, Van Hoof J, Zitman F. Retardation and antidepressant treatment: changes in fine motor retardation in depressed patients treated with fluoxetine. *J Affect Disord* (1999) **40**:149–57. doi:10.1016/0165-0327(96)00052-3
63. Pier MP. *Psychomotor Retardation in Subtypes of Depression*. Enschede: Printpartners Ipskamp (2006).
64. Destoop M. Multimodal perspectives on affective disorders. From clinics to imaging [Doctoral thesis]. Antwerpen: Universiteit Antwerpen, Faculteit geneeskunde en gezondheidswetenschappen (2013).
65. Smith PL, Ratcliff R. Psychology and neurobiology of simple decisions. *Trends Neurosci* (2004) **27**(3):161–8. doi:10.1016/j.tins.2004.01.006
66. Walther S, Hügli S, Höfle O, Federspiel A, Horn H, Bracht T, et al. Frontal white matter integrity is related to psychomotor retardation in major depression. *Neurobiol Dis* (2012) **47**:13–9. doi:10.1016/j.nbd.2012.03.019
67. Rypma B, Berger JS, Prabhakaram V, Bly BM, Kimberg DY, Biswal BB, et al. Neural correlates of cognitive efficiency. *J Neuroimage* (2006) **33**:969–79. doi:10.1016/j.neuroimage.2006.05.065
68. Bracht T, Federspiel A, Schnell S, Horn H, Höfle O, Wiest R, et al. Cortico-cortical white matter motor pathway microstructure is related to psychomotor retardation in major depressive disorder. *PLoS One* (2012) **7**(12):e52238. doi:10.1371/journal.pone.0052238
69. Zuromski CF, Rubin EH. *Psychiatry and Clinical Neuroscience: A Primer*. New York: Oxford University Press (2011).
70. Walther S, Höfle O, Federspiel A, Horn H, Hügli S, Wiest R, et al. Neural correlates of disbalanced motor control in major depression. *J Affect Disord* (2012) **136**:124–33. doi:10.1016/j.jad.2011.08.020
71. Dyck van CH, Avery RA, Mac Avoy MG, Marek KL, Quinlan DM, Baldwin RM, et al. Striatal dopamine transporters correlate with simple reaction time in elderly subjects. *Neurobiol Aging* (2008) **29**:1237–46. doi:10.1016/j.neurobiolaging.2007.02.012
72. Harper Mozley L, Gur RC, Mozley RD, Gur RE. Striatal dopamine transporters and cognitive functioning in healthy men and women. *Am J Psychiatry* (2001) **158**(9):1492–9. doi:10.1176/appi.ajp.158.9.1492
73. Wise RA. Dopamine, learning and motivation. *Nat Rev Neurosci* (2004) **5**:483–94. doi:10.1038/nrn1406
74. Treadway MT, Zald D. Reconsidering anhedonia in depression: lessons from translational neuroscience. *Neurosci Biobehav Rev* (2011) **35**(3):537–55. doi:10.1016/j.neubiorev.2010.06.006

75. Mingote S, Font L, Farrar AM, Vontell R, Worden LT, Stopper CM, et al. Nucleus accumbens adenosine A2A receptors regulate exertion of effort by acting on the ventral striatopallidal pathway. *J Neurosci* (2008) **28**(36):9037–46. doi:10.1523/JNEUROSCI.1525-08.2008
76. Morrens M, Hulstijn W, Sabbe B. Psychomotor slowing in schizophrenia. *Schizophr Bull* (2007) **33**(4):1038–53. doi:10.1093/schbul/sbl051
77. Moore AR, O'Keeffe ST. Drug-induced cognitive impairment in the elderly. *Drugs Aging* (1999) **15**(1):15–28. doi:10.2165/00002512-199915010-00002
78. Robles Bayón A, Gude Sampedro F. Prescripciones inconvenientes en el tratamiento del paciente con deterioro cognitivo [Inappropriate treatments for patients with cognitive decline]. *Neurologia* (2014) **29**(9):523–32 [Original article in Spanish]. doi:10.1016/j.nrleng.2012.05.009
79. Hickie IB, Naismith SL, Ward PB, Little CL, Pearson M, Scott EM, et al. Psychomotor slowing in older patients with major depression: relationships with blood flow in the caudate nucleus and white matter lesions. *Psychiatry Res* (2009) **155**(3):211–20. doi:10.1016/j.pscychresns.2007.01.006
80. Soumaré A, Elbaz A, Zhu Y, Maillard P, Crivello F, Tavernier B, et al. White matter lesions volume and motor performances in the elderly. *Ann Neurol* (2009) **65**(6):706–15. doi:10.1002/ana.21674
81. Rabbitt P, Scott M, Lunn M, Thacker N, Lowe C, Pendleton N, et al. White matter lesions account for all age-related declines in speed but not in intelligence. *Neuropsychology* (2007) **3**:363–70. doi:10.1037/0894-4105.21.3.363

Permissions

All chapters in this book were first published in PSPI&CAPDSFMHCD, by Frontiers; hereby published with permission under the Creative Commons Attribution License or equivalent. Every chapter published in this book has been scrutinized by our experts. Their significance has been extensively debated. The topics covered herein carry significant findings which will fuel the growth of the discipline. They may even be implemented as practical applications or may be referred to as a beginning point for another development.

The contributors of this book come from diverse backgrounds, making this book a truly international effort. This book will bring forth new frontiers with its revolutionizing research information and detailed analysis of the nascent developments around the world.

We would like to thank all the contributing authors for lending their expertise to make the book truly unique. They have played a crucial role in the development of this book. Without their invaluable contributions this book wouldn't have been possible. They have made vital efforts to compile up to date information on the varied aspects of this subject to make this book a valuable addition to the collection of many professionals and students.

This book was conceptualized with the vision of imparting up-to-date information and advanced data in this field. To ensure the same, a matchless editorial board was set up. Every individual on the board went through rigorous rounds of assessment to prove their worth. After which they invested a large part of their time researching and compiling the most relevant data for our readers.

The editorial board has been involved in producing this book since its inception. They have spent rigorous hours researching and exploring the diverse topics which have resulted in the successful publishing of this book. They have passed on their knowledge of decades through this book. To expedite this challenging task, the publisher supported the team at every step. A small team of assistant editors was also appointed to further simplify the editing procedure and attain best results for the readers.

Apart from the editorial board, the designing team has also invested a significant amount of their time in understanding the subject and creating the most relevant covers. They scrutinized every image to scout for the most suitable representation of the subject and create an appropriate cover for the book.

The publishing team has been an ardent support to the editorial, designing and production team. Their endless efforts to recruit the best for this project, has resulted in the accomplishment of this book. They are a veteran in the field of academics and their pool of knowledge is as vast as their experience in printing. Their expertise and guidance has proved useful at every step. Their uncompromising quality standards have made this book an exceptional effort. Their encouragement from time to time has been an inspiration for everyone.

The publisher and the editorial board hope that this book will prove to be a valuable piece of knowledge for researchers, students, practitioners and scholars across the globe.

List of Contributors

Pascal Sienaert
Department of Mood Disorders and Electroconvulsive Therapy, University Psychiatric Center, KU Leuven, Leuven, Belgium
Department of Neurosciences, KU Leuven, Leuven, Belgium

Dirk M. Dhossche
Department of Psychiatry, University of Mississippi Medical Center, Jackson, MS, USA

Davy Vancampfort and Marc De Hert
University Psychiatric Center, KU Leuven, Leuven, Belgium

Gábor Gazdag
Center for Psychiatry and Addiction Medicine, Szent István and Szent László Hospitals, Budapest, Hungary
Department of Psychiatry and Psychotherapy, Faculty of Medicine, Semmelweis University, Budapest, Hungary

Dusan Hirjak, Laura Mehl, Janna K. Kelbel, Katharina Maria Kubera, Thomas Fuchs and Philipp Arthur Thomann
Department of General Psychiatry, Center for Psychosocial Medicine, University of Heidelberg, Heidelberg, Germany

Robert Christian Wolf
Department of General Psychiatry, Center for Psychosocial Medicine, University of Heidelberg, Heidelberg, Germany
Department of Psychiatry, Psychotherapy and Psychosomatics, Saarland University, Homburg, Germany

Sabine C. Koch
Department of Dance Movement Therapy, Faculty of Therapeutic Sciences, SRH University Heidelberg, Heidelberg, Germany

Tanja Traeger
Personality, Psychological Assessment, and Psychological Methods, Department of Psychology, University of Koblenz Landau, Landau, Germany

Gian Mauro Manzoni and Gianluca Castelnuovo
Psychology Research Laboratory, Istituto Auxologico Italiano IRCCS, Verbania, Italy
Department of Psychology, Catholic University of Milan, Milano, Italy

Angelo Compare
Department of Psychology, University of Bergamo, Bergamo, Italy

Francesco Pagnini
Department of Psychology, Catholic University of Milan, Milano, Italy

Vidal Essebag
McGill University Health Center, Montreal, QC, Canada

Riccardo Proietti
Cardiology Department, Luigi Sacco Hospital, Milano, Italy

Phillip Grant, Mona Balser, Aisha Judith Leila Munk, Jens Linder and Juergen Hennig
Personality Psychology and Individual Differences, Department of Psychology, Justus-Liebig-University Giessen, Giessen, Germany

Talitha C. Ford and David P. Crewther
Centre for Human Psychopharmacology, Faculty of Health, Arts and Design, School of Health Sciences, Swinburne University of Technology, Melbourne, VIC, Australia

Sebastian Walther, Katharina Stegmayer, Helge Horn, Luca Rampa, Nadja Razavi, Thomas J. Müller and Werner Strik
University Hospital of Psychiatry, University of Bern, Bern, Switzerland

Christina Daniel and Oliver John Mason
Research Department of Clinical, Educational and Health Psychology, University College London, London, UK

Anna Lovatt
Cheshire andWirral Partnership NHS Foundation Trust, Chester, UK

Claudia Cornelis, Livia J. De Picker, Glenn Dumont and Bernard G. C. Sabbe
Collaborative Antwerp Psychiatric Research Institute, University of Antwerp, Antwerp, Belgium
University Psychiatric Center St. Norbertushuis, Duffel, Belgium

Wouter Hulstijn
Collaborative Antwerp Psychiatric Research Institute, University of Antwerp, Antwerp, Belgium
Donders Institute for Brain, Cognition and Behaviour, Radboud University Nijmegen, Nijmegen, Netherlands

Maarten Timmers and Luc Janssens
Janssen Research and Development, Janssen Pharmaceutica N.V., Beerse, Belgium

Manuel Morrens
Collaborative Antwerp Psychiatric Research Institute, University of Antwerp, Antwerp, Belgium
Psychiatric Hospital Broeders Alexianen, Boechout, Belgium

Nadja Urbanowitsch and Christina Degen
Section of Geriatric Psychiatry, University of Heidelberg, Heidelberg, Germany

Pablo Toro
Department of Psychiatry, Centro Interdisciplinario de Neurociencias, School of Medicine, Pontificia Universidad Católica de Chile, Santiago, Chile

Johannes Schröder
Section of Geriatric Psychiatry, University of Heidelberg, Heidelberg, Germany
Institute of Gerontology, University of Heidelberg, Heidelberg, Germany

Christine Mohr
Institute of Psychology, University of Lausanne, Lausanne, Switzerland

Ulrich Ettinger
Department of Psychology, University of Bonn, Bonn, Germany

Erik Fransen
StatUA, University of Antwerp, Antwerp, Belgium

Kyran T. Graham and Mathew T. Martin-Iverson
Pharmacology, Pharmacy and Anaesthesiology Unit, School of Medicine and Pharmacology, Faculty of Medicine, Dentistry and Health Sciences, The University of Western Australia, Perth,WA, Australia
Statewide Department of Neurophysiology and Clinical Research Centre, Graylands Hospital, North Metropolitan Health Services - Mental Health, Perth,WA, Australia

Nicholas P. Holmes
Centre for Integrative Neuroscience and Neurodynamics, School of Psychology and Clinical Language Sciences, University of Reading, Reading, UK

Assen Jablensky
Centre for Clinical Research in Neuropsychiatry, School of Psychiatry and Clinical Neurosciences, The University ofWestern Australia, Perth,WA, Australia

Flavie Waters
Statewide Department of Neurophysiology and Clinical Research Centre, Graylands Hospital, North Metropolitan Health Services - Mental Health, Perth,WA, Australia

Centre for Clinical Research in Neuropsychiatry, School of Psychiatry and Clinical Neurosciences, The University ofWestern Australia, Perth,WA, Australia

Mirella Stuivenga
Collaborative Antwerp Psychiatric Research Institute (CAPRI), University of Antwerp, Antwerp, Belgium

Ellen-ge D. Denton and Karina W. Davidson
Department of Medicine, Columbia University Medical Center, NewYork, NY, USA

Nina Rieckmann
Berlin School of Public Health, Charité Universitätsmedizin Berlin, Berlin, Germany

William F. Chaplin
Department of Psychology, St. John's University, Jamaica, NY, USA

Jessica A. Bernard
Department of Psychology and Neuroscience, University of Colorado Boulder, Boulder, CO, USA

Vijay A. Mittal
Department of Psychology and Neuroscience, University of Colorado Boulder, Boulder, CO, USA
Center for Neuroscience, University of Colorado Boulder, Boulder, CO, USA

Benny Liberg
Department of Psychiatry, Melbourne Neuropsychiatry Centre, The University of Melbourne, Melbourne, VIC, Australia
Section of Psychiatry, Department of Clinical Neuroscience, Karolinska Institutet, Stockholm, Sweden
Department of Clinical Science, Intervention and Technology (CLINTEC), Division of Medical Imaging and Technology, Karolinska Institutet, Stockholm, Sweden

Ian H. Harding
Department of Psychiatry, Melbourne Neuropsychiatry Centre, The University of Melbourne, Melbourne, VIC, Australia

Paul Klauser
Department of Psychiatry, Melbourne Neuropsychiatry Centre, The University of Melbourne, Melbourne, VIC, Australia
Monash Clinical and Imaging Neuroscience, School of Psychology and Psychiatry, Monash University, Clayton, VIC, Australia
School of Psychological Sciences, Monash University, Melbourne, VIC, Australia

Mats Adler, Johan Lundberg and Thomas Masterman
Section of Psychiatry, Department of Clinical Neuroscience, Karolinska Institutet, Stockholm, Sweden

Christoffer Rahm
Department of Psychiatry, Melbourne Neuropsychiatry Centre, The University of Melbourne, Melbourne, VIC, Australia
Department of Medicine Huddinge, Karolinska Institutet, Stockholm, Sweden

Caroline Wachtler
Primary Care Research Unit, Department of General Practice, The University of Melbourne, Melbourne, VIC, Australia
Centre for Family Medicine (CeFAM), Department of Neurobiology, Care Sciences and Society, Karolinska Institutet, Stockholm, Sweden

Tomas Jonsson
Department of Clinical Science, Intervention and Technology (CLINTEC), Division of Medical Imaging and Technology, Karolinska Institutet, Stockholm, Sweden
Department of Medical Physics, Karolinska University Hospital Huddinge, Stockholm, Sweden

Maria Kristoffersen-Wiberg
Department of Clinical Science, Intervention and Technology (CLINTEC), Division of Medical Imaging and Technology, Karolinska Institutet, Stockholm, Sweden
Department of Radiology, Karolinska University Hospital, Stockholm, Sweden

Christos Pantelis
Department of Psychiatry, Melbourne Neuropsychiatry Centre, The University of Melbourne, Melbourne, VIC, Australia

Björn Wahlund
Department of Energy and Engineering, Swedish University of Agricultural Sciences, Uppsala, Sweden

Daniela A. Herzig
Department of Experimental Psychology, University of Bristol, Bristol, UK
Institute for Response-Genetics, University of Zurich, Kilchberg, Switzerland
Clienia AG Littenheid, Littenheid, Switzerland

David J. Nutt
Neuropsychopharmacology Unit, Imperial College London, London, UK

Christine Mohr
Department of Experimental Psychology, University of Bristol, Bristol, UK
Faculté des Sciences Sociales et Politiques, Institut de Psychologie, Université de Lausanne, Lausanne, Switzerland

Rachel A. Batty
Brain and Psychological Sciences Research Centre (BPsyC), Faculty of Health, Arts and Design, Swinburne University of Technology, Melbourne, VIC, Australia
School of Health Science, Psychology, RMIT University, Bundoora, VIC, Australia

Andrew J. P. Francis
School of Health Science, Psychology, RMIT University, Bundoora, VIC, Australia

Hamish Innes-Brown
The Bionics Institute, Melbourne, VIC, Australia

Nicole R. Joshua
Pearson Clinical Assessment, Melbourne, VIC, Australia

Susan L. Rossell
Brain and Psychological Sciences Research Centre (BPsyC), Faculty of Health, Arts and Design, Swinburne University of Technology, Melbourne, VIC, Australia
Cognitive Neuropsychiatry Laboratory, Monash-Alfred Psychiatry Research Centre (MAPrc), The Alfred Hospital and Central Clinical School Monash University, Melbourne, VIC, Australia
Psychiatry, St. Vincents Hospital, Melbourne, VIC, Australia

Caterina Gawrilow
Faculty of Science, Department of Psychology, Eberhard Karls Universität Tübingen, Tübingen, Germany
German Institute for International Educational Research (DIPF), Frankfurt, Germany
Center for Research on Individual Development and Adaptive Education of Children at Risk (IDeA), Frankfurt, Germany
LEAD Graduate School, Eberhard Karls Universität Tübingen, Tübingen, Germany

Jan Kühnhausen
German Institute for International Educational Research (DIPF), Frankfurt, Germany
Center for Research on Individual Development and Adaptive Education of Children at Risk (IDeA), Frankfurt, Germany

Johanna Schmid
Faculty of Science, Department of Psychology, Eberhard Karls Universität Tübingen, Tübingen, Germany
LEAD Graduate School, Eberhard Karls Universität Tübingen, Tübingen, Germany

Gertraud Stadler
Psychology Department, Columbia University, NewYork, NY, USA

Katherine S. Young
Department of Psychiatry, Warneford Hospital, Oxford, UK
MindLab/Center of Functionally Integrative Neuroscience (CFIN), Aarhus University, Aarhus, Denmark
Department of Psychology, University of California, Los Angeles (UCLA), Los Angeles, USA

Christine E. Parsons and Morten L. Kringelbach
Department of Psychiatry, Warneford Hospital, Oxford, UK
MindLab/Center of Functionally Integrative Neuroscience (CFIN), Aarhus University, Aarhus, Denmark

Alan Stein
Department of Psychiatry, Warneford Hospital, Oxford, UK

Silke Bachmann
Clienia Littenheid AG, Littenheid, Switzerland
Department of Psychiatry, Psychotherapy, and Psychosomatics, University of Halle, Halle, Germany

Franz Josef Geider
Section of Geriatric Psychiatry, Institute of Gerontology, University of Heidelberg, Heidelberg, Germany

Lieve Lia Beheydt, Didier Schrijvers and Lise Docx
Collaborative Antwerp Psychiatric Research Institute (CAPRI), Antwerp University, Antwerp, Belgium

Filip Bouckaert
University Psychiatric Center KU Leuven, Kortenberg, Belgium

Index

www.ingramcontent.com/pod-product-compliance
Lightning Source LLC
LaVergne TN
LVHW060536210926
848485LV00005B/1206
9781639894505